FETAL AND NEONATAL HEMATOLOGY, ONCOLOGY AND IMMUNOLOGY

FETAL AND NEONATAL HEMATOLOGY, ONCOLOGY AND IMMUNOLOGY

Editors-in-Chief

MR Lokeshwar
MD DCH
Consultant Pediatrician and
Pediatric Hematologist
Shushrusha Citizens' Co-operative Hospital
Lilavati Hospital and Research Center
Mumbai, Maharashtra, India

Anupam Sachdeva
MD DCH
Director
Pediatric Hematology-Oncology and
Bone Marrow Transplantation
Institute for Child Health
Sir Ganga Ram Hospital
New Delhi, India
Recipient, Dr BC Roy Award
Recipient, Silver Jubilee Research Award

Editors

Nitin K Shah
MD DCH
Professor
DNB Pediatrics and Consultant Pediatrician
PD Hinduja National Hospital and
Medical Research Center
Professor
FNB Pediatric Hematology-Oncology
BJ Wadia Hospital for Children
Mumbai, Maharashtra, India
Past President
Indian Academy of Pediatrics, 2006

Bharat Agarwal
MD DCH (Bom) DNB (MNAMS)
Head
Department of Pediatric
Hematology and Oncology
BJ Wadia Hospital for Children
Institute of Child Health and
Research Center
Mumbai, Maharashtra, India

Mamta Manglani
MD (Ped) DCH
Director
Comprehensive Thalassemia Care Centre and
Bone Marrow Transplantation Centre
Magathane, Borivli (East)
(A Satellite Centre of LTM Medical College and
General Hospital, Sion
Mumbai, Maharashtra, India)

Executive Editor

Asha Pillai

Forewords

Santosh T Soans

Raj Warrier

JAYPEE The Health Sciences Publisher
New Delhi | London | Panama

Jaypee Brothers Medical Publishers (P) Ltd.

Headquarters
Jaypee Brothers Medical Publishers (P) Ltd.
4838/24, Ansari Road, Daryaganj
New Delhi 110 002, India
Phone: +91-11-43574357
Fax: +91-11-43574314
E-mail: jaypee@jaypeebrothers.com

Overseas Offices
J.P. Medical Ltd.
83, Victoria Street, London
SW1H 0HW (UK)
Phone: +44 20 3170 8910
Fax: +44(0) 20 3008 6180
E-mail: info@jpmedpub.com

Jaypee Highlights Medical Publishers Inc.
City of Knowledge, Building 235, 2nd Floor
Clayton, Panama City, Panama
Phone: +1 507-301-0496
Fax: +1 507-301-0499
E-mail: cservice@jphmedical.com

Jaypee Brothers Medical Publishers (P) Ltd.
17/1-B, Babar Road, Block-B, Shaymali
Mohammadpur, Dhaka-1207
Bangladesh
Mobile: +08801912003485
E-mail: jaypeedhaka@gmail.com

Jaypee Brothers Medical Publishers (P) Ltd.
Bhotahity, Kathmandu, Nepal
Phone: +977-9741283608
E-mail: kathmandu@jaypeebrothers.com

Website: www.jaypeebrothers.com
Website: www.jaypeedigital.com

Inquiries for bulk sales may be solicited at: jaypee@jaypeebrothers.com

Fetal and Neonatal Hematology, Oncology and Immunology

First Edition: **2017**

ISBN: 978-93-86322-76-0

Printed at Sanat Printers

Dedicated to

All children—Born and to be Born in the World!

Contributors

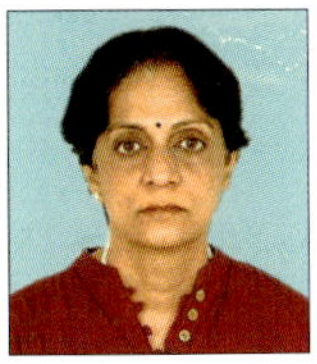

Aarathi R Rau MD
Professor
Department of Pediatrics
MS Ramaiah Medical College
Bengaluru, Karnataka, India

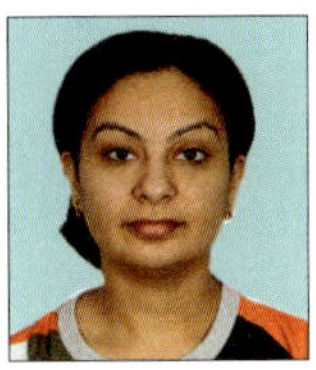

Akanksha Chichra
MBBS DNB (Pediatrics) FNB (Pediatric Hematology/Oncology)
Pediatric Hematologist/Oncologist
Asian Cancer Institute
Kohinoor Hospital
Surya Children Hospital
Mumbai, Maharashtra, India

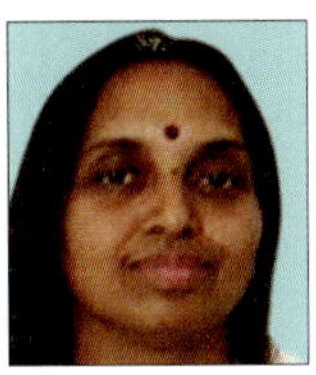

Amita Aggarwal MD DM FASc FNASc FAMS
Professor
Department of Clinical Immunology
Sanjay Gandhi Postgraduate Institute of
Medical Sciences
Lucknow, Uttar Pradesh, India

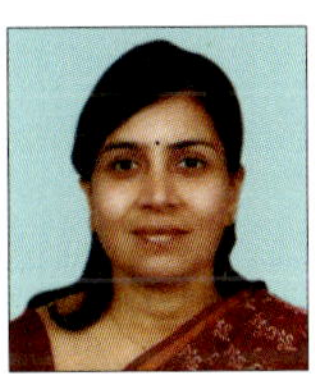

Amita Mahajan MD MRCPCH CCST
Senior Consultant Pediatric
Hematology and Oncology
Indraprastha Apollo Hospital
New Delhi, India

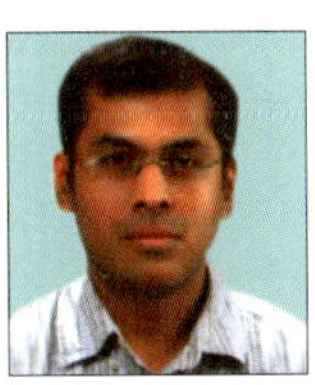

Amit Rawat MD (Pathology) PDCC (Laboratory Immunology)
PDCC (Nephropathology) MAMS
Additional Professor
Department of Pediatric Allergy and Immunology
Pediatric Allergy Immunology Unit
Postgraduate Institute of Medical
Education and Research
Chandigarh, India
Investigator
ICMR Center for Advanced Research in Primary
Immunodeficiency Diseases

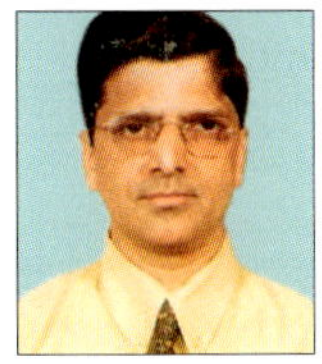

Anand Deshpande MD (Pathology)
Consultant
Transfusion Medicine and Hematology
Consultant Hematopathologist and
In-Charge Transfusion Medicine
PD Hinduja National Hospital and
Medical Research Center
Mumbai, Maharashtra, India

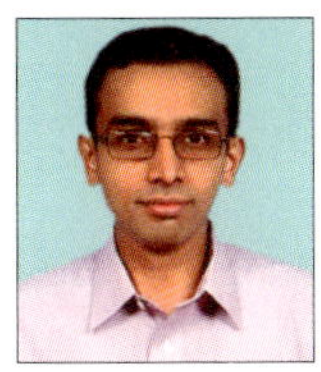

Anand Prakash MD DNB FNB (Ped Hem Onc)
Associate Professor
Department of Pediatrics
St Johns Medical College Hospital
Bengaluru, Karnataka, India

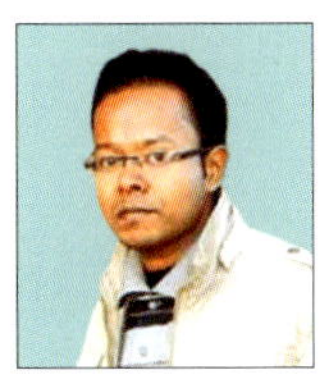

Anirban Das
MD (Pediatrics) DM (Pediatric Hematology-Oncology)
Consultant
Department of Pediatrics Hematology-Oncology
Tata Medical Center
Kolkata, West Bengal, India

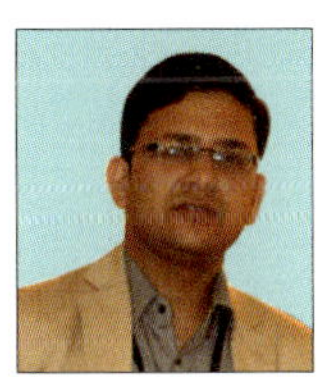

Ankur Jindal MD (Pediatrics)
Senior Resident (DM)
Pediatric Immunology and Rheumatology Unit
Advance Pediatric Center
Postgraduate Institute of Medical
Education and Research
Chandigarh, India

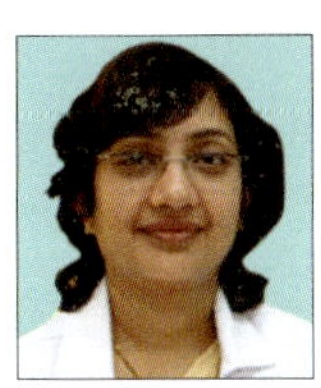

Anupama S Borker MD DCH
Consultant
Department of Pediatric Oncology
Asian Cancer Institute
Somaiya Ayurvihar
Mumbai, Maharashtra, India

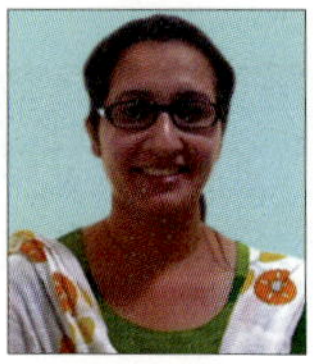

Anupa Mishra MD (Pediatrics and FIAP Pediatric Hematology Oncology)
Consultant Pediatric Hematologist Oncologist
HCG Cancer Center
Ahmedabad, Gujarat, India

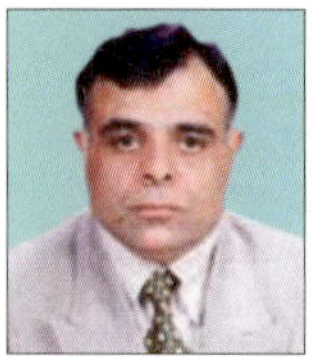

Anupam Sachdeva MD DCH
Director
Pediatric Hematology Oncology and Bone Marrow Transplantation
Institute for Child Health
Sir Ganga Ram Hospital
New Delhi, India
Recipient, Dr BC Roy Award
Recipient, Silver Jubilee Research Award

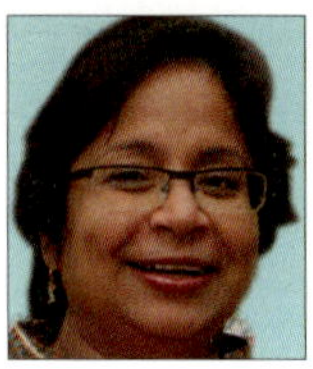

Arpita Bhattacharya MRCP (Pediatrics)
Senior Consultant
Department of Pediatric Oncology
Tata Medical Center
Kolkata, West Bengal, India

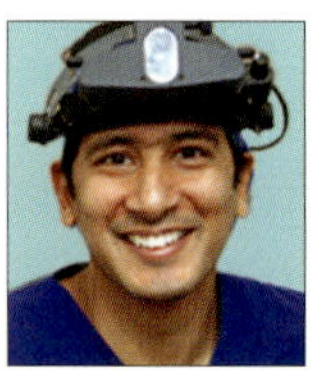

Ashwin Mallipatna MS DNB
Pediatric Ophthalmologist
Battu Eye Center
Bengaluru, Karnataka, India

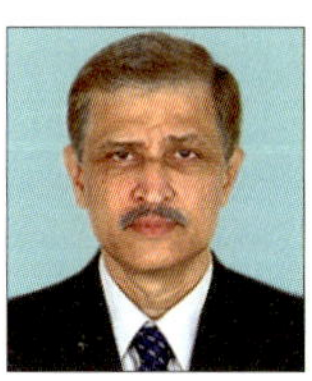

(Col) ATK Rau MD DHA
Professor and In-Charge
Pediatric Hematology-Oncology Unit
Department of Pediatrics
MS Ramaiah Medical College
Bengaluru, Karnataka, India
Former Chairperson
PHO Chapter of the IAP

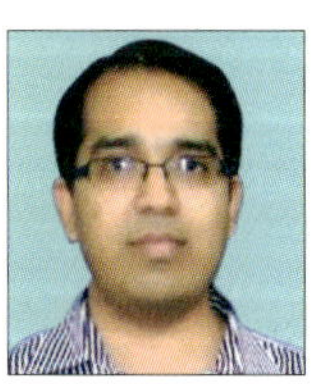

Avijeet Yadav MD (Pediatrics)
Consultant Neonatologist and Pediatrician
Dr BL Kapur Memorial Hospital
New Delhi, India

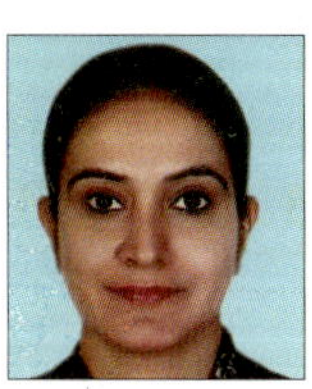

Avneet Kaur MBBS DCH DNB (Pediatrics) DNB (Neonatology-Gold medalist) FAGE
Consultant Neonatologist
Apollo Cradle
New Delhi, India

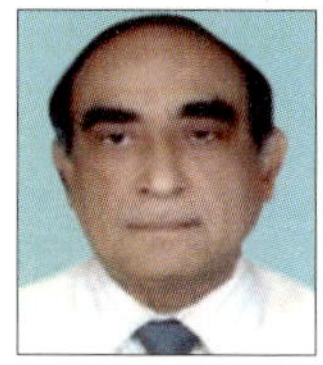

BD Bhatia MD DCH FAMS FICN FIAP FNNF
Professor and Head
Department of Pediatrics
Heritage Institute of Medical Sciences
Varanasi, Uttar Pradesh, India

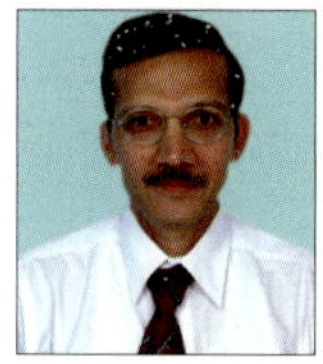

Bharat Agarwal MD DCH (Bom) DNB (MNAMS)
Head
Department of Pediatric Hematology and Oncology
BJ Wadia Hospital for Children
Institute of Child Health and Research Center
Mumbai, Maharashtra, India

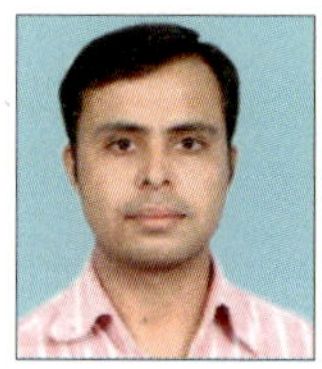

Bharat Choudhary MBBS MD (Pediatrics)
Senior Resident
Department of Pediatrics
All India Institute of Medical Sciences
Bhopal, Madhya Pradesh, India

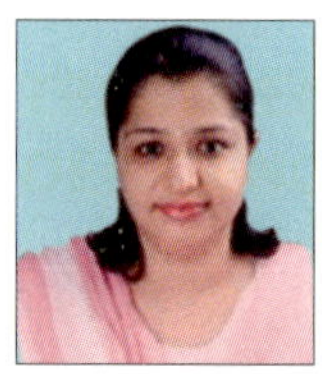

Bhavna Dhingra MD DNB (Pediatrics)
Assistant Professor
All India Institute of Medical Sciences
Bhopal, Madhya Pradesh, India

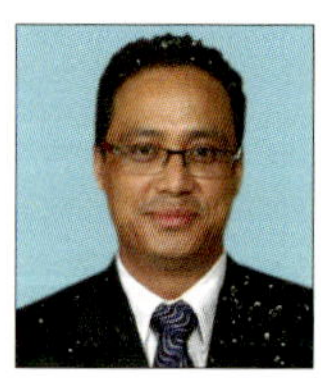

Biman Saikia MD (Pathology) MNAMS
Professor
Department of Immunopathology
Postgraduate Institute of Medical Education and Research
Chandigarh, India

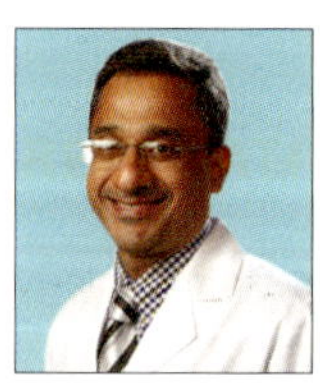

Deepak Bansal MD DNB MAMS
Professor
Pediatric Hematology Oncology Unit
Department of Pediatrics
Advanced Pediatric Center
Postgraduate Institute of Medical Education and Research
Chandigarh, India

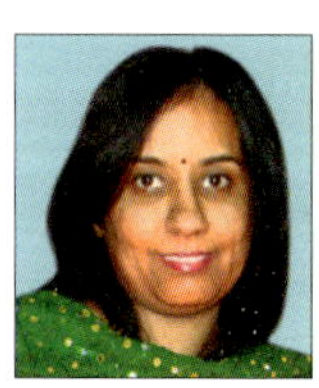

Deepti Suri MD (Pediatrics) DNB
Associate Professor
Division of Pediatric Allergy and Immunology
Advanced Pediatrics Center
Postgraduate Institute of Medical Education and Research
Chandigarh, India

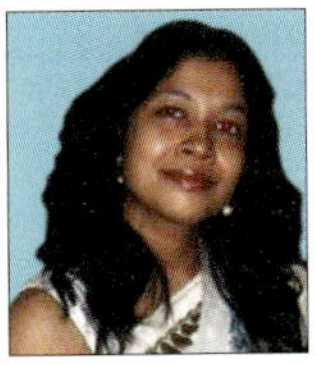

Dipshikha Maiti MD (Pediatrics)
Fellowship Pediatric Oncology
Senior Fellow
Tata Medical Center
Kolkata, West Bengal, India

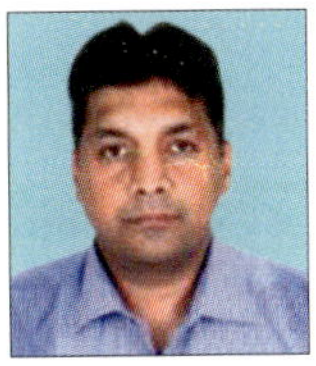

Gaurav Tripathi MD (Ped) Fellowship IAP (PHO)
Consultant Pediatric Hemato-oncologist
KBT Government Hospital
Rewa, Madhya Pradesh, India

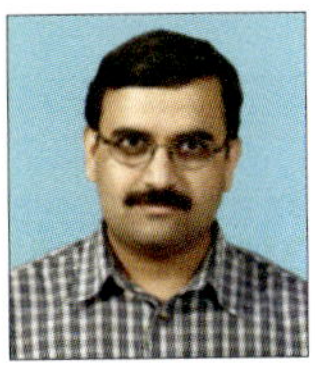

Girish Chinnaswamy MD MRCP (Pediatrics)
Associate Professor (Pediatric Oncology)
Department of Medical Oncology
Tata Memorial Hospital
Mumbai, Maharashtra, India

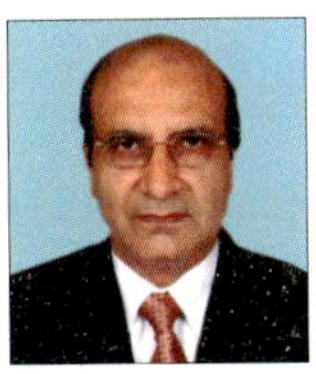

Jagdish Chandra MD FIAP
Director and Professor
Department of Pediatrics
In-Charge
Pediatric Hematology and
Thalassemia Day Care Center
Programme Director
Pediatric Center of Excellence (HIV)
Kalawati Saran Children's Hospital and
Lady Hardinge Medical College
New Delhi, India

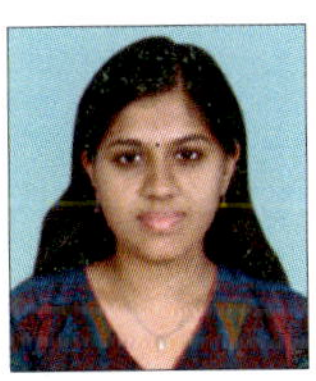

Jahnavi Aluri MTech (Biotechnology) PhD student
National Institute of Immunohematology
Padmashree Dr DY Patil University
Mumbai, Maharashtra, India

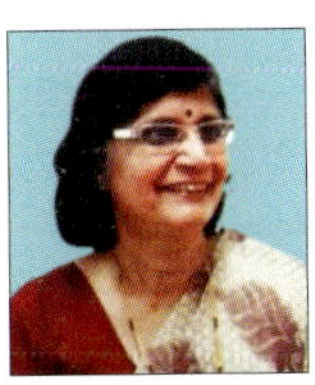

Jayashree Mondkar MD DCH
Professor and Head
Department of Neonatology
Lokmanya Tilak Municipal Medical College and
General Hospital
Mumbai, Maharashtra, India

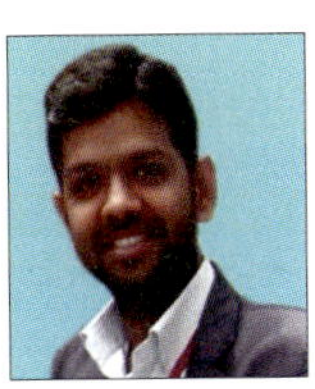

Jitendra K Shandilya PhD student
Pediatric Allergy and Immunology Unit
Department of Pediatrics
Advanced Pediatrics Center
Postgraduate Institute of Medical
Education and Research
Chandigarh, India

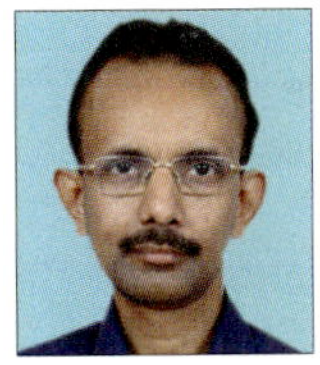

Julius Xavier Scott DCH DNB MD (Pediatrics)
Fellowship in Pediatric Hemato-oncology (Australia)
Head
Division of Pediatric Hemato-oncology
Sri Ramachandra University
Chennai, Tamil Nadu, India

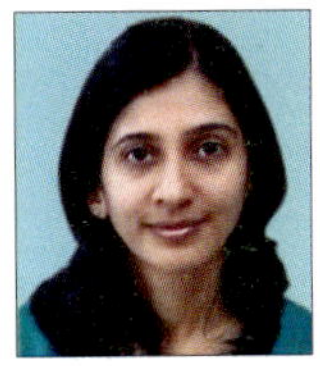

Khushnooma Italia MSc PhD
Research Associate
National Institute of Immunohematology
Mumbai, Maharashtra, India

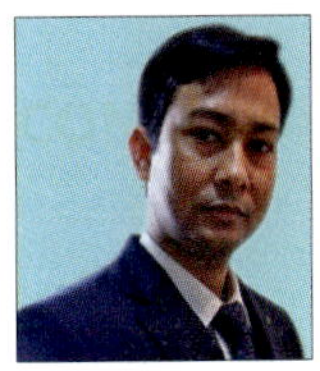

Kumar Ankur MBBS MD DNB (Neonatology)
Consultant In-Charge
Neonatal Intensive Care Unit
Dr BL Kapur Memorial Hospital
New Delhi, India

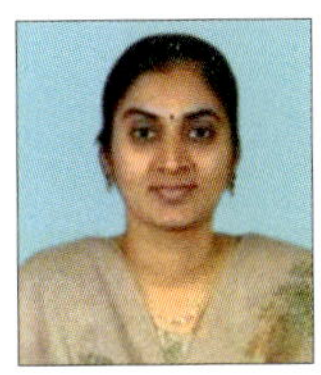

Latha M Sneha MD (Pediatrics)
Assistant Professor
Division of Pediatric Hemato-oncology
Sri Ramachandra University
Chennai, Tamil Nadu, India

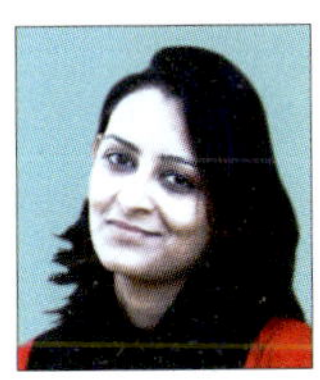

Latika Gupta MD
Senior Resident
Department of Clinical Immunology
Sanjay Gandhi Postgraduate Institute of
Medical Sciences
Lucknow, Uttar Pradesh, India

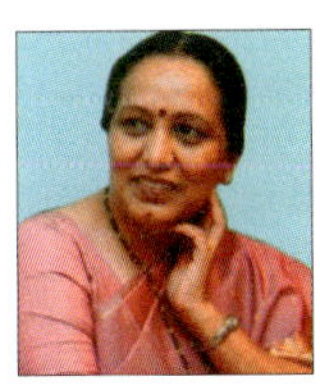

Mamta Manglani MD (Pediatrics) DCH
Director
Comprehensive Thalassemia Care
Centre and Bone Marrow Transplantation
Centre, Magathane, Borivli (East)
(A Satellite Centre of LTM Medical College and
General Hospital, Sion
Mumbai, Maharashtra, India)

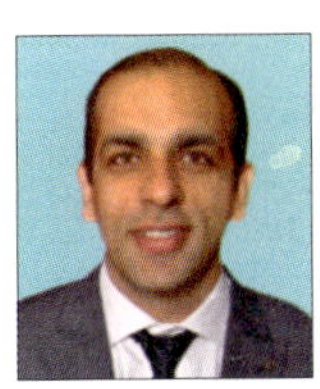

Manas Kalra MD DNB FNB (Fellowship Westmead Hospital)
Consultant
Pediatric Hematology and Oncology
Indraprastha Apollo Hospital
New Delhi, India

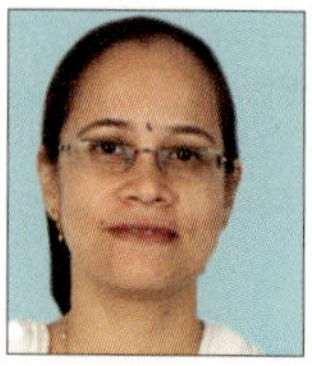

Manisha Madkaikar MD
Director-In-Charge and Scientist F
Department of Pediatric Immunology and Leukocyte Biology
National Institute of Immunohematology (ICMR)
Mumbai, Maharashtra, India

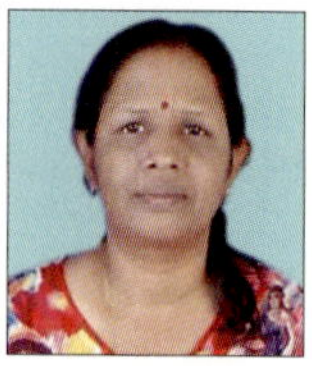

Maya Gupta MSc (Applied Biology)
Technical Assistant
National Institute of Immunohematology
Mumbai, Maharashtra, India

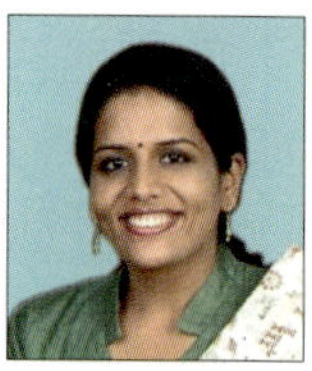

Maya Prasad MD (Pediatrics)
Fellowship in Pediatric Oncology
Assistant Professor
Pediatric Oncology
Tata Memorial Hospital
Mumbai, Maharashtra, India

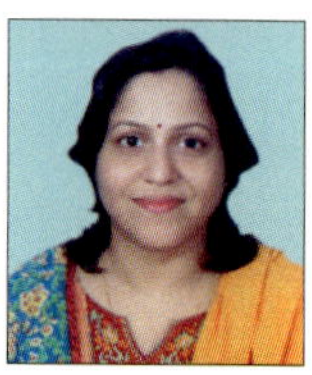

Meenal Agarwal
MD (Obs and Gyne) DM (Medical Genetics)
Head
Clinical Genetics
GenePath Dx
Causeway Health Care Private Ltd
Pune, Maharashtra, India

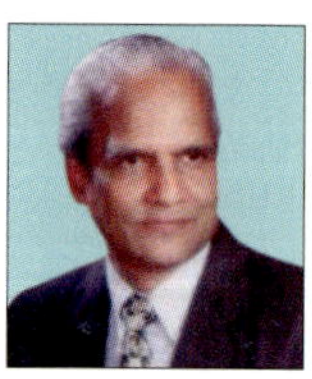

MR Lokeshwar MD DCH
Consultant Pediatrician and Pediatric Hematologist
Shushrusha Citizens' Co-operative Hospital
Lilavati Hospital and Research Center
Mumbai, Maharashtra, India

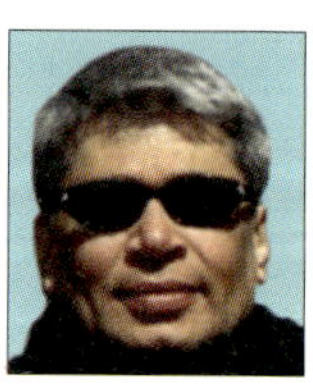

Mukesh Desai MBBS DCH MD (Pediatrics)
Professor
Department of Pediatric Hematology Oncology
DNB Board
Head
Division of Immunology
BJ Wadia Hospital for Children
Mumbai, Maharashtra, India

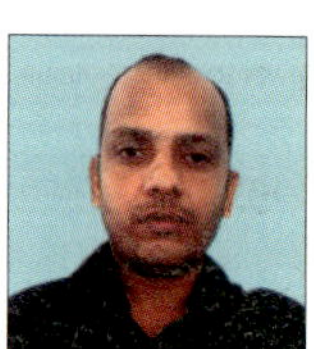

Nagendra Chaudhary MBBS MD (Pediatrics)
Assistant Professor
Department of Pediatrics
Universal College of Medical Sciences
Bhairahawa, Nepal

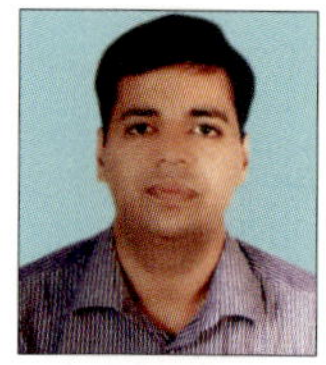

Naveen Gupta MD DNB Neonatology Fellowship in Neonatal and Perinatal Medicine (BC Children Hospital, Vancouver, Canada)
Consultant Neonatologist and In-Charge
Neonatal Intensive Care Unit (NICU)
Max Super Speciality Hospital
New Delhi, India

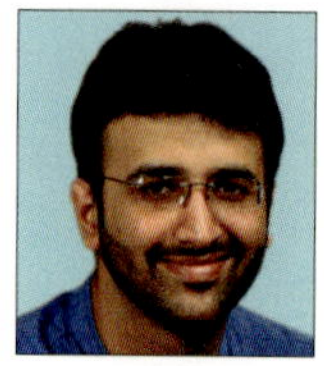

Nimish Kulkarni
MD (Pediatrics) Fellow Pediatric Hematology and Oncology
Department of Pediatrics
Lokmanya Tilak Municipal Medical College and General Hospital
Mumbai, Maharashtra, India

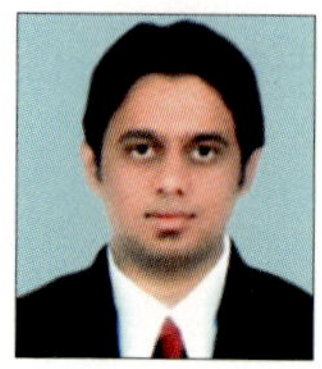

Nirav Thacker MD DM
Specialist Registrar
Department of Pediatric Oncology
Tata Memorial Center
Mumbai, Maharashtra, India

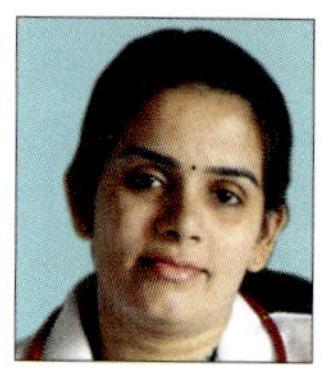

Nita Radhakrishnan MD FNB
Consultant
Department of Pediatric Hematology-Oncology
Institute of Child Health
Sir Ganga Ram Hospital
New Delhi, India

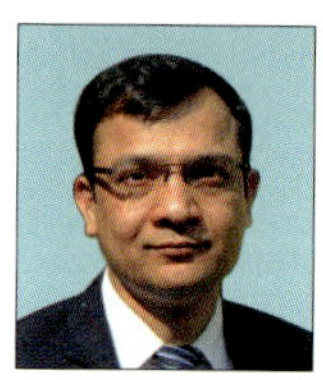

Nitin Gupta DM Clinical Hematology (AIIMS, Delhi)
Fellowship Leukemia/BMT, Vancouver, Canada
Consultant
Clinical Hematology and Bone Marrow/ Stem Cell Transplantation
Sir Ganga Ram Hospital
New Delhi, India

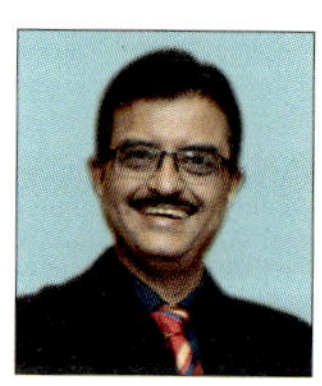

Nitin K Shah MD DCH
Professor
DNB Pediatrics and Consultant Pediatrician
PD Hinduja National Hospital and Medical Research Center
Professor
FNB Pediatric Hematology-Oncology
BJ Wadia Hospital for Children
Mumbai, Maharashtra, India
Past President
Indian Academy of Pediatrics, 2006

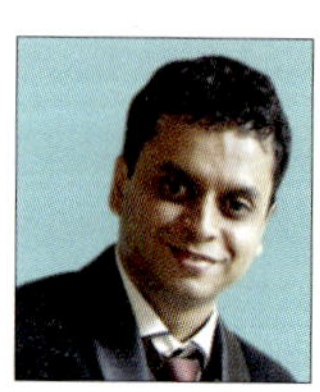

Omkar Nagesh Khandkar
DNB (Pediatrics) Fellow in Pediatric Hematology-Oncology
Department of Pediatrics
Lokmanya Tilak Municipal Medical College and General Hospital
Mumbai, Maharashtra, India

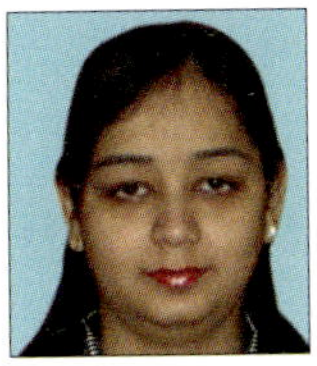

Parikshaa Gupta MD DNB (Pathology)
MNAMS Postdoctoral Fellow (Cytopathology)
Assistant Professor
Department of Cytology and
Gynecological Pathology
Postgraduate Institute of Medical
Education and Research
Chandigarh, India

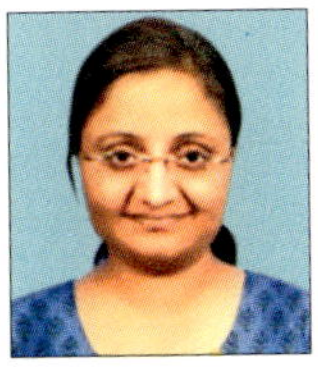

Parvati Joshi MBBS MD (Pathology)
Senior Resident
Department of Immunopathology
Postgraduate Institute of Medical
Education and Research
Chandigarh, India

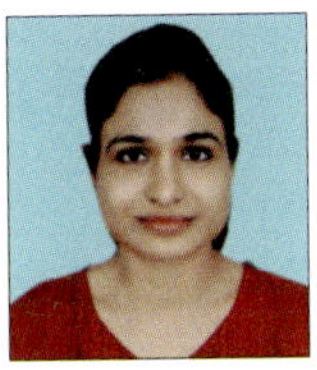

Piali Mandal MD (Pediatrics)
Assistant Professor
Department of Pediatrics
Lady Hardinge Medical College and
Kalawati Saran Children's Hospital
New Delhi, India

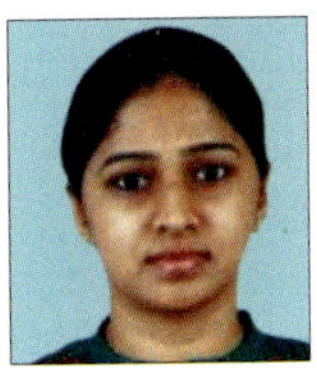

Pooja Balasubramanian MD (Pediatrics)
Fellow in Pediatric Hematology-Oncology
Lokmanya Tilak Municipal Medical College and
General Hospital
Mumbai, Maharashtra, India

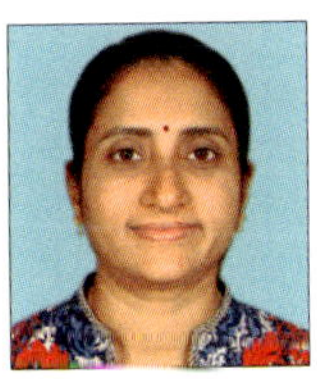

Prajnya Ranganath
MD (Pediatrics) DM (Medical Genetics)
Associate Professor and Head
Department of Medical Genetics
Nizam's Institute of Medical Sciences
Adjunct Scientist
Diagnostics Division
Center for DNA Fingerprinting and Diagnostics
Hyderabad, Telangana, India

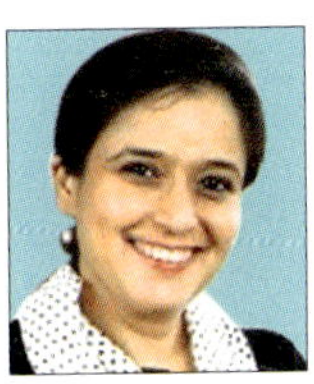

Prathima Radhakrishnan MD
Director
Bangalore Fetal Medicine Center
Bengaluru, Karnataka, India

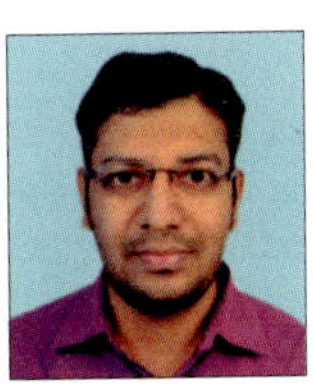

Praveen Narsaria MD (Pediatrics)
NICU/PICU In-Charge
Nagarmal Modi Seva Sadan
Ranchi, Jharkhand, India

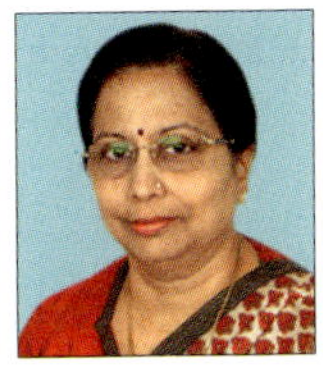

Purna Kurkure MD (Pediatrics) DCH FIAP
Chairperson
Division of Pediatric Oncology
Chief
Academic Division
Asian Cancer Institute
Somaiya Ayurvihar
Mumbai, Maharashtra, India

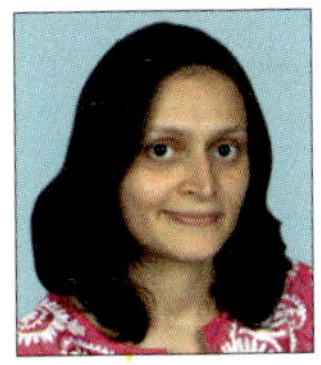

Purvi Kadakia Kutty
MD (Pediatrics) DCH FIAP (Pediatric Hematology and Oncology)
FNB (Pediatric Hematology and Oncology)
Assistant Professor
Department of Oncology
Topiwala National Medical College and
BYL Nair Charitable Hospital
Mumbai, Maharashtra, India

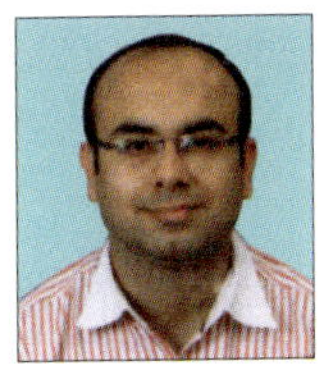

Rahul Arora DNB (Hematology (SGRH, Delhi))
Senior Resident
Clinical Hematology and Bone Marrow/
Stem Cell Transplantation
Sir Ganga Ram Hospital
New Delhi, India

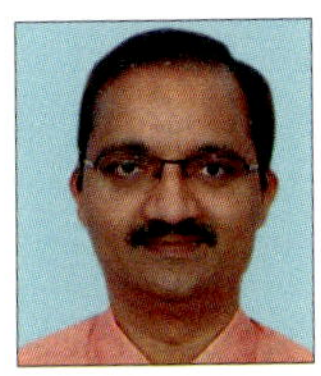

Rajesh B Sawant MD (Pathology)
Consultant Transfusion Medicine
Kokilaben Dhirubhai Ambani Hospital
Mumbai, Maharashtra, India

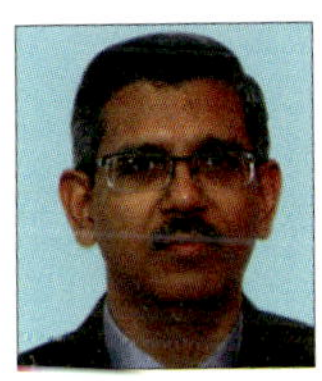

Rakesh Lodha MD
Professor
Department of Pediatrics
All India Institute of Medical Sciences
New Delhi, India

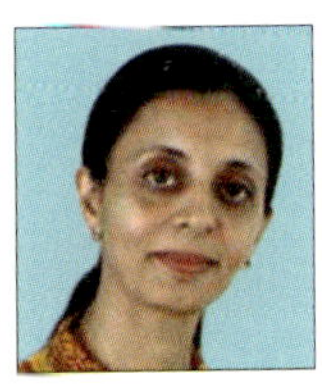

Ratna Sharma
MD (Pediatrics) DNB (Fellowship Ped Hem-Onc, Mumbai)
Consultant
Department of Pediatrics Hematology-Oncology
Lokmanya Tilak Municipal Medical College and
General Hospital, Mumbai
Jupiter Hospital
Mumbai, Maharashtra, India

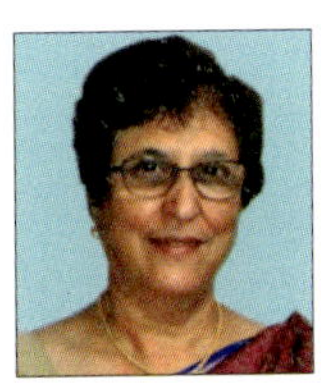

Roshan Colah MSc PhD
Former Director-in-Charge
National Institute of Immunohematology
Mumbai, Maharashtra, India

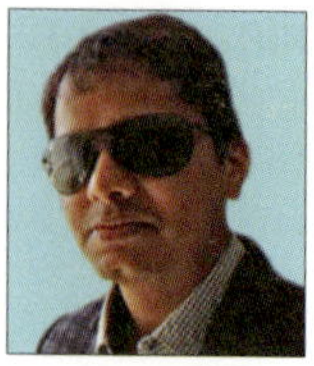

Sagar Bhattad MD DM (Ped C Imm and Rheum)
Senior Resident
Allergy Immunology Unit
Advanced Pediatrics Center
Postgraduate Institute of Medical
Education and Research
Chandigarh, India

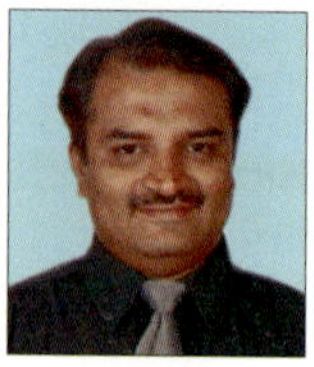

Sajid Qureshi MS DNB FICS FAIS
Professor and Head
Division of Pediatric Surgical Oncology
Department of Surgical Oncology
Tata Memorial Center
Mumbai, Maharashtra, India

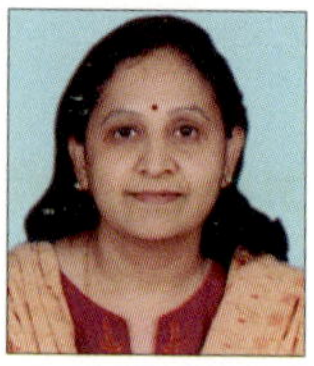

Sangeeta Mudaliar DNB MRCPCH
Consultant
Department of Hematology and Oncology
BJ Wadia Children Hospital, Mumbai
Honorary Consultant
SL Raheja Hospital
Gurunanak Hospital
Mumbai, Maharashtra, India

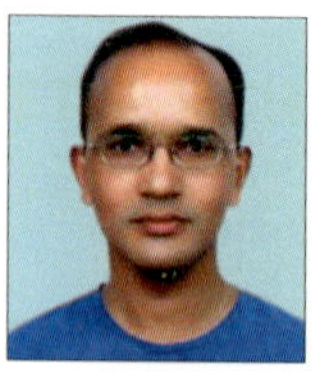

Sanjeev Chetry MD (Ped) DNB (Neonatology)
Neonatologist
BLK Superspecialty Hospital
New Delhi, India

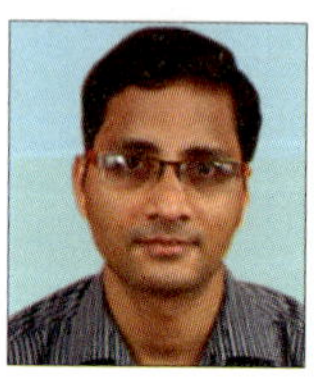

Saroj P Panda
MD (Ped) Fellow (Ped H and O) DM (Ped Onco)
Specialist Senior Registrar
Department of Pediatric Oncology
Tata Memorial Hospital
Mumbai, Maharashtra, India

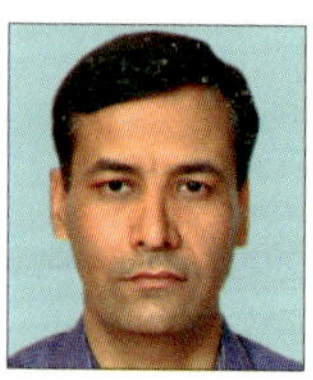

Satyendra Katewa
MBBS DCH DNB (Peds Fellowship in Peds Hem-Onco and BMT)
Head
Department of Pediatric Hemato-oncology
and Bone Marrow Transplant
Manipal Hospital
Jaipur, Rajasthan, India

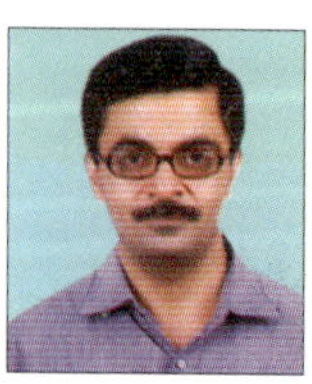

Satyen K Hemrajani MD (Pediatrics) DNB (Neonatology)
Fellowship in Neonatology
Senior Consultant and In-Charge
Neonatal Intensive Care Unit
Fortis Escorts Hospital
Jaipur, Rajasthan, India

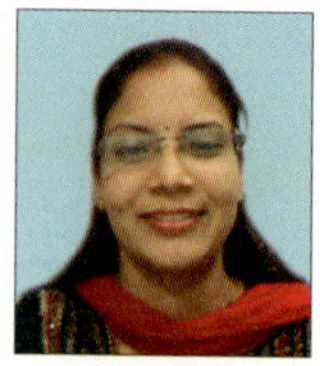

Savita Khadse MD (Pediatrics)
Assistant Professor
Department of Pediatrics
Lokmanya Tilak Municipal Medical College and
General Hospital
Mumbai, Maharashtra, India

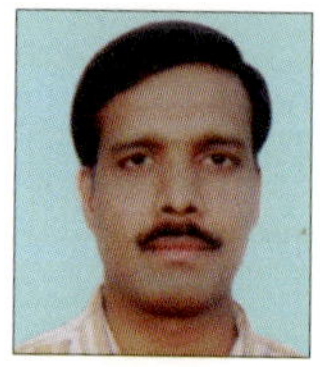

Sheikh Minhaj Ahmed MD DNB MNAMS (Pediatrics)
Consultant
Pediatric Intensive Care Unit
Lilavati Hospital and Research Center
Mumbai, Maharashtra, India

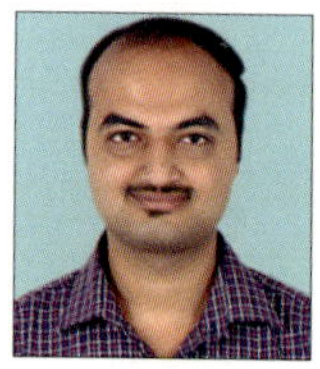

Shashidhar A MD DM (Neonatology)
Assistant Professor
Department of Neonatology
St Johns Medical College
Bengaluru, Karnataka, India

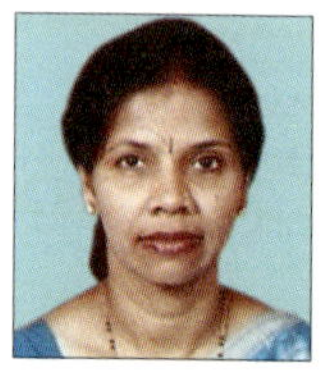

Shrimati Shetty MSc PhD
Scientist E
National Institute of Immunohematology
Mumbai, Maharashtra, India
Indian Council of Medical Research
New Delhi, India

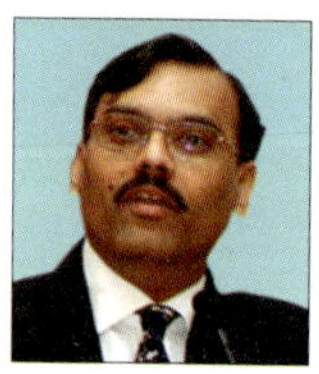

Shripad D Banavali MD (Med, Bom) BC (Ped, USA)
BE (Hem-Onc, USA)
Professor and Head
Department of Medical and Pediatric Oncology
Tata Memorial Center
Mumbai, Maharashtra, India

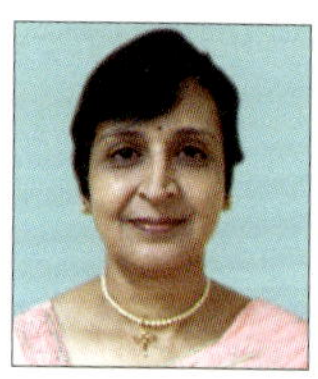

Shubha R Phadke MD (Pediatrics) DM (Medical Genetics)
Professor and Head
Department of Medical Genetics
Sanjay Gandhi Postgraduate Institute of
Medical Sciences
Lucknow, Uttar Pradesh, India
Founding President of Society for Indian
Academy of Medical Genetics

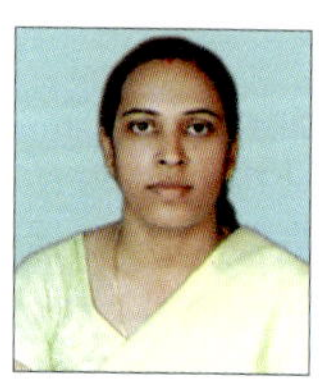

Shweta Singh MD
Assistant Professor
Department of Pediatrics
Heritage Institute of Medical Sciences
Varanasi, Uttar Pradesh, India

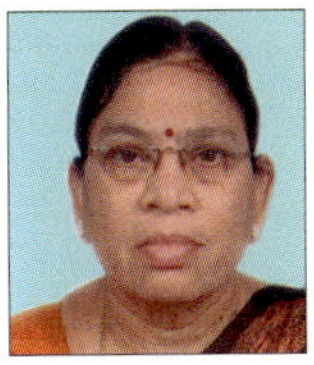

Snehalata C Gupte MSc PhD
Ex-Director
Surat Raktadan Kendra and Research Center
Ex-Deputy Director
National Institute of Immunohematology
Mumbai, Maharashtra, India

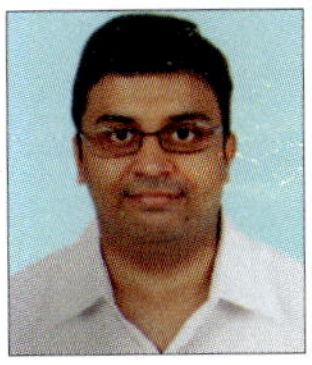

Snehavardhan Pandey DCH DNB
Specialty Medical Officer
Division of Hematology-Oncology
Lokmanya Tilak Municipal Medical College and General Hospital
Mumbai, Maharashtra, India

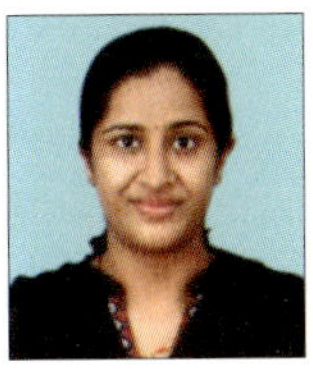

Soundarya M MD
Associate Professor
Department of Pediatrics
Kasturba Medical College, Mangaluru
Manipal University
Manipal, Karnataka, India

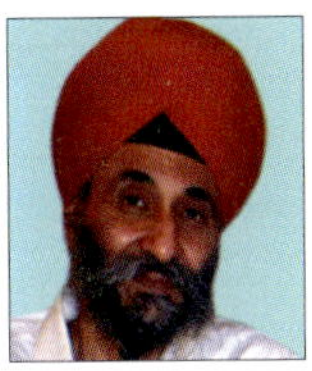

Surjit Singh MD DCH FRCP FRCPCH (Lon) FAMS
Professor
Department of Pediatrics
In-Charge
Allergy Immunology Unit
Advanced Pediatrics Center
Postgraduate Institute of Medical Education and Research
Chandigarh, India
Principal Investigator
ICMR Center for Advanced Research in Primary Immunodeficiency Diseases

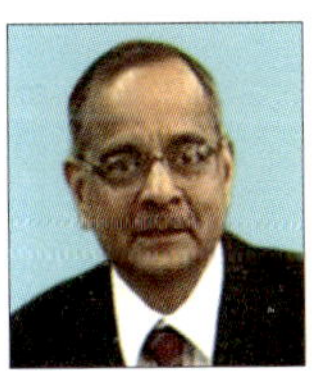

Sushil K Kabra MD DNB
Professor
Department of Pediatrics
All India Institute of Medical Sciences
New Delhi, India

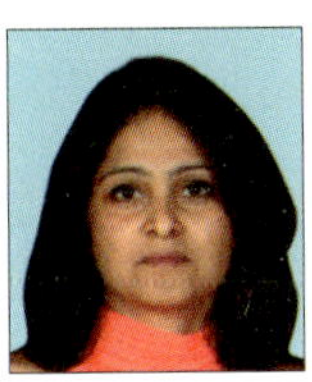

Swathi Shetty MSc
Research Faculty
Center for Human Genetics
Bengaluru, Karnataka, India

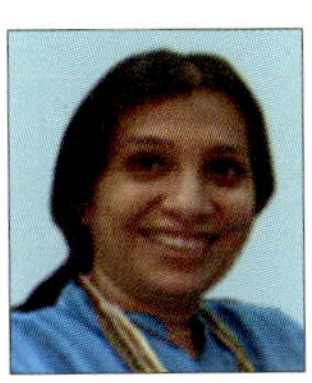

Swati Kanakia MD DCH PHD
Pediatric Hematologist Oncologist
Lilavati Hospital and Research Center
Kanakia Health Care
Mumbai, Maharashtra, India

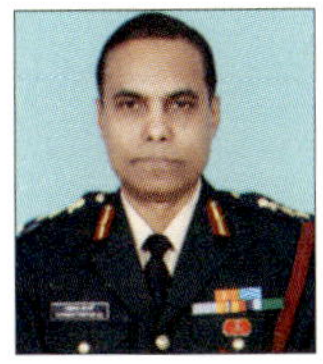

(Col) Tathagata Chatterjee MD MNAMS DM
Professor and Head
Department of Immunohematology and Transfusion Medicine
Armed Forces Medical College
Pune, Maharashtra, India

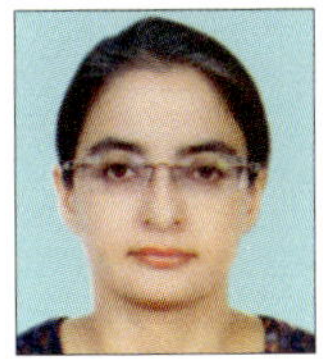

Tulika Seth MD American Board Certified Fellowship in Hematology Oncology (USA)
Professor
Department of Hematology
All India Institute of Medical Sciences
New Delhi, India

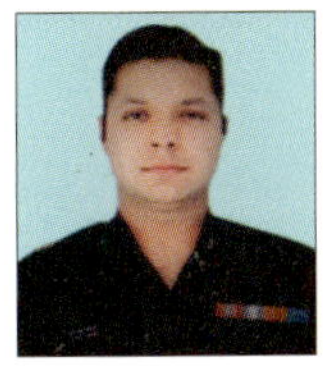

(Maj) Ujjwal Dimri MD (IH & BT)
OIC Blood Bank
Armed Forces Transfusion Center
New Delhi, India

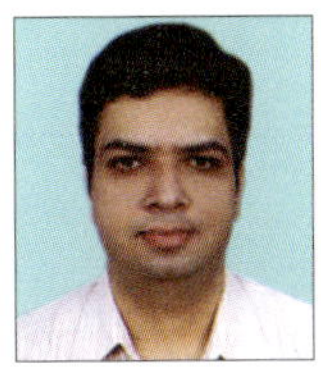

Venkatraman Radhakrishnan MD DM
Associate Professor
Department of Medical and Pediatric Oncology
Cancer Institute
Chennai, Tamil Nadu, India

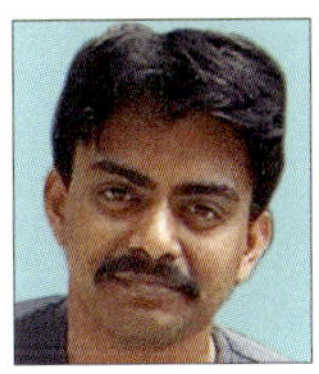

Vignesh P MD
DM Resident
Division of Pediatric Allergy and Immunology
Advanced Pediatrics Center
Postgraduate Institute of Medical Education and Research
Chandigarh, India

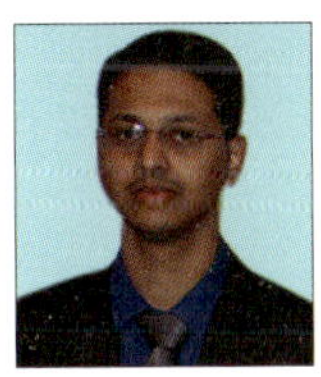

Vinod Gunasekaran
MD FNB IAP Fellowship (Ped Hemato-onco)
Clinical Assistant
Pediatric Hemato Oncology and Bone Marrow Transplantation Unit
Sir Ganga Ram Hospital
New Delhi, India

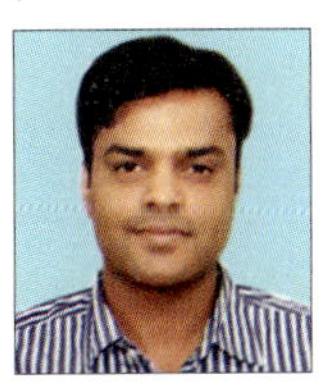

Vivek Choudhury
MBBS MD (Pediatrics) DNB (Neonatology)
Consultant Neonatologist
Apollo Cradle
New Delhi, India

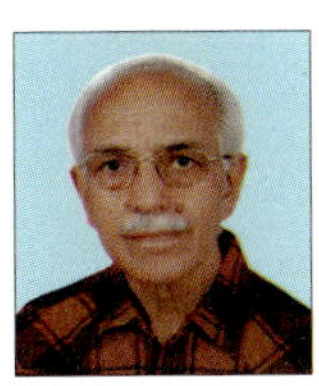

VP Choudhry MD FIAP FIMSA FIACM FISHTM
Senior Consultant Hematology
Batra Hospital and Medical Research Center
New Delhi, India
Fortis Escorts Hospital
Faridabad, Haryana, India

Foreword

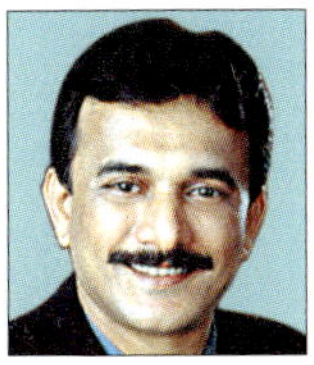

Compiling an authoritative book on a technically complex subject calls for a considerable team work. The *Fetal and Neonatal Hematology, Oncology and Immunology* is an outstanding example of such a quest. It is an encyclopedic work boasting of the combined talents of 95 experts in the field who have contributed to its making. The editorial team has been able to bring together so many professionals to write on the diverse subjects and present the output in a cohesive and comprehensible format. This itself is impressive.

The book spanning 450 plus pages is neatly organized into 57 chapters with attractive design, and illustrated with color, black and white photographs, line art and flow charts, tables and boxes. The very narrow focus of the book implies the intensity of expertise, which can be accessed between its covers. Issues concerning fetal and neonatal hematology and oncology are by their very nature very rare occurrences. Hence, even experienced pediatricians can find themselves challenged, when confronted with such complaints in a clinical setting. Books like these come in handy precisely at such a juncture and are instrumental in helping the pediatricians to meet the demands of the moment.

The editorial board under the stewardship of Dr MR Lokeshwar, who is a father figure in the field of pediatric hemato-oncology, comprises of stalwarts such as Dr Anupam Sachdeva, Dr Nitin K Shah, Dr Bharat Agarwal and Dr Mamta Manglani. They deserve our gratitude and congratulations for dedicating their time, and effort in putting this book together. It is a valuable addition to the available body of literature concerning the subjects. I am sure that they will feel sufficiently motivated by the response and support attracted by the present edition, and will continue their endeavor to bring out follow-up subsequent editions in the future.

I express my best wishes to the authors and the readers alike. I hope that the information contained in this book will be beneficial in providing timely relief to the patient community at large.

Santosh T Soans MD DCH
Pediatrician and Intensivist
Medical Chambers
Mangaluru, Karnataka, India
President Elect 2017
Central IAP

Foreword

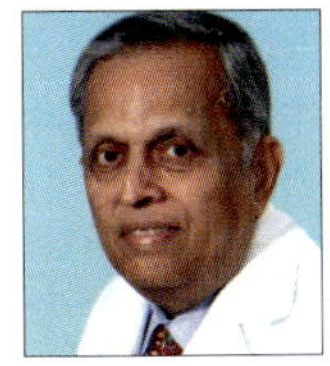

I feel privileged to write a foreword to *Fetal and Neonatal Hematology, Oncology and Immunology* being edited and published by some of the leaders in the field in the country as well as many future leaders. The field of pediatric hematology has seen immense development over the last few decades. It was with heartbreaking sadness that I left India to USA in 1975 to get training in Pediatric Hematology Oncology. Now, we have multiple centers of excellence in care and education for the specialty with significant clinical and even basic research programs. The level of interest for the field among students, residents and primary care doctors is immense, the book will go a long way in educating them, and also offer the options for initial care and follow-up. My special thanks to Drs MR Lokeshwar, Anupam Sachdeva, Nitin K Shah, Bharat Agarwal, and Mamta Manglani and among others for fostering and developing the specialty and now publishing this comprehensive review which will benefit the children along with the doctors.

Proud to be an Indian Pediatric Hematologist/Oncologist!

Raj Warrier MD FAAP FIAP

Pediatric Hematology/Oncology
Ochsner Hospital for Children

Professor Emeritus and Clinical Professor
LSU Health Sciences Center and Children's Hospital

Professor
Department of Pediatrics
Tulane University School of Medicine
New Orleans, Louisiana, USA

Professor
Department of Pediatrics
University of Queensland
Brisbane, Queensland, Australia

Adjunct Professor of Pediatrics

Former Vice-Chancellor
Manipal University
Manipal, Karnataka, India

Preface

After a highly successful textbook on Pediatric Hematology-Oncology, we are extremely pleased to present this first of its kind and a unique textbook on *Fetal and Neonatal Hematology, Oncology and Immunology*. The book covers the problems related to fetal and neonatal hematology, oncology, something that we encounter often in our day-to-day practice and do not have enough resources for help, as such a book is rare to find.

This book is extensively written with 57 chapters contributed by a galaxy of 95 pioneering authors across the country and abroad. It is spread over 450 plus pages, making it elaborate enough to cover all aspects of *Fetal and Neonatal Hematology, Oncology and Immunology* and yet concise enough to make reading easy and interesting. The chapters are lucidly written and simplified by having tables and boxes to illustrate salient features of the article, making it easy to revise it at a glance. There are 65 colored photographs, 21 black and white photographs, 37 line arts and 44 flow charts, which makes the reading non-monotonous and captivating.

Looking at the size of the book, the number of important topics covered, a galaxy of authors and colorful illustrations with the help of photographs, tables and flow charts, we are confident that this book will become a table companion for Pediatricians, Pediatric Hematologists/Oncologists/Immunologists and Neonatologists alike, when faced with problems related to Fetal and Neonatal Hematology, Oncology and Immunology. Do write back to us with your suggestions and criticism that will help us to improve the subsequent edition of the book.

Editors

Acknowledgments

We would like to express our gratitude to all who enabled us to publish this book, without whose help this book would not have seen the light of the day:

Our sincere and grateful thanks to the family of M/s Jaypee Brothers Medical Publishers (P) Ltd, New Delhi, India, Ms Chetna Malhotra (Associate Director–Publishing) and Mr Manish Pahuja (General Manager) without whom publishing this book would not have been possible.

We are grateful to all our contributors for meeting deadlines and excellent work delivered.

Our special thanks to Mr Harish Raut, Mr Sunil Kumar Dogra (Production Executive), Mr Binay Kumar (Proofreader), Mr Manver Singh (Typesetter), and Mr Amit Mathur (Graphic Designer) for assisting us in the editing, proofreading and designing skills.

All the patients and families for allowing us to continue to learn the subject.

We would also like to thank our family members for their support during the making of this book when we might have not been available to them due to the pressures of our work.

Last but not least, we beg forgiveness of all those whose names might have been inadvertently missed though they have been a part of our journey with the book.

Editorial Board

Contents

SECTION 1

FETAL HEMATOLOGY AND ANTENATAL DIAGNOSIS OF HEMATOLOGICAL DISORDERS

Section Editors: **Anupam Sachdeva, Shubha R Phadke**

SECTION 3
COAGULATION DISORDERS IN NEWBORN

Section Editors: **Mamta Manglani, Jagdish Chandra**

SECTION 7

BLOOD TRANSFUSION (COMPONENT THERAPY) AND SUPPORTIVE THERAPY

***Section Editors:* Anand Deshpande, Avneet Kaur**

SECTION 1

Fetal Hematology and Antenatal Diagnosis of Hematological Disorders

Section Editors

Anupam Sachdeva, Shubha R Phadke

CHAPTER

1

Physiology of Hematopoiesis

Vinod Gunasekaran, Anupam Sachdeva

INTRODUCTION

Hematopoiesis is an integral part in the growth process of embryo into fetus and later into an adult. It is essential for survival of fetus and to produce hematopoietic stem cells, which later contributes to hematopoiesis throughout the life. In the fetus, the blood cells are the first among the different cell types to become functionally mature. Erythroid cells are the first among the blood cells to be seen in the conceptus. Throughout the fetal development, hematopoiesis occurs in multiple sites before getting shifted to the final sites (bone marrow and thymus).[1] The synthesis occurs in waves beginning in the extraembryonic yolk sac early in the fetal life, later involving arterial cell clusters before migrating to fetal liver and finally seeding the bone marrow. The initial blood cells synthesized have limited progenitor activity, while the definitive adult-type hematopoietic stem cells (HSCs) have multi-lineage differentiation. The hemoglobin produced in early fetal development also differs from that of adult hemoglobin. This chapter discusses these physiological processes in detail.

STEPS IN FETAL HEMATOPOIESIS

The fetal hematopoiesis occurs sequentially in four structures as follows and is illustrated in **Flow chart 1.1**:

1. Extraembryonic yolk sac
2. Embryonic arterial cell clusters
3. Fetal liver
4. Bone marrow.

Yolk Sac Hematopoiesis (Mesoblastic Phase)

Fetal hematopoiesis first starts in the mesoderm of extra embryonic yolk sac (seen as blood islands attached to vascular endothelium).[2] These are seen as early as 16 days of embryonic development. The cells initially produced here are primitive erythroid cells, macrophages and megakaryocytes.[1] At 4.5 weeks of development, various clonogenic progenitors of these series of cells have been documented. Fetal cardiac activity and blood circulation starts at day 21 of development. Yolk sac hematopoiesis totally disappears after 6–8 weeks of gestation. Thus, this phase is short lived (16 days–8 weeks of gestation) as compared to birds and rodents.[2]

Embryonic Arterial Cell Clusters

Previously, it was thought that the yolk sac generated stem cells seed fetal liver and bone marrow and is the sole source of hematopoiesis throughout the adult life. But, it has been observed that as the embryo matures, the major arteries in embryo, yolk sac and placenta produce HSCs.

At 27th day, these are first detected attached to aorta, and are seen in increased numbers by 35th day to finally disappear by 40th day.[2] Precursors of aorta (splanchnopleura) are intrinsically found to be capable of generating HSCs on 19th day (i.e. prior to onset of blood circulation), thereby confirming the embryonic origin rather than the migratory

Flow chart 1.1 Ontogeny of hematopoiesis in humans from embryo to adult life

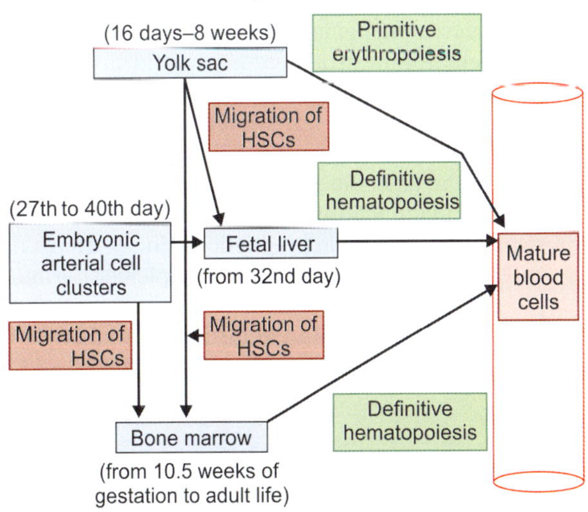

Abbreviation: HSCs: hematopoietic stem cells

HSCs from yolk sac. Also these cells are exclusively capable of generating B- and T-lymphocytes unlike the yolk sac derived cells. The HSCs do not differentiate further in these sites rather they migrate to fetal liver, bone marrow and thymus for further differentiation.[2]

In both yolk sac and embryonic origin of HSCs, these arise in proximity to vascular endothelium, thereby leading to a postulation that a common precursor angiohematopoietic cell (hemangioblast) differentiates into hematopoietic as well as vascular endothelial cells. Recently, human placenta in first trimester has been found to be niche which supports the terminal differentiation of primitive erythroid cells along with interactions from macrophages.

Liver Hematopoiesis (Hepatic Phase)

As the blood circulation is established, these HSCs from yolk sac reaches the embryo and seed the fetal liver first from where hematopoiesis occur till the seeding of bone marrow occurs later. Liver is embryologically derived from the endodermal diverticulum of foregut and the mesodermal structure septum transversum (starting from 22nd day of gestation). At 23rd day, first hepatic colonization is said to occur by CD34 negative erythromyeloid cells. A 2nd colonization occurs at 30th day by CD34+ late stage progenitors (derived from embryonic arterial cell clusters), after which liver is able to sustain hematopoiesis (by 32nd day). Embryo-to-fetal hemoglobin switch including the shift in synthesis of ζ and ε chains to α and γ chains occur in the liver. However, recent studies have shown that definitive erythropoiesis occurs as a second wave in yolk sac as well.[1]

Bone Marrow Hematopoiesis (Myeloid Phase)

In bone marrow, hematopoiesis starts from 11th week (10.5 weeks) of gestation. *Primary logettes* are specialized mesenchymal structures in marrow from where it occurs. The niche supporting these cells comprises of fibrillar material and osteoblasts. Myeloid series are the earliest to differentiate followed by erythroid cells. CD34+ HSCs are however initially absent in the bone marrow and are acquired later which are capable of sustaining hematopoiesis all through the life. At birth, the hematopoiesis is predominant in marrow.[3] The fetus contains HbF$\alpha_2\gamma_2$ (90%) and HbA$\alpha_2\beta_2$ (5–10%).[4] Fetal hemoglobin (HbF) has a left-shifted oxygen dissociation curve (high affinity to oxygen), facilitating oxygen delivery to fetus from the placenta.[3] Adult hemoglobin (HbA) is first detected in fetal circulation at 13th week.[3] But the fetal-to-adult switch in hemoglobin production (HbF → HbA) starts at around 32 weeks of gestation and is completed shortly after birth.[1] In circulation, this process is largely complete by 6 months of postnatal life.[4] HbA at birth is around 20–30% of the total Hb.[3] A normal adult has HbA (97%), HbA2$\alpha_2\delta_2$ (2.5%) and HbF (0.5%).[4]

NORMAL BLOOD COUNTS IN FETUS

Over a period of time (from 18th week to 30th week of gestation), parameters including white cell count (4.68 × 10^9/L–7.71 x 10^9/L), hemoglobin (11.69–13.64 g%), hematocrit (HCT) and red blood cell (RBC) count progressively increases whereas mean corpuscular volume decreases from 131 fL to 114 fL. Platelet count remains comparable to adult values throughout this time. The platelet counts are also found to increase from 32 weeks of gestation till birth and continues to rise during the first 9 weeks after birth to a level of around 7,50,000/μL. These platelets in neonates are however found to be hyporesponsive to agonists with decreased granule secretion and expression of fibrinogen binding sites for the initial 2–4 weeks of life.[5] Differential count shows lymphocyte predominance (80%) throughout this time.[6] The time points of significant events in fetal hematopoiesis are summarized in **Table 1.1**.

Table 1.1 Important time points in fetal hematopoiesis

Gestational age	*Event*
16 days	Yolk sac hematopoiesis starts
19 days	Splanchnopleura capable of initiating hematopoiesis
21 days	Fetal cardiac activity starts
22 days	Liver development starts
23 days	First hepatic colonization occurs (CD34–cells)
27 days	Embryonic arterial cell clusters first detected around aorta
30 days	Second hepatic colonization occurs (CD34+ late stage progenitors)
32 days	Liver can sustain hematopoiesis
4–5 weeks	Peak yolk sac hematopoiesis seen
35 days	Embryonic arterial cell clusters seen in maximum
40 days	Embryonic arterial cell clusters totally disappears
6–8 weeks	Yolk sac hematopoiesis disappears
8–9 weeks	Platelets first seen in circulation
10.5 weeks	Bone marrow hematopoiesis starts (from primary logettes)
13 weeks	HbA first detected in circulation
32 weeks	Fetal-to-adult Hb switch (HbF → HbA) starts

REGULATION OF HEMATOPOIESIS

Unlike most other organs, bone marrow has to continuously regenerate hematopoietic elements throughout the life, even when introduced into another host. This capacity of the bone marrow forms the basis for blood donations and administration of myelosuppressive chemotherapy in malignancies. It is also this phenomenon which has formed the basis of hematopoietic stem cell transplantation in the recent years. This continuous renewal occurs in sequential steps of maturation and differentiation from a multipotent stem cell. During progressive steps, this cell gets committed to definite cell lineages. This process occurs in stroma and is regulated by a variety of growth factors and hormones. Hematopoietic stem cells (HSCs) are also regulated by signals from neighboring cells during the continuous self-renewal process. This microenvironment is called the *niche*. HSCs differentiate to wide variety of hematopoietic elements including erythrocytes, platelets, granulocytes (eosinophil, basophils and neutrophils), lymphocytes (T, B and NK cells), monocyte-macrophage system, dendritic cells and mast cells. Any derangements in the niche of hematopoiesis lead to wide range of pathological conditions including anemia, neutropenia, thrombocytopenia, pancytopenia and leukemia.

Regulation of Yolk Sac Hematopoiesis

The visceral endoderm layer of yolk sac regulates mesoblastic phase of hematopoiesis by secreting certain factors including Indian Hedgehog and vascular endothelial growth factor (VEGF). GATA4, a transcription factor is essential for differentiation of visceral endoderm.[7] Absence of this factor leads to inability to form blood cell islands in this phase. The primitive erythroid progenitors express receptors for stem cell factor (named c-Kit), transforming growth factor-β, erythropoietin, angiopoietin and VEGF, thereby making these factors regulate hematopoiesis.

Regulation of Embryonic Arterial Cell Clusters

The tissues located ventrally to dorsal aorta are found to support HSCs. This niche supports hematopoiesis through cytokines, soluble factors and physical anchorage. Some of these factors include Flt3 ligand, stem cell factor and interleukin-3 (IL-3).[7] Catecholamines also exert influence via sympathetic nerves around arteries located here.

Regulation of Liver Hematopoiesis

The HSCs in fetal liver is supported by a niche consisting of sinusoidal endothelial cells, stromal fibroblasts, macrophages and hepatoblasts. Secretory factors including stem cell factor, IL-6, IL-7, erythropoietin and thrombopoietin secreted by hepatoblasts regulate this phase.[7] HSCs adhere to sinusoidal endothelial cells which help in orientation of HSCs and in mitosis. Liver macrophages form a microenvironment called erythroblastic island and help in engulfing the nuclei expelled by the erythroid precursors. A central macrophage is surrounded by a mixed type of cells along with erythroid precursors to form this erythroblastic island, providing a niche for erythropoiesis.

Regulation of Fetal Bone Marrow Hematopoiesis

The long bones develop from mesodermal progenitors initially as cartilaginous bone templates that later get vascularized and form epiphyseal plates. Along with vascular endothelial cells (that form blood vessels), osteoblasts also occupy the bone marrow cavity and play a key role in the establishment of fetal bone marrow niche for HSCs. The process of HSCs homing the marrow and starting hematopoiesis is regulated by chemotactic factors (CXCL12 and its receptor CXCR4 along with other associated molecules).[7] Animal studies have shown that mutation of these factors leads to clinical condition with normal liver hematopoiesis but defective homing of bone marrow with HSCs.

Regulation of Neonatal and Juvenile Bone Marrow Hematopoiesis

Like any other organ, bone marrow also needs to adapt to the profound physiological changes that occur after birth. Onset of breathing leading to changes in oxygen content of blood and exposure to external environment leading to immune system activation are the major changes to tackle by the neonatal bone marrow. The exact changes in bone marrow niche are not exactly delineated yet.[7] Recognition of increased calcium ions released by the bone matrix is a crucial step. As the ossification process ensues with age, preserving a niche for lifelong hematopoiesis is essential which is regulated by transcription factors.

Regulation of Adult Bone Marrow Hematopoiesis

In an adult bone, HSCs are seen predominantly in metaphyseal regions, but also in diaphyseal and epiphyseal regions. They are localized in two distinct niches in endosteal region (close to bone) and in perivascular region (close to arterioles). HSCs are adherent to osteoblasts which supports hematopoiesis. The role of osteoclasts in hematopoiesis is controversial. The endosteal niche is regulated by various cytokine signaling and cell adhesion molecules. The HSCs in perivascular niche is supported by the surrounded mesenchymal type cells. These mesenchymal cells secrete stem cell factor, CXCL12 thereby regulating hematopoiesis. Megakaryocytes and thrombopoietin are also found to be essential for normal hematopoiesis.[7] As aging occurs, hematopoietic cells in the bone marrow are gradually replaced by yellow adipose tissue in selected areas. This adipose tissue has been found to have an inhibitory effect on the HSCs.

STRESS ERYTHROPOIESIS

In the postnatal life, erythropoiesis is usually restricted to bone marrow. But under anemic stress including blood loss, hemolysis (sickle cell anemia, thalassemia), infiltrative conditions (leukemia, myelofibrosis), the erythroid precursors home the extramedullary organs (spleen and liver) and begins erythropoiesis. Erythroblastic islands are formed here. This clinically manifests with splenomegaly and hepatomegaly.

ERYTHROID LINEAGE DIFFERENTIATION

Primitive Erythropoiesis

For a short duration of around 48 hours, the hematopoiesis in yolk sac is predominated by primitive erythroid cells.[1] These are large nucleated cells. The differentiated elements of these cells are detected in the circulation even after birth though in a minority. Gastrulation is a developmental step in

CHAPTER

2 Developmental Hemostasis and Physiology of Hemostasis in the Fetus and the Newborn

Shrimati Shetty

INTRODUCTION

Hemostasis in humans is a dynamic process and the levels of coagulation factors, inhibitors and the fibrinolytic proteins vary throughout different gestational ages, neonatal and the pediatric age groups.[1,2] It is the complex interaction between different components of the blood coagulation system and the cellular and endothelial components resulting in both positive and negative feedback maintaining a tightly regulated hemostatic balance. Thus, despite age-specific differences in the levels of blood coagulation proteins, the hemostatic balance is always maintained. Besides maintaining thrombohemorrhagic balance, many of the blood coagulation proteins also have nonhemostatic functions like angiogenesis, inflammation, immune responses and wound healing **(Flow chart 2.1)**.

The dynamic changes that take place throughout the gestational period and get continued in the neonatal period till the adult life, maintaining the thrombohemorrhagic balance is termed as developmental hemostasis. Understanding this process is important not only for the treating clinicians but also for the laboratory personnel, for an optimal diagnostic and treatment strategies. As the coagulation proteins cannot cross the placental barrier, the hemostatic system in a neonate is independent of maternal hemostatic system.[3] Hemostasis in the fetus as well as the neonate evolves at a much faster rate than that of the adult and it is important to establish age-specific normal ranges in these groups. The treatment strategies also differ between neonates and adults. A better understanding of the physiology of neonates is thus important for optimal care.

Flow chart 2.1 Hemostasis in humans

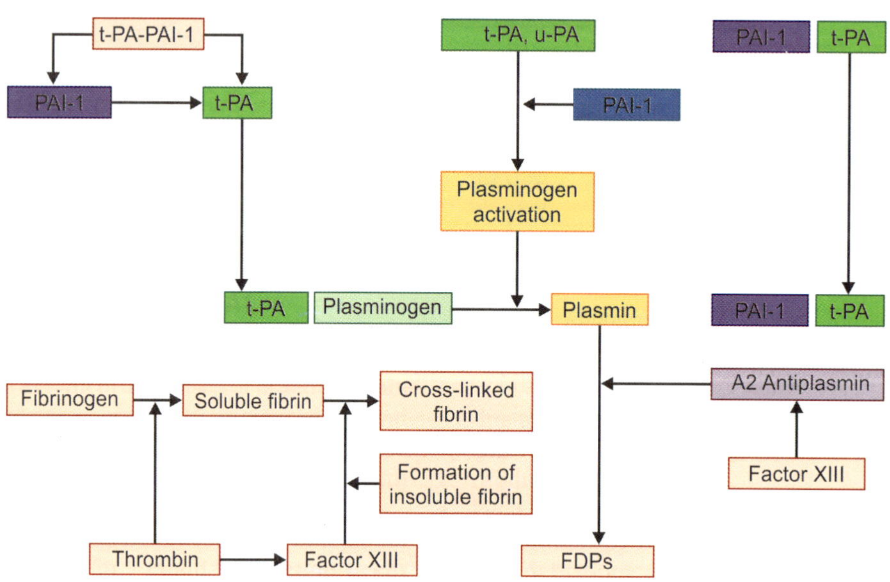

Abbreviations: t-PA, tissue plasminogen activator; PAI-1, plasminogen activator inhibitor-1; u-PA, urinary plasminogen activator; FDPs, fibrin degradation product

Changes in the hemostatic system with age may mainly be attributed to the multifunctional role of the coagulation proteins rather than the hemostatic function itself. Many of the coagulation proteins for instance antithrombin (AT), are also involved in angiogenesis, wound healing and inflammation. At different developmental stages, the demand of these systems is different and as such we get variations in the levels of these factors during fetal and neonatal period.

As hemorrhagic disease of the newborn (HDN) is the most common bleeding manifestation in neonates, lot of reports are available on the levels of vitamin K-dependent factors[4,5] in neonates. Apart from this, knowledge about fetal or neonatal hemostasis is always inadequate. The main reasons for this are the difficulties in sampling and the methodological and reagent differences across different laboratories.[6,7] Another important point to be noted is that unlike adults, one needs multiple reference ranges in the fetal or neonatal period due to the rapidly evolving hemostatic system during this period.

PRIMARY HEMOSTASIS

Primary hemostasis refers to the formation of hemostatic plug at the site of injury by the interaction of platelets with the endothelial components. Platelets are formed in the human fetus as early as 5 weeks of gestation and they steadily increase till they attain a count of 150×10^9/L at the end of first trimester of pregnancy. Once the normal platelet count is attained, the same level is retained till full term.[8]

In the first 9 weeks of neonatal period, there is an increase in the platelet count up to 750×10^9/L and thereafter gets reduced to the adult normal range.[9] In a large series of 47,291 neonates treated in a multihospital system, reference ranges for platelet counts at different gestational and postconceptional ages were determined and platelet counts for infants less than or equal to 32 weeks gestation was found to be 104×10^9/L, compared with 123×10^9/L for neonates greater than 32 weeks of age.[10]

Even though platelet numbers are normal or increased, platelet function analysis suggests that neonatal platelets are hyporeactive compared with adults. It is surprising, therefore, to see a shortened bleeding time in normal healthy neonates.[11] The explanation for this observation has been the presence of large multimers and the increased packed cell volume in neonates.[12] The platelet aggregation response to different agonists like collagen, adenosine 5′-diphosphate (ADP), and epinephrine is also reduced in neonates as compared to adults.[13] It is also shown that bleeding time in infants born preterm (<33 weeks of gestation) have longer bleeding times as compared to full term infants.[14] Decreased platelet adhesion has also been observed in preterm infants as compared to full term infants.[15] The platelet function analyzer-100 closure time with ADP was found to be inversely correlated with the gestational age.[16] Thus overall, by all investigations, it is clear that the primary hemostasis is less developed in premature infants as compared to full term infants.

SECONDARY HEMOSTASIS

The secondary hemostasis refers to the sequential activation of blood coagulation factors resulting in the formation of fibrin clot, which is also strictly regulated by inhibitors to each of these factors. The physiology of hemostasis in fetus, neonate and the adult is different with the normal ranges of all coagulation factors being reduced but the fine balance between procoagulant and anticoagulant factors is always maintained.

Very little is known about the coagulation system during the intrauterine life. Whatever reports are available there are wide differences in the range of different factors. The variable results are due to the difficulties in the fetal blood sampling. Fetal hemostasis is unique in several ways and many of the coagulation proteins developed during early gestational period have nonhemostatic functions like cell growth and cell differentiation.[17] Fetal hemostasis is significantly different from the adult and has some distinct features. Both qualitative and quantitative differences have been observed in the fetal blood samples as compared to the adults. All the procoagulants and anticoagulants in the fetal blood samples are of fetal origin as they do not cross the placenta. Though it is difficult to ascertain the exact time at which the different coagulation factors are synthesized, the hemostatic function of fetal blood is known to be initiated around 11th week of pregnancy.[18]

About 20 weeks of gestational age, the levels of almost all procoagulants and anticoagulants is one-fifth of the adult value.[19] In 19–29-week gestational age, the prothrombin time (PT) is almost six times and activated partial thromboplastin time (APTT) is five times the control value which can be clearly related to the low levels of all coagulation factors, i.e. vitamin K-dependent proteins contact factors namely, V and VIII, and fibrinogen.[2] This is expected as there is a drastic reduction of almost all the coagulation factors. But even the natural inhibitors of these factors, i.e. protein C (PC), protein S (PS), AT, tissue factor pathway inhibitor (TFPI) and heparin cofactor II (HCII) are reduced, there exists a thrombohemorrhagic balance.[19]

Between 30 weeks and 38 weeks of gestation, a significant shortening of PT and APTT was recorded. At the same time, most coagulation factors increased slightly (up to 25–30%), whereas factors V, VII, and VIII were between 45% and 50% of adult values. All coagulation inhibitors, i.e. AT, HCII, PC, PS and TFPI, are also greatly reduced, and we can thus assume that at this age a well-balanced hemostatic equilibrium is maintained. All coagulation inhibitors remain at levels near or less than 20%, except AT, which reaches a mean value of 37% at the end of pregnancy.

It is only between 30 weeks and 38 weeks, there is an accelerated increase in all these factors and only three clotting proteins, i.e. factors V, VII and XIII reach the adult values at birth. The levels of all blood coagulation inhibitors also increase during this period, but it is still low, i.e. around 50% during delivery except AT and HCII which are

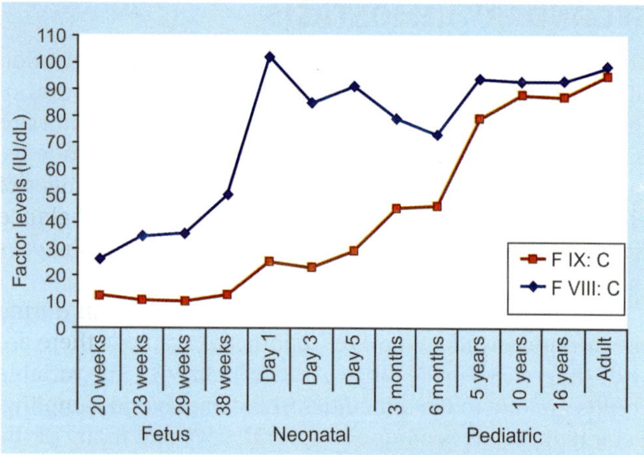

Figure 2.1 Factor VIII and IX at different gestational weeks, neonatal, pediatric and up to 6 months of age

around 60% of the adult values. Except PC, the levels of the anticoagulants reach the adult values only around 6th month of life. Despite the low thrombin generation potential, the thrombohemorrhagic balance is never compromised in fetal life. Thrombin generation potential of fetal blood has been found to be lower, i.e. 30–50% of that of the adult. This is expected due to the low levels of all the clotting factors.[19]

Reference ranges for coagulation factors according to different age groups, specifically in the gestational and the neonatal period, are of utmost importance for an accurate diagnosis. The reference range for different coagulation factors during different gestational ages specifically between 18 weeks and 20 weeks enables the geneticists to offer prenatal diagnosis of affected families by performing phenotypic assays in the cord blood sample.[20] This would facilitate the second trimester antenatal diagnosis, wherein the families are either noninformative for the genetic markers or they have turned out late for diagnosis during which chorionic villus sampling will not be feasible. **Figure 2.1** shows the different levels factor VIII and IX at different gestational weeks, neonatal, pediatric and up to 6 months of age.

NEONATAL HEMOSTASIS

The hemostatic system in a neonate is much different from the pediatric as well as the adult cases. Except factors V, VIII and von Willebrand Factor, all the remaining procoagulant factors are decreased as compared to the adults. Among the natural anticoagulants, except alpha 2 macroglobulin, all the remaining factors are decreased. Though most of the coagulation factors are still lower in the neonatal period, FVIII has been found to be higher on day 1 of the neonate but comes back to the adult value in day 3. Whether this is a transient increase due to stress of delivery or a protective mechanism to prevent excessive bleeding is not clear. In the neonates, the levels of coagulation factors also depend on the birth weight of the baby or whether the child is born full term or small for gestational age.[21] This goes in line with the observation that premature babies have higher morbidity and mortality due to bleeding or thrombotic manifestations.[22] Varied reports are available in literature with regard to different factor levels in full term and premature infants. Alpha-2-macroglobulin is increased both in neonates and pediatric cases, which has often been considered as a protective mechanism from thromboembolic events in neonates. As such the incidence of thrombosis is quite rare in neonates compared to adults.[23]

Qualitative Abnormalities in Coagulation Factors in Fetal and Neonatal Period

Most of the reports available in literature are on the quantitative variations of hemostatic protein, but there are no reports on the qualitative age-specific differences. It has been reported that fibrinogen is functionally abnormal during both fetal and neonatal period in that the polymerizing ability.[24] In addition, the fetal fibrinogen has also been found to have increased sialic acid content as compared to adult fibrinogen, the significance of which, however, is not clear.[25] The phosphorous content of the fetal fibrinogen has also been found to be highly increased[26,27] as compared to adult fibrinogen. The molecular weight of alpha, beta and gamma chains of fibrinogen protein has been found to be increased in fetal fibrinogen,[28] mainly due to the increased sialic acid content. Qualitative differences have also been observed in PC from neonates, but none of the other coagulation factors have been analyzed for the functional differences between different age groups.[29]

Laboratory Diagnosis of Hemostasis in a Neonate

Whenever a neonate presents with bleeding manifestations, it is important to take a good history. If the bleeding is presented in otherwise a healthy neonate, it may either be an acquired condition like immune thrombocytopenia or it may be due to hereditary bleeding disorders. If bleeding occurs in a sick neonate it may most probably be due to disseminated intravascular coagulation. The hemostatic system matures rapidly during the first few days, weeks and months of life, and the levels of most hemostatic proteins reach adult values by 6 months of life. The laboratory diagnosis of hemostatic parameters in a neonate is difficult because of the sample quality. Therefore, repeating the tests to look for reproducibility of the results is important before the final diagnosis is offered. One of the important points to be considered while establishing an age-specific reference range is the use of specific assays and specific manufacturers. For instance, the reference range for PC antigen may be different than that of PC activity.[30] Similarly, the reference range also may vary between different manufacturers. The final diagnosis in a neonate should be exercised with caution. The normal age-specific reference range should always be established in the same laboratory where the tests are performed. Abnormal results should always be repeated as there are higher chances of sampling errors in a neonate.

ROLE OF MICRO-RNA IN DEVELOPMENTAL HEMOSTASIS

MicroRNAs (miRNAs) are short, single-stranded RNA segments having an important role in gene regulation which generally act at the post-transcriptional level. Continuing work in the area of miRNAs suggests that they regulate almost every physiological process in human body.[31,32] Among the hemostatic proteins, there are only two proteins, i.e. fibrinogen and plasminogen activator inhibitor-1, wherein the functional roles of miRNA has been investigated.[33,34] Several authors have also proposed that miRNAs may be regulating the differential expression of blood coagulation proteins during embryonic development.[35] It is of immense importance to understand the role of miRNAs in the regulation of blood coagulation proteins because even small differences in the levels of coagulation factors can prove a risky factor for bleeding or thrombosis. Identification of the regulators of synthesis of other coagulation proteins can provide an explanation for the age-specific differences of coagulation proteins.

SIGNIFICANCE OF UNDERSTANDING FETAL AND NEONATAL HEMOSTASIS

- Reference ranges in the second trimester of pregnancy are essential to offer prenatal diagnosis of coagulation disorders
- Understanding the physiology of hemostasis and the reference ranges are essential for clinical monitoring
- Preoperative analysis of neonates with or without bleeding disorders
- To monitor the efficacy of drugs with specific targets, for instance, the oral thrombin inhibitor dabigatran is a specific inhibitor of thrombin. Knowing the basal levels of thrombin in different age groups is essential for optimal impact and to prevent adverse side effects.

CONCLUSION

- The hemostatic indices gradually evolve during early life and attain adult values by 6 months of age
- It is important that both the laboratory personnel and the treating physicians be aware of the reference ranges for different age groups for different coagulation parameters
- The levels of coagulation factors increase with age; besides there also exists statistically significant interindividual variability
- In a neonate, it is essential to understand the clinical setting at which the neonate bleeds. Family history, parental consanguinity all are pointers to congenital bleeding disorders and bleeding in a sick child may be due to consumptive coagulopathy.

REFERENCES

1. Shetty S, Ghosh K, Anbhavne S, Mohanty D. Requiem to prenatal diagnosis of haemophilia A and B using coagulation activity and antigen based assays: not yet! Eur J Haematol. 2003;70(4):253-4.
2. Reverdiau-Moalic P, Delahousse B, Body G, Bardos P, Leroy J, Gruel Y. Evolution of blood coagulation activators and inhibitors in the healthy human fetus. Blood. 1996;88(3):900-6.
3. Pichler E, Pichler L. The neonatal coagulation system and the vitamin K deficiency bleeding - a mini review. Wien Med Wochenschr. 2008;158(13-14):385-95.
4. Gruel Y, Boizard B, Daffos F, Forestier F, Caen J, Wautier JL. Determination of platelet antigens and glycoproteins in the human fetus. Blood. 1986;68(2):488-92.
5. Whaun JM, Smith GR, Sochor VA. Effect of prenatal drug administration on maternal and neonatal platelet aggregation and PF4 release. Haemostasis. 1980;9(4):226-37.
6. Monagle P, Barnes C, Ignjatovic V, Furmedge J, Newall F, Chan A, et al. Developmental haemostasis. Impact for clinical haemostasis laboratories. Thromb Haemost. 2006;95(2):362-72.
7. Ignjatovic V, Kenet G, Monagle P. Perinatal and Paediatric Haemostasis Subcommittee of the Scientific and Standardization Committee of the International Society on Thrombosis and Haemostasis. Developmental haemostasis: recommendations for laboratories reporting pediatric samples. J Thromb Haemost. 2012;10(2):298-300.
8. Forestier F, Daffos F, Catherine N, Renard M, Andreux JP. Developmental hematopoiesis in normal human fetal blood. Blood. 1991;77(11):2360-3.
9. Sitaru AG, Holzhauer S, Speer CP, Singer D, Obergfell A, Walter U, et al. Neonatal platelets from cord blood and peripheral blood. Platelets. 2005;16(3-4):203-10.
10. Wiedmeier SE, Henry E, Sola-Visner MC, Christensen RD. Platelet reference ranges for neonates, defined using data from over 47,000 patients in a multihospital healthcare system. J Perinatol. 2009;29(2):130-6.
11. Andrew M, Paes B, Bowker J, Vegh P. Evaluation of an automated bleeding time device in the newborn. Am J Hematol. 1990;35(4):275-7.
12. Michelson AD. Platelet function in the newborn. Semin Thromb Hemost. 1998;24(6):507-12.
13. Israels SJ, Rand ML, Michelson AD. Neonatal platelet function. Semin Thromb Hemost. 2003;29:363-72.
14. Del Vecchio A, Latini G, Henry E, Christensen RD. Template bleeding times of 240 neonates born at 24 to 41 weeks gestation. J Perinatol. 2008;28(6):427-31.
15. Levy-Shraga Y, Maayan-Metzger A, Lubetsky A, Shenkman B, Kuint J, Martinowitz U, et al. Platelet function of newborns as tested by cone and plate(let) analyzer correlates with gestational age. Acta Haematol. 2006;115(3-4):152-6.
16. Saxonhouse MA, Garner R, Mammel L, Li Q, Muller KE, Greywoode J, et al. Closure times measured by the platelet function analyzer PFA-100 are longer in neonatal blood compared to cord blood samples. Neonatology. 2010;97(3):242-9.
17. Manco-Johnson MJ. Development of hemostasis in the fetus. Thromb Res. 2005;115 Suppl 1:55-63.
18. Kuhle S, Male C, Mitchell L. Developmental hemostasis: pro- and anticoagulant systems during childhood. Semin Thromb Haemost. 2003;29(4):329-38.
19. Uszyński M, Uszyński W, Szymański M. Procoagulants and anticoagulants in fetal blood. A literature survey. Folia Histochem Cytobiol. 2009;47(4):545-50.
20. Mota L, Ghosh K, Shetty S. Second trimester antenatal diagnosis in rare coagulation factor deficiencies. J Pediatr Hematol Oncol. 2007;29(3):137-9.

21. Abdollahi A, Sheikhbahaei S, Hafezi-Nejad N, Mahdaviani B. Hemostatic profile in healthy premature neonates; does birth weight affect the coagulation profile? J Clin Neonatol. 2014;3(2):89-92.
22. Gurgey A, Tekinalp G, Cinar A, Cakmak F. Symptomatic thrombosis in Turkish neonates. J Pediatr Hematol Oncol. 2004;26:417-20.
23. Ignjatovic V, Lai C, Summerhayes R, Mathesius U, Tawfilis S, Perugini MA, et al. Age-related differences in plasma proteins: how plasma proteins change from neonates to adults. PLoS One. 2011;6(2):e17213.
24. Hamulyák K, Nieuwenhuizen W, Devilée PP, Hemker HC. Reevaluation of some properties of fibrinogen, purified from cord blood of normal newborns. Thomb Res. 1983;32(3):301-10.
25. Ignjatovic V, Ilhan A, Monagle P. Evidence for age-related differences in human fibrinogen. Blood Coagul Fibrinolysis. 2011;22(2):110-7.
26. Guttilla IK, White BA. Coordinate regulation of FOXO1 by miR-27a, miR-96, and miR-182 in breast cancer cells. J Biol Chem. 2009;284(35):23204-16.
27. Witt I, Müller H. Phosphorus and hexose content of human foetal fibrinogen. Biochim Biophys Acta. 1970;221(2):402-4.
28. Dang C, Shin CK, Bell WR, Nagaswami C, Weisel JW. Fibrinogen sialic acid residues are low affinity calcium binding sites that influence fibrin assembly. J Biol Chem. 1989;264(25):15104-8.
29. Manco-Johnson M, Spedale S, Peters M. Identification of a unique form of protein C in the ovine fetus: developmentally linked transition to the adult form. Pediatr Res. 1995;37(3): 365-72.
30. Attard C, van der Straaten T, Karlaftis V, Monagle P, Ignjatovic V. Developmental haemostasis: age-specific differences in the quantity of hemostatic proteins: reply to a rebuttal. J Thromb Haemost. 2014;12(2):286.
31. Brodersen P, Voinnet O. Revisiting the principles of microRNA target recognition and mode of action. Nat Rev Mol Cell Biol. 2009;10(2):141-8.
32. Guo H, Ingolia NT, Weissman JS, Bartel DP. Mammalian microRNAs predominantly act to decrease target mRNA levels. Nature. 2010;466(7308):835-40.
33. Fort A, Borel C, Migliavacca E, Antonarakis SE, Fish RJ, Neerman-Arbez M. Regulation of fibrinogen production by microRNAs. Blood. 2010;116(14):2608-15.
34. Muth M, Theophile K, Hussein K, Jacobi C, Kreipe H, Bock O. "Hypoxia-induced down-regulation of microRNA-449a/b impairs control over targeted SERPINE1 (PAI-1) mRNA - a mechanism involved in SERPINE1 (PAI-1) overexpression". J Transl Med. 2010;8:33.
35. Tzur G, Israel A, Levy A, Benjamin H, Meiri E, Shufaro Y, et al. Comprehensive gene and microRNA expression profiling reveals a role for microRNAs in human liver development. PLoS One. 2009;4(10):e7511.

CHAPTER 3

Granulocytes: Development and Physiology

Tulika Seth

PRESENT KNOWLEDGE

Neonates are at a higher risk for bacterial infections than older children and adults. This is due to both quantitative and qualitative insufficiencies of their innate immunity. It is important to understand the basis of these defects in order to try to develop newer strategies for management. Though antibiotics remain the mainstay of treatment, adjuvant therapies which enhance immune function have a possible role in treating sepsis in neonates.

Flow chart 3.1 Earliest appearance of neutrophil precursors and their fate

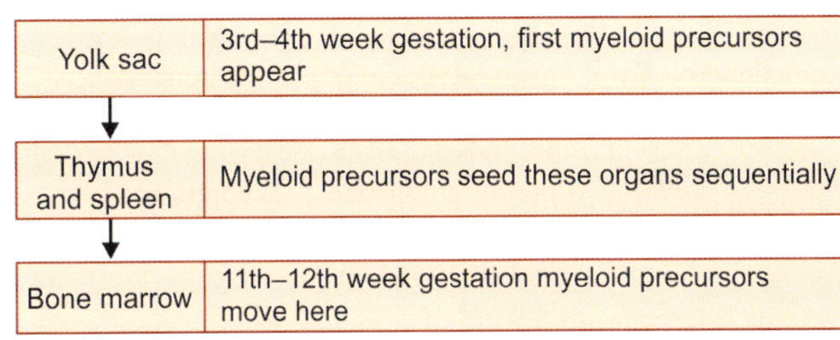

Flow chart 3.2 Granulopoiesis and terminal neutrophil maturation

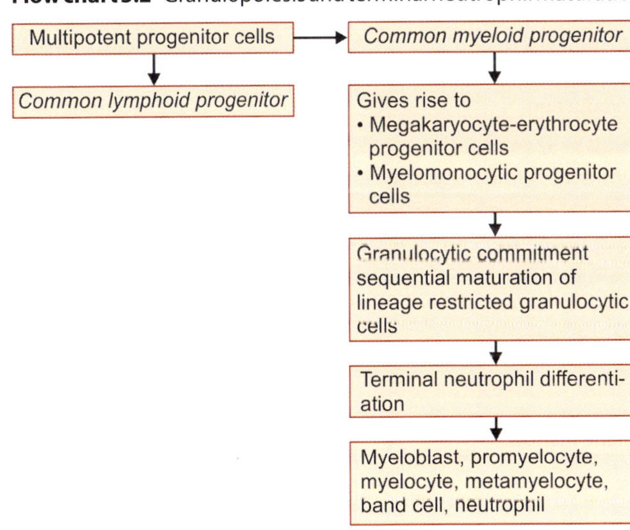

GRANULOPOIESIS

All granulocytic cells and other mature hematopoietic cells are derived from the pluripotent hematopoietic stem cells, which emerge from the yolk sac, chorioallantoic placenta and aorta-gonad-mesonephros (AGM) region.[1] The first myeloid progenitor cells are present in the yolk sac at 3rd to 4th week of gestation. They sequentially seed the liver, thymus, spleen and eventually move to populate the bone marrow at 11th to 12th week of gestation **(Flow chart 3.1)**. The production of mature granulocytes is very limited in the fetus until the end of the 2nd trimester, after which the fetal bone marrow takes over hematopoietic production.[1,2]

The multipotent progenitor cells differentiate **(Flow chart 3.2)** into either a lymphoid or myeloid lineage pathway by the production of common lymphoid progenitor cells or common myeloid progenitor (CMP) cells.[3] The CMP cells can give rise to megakaryocyte-erythrocyte progenitor cells or granulocyte/macrophage progenitor (GMP) cells. The GMPs commit to granulocyte lineage development, terminal neutrophil differentiation occurs, which results in the sequential maturation of lineage restricted granulocytic progenitor cells. This results in the terminal neutrophil differentiation including myeloblast, promyelocyte, myelocyte, metamyelocyte, band cell and mature neutrophil stages. Each stage is marked by a specific transcriptional program, cell cycle status, cytokine receptor expression, phagocytosis capacity, granule and bactericidal content, reactive oxygen intermediate production, and varying ability to degrade phagocytosed material.[4,5] We can identify the cells and their maturation levels by flow cytometry, cell sorting and molecular biological analysis. Now researchers can study the transcriptional control of neutrophil lineage differentiation at various stages.[4]

Mature neutrophils must also produce chemokines and cytokines **(Box 3.1)** that regulate other immune effect

Table 3.2 Quantitative neutrophil defects in the neonate

Colony-forming unit-granulocyte: macrophage (CFU-GM)	*Adults*	*Neonates*
Myeloid progenitor pool (%)		
1. At rest	100	10
2. Sepsis	2–3 fold increase	Decrease
Neutrophil storage pool (%)		
1. At rest	100	20
2. Sepsis	Initial decrease	Decrease
Peripheral neutrophil count during sepsis	Transient neutropenia, followed by neutrophilia	Prolonged neutropenia
Proliferative rate (%)		
1. At rest	Low	High
2. Sepsis	Increase	No change (maximal already)

Source: Adapted from Seth T, Cairo MS. Monograph: The role of cytokines in the prevention and treatment of neonatal sepsis. In: Bellanti JA, Bracci R, Prindull G, Xanthou M (Eds). Neonatal Hematology and Immunology. Amsterdam: Elsevier; 1997. pp. 49-53.

Table 3.3 Deficiencies in pathogen recognition present in neonatal granulocytes

Receptor or property	*Neonatal status*	*Study*
TLRs	*Deficient:* • TLRs bind to conserved molecular patterns on pathogens and initiate key events of the innate immune response • TLR4 is a transmembrane receptor for the gram negative bacterial product LPS • Studies shown activation of intracellular signaling factors MyD88 and p38 is insufficient following LPS binding to TLR4 on neonatal neutrophils • Decreased production of TNF-α in response to LPS • Neonatal blood has high concentrations of circulating adenosine—this adenosine activity increases cytosolic cAMP concentrations which subsequently inhibit LPS induced TNF-α production	Förster-Waldl (2005)[30]
Adherence	• Selectins mediate contact between neutrophils and the vascular endothelium • Analysis of cord blood from neonates less than one month old has demonstrated lower levels of L-selectin than seen in adults, insufficiency in the ability of neonatal neutrophils to adhere to the vascular endothelium • Mac-1 (CD11b/CD18), is important in neutrophil adhesion • 50% reduction in transmigration	Anderson (1986)[31]
Chemotaxis	• Deficiency in neonatal neutrophil adherence and migration • Neonatal chemotaxis reduced 60% during the 1st week of postnatal life • Defective actin polymerization prevents neutrophils motile functions and leads to recurrent, severe bacterial and fungal infections	Eisenfeld (1990)[32]
Phagocytosis	• Neonates are less able to phagocytose *Candida*, due to deficit of neonatal neutrophils to engulf larger particles	Falconer (1995)[33]
Intracellular killing	• Balanced changes result in oxidative function of neonatal neutrophils similar to that seen in adults • Under prolonged periods of infection, however, specific deficiencies in cytosolic components and granules might restrict neutrophil response	Ambruso (2004)[34]
Clearance or apoptosis	• Decreased response of neonatal neutrophils to proapoptotic signals to decreased surface receptor expression of the FAS receptor, decreased proapoptotic intracellular signaling molecule caspase-3, and decreased activity of the pro-apoptotic proteins Siglec-9 and SHP-1	Hanna (2005)[35]
NETosis	• Term and premature neonates have deficient neutrophil NET formation and NET-mediated extracellular killing	Fuchs (2007)[36]
NETs provide high concentrations of microbicidal products to disarm and kill bacteria extracellularly	• This defect is also found in neutrophils isolated from CGD patients.	

Abbreviations: cAMP, cyclic adenosine monophosphate; CGD, chronic granulomatous disease; LPS, lipopolysaccharide; Mac-1, macrophage-1; MyD88, myeloid differentiation antigen 88; NETs, neutrophil extracellular traps; TLRs, toll-like receptor; TNF-α, tumor necrosis factor-α defects in all of their functions such as pathogen recognition, adherence, chemotaxis, phagocytosis, intracellular killing, clearance or apoptosis and NETosis **(Table 3.3)**.

Adjuvant Therapies for Treating Neonatal Sepsis

During the last 3 decades, physicians and researchers have been investigating therapeutic approaches to strengthen neonatal immunity while they concurrently treat patients with antibiotics. A number of adjuvant strategies to improve neonatal immune function during sepsis have been explored.

Colony Stimulating Factors

Colony stimulating factors play a vital role in the development of a hematopoietic stem cell into mature blood cells. They also modulate granulocyte function including phagocytosis and cell mediated killing. Two extensively studied CSFs for the treatment of neonatal sepsis are G-CSF and GM-CSF. Both G-CSF and GM-CSF regulate the production and release of neutrophils from the bone marrow.[37-39] Investigators have applied their use in two strategies to combat neonatal sepsis.

Prophylactically stimulating neutrophil production and enhancing bactericidal function of existing granulocytes. Roberts et al. demonstrated increased neutrophil production as a result of G-CSF administration to a neutropenic neonate.[40] Recently a multicenter trial by Kuhn et al. including 200 infants, studied the benefit of prophylactic recombinant G-CSF (rG-CSF) treatment in preterm neonates with neutropenia in preventing nosocomial infections during 4 weeks of treatment. Although rG-CSF increased the number of neutrophils in these patients during the initial two weeks of treatment, this difference did not persist to the conclusion of the study.[41] Kuhn et al. concluded that prophylactic rG-CSF did not increase infection free survival 4 weeks after initiating treatment.[41] rG-CSF prophylaxis, however, may prove beneficial in bolstering neutrophil number and preventing infection in some subsets of neonates including those that are small for gestational age and those with early established postnatal neutropenia.

Granulocyte-macrophage-colony forming unit is upregulated in response to inflammatory stimuli. The effects of GM-CSF are broader spectrum than G-CSF as it is produced by many different cell types and promotes the growth of precursors for multiple myeloid and megakaryocytic lineages.[37,38] When administered prophylactically recombinant GM-CSF (rGM-CSF) can significantly increase neutrophil counts in at-risk neonates. GM-CSF can also improve neonatal neutrophil function.

However, in spite of proliferative and functional benefits of GM-CSF on the neonatal neutrophil population, rGM-CSF administration does not significantly increase sepsis free survival and there is insufficient evidence to support its use both as a prophylactic and treatment strategy.[42]

FUTURE PERSPECTIVES

Understanding more about cell cycle signaling and transcriptional control of granulopoiesis may lead to further breakthroughs.

REFERENCES

1. Melvan JN, Bagby GJ, Welsh DA, Nelson S, Zhang P. Neonatal sepsis and neutrophil insufficiencies. Int Rev Immunol. 2010;29(3):315-48.
2. Dzierzak E, Speck NA. Of lineage and legacy: the development of mammalian hematopoietic stem cells. Nat Immunol. 2008;9(2):129-36.
3. Migliaccio G, Migliaccio AR, Petti S, Mavilio F, Russo G, Lazzaro D, et al. Human embryonic hemopoiesis, kinetics of progenitors and precursors underlying the yolk sac—liver transition. J Clin Invest. 1986;78(1):51-60.
4. Kondo M, Wagers AJ, Manz MG, Prohaska SS, Scherer DC, Beilhack GF, et al. Biology of hematopoietic stem cells and progenitors: implications for clinical application. Annu Rev Immunol. 2003;21:759-806.
5. Iwasaki H, Akashi K. Myeloid lineage commitment from the hematopoietic stem cell. Immunity. 2007;26(6):726-40.
6. Theilgaard-Mönch K, Porse BT, Borregaard N. Systems biology of neutrophil differentiation and immune response. Curr Opin Immunol. 2006;18(1):54-60.
7. Radomska HS, Huettner CS, Zhang P, Cheng T, Scadden DT, Tenen DG. CCAAT/enhancer binding protein alpha is a regulatory switch sufficient for induction of granulocytic development from bipotential myeloid progenitors. Mol Cell Biol. 1998;18(7):4301-14.
8. Koschmieder S, Halmos B, Levantini E, Tenen DG. Dysregulation of the C/EBPalpha differentiation pathway in human cancer. J Clin Oncol. 2009;27(1):619-28.
9. Metcalf D. Control of granulocytes and macrophages: molecular, cellular, and clinical aspects. Science. 1991;254(5031):529-33.
10. Panopoulos AD, Watowich SS. Granulocyte colony-stimulating factor: molecular mechanisms of action during steady state and 'emergency' hematopoiesis. Cytokine. 2008;42(3):277-88.
11. Nicola NA, Metcalf D. Binding of 125I-labeled granulocyte colony-stimulating factor to normal murine hemopoietic cells. J Cell Physiol. 1985;124(2):313-21.
12. Demetri GD, Griffin JD. Granulocyte colony stimulating factor and its receptor. Blood. 1991;78(11):2791-808.
13. Yan SR, Byers DM, Bortolussi R. Role of protein tyrosine kinase p53/56lyn in diminished lipopolysaccharide priming of formylmethionylleucyl-phenylalanine-induced superoxide production in human newborn neutrophils. Infect Immun. 2004;72(11):6455-62.
14. Maródi L. Deficient interferon-gamma receptor-mediated signaling in neonatal macrophages. Acta Paediatr Suppl. 2002;91(438):117-9.
15. Maródi L, Goda K, Palicz A, Szabó G. Cytokine receptor signalling in neonatal macrophages: defective STAT-1 phosphorylation in response to stimulation with IFN-gamma. Clin Exp Immunol. 2001;126(3):456-60.
16. Demetri GD, Griffin JD. Granulocyte colony-stimulating factor and its receptor. Blood. 1991;78(11):2791-808.
17. Semerad CL, Liu F, Gregory AD, Stumpf K, Link DC. G-CSF is an essential regulator of neutrophil trafficking from the bone marrow to the blood. Immunity. 2002;17(4):413-23.

18. Ueda Y, Kondo M, Kelsoe G. Inflammation and the reciprocal production of granulocytes and lymphocytes in bone marrow. J Exp Med. 2005;201(11):1771-80.
19. Adams GB, Scadden DT. The hematopoietic stem cell in its place. Nat Immunol. 2006;7(4):333-7.
20. Osawa M, Nakamura K, Nishi N, Takahasi N, Tokuomoto Y, Inoue H, et al. In vivo self-renewal of c-Kit+ Sca-1+ Lin(low/-) hemopoietic stem cells. J Immunol. 1996;156(9):3207-14.
21. Essers MA, Offner S, Blanco-Bose WE, Waibler Z, Kalinke U, Duchosal MA, et al. IFNalpha activates dormant haematopoietic stem cells in vivo. Nature. 2009;458(7240):904-8.
22. Lothian C, Dahlgren C, Lagercrantz H, Lundahl J. Different expression and mobilisation of the complement regulatory proteins CD35, CD55 and CD59 in neonatal and adult neutrophils. Biol Neonate. 1997;72(1):15-21.
23. Rudolph AM, Barnett HL, Einhorn AH. In: Rudolph AM, Barnett HL, Einhorn AH. Pediatrics, 16th edition. New York: Appleton-Century-Crofts; 1977.
24. Manroe BL, Weinberg AG, Rosenfeld CR, Browne R. The neonatal blood count in health and disease. I. Reference values for neutrophilic cells. J Pediatr. 1979;95(1):89-98.
25. Mouzinho A, Rosenfeld CR, Sánchez PJ, Risser R. Revised reference ranges for circulating neutrophils in very-low-birth-weight neonates. Pediatrics. 1994;94(1):76-82.
26. Christensen RD, Calhoun DA, Rimsza LM. A practical approach to evaluating and treating neutropenia in the neonatal intensive care unit. Clin Perinatol. 2000;27(3):577-601.
27. al-Mulla ZS, Christensen RD. Neutropenia in the neonate. Clin Perinatol. 1995;22(3):711-39.
28. Ohls RK, Li Y, Abdel-Mageed A, Buchanan G Jr, Mandell L, Christensen RD. Neutrophil pool sizes and granulocyte colony-stimulating factor production in human mid-trimester fetuses. Pediatr Res. 1995;37(6):806-11.
29. Carr R, Modi N. Haemopoietic colony stimulating factors for preterm neonates. Arch Dis Child Fetal Neonatal Ed. 1997;76(2):F128-33.
30. Waldl E, Sadeghi K, Tamandl D, Gerhold B, Hallwirth U, Rohrmeister K, et al. Monocyte toll-like receptor 4 expression and LPS-induced cytokine production increase during gestational aging. Pediatr Res. 2005;58(1):121-4.
31. Anderson DC, Miller LJ, Schmalstieg FC, Rothlein R, Springer TA. Contributions of the Mac-1 glycoprotein family to adherence-dependent granulocyte functions: structure-function assessments employing subunit-specific monoclonal antibodies. J Immunol. 1986;137(1):15-27.
32. Eisenfeld L, Krause PJ, Herson V, Savidakis J, Bannon P, Maderazo E, et al. Longitudinal study of neutrophil adherence and motility. J Pediatr. 1990;117(6):926-9.
33. Falconer AE, Carr R, Edwards SW. Impaired neutrophil phagocytosis in preterm neonates: lack of correlation with expression of immunoglobulin or complement receptors. Biol Neonate. 1995;68(4):264-9.
34. Ambruso DR, Cusack N, Thurman G. NADPH oxidase activity of neutrophil specific granules: requirements for cytosolic components and evidence of assembly during cell activation. Mol Genet Metab. 2004;81(4):313-21.
35. Hanna N, Vasquez P, Pham P, Heck DE, Laskin JD, Laskin DL, et al. Mechanisms underlying reduced apoptosis in neonatal neutrophils. Pediatr Res. 2005;57(1):56-62.
36. Fuchs TA, Abed U, Goosmann C, Hurwitz R, Schulze I, Wahn V, et al. Novel cell death program leads to neutrophil extracellular traps. J Cell Biol. 2007;176(2):231-41.
37. Cairo MS, Agosti J, Ellis R, Laver JJ, Puppala B, deLemus R, et al. A randomized, double-blind, placebo-controlled trial of prophylactic recombinant human granulocyte-macrophage colony-stimulating factor to reduce nosocomial infections in very low birth weight neonates. J Pediatr. 1999;134(1):64-70.
38. Seth T, Cairo MS. Monograph-The role of cytokines in the prevention and treatment of neonatal sepsis. In: Bellanti JA, Bracci R, Prindull G, Xanthou M (Eds). Neonatal Hematology and Immunology. Amsterdam: Elsevier; 1997. pp. 49-53.
39. Molloy EJ, O'Neill AJ, Grantham JJ, Sheridan-Pereira M, Fitzpatrick JM, Webb DW, et al. Granulocyte colony-stimulating factor and granulocyte-macrophage colony-stimulating factor have differential effects on neonatal and adult neutrophil survival and function. Pediatr Res. 2005;57(6):806-12.
40. Roberts RL, Szelc CM, Scates SM, Boyd MT, Soderstrom KM, Davis MW, et al. Neutropenia in an extremely premature infant treated with recombinant human granulocyte colony-stimulating factor. Am J Dis Child. 1991;145(7):808-12.
41. Kuhn P, Messer J, Paupe A, Espagne S, Kacet N, Mouchnino G, et al. A multicenter, randomized, placebo-controlled trial of prophylactic recombinant granulocyte-colony stimulating factor in preterm neonates with neutropenia. J Pediatr. 2009;155(3):324-30.
42. Carr R, Modi N, Doré C. G-CSF and GM-CSF for treating or preventing neonatal infections. Cochrane Database Syst Rev. 2003;(3):CD003066.

CHAPTER 4

Developmental Aspects of Platelets

Sangeeta Mudaliar

DEVELOPMENTAL ASPECTS OF PLATELETS

Platelets are small anucleate cell fragments with a size of about 1–3 µm in diameter and a discoid shape. They are produced in the bone marrow from cytoplasm of large cells called megakaryocytes (MKs). The MKs have a size of 50–100 µm and are the largest cells in the marrow **(Figs 4.1A and B)**. Each giant MK approximately releases 1,000 platelets. MKs reside mainly in bone marrow but are also found in peripheral blood and lung. Most MKs are large cells which can be identified with low power **(Fig. 4.1B)**.

Platelets have an important role in hemostasis, angiogenesis (vessel repair), wound healing and inflammation.

The proteins on the platelet surface allow them to stick to breaks in blood vessel and one another and thus help to stop bleeding. The granules in platelets produce other proteins, which are required to create a firm platelet plug to seal blood vessel.

In this chapter, we will discuss about the incredible journey of development of platelets from MKs and about various aspects of platelet production in fetal and neonatal period.

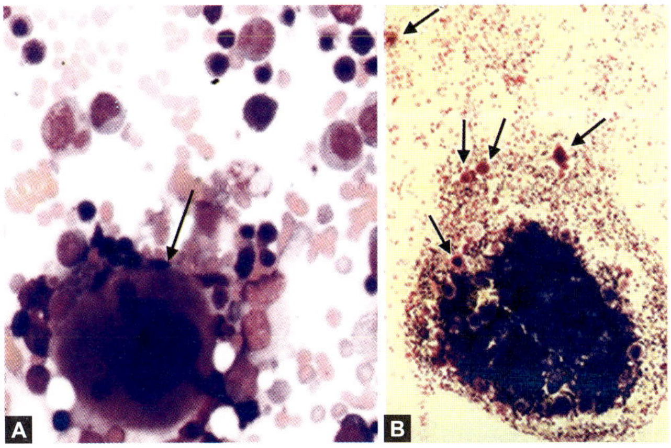

Figures 4.1A and B Megakaryocyte in marrow. (A) Megakaryocyte in high power field; (B) Increased megakaryocyte numbers

MEGAKARYOCYTES DURING FETAL DEVELOPMENT

Megakaryocytes are first detectable at 10 weeks of gestation in liver and spleen. By 30 weeks, they are seen in bone marrow. Active thrombopoiesis from MKs in marrow is seen at 30 weeks.

Platelets: Size, Numbers and Survival during Fetal Development

Circulating platelets are first detected by 11 weeks of gestation. The adult range of platelets ($150–450 \times 10^9$/L) is reached by 18 weeks of gestation. Mean platelet volume (MPV) is larger in the earlier phase and soon reaches adult range of 7–9 fL.

The platelets have variable size with about 0.5–1 µm thickness and 1.5 µm diameter. Numerous factors regulate the platelet size during their biogenesis with critical role being played by cell surface GlycoProtein Ib (GPIb) and non-muscle Myosin Heavy chain IIA (MYHIIA). Thus, in failure of GPIb expression (underlying molecular disorder of Bernard-Soulier syndrome), platelets are as large as lymphocytes. Mutations in *MYH9* gene interferes with contractile events in formation of platelet, the gene encodes nonmuscle MYHIIA. Disorders related to *MYH9* are characterized by macrothrombocytopenia. These disorders include May-Hegglin anomaly, Fechtner syndrome, Sebastian syndrome, Epstein syndrome and Alport syndrome. Patients may also experience cataract, hearing loss and nephritis and/or granulocyte inclusion body formation. The low platelet count seen in *MYH9* gene disorder results because of defective platelet production.[1]

Platelet size correlates with platelet reactivity. Higher MPV is associated with increased expression of adhesion molecules, increased platelet aggregation and higher risk of peripheral arterial and cardiovascular diseases. Still all the factors regulating the platelet size are yet to be revealed. About 68 genomic loci are found to have association with platelet volume.

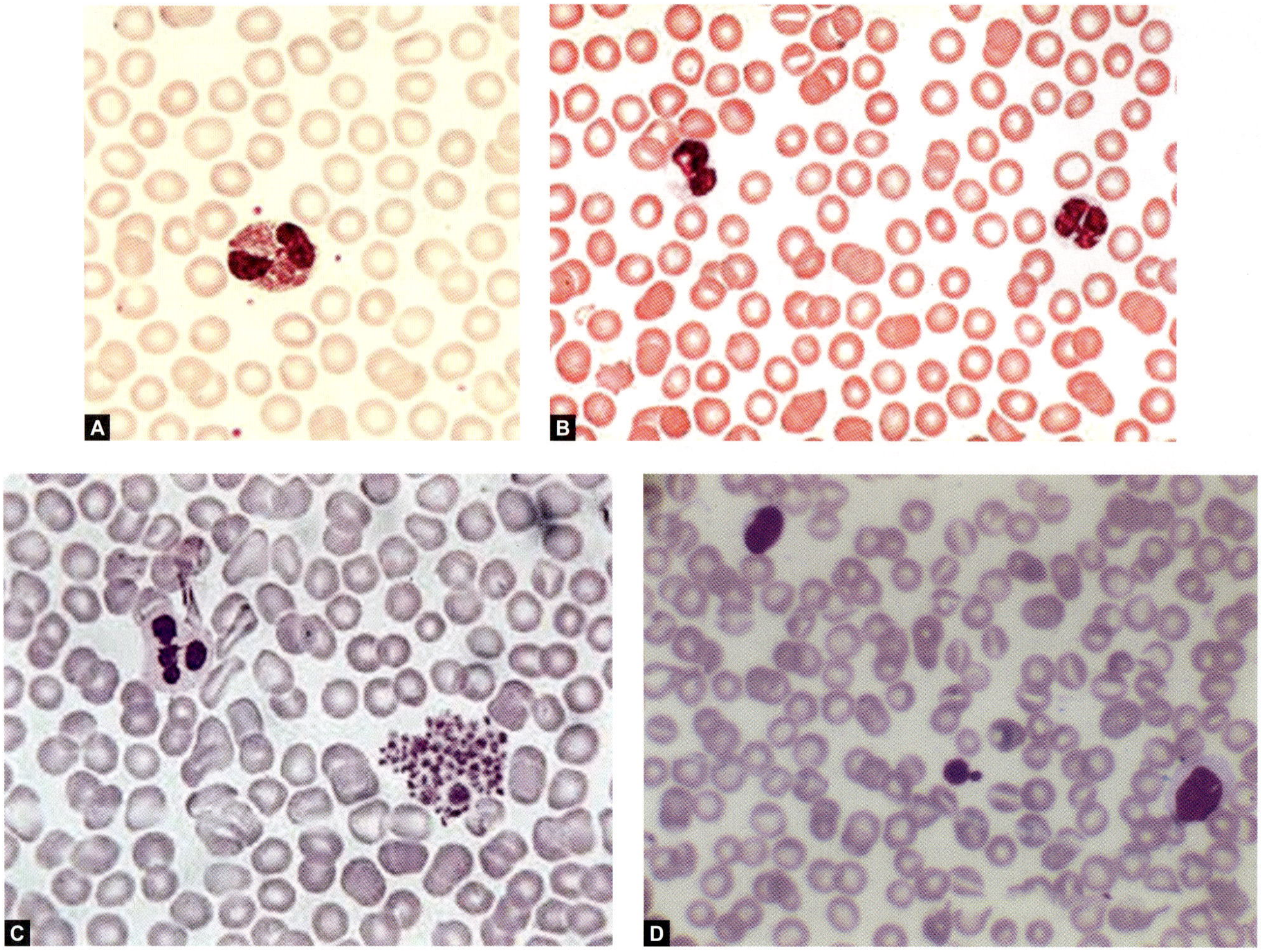

Figures 4.2A to D Platelets in peripheral smear. (A) Normal platelets in smear; (B) Absent platelets in peripheral smear; (C) Spurious thrombocytopenia due to platelet aggregates; (D) Giant Platelet in a case of Bernard-Soulier syndrome
Courtesy: Dr Ankit Parmar

Figures 4.2A to D show to appreciate the normal and abnormal size and numbers of platelet in peripheral smear.

Platelet Structure

The resting platelets have a discoid shape because of circumferential coils of microtubules. The platelets are packed with alpha granules, lysosomes, few dense granules, a few Golgi remnants and several mitochondria. Also they contain occasional vestiges of rough endoplasmic reticulum. Platelets also have two specialized membrane systems not seen in any other cells. These are dense tubular system (DTS) and surface-connected open canalicular system (OCS).[2]

The OCS serves as an internal reservoir of plasma membrane. The OCS is a series of tortuous invagination of plasma membrane, and increases the surface area of exposed plasma membrane by more than 400% when platelets round up, extend filopods and lamellipods and spread during platelet activation. The OCS channel also function as a conduit for the rapid expulsion of dense and alpha granules during platelet activation.

The DTS is present throughout the cytoplasm and is a remnant of smooth endoplasmic reticulum. The DTS harbors high concentration of calcium. It contains Sarcoplasmic or Endoplasmic Reticulum Ca^{2+} pump (SERCA) 2b, which is 100 kDa calcium adenosine triphosphatase, which functions to sequester and store cytosolic calcium in resting cells.[2]

Circulating platelets in newborns have similar platelet specific granules as adults and older children. But concentration of adenosine diphosphate (ADP) and serotonin stored in dense granules is half as compared to adults. The levels of receptor GPIb, GPIa/IIa, P-selectin and PIA1 are normal in newborn platelets.[2]

Platelet Function

Neonatal and cord blood platelets show hyporesponsiveness to ADP, epinephrine, collagen and thrombin on platelet aggregometry studies as compared to older children and adults. This resolves by 2–9 days spontaneously in full-term babies. But response to low concentrations of ristocetin is enhanced significantly in fetal and newborn platelet rich plasma, as compared to that of adults. This is probably due to high von Willebrand factor (vWF) levels in newborn plasma.[2]

The hyporesponsiveness to some platelet agonists and hyper-responsiveness to vWF balance each other in healthy term infants and hence they do not experience bleeding or thrombotic complications.

MEGAKARYOCYTE MATURATION AND DEVELOPMENT

Megakaryocytes are derived from hematopoietic stem cells (HSCs). HSCs reside mainly in bone marrow, but also are present in the yolk sac, fetal liver, and spleen during early development. The HSCs evolve from blood and blood vessel precursor cells, hemangioblasts, as described in **Flow chart 4.1**.

From the HSCs, early common myeloid progenitors (CMPs) are formed. From these early CMPs, a common MK-erythroid progenitors arise which lead to erythroid and MK lineages. Depending on the cytokines, chemokines and environmental factors, the bipotential megakaryocyte-erythrocyte progenitor develops into either early erythroid progenitors or late erythroid progenitors (BFU-E and CFU-E) or early MK burst forming unit (BFU-MK) or colony forming unit megakaryocyte (CFU-MK).[3]

The MK progenitors have two subcategories, primitive MK progenitors, BFU-MK, which produce large multifocal colonies containing 50 or more MKs, they express CD34 and not human leukocyte antigen (HLA)-DR and more differentiated cells, CFU-MK, which generate smaller (3–50 cells/colony) unifocal colonies, express CD34 and HLA-DR.

The MK progenitors lose their capacity to divide but retain the ability for DNA replication and cytoplasmic maturation. Early megakaryoblasts have the highest nuclear or cytoplasmic ratio and contain prominent ribosomes, rough endoplasmic reticulum, elevated ribonucleic acid (RNA) levels, alpha granules, dense bodies, primitive demarcation membrane and express platelet peroxidase. With the maturation of MK, expansion of cytoplasm occurs, the nucleus becomes horseshoe shaped, and amplification of demarcation membrane system and platelet organelles occur. High concentration of ribosomes is filled in to facilitate production of platelet specific proteins.

The MKs become polyploid by endomitosis (only DNA replication occurs without cell division), this is followed by maturation in which multiple long processes of cytoplasm is packed to form 10–20 proplatelets and the nucleus is extruded. The polyploidization (endoreduplication) and expansion of the cytoplasmic mass are the hallmarks of MK maturation.

The proplatelets start as a blunt protrusion which elongate, thin out and branch multiple times. At the tips of these proplatelets, platelets are formed.

The proplatelets are formed of platelet-sized swellings in tandem arrays which are connected by thin cytoplasmic bridges. The principle machinery for platelet production is the cytoskeleton. For proplatelet formation, beta1 tubulin is essential. It has been shown in mice that in absence of beta-1

Flow chart 4.1 Developmental pathway of platelets

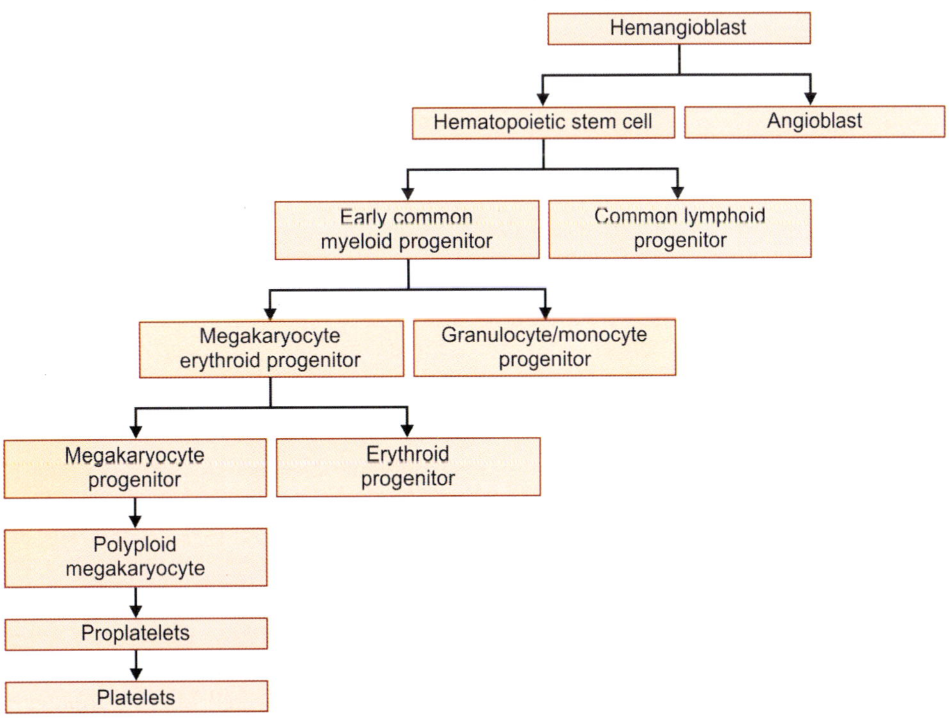

tubulin 60% fewer platelets are formed and the platelets which are produced have functional and structural defects. In humans, autosomal dominant macrothrombocytopenia results from mutation of beta-1 tubulin.

The assembly points required by proplatelets to bend and bifurcate are formed by F-actin. *MYH9* mutation causes reduced activity of myosin II and have been shown to be associated with premature initiation of proplatelet formation and reduced number of circulating platelets. Runt-related transcription factor 1 (RUNX1) also affects proplatelet formation by regulating *MYH9, myosin light chain 9 (MYL9)* and *MYH10* explaining the presentation of thrombocytopenia in germline heterozygous RUNX1 alterations.

PLATELET FORMATION

The platelets are produced from the bone marrow MKs in a sequential well-regulated process. The primary growth factor for megakaryocytic lineage is the circulating level of thrombopoietin (TPO). TPO binds to c-Mpl receptor and signals induction of concentration dependent proliferation and maturation of MK progenitors. TPO has half-life of 45 minutes and takes 24 hours to rise maximally. The levels of TPO are inversely and exponentially proportional to the platelet mass. The platelets bind and clear TPO from the circulation but hepatic TPO production is not altered by changes in the platelet mass. Concentrations of TPO are about double in fetal as compared to adult plasma. These may suggest possible increased turnover of platelets in fetuses than adults.

Formation of platelets is arbitrarily divided into two phases. The first phase requires MK specific growth factors and few days to complete, and involves MK maturation and development **(Fig. 4.3)**.

During the second phase, MKs generate platelets. It is a rapid phase taking few hours and involves remodeling of cytoplasm into proplatelets and then preplatelets which undergo fission to produce platelets. Preplatelets are 2–10 mm in diameter, anucleate and discoid particles which can reversibly convert into barbell-shaped proplatelets. The platelets receive their organelle content and granules as streams of individual particles transported from the MK cell body. A heterogeneous mix is released into the blood from MK cells and terminal platelet formation continues in the peripheral blood.[4]

Transcriptional Control of Platelet Formation

Identification of cellular controls at each step will give a complete understanding of platelet formation. Only a few signaling and transcriptional factors have been implicated in platelet generation till date as mentioned in **Table 4.1**.

The two factors that play major role in thrombopoiesis are GATA1 and FOG (friend of GATA). GATA1 are involved in lineage commitment of erythrocytes and MK from their progenitors. It also functions in MK development and controlling of proliferation. Missense mutation in GATA1 leads to low platelet count and abnormal bone marrow MKs because of disrupted interaction with FOG. In acute myeloid leukemia and transient myeloproliferative disorder, a truncated version of GATA1 is expressed, which is able to interact with FOG but lacks an N terminal activation domain, resulting in decreased transcriptional activation.[5]

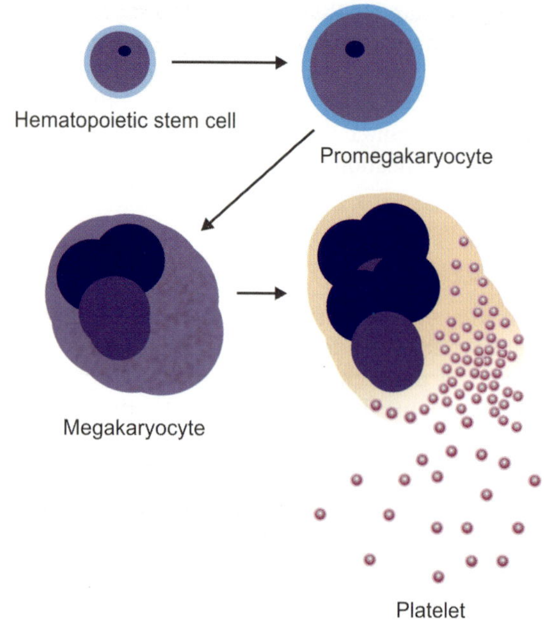

Figure 4.3 Platelet formation from precursor cell

NF-E2 is another transcription factor identified as a major regulator of platelet biosynthesis. NF-E2 interacts with promoter of Rab27b, a small GTPase in platelet, which regulate proplatelet production.

MEGAKARYOCYTE MATURATION

As the MK matures, cytoplasm expands, the polyploid nucleus becomes horseshoe shaped, become full of platelet specific granules, the demarcation membrane and platelet organelles are amplified and a highly tortuous invaginated membrane system is formed.

ENDOMITOSIS

It is mainly a TPO driven process in which MK becomes polyploid through cycles of replication of DNA without cell division. The MKs become polyploid to package large quantities of mRNA and protein in the platelet without undergoing stress of mitosis and cytokinesis yet retaining their ability to perform multiple functions. Nicotinamide (form of vitamin B3) increases ploidy in human MKs in culture. But its effect on platelet formation is controversial.

Thrombopoietin

Thrombopoietin stimulates the maturation and proliferation of MK progenitor cell. These cytokines have about 2-fold levels in fetuses as compared to adults, suggesting higher turnover of platelets during fetal life. Increase in the MK cell

Table 4.1 Thrombocytopenia and thrombocytosis due to disruption of signaling molecules or transcription factor

Genetic mutation	*Protein dysfunction*	*Disease type*
c-Mpl mutation in extracellular or external intramembrane domain	C-Mpl	Congenital amegakaryocytic thrombocytopenia
GATA 1 N V205G mutation	Major disruption of GATA 1 FOG 1 interaction	X-linked severe congenital dyserythropoietic anemia and thrombocytopenia
GATA 1 N V208S mutation	Disruption of GATA 1 FOG 1 interaction	X-linked macrothrombocytopenia mild dyserythropoiesis
GATA 1 N D218G mutation	Minor disruption of GATA 1 FOG 1 interaction	X-linked macrothrombocytopenia without anemia
GATA 1 N R216Q mutation	Reduced DNA binding of FOG domain	X-linked thrombocytopenia with thalassemia
Terminal 11q deletion	Loss or ETS protein	Jacobsen and Paris-Trousseau syndrome, dysmegakaryopoiesis
RUNX 1/AML 1 mutation	Loss of DNA binding	Familial platelet disorder with predisposition to AML
TPO mutation	Sustained signaling causes enhanced progenitor proliferation and thrombopoiesis	Inherited thrombocytosis
c-Mpl mutations in transmembrane domain	Enhanced megakaryocyte progenitor proliferation	Familial essential thrombocythemia
JAK2 V617F		
Down syndrome GATA 1S truncated isoforms	Proliferation or accumulation of MK progenitors with reduced maturation	AMK leukemia and transient MPD

Abbreviations: AML 1, acute myeloid leukemia 1, FOG, friend of GATA; MPD, myeloproliferative disease; ETS, erythroblast transformation-specific

size, ploidy and formation of proplatelets are stimulated by TPO. TPO is also known as c-Mpl ligand.

The gene that encodes TPO is located on long arm of chromosome 3. The TPO-mRNA is expressed mainly in kidney and liver, also in lesser extent in marrow stroma. TPO is the main but not sole regulator of platelet production. Apart from regulation and stimulation of MK progenitors, TPO also has role in myeloid, erythroid and multipotential progenitors. TPO production occurs at the site of hematopoiesis, unlike erythropoietin (EPO), which is not at all produced in marrow stroma. TPO is the major regulator of circulating platelet levels like the EPO for erythroid lineage, but expression of TPO gene expression is not transcriptionally regulated or significantly influenced by platelet levels in contrast to EPO. In normal circumstances, TPO is constantly produced and released in the circulation, and also removed rapidly by the circulating platelets and also possibly by MKs. So, during thrombocytopenia, TPO does not get removed due to platelet shortage, this results in rise in the levels of TPO, which in turn stimulates platelet production.

Thrombopoietin is the main but not exclusive regulator of process of MK production. The other factors, which stimulate megakaryocytopoiesis alone or in combination with TPO, are IL-3, IL-6, IL-11, granulocyte-macrophage colony stimulating factor (GM-CSF), stem cell factor, FLT ligand, fibroblast growth factor and EPO.[6]

There are certain factors which inhibit development of MK, these are IL4, PF4, transforming growth factor beta1and Src kinase inhibitors. Knowledge of this may be useful for developing therapeutic modalities for treatment of thrombocytosis.

Recombinant TPO to treat thrombocytopenia was first evaluated in 1995. But a few patients developed antibodies to TPO which resulted in paradoxical thrombocytopenia.

Thrombopoietin mimetic such as eltrombopag and romiplostim were then created and found effective in raising platelet counts in idiopathic thrombocytopenic purpura (ITP) but they take up to 5 days to increase platelet count and 12 days to reach maximum effect. TPO mimetic may sometimes cause a serious side effect of bone marrow myelofibrosis. For acute conditions wherein instantaneous elevation of platelet counts is necessary such as sepsis, disseminated intravascular coagulation (DIC), trauma or surgery, other alternatives to platelet transfusion is needed. Several groups are working on to create in vitro MK cultures derived from either induced pluripotent stem cells or embryonic stem cells. Also progress is being made at differentiating different types of cell into MK.

c-Mpl

The c-Mpl, which is the TPO receptor, is expressed on platelets, all stages of MKs, hemangioblasts and hematopoietic tissues. The c-Mpl receptors on MKs and platelets undergo conformational changes to initiate signal transduction after TPO binds the receptors. TPO binds to its specific receptor through the JAK-STAT (members of the Janus tyrosine kinase family and members of the Stat family of transcription factors) signal transduction pathway.

The TPO-receptor was identified some years before TPO was identified as its ligand, and was named with the acronym c-Mpl (for cellular homolog of a retrovirus complex inducing myeloproliferative leukemia). The functional c-Mpl gene in humans is located on chromosome 1p34. Multiple mutations have been identified in this gene, this results in total absence of the c-Mpl receptor or functionally defective TPO-binding and/or signaling, the course of disease is predicted by the type of mutation.

c-Mpl belongs to the cytokine receptor family. It is composed of a 466-amino acid extracellular ligand-binding domain. The distal cytokine receptor motif of the extracellular domain is responsible for ligand binding. In the absence of TPO, it inhibits the constitutive signaling activity of the membrane proximal cytokine receptor motif.

PRACTICAL ASPECTS OF MEGAKARYOCYTE CELL BIOLOGY AND CLINICAL USE OF THROMBOPOIETIC AGENTS

For hemostasis, platelets are essential. Thrombocytopenia poses major clinical problem in several conditions such as ITP, aplastic anemia, chemotherapy, etc.

It was expected that exogenous stimulation of platelet production by recombinant human thrombopoietin (rHuTPO) or truncated cloned recombinant human megakaryocyte growth and development factor (rHuMGDF) may be effective. But because of the observation in some patients of antibody formation the trials had to be closed. The rHuTPO facilitated the collection of platelets in normal donors but were not found effective in platelet recovery postaggressive chemotherapy.

In a phase 1 study by children's oncology group with rHuTPO and granulocyte colony-stimulating factor (GCSF) in solid tumors after combination chemotherapy showed improvement in hematological recovery and median number of platelet transfusion.

In chronic bone marrow failure states, patients receiving thrombopoietic factors showed slow but durable response suggesting useful role of TPO in thrombocytopenic states where there is no severe depletion of platelets and marrow microenvironment can support platelet formation.

Trial with IL-6 and IL-11 has been done. IL-6 were found to have potent thrombopoietic activity, but was associated with severe toxicities. IL-11 (neumega) was found to be useful for chemotherapy-induced thrombocytopenia and in some patients with bone marrow failure. It has limited effects with no cost benefit over platelet transfusion.[3]

Thrombopoietin mimetic agents, romiplostim and eltrombopag, are effective in chronic ITP but have no role in acute thrombocytopenia.[4] The ability to make platelets from MK culture would be useful, but cultured MK from embryonic or induced pluripotent stem cells yield only about 20–400 platelets/MK.

Still due to dearth of knowledge about regulators of proplatelets, there is no direct control of platelet formation.

As we learn more about thrombopoiesis, we may be able to create MKs that is ideal for platelet formation that is optimized for their job.

REFERENCES

1. Smith OP, Arceci RJ, Hann IM. Inherited and congenital thrombocytopenia. Pediatric Hematology, 3rd edition. New Jersey: Wiley-Blackwell; 2006.
2. Cantor AB. Developmental haemostasis: Relevance to newborns and infants. In: Orkin SH, Nathan DG, Ginsburg D, Look AT, Fisher DE. Lux SE (Eds). Nathan and Oskis Haematology of Infancy and Childhood, 7th edition. Philadelphia: Saunders Elsevier; 2009.pp.147-92.
3. Deutsch VR, Tomer A, Megakaryocyte development and platelet production. Br J Haematol. 2006;134(5):453-66.
4. Machlus KR, Italiano JE Jr. The incredible journey: From megakaryocyte development to platelet formation. J Cell Biol. 2013;201(6):785-96.
5. Patel SR, Hartwig JH, Italiano JE Jr. The biogenesis of platelets from megakaryocyte proplatelets. J Clin Invest. 2005;115(12):3348-54.
6. Chang M, Suen Y, Meng G, Buzby JS, Bussel J, Shen V, et al. Differential mechanisms in the regulation of endogenous levels of thrombopoietin and interleukin-11 during thrombocytopenia: insight into the regulation of platelet production. Blood. 1996;88(9):3354-62.

CHAPTER

5

Fetal Anemia

Meenal Agarwal

DEFINITION

When fetal hemoglobin (Hb) or hematocrit is less than two standard deviations below the mean for that gestational age (GA), it is called fetal anemia.[1] Hematocrit less than 30% or Hb deficit more than 5–6 g/dL results in fetal hydrops, which is lethal if not treated except in few cases of intrauterine infection when it is transient and self-limiting.The normal values of Hb and hematocrit are represented in **Table 5.1**.[2]

CAUSES OF FETAL ANEMIA

The causes of fetal anemia may be described in different ways.[1] On the basis of pathophysiology, it can broadly be categorized into following headings:

- *Decreased production of red blood cells (RBCs):*
  - Parvovirus B19 infection during pregnancy
  - Less commonly occurring other intrauterine fetal infection like cytomegalovirus, toxoplasmosis and syphilis

Table 5.1 Normal range of hemoglobin and hematocrit from 18 weeks of gestational age to 40 weeks

Gestational age (weeks)	*Hematocrit (%)*	*Hemoglobin (g/dL)*
18–20	36 ± 3	11.5 ± 0.8
21–22	39 ± 3	12.3 ± 0.9
23–25	39 ± 2	12.4 ± 0.8
26–27	62 ± 8	19.0 ± 2.5
28–29	60 ± 7	19.3 ± 1.8
30–31	60 ± 8	19.1 ± 2.2
32–33	60 ± 6	18.5 ± 2.0
34–35	61 ± 7	19.6 ± 2.1
36–37	64 ± 7	19.2 ± 1.7
38–40	61 ± 7	19.3 ± 2.2

Source: Bizzarro MJ, Colson E, Ehrenkranz RA. Differential diagnosis and management of anemia in the newborn. Pediatr Clin North Am. 2004;51:1087-107.

- *Increased destruction or hemolysis or ineffective erythropoiesis:*
  - Maternal alloimmunization for RBC antigens present on fetal RBCs
  - Alpha thalassemia
  - Hereditary spherocytosis
  - Congenital dyserythropoietic anemia
  - Glucose-6-phosphate dehydrogenase deficiency
  - Pyruvate kinase deficiency
- *Fetal hemorrhage:*
  - Twin-to-twin transfusion syndrome
  - Fetomaternal hemorrhage
  - Internal bleeding into fetal organs such as intracranial or intrathoracic hemorrhage
  - Large arteriovenous fistula, hemangioma, placental chorioangioma, etc.

In most of these scenarios, however, multiple mechanisms are collectively responsible for final phenotype of fetal anemia.

The most common causes in Indian scenario are rhesus (Rh) alloimmunization, fetal hemorrhage and parvovirus B19 infection. The detailed discussion for pathophysiology and management of all the above causes are beyond the scope in this chapter and it will be focused on overall management of fetal anemia and Rh alloimmunization.

Brief Pathophysiology of Red Blood Cell Alloimmunization

This situation arises when mother's circulation has antibodies for a specific RBC surface antigen present on fetal RBCs.[3] These antibodies may be present in maternal circulation before exposure of RBCs bearing the particular antigen (ABO incompatibility) or may arise after exposure to RBCs (RhD, C, c, E, e, Kell, Kidd and Duffy antigens). There are about 50 RBC antigens for which such maternal alloimmunization can cause fetal anemia of varying severity. ABO incompatibility usually affects the first pregnancy and results in mild fetal anemia or neonatal hyperbilirubinemia. In case of incompatibility for

RhD antigen, the risk is to those mothers who themselves are RhD negative and their fetus is RhD positive. During antenatal period small number of fetal RBCs may enter into maternal circulation (1–2% of cases). The chance of mixing of fetal blood with maternal blood is larger at the time of antepartum hemorrhage, antenatal invasive procedure or labor. This sensitizes the maternal immune system for the RhD antigen and produces antibodies in response. These antibodies initially are of immunoglobulin M (IgM) type. Being pentameric structure, these antibodies are unable to pass through placental barrier. In subsequent pregnancies, even small leakage of fetal RBCs causes clonal proliferation of committed maternal plasma cells. These antibodies are of IgG type which cross placental barrier and react with fetal RBCs bearing RhD antigen causing destruction of fetal RBCs in reticuloendothelial system. This results in varying degree of fetal anemia and hyperbilirubinemia. Usually, the first pregnancy with Rh-incompatible fetus remains unaffected while in subsequent pregnancies, fetus gets affected at earlier gestational age (GA) and to more severe degree.

Clinical Presentation and Diagnosis

The diagnosis of fetal anemia is suspected mainly on the basis of maternal history and ultrasonographic features in present pregnancy. Previous history of multiple stillbirths, hydrops in previous pregnancies, neonatal jaundice, need of neonatal exchange transfusion may point toward the possibility of hemolytic disease of fetus and newborn. History of exposure to a child with erythema infectiosum or fifth disease or slapped cheek disease point toward the possibility of fetal parvovirus B19 infection and fetus needs to be followed up by serial ultrasonography and Doppler evaluation for the development of anemia. High maternal serum alpha-fetoprotein, done as a part of routine serum screening of aneuploidy, increases the risk of possibility of placental chorioangioma. In majority of cases, fetal anemia or hydrops are accidentally detected in antenatal ultrasonographic and Doppler evaluation.

Complete family, personal and obstetric history needs to be taken including history of present pregnancy.

Important points include ethnic origin, consanguinity, family history of any genetic disorder especially hemolytic anemia or recurrent jaundice during illness or after ingestion of drugs, previous history of blood transfusion and transfusion reactions if any, previous history of hydrops in pregnancy, neonatal jaundice or neonate requiring blood transfusion or exchange transfusion, history of exposure to parvovirus B19/fifth disease in present pregnancy, USG reports of previous and present pregnancy if available.

The final way of diagnosing fetal anemia is percutaneous umbilical fetal blood sampling (PUBS) and fetal hemoglobin (Hb) estimation. As PUBS is associated with fetal loss rate of 1–2%, various noninvasive and invasive methods have been evolved to diagnose fetal anemia and to predict the need of invasive fetal sampling. As the most common causes of fetal anemia in clinical scenario is Rh alloimmunization the further discussion will be focused on fetal anemia due to Rh incompatibility.

NONINVASIVE PREDICTORS OF FETAL ANEMIA

Antibody Titers in the Mother

In the cases of Rh alloimmunization, before the introduction of serial amniocentesis and ultrasonography based criteria, the degree of fetal anemia used to be predicted on basis of rising maternal Rh antibody titer. Maternal Rh antibody titer more than 1:16 to 32 (depending upon individual laboratory standards) is usually suggestive of moderate-to-severe hemolysis in the fetus and hence the indication of invasive fetal sampling. In case of alloimmunization for Kell antigen, titers of 1:8 may result in fetal anemia as it causes erythropoietic suppression also. The monitoring by maternal titers is useful only in first alloimmunized pregnancy and not in subsequent ones.

ULTRASONOGRAPHY-BASED PREDICTORS OF FETAL ANEMIA

Measurement of Peak Systolic Velocity of Middle Cerebral Artery

This is based on the hypothesis that fetal anemia and decreased fetal hematocrit decreases the blood viscosity and hence increases the systolic velocity in middle cerebral artery.[4] This technique can be followed up for the onset and degree of fetal anemia in a noninvasive manner. Regardless of the cause of fetal anemia, the screening in high-risk cases can be started from 16 weeks to 18 weeks of GA onwards. The positive and negative predictive value for detection of moderate or severe anemia is estimated to be 70% and 100%, respectively, with false positive rate of 10–12%. Doppler measurement of middle cerebral artery (MCA) peak systolic velocity (PSV) is also found to be useful in predicting the timing for repeated intrauterine transfusion. However, it is not found to be useful at GA of more than 35 weeks. There are certain guidelines to measure MCA PSV as shown in **Figure 5.1**. These include:

- It should be taken in axial section of fetal head at the level of circle of Willis
- The proximal or distal MCA can be sampled
- The Doppler gate should be kept close to origin of MCA from circle of Willis
- The angle of insonation should be close to zero without angle correction
- The probe should not be pressed too much. It will give falsely high values.

Middle cerebral artery PSV is then compared with standard graphs. The values lying at more than 1.29 multiple of median (MoM) for that particular GA is suggestive of mild anemia and PSV more than 1.5 MoM value is suggestive of severe fetal anemia and is an indication of fetal intervention in form of PUBS and decision for intrauterine fetal blood transfusion (IUT) if required. The standard charts are available to convert PSV to MoM (Mari et al). The thumb rule is, however, if

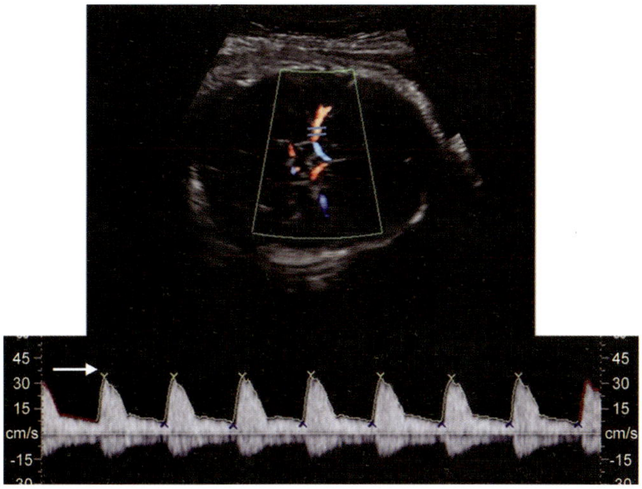

Figure 5.1 Measurement of peak systolic velocity of middle cerebral artery and its Doppler waveform. The "=" sign shows the position of gate while white arrow shows the peak systolic velocity in cm/sec. (*Courtesy*: Dr K Subapriya, Fetal Medicine Consultant, Fetoscan Fetal Medicine Center, Chennai)

the PSV of MCA is closer to twice the value of GA, fetus is having moderate to severe anemia. The online calculator is also available to convert MCA PSV value to MoM (*http://perinatology.com/calculators/MCA.htm*).

Apart from MCA PSV, other ultrasonographic parameters including sizes of liver and spleen, placental thickness, size and contractility of cardiac chambers, diameter of hepatic veins, Doppler study of abdominal aorta and severity of hydrops have also been studied as methods of predicting fetal anemia but these have not been found to be sensitive enough to differentiate moderate from severe anemia. Fetal hydrops usually is a terminal event in cases of fetal anemia and outcome becomes less satisfactory even after IUT. MCA PSV remains to be most useful and recommended procedure with better sensitivity, specificity and reproducibility to screen, diagnose and to follow the suspected and high-risk cases of fetal anemia.

The Invasive Predictor of Fetal Anemia

It includes amniocentesis and measurement of deviation of optical density of amniotic fluid by spectrophotometer at 450 nm (Delta OD 450).[5] This method indirectly predicts fetal anemia as a result of hemolysis and subsequent hyperbilirubinemia. This method was first described in 1961 by Liley who proposed the serial amniocentesis and measurement of delta OD level. Liley correlated the delta OD 450 level with the degree of fetal anemia and extrapolated a graph. The graph was divided in three zones. If the delta OD is lying in upper half of second zone or third zone, the fetus was predicted to have moderate or severe anemia and hence becomes an indication of fetal blood sampling or early delivery depending upon GA. The sensitivity and specificity of this method was predicted to have 80% and 90–95%, respectively. Every attempt of amniocentesis is associated with 0.5–1% risk of fetal loss and up to 2–5% of fetomaternal hemorrhage and hence increasing the maternal production of alloantibodies and more hemolysis. Queenan later modified and extrapolated the Liley's chart to 2nd trimester. But in era of noninvasive ultrasonography-based predictors of fetal anemia serial amniocentesis is almost abandoned.

Investigations if Suspecting Fetal Anemia or Hemolytic Disease of Fetus and Newborn

The recommended investigations in mother include Rh ABO, indirect Coombs test, Rh antibody titer in case of Rh incompatibility, PCR for parvovirus B19, if history is suggestive of exposure.[1,3,6] Detailed ultrasonographic evaluation including examination of placenta, liquor, fetal malformations including echocardiography, Doppler for MCA PSV, size of liver and spleen and extent of hydrops if present should be done. Ultrasonography can also detect fetal vascular mass, intracranial hemorrhage or evidence of twin-to-twin transfusion syndrome. Fetal coagulopathy including alloimmune thrombocytopenia should be suspected in case of internal fetal hemorrhage and detailed work up should be done if no vascular malformation is found in USG.

Prevention of Rh Alloimmunization

Prophylactic anti-D-immunoglobulins administration to the mother bearing the Rh-positive fetus is an effective way to prevent the development of fetal hemolysis in subsequent pregnancies. Any pregnant woman should be tested for Rh ABO in first antenatal visit as shown in **Flow chart 5.1**. Anti-D-immunoglobulins should also be given to mother in cases of threatened abortion or any invasive prenatal testing during antenatal period. If gestational age is less than 12 weeks, then 50 µg, and if GA is more than 12 weeks then 300 µg should be given to mother intramuscularly. At 28 weeks of GA, if mother's Rh antibody titers are negative, then she should be given 300 µg of Anti-D immunoglobulins.

After delivery, neonate should be tested for Rh, ABO and direct Coombs test. If fetus is Rh positive and Coombs test is negative, then within 24–72 hours of delivery; mother again should be given 300 µg of anti-D immunoglobulins intramuscularly. Anti-D prophylaxis significantly reduces the maternal alloimmunization. Immunoglobulins for RBC antigens other that RhD antigens are not available. The overall management of fetal anemia and Rh incompatibility have been summarized in **Flow charts 5.1 to 5.3**.

PLAN FOR CONSERVATIVE MANAGEMENT OR INVASIVE SAMPLING

- If maternal Rh antibody titer is less than 1:16, MCA PSV is less than 1.29 MoM and no signs of hydrops: Follow 2–4 weekly
- If maternal Rh antibody titer is more than 1:16–32 or if MCA PSV is more than 1.29, MoM: Follow 1–2 weekly

Flow chart 5.1 Management of Rh-alloimmunization in case of nonimmunized pregnancy

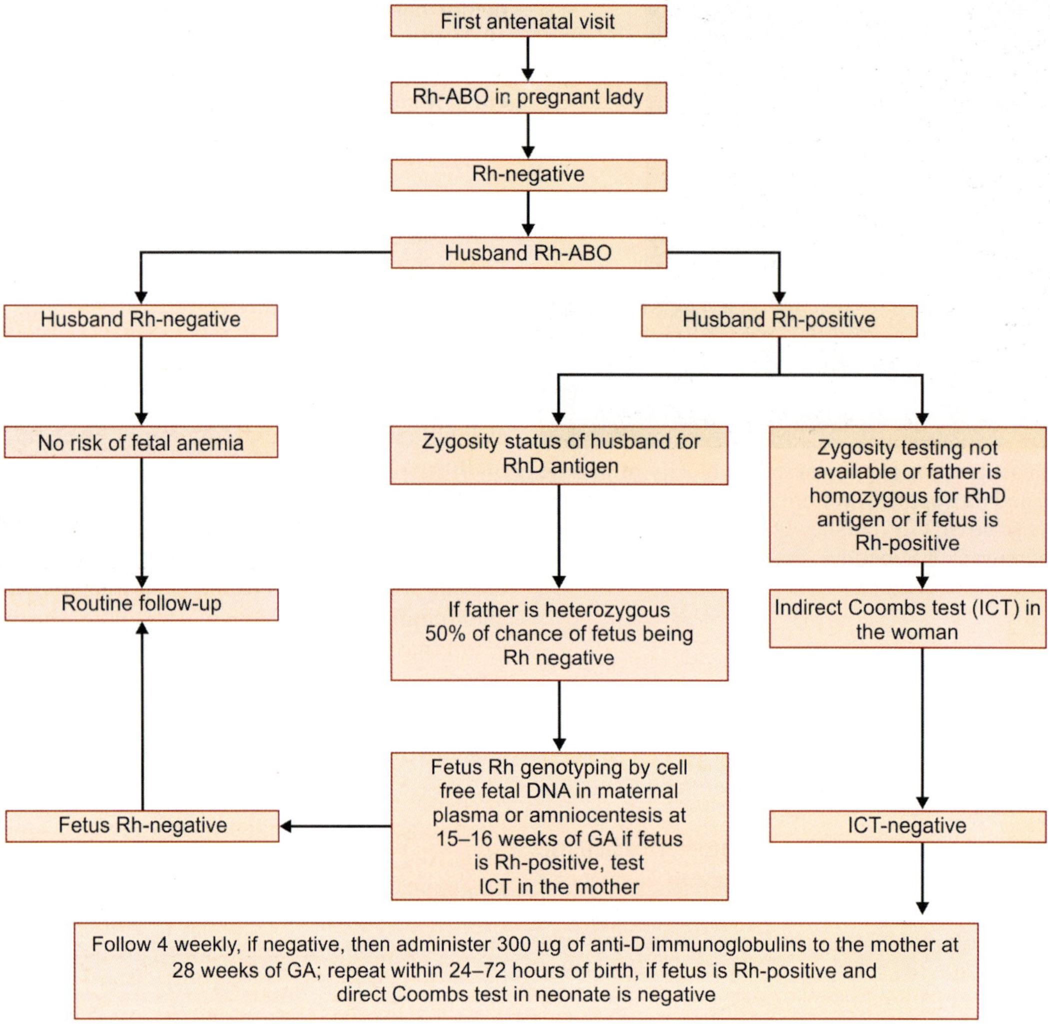

Abbreviations: Rh, Rhesus; RhD, Rhesus blood group D; GA, gestational age

- If MCA-PSV is more than 1.5 MoM or signs of hydrops, and GA is less than 34–35 weeks, then perform PUBS. IUT may be done depending on the severity of anemia, fetal weight and GA. If GA is more than 35 weeks, then delivery can be planned with good neonatal care.

Investigations to be Ordered in Fetal Blood in Case Cord Blood Sampling is Done

- Hemoglobin, hematocrit, Rh ABO blood grouping, direct Coombs test, reticulocyte count, serum bilirubin, should be done in fetal blood. Also remaining blood should be kept safe in ethylenediaminetetraacetic acid (EDTA) vial
- Sample can be sent for PCR for parvovirus B19, if history is suggestive
- Work up for other genetic hemolytic anemia can be planned; it can be done in case investigations are not suggestive of RBC alloimmunization
- If fetal hematocrit is less than 30% plan for IUT in treatable causes which include RBC alloimmunization, parvovirus B19 infection and few cases of placental chorioangiomata, twin-to-twin transfusion syndrome and genetic hemolytic anemia. IUT is generally not recommended in Hb Bart syndrome or homozygous alpha thalassemia because of poor prognosis postnatally.

INTRAUTERINE FETAL TRANSFUSION: THE TECHNIQUE

Pretransfusion

Informed consent should be obtained from the family after explaining the potential risks to mother and fetus. Preprocedure antibiotics should be given to mother to reduce the risk of maternal infection. Antenatal administration of steroids to mother may be considered for fetal lung maturity

Flow chart 5.2 Management in case of Rh alloimmunization with mother being positive of indirect Coombs test

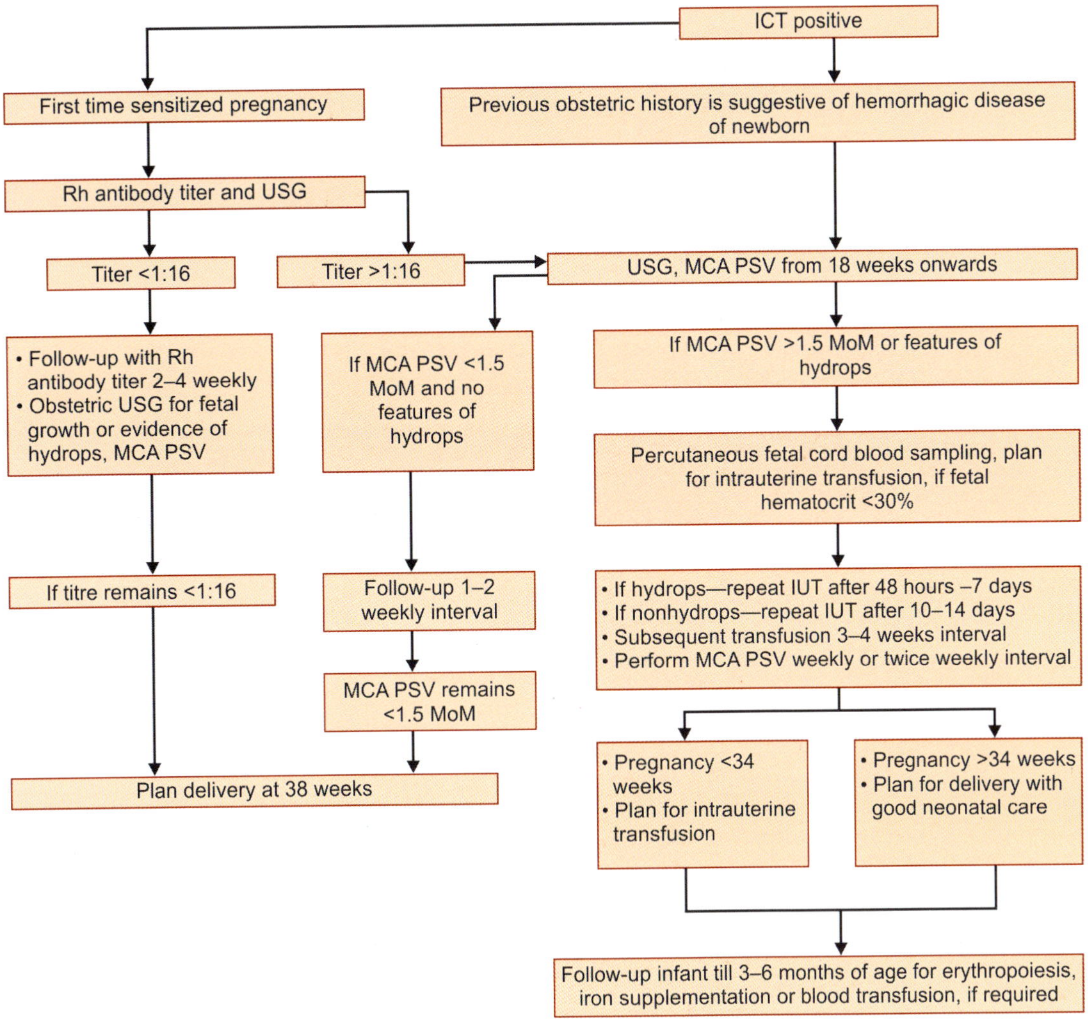

Abbreviations: USG, ultrasonography; Rh, Rhesus; MCA, middle cerebral artery; PSV, peak systolic velocity; MoM, multiple of median; IUT, intrauterine fetal blood transfusion

if indicated. USG should be performed to calculate estimated fetal weight, degree of anemia based on MCA PSV and severity of hydrops.

About the Blood

The unit to be transfused should be O negative, cross-matched with maternal blood sample, irradiated, leukopoor, less than 5 days old and concentrated to have final hematocrit of 75–85% to minimize the final volume to be transfused.

About the Technique

Things to be Kept Ready

Assistance by two persons, sterile gloves, spinal needle 20 gauze, triway with long tubing, sterile probe cover and jelly, EDTA vials to check pretransfusion and post-transfusion fetal Hb and hematocrit, blood unit, syringes 10 mL and 20 mL, vecuronium 0.1 mg/kg of fetal weight and furosemide 0.1 mg/kg of fetal weight blood preloaded in a syringe.

Total amount of blood to be transfused can be calculated from various methods. The most commonly used formula is:

$$\frac{(\text{Required hematocrit} - \text{fetal hematocrit}) \times \text{fetal weight in grams} \times 0.15}{\text{Donor hematocrit}}$$

The desired hematocrit is usually kept at 45–55% and around 25–30% if fetal hydrops is present.[1,7]

Procedure

Ultrasonographically guided intrauterine intravascular transfusion is the treatment of choice. Intraperitoneal transfusion has a role in certain scenarios like fetal hydrops at less than 18 weeks of GA when access to a fetal umbilical cord

Flow chart 5.3 Management of nonalloimmunized case of fetal anemia

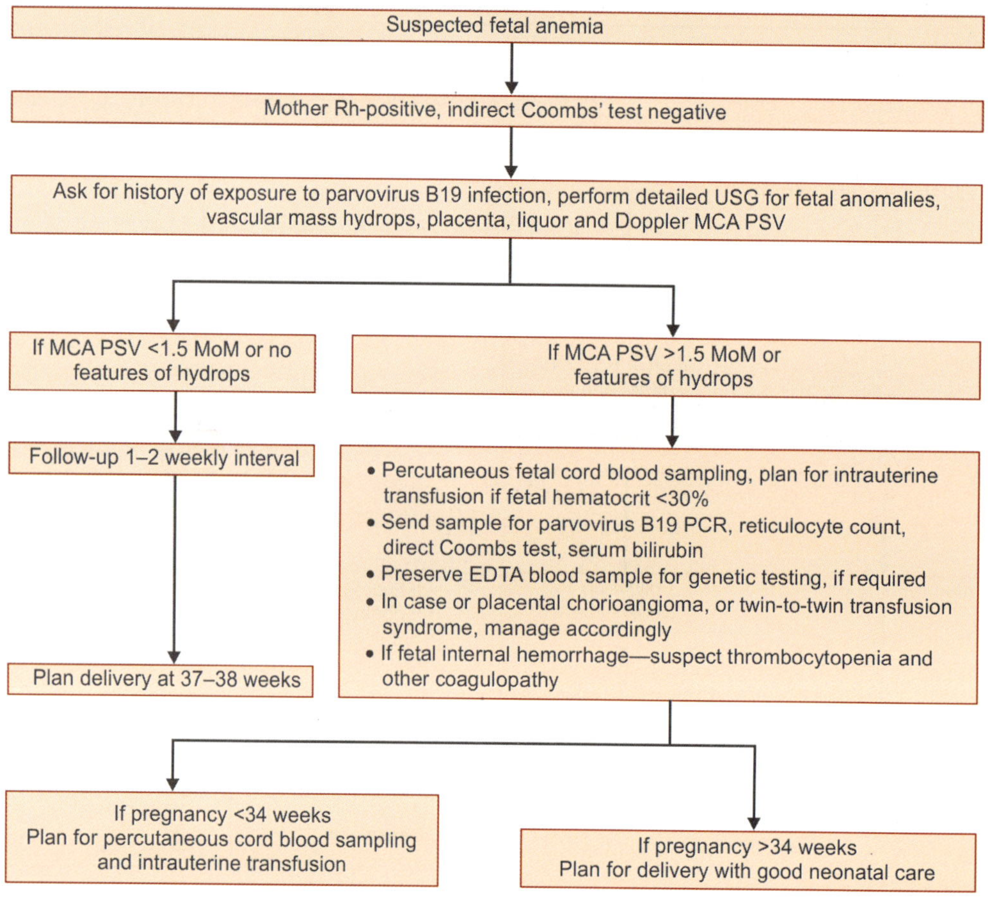

Abbreviations: Rh, Rhesus; MCA, middle cerebral artery; PSV, peak systolic velocity; MoM, multiple of median; USG, ultrasonography; PCR, polymerase chain reaction; EDTA, ethylenediaminetetraacetic acid

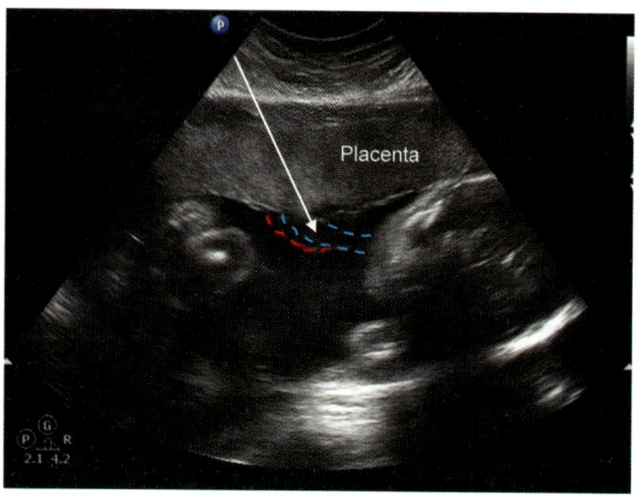

Figure 5.2 Ultrasonographic image of cordocentesis. Needle path is being shown by white arrow, blue dotted line represents the umbilical vein and red dotted line represents the umbilical artery. (*Courtesy*: Dr Girisha KM, Professor and Head, Department of Medical Genetics, Kasturba Medical College, Manipal)

is difficult. Umbilical vein near placental insertion site is the most common site of fetal vascular access **(Fig. 5.2)**. Umbilical artery, intrahepatic portion of umbilical vein, intracardiac and free cord loops are other sites for vascular access but are associated with higher rate of fetal complications.

As soon as cord is punctured, take 1 mL of fetal blood and check for Hb and hematocrit if not done before. Vecuronium in desired dosage is pushed inside cord. Furosemide can also be given at this time. Blood should be transfused at a rate of not more than 5–10 mL/minute. Fetal heart rate should be monitored frequently. If fetal bradycardia is noted, stop the procedure for few seconds and observe the fetal heart rate.

Risk Associated with Intrauterine Fetal Blood Transfusion

The procedure may be associated with fetal loss in 1–2% of cases. Other reported complications are maternal infection, preterm rupture of membranes and preterm labor, but overall risk appears to be very low in expert hands. During procedure, fetal bradycardia may develop because of vascular spasm, sudden volume expansion, cord hematoma and leakage of blood from cord puncture site. In most of the time, bradycardia improves when the transfusion is slowed or stopped, but in few cases procedure need to be abandoned.

Follow-up of Pregnancy after Intrauterine Fetal Blood Transfusion

The usual interval between first IUT and second IUT is 10–14 days. In case of fetal hydrops, the second transfusion may be planned even after 48 hours–7 days of first transfusion to allow fetal cardiovascular system adjustment according to increased fetal blood volume. A decline in hematocrit should be expected by rate of 1% per day. MCA PSV can be monitored weekly and can be useful in guiding the timing of subsequent transfusion. After the second transfusion, subsequent transfusion is usually required at the interval of 3–4 weeks. In case of parvovirus B19 infection, repeated IUTs are usually not required.

Planning for Delivery and Neonatal Management

If the pregnancy is being followed up conservatively then delivery should be planned at 37–38 weeks. In case fetus has received one or more IUTs, then decision should be taken after giving considerable thoughts to the risk of IUT and perinatal morbidity and mortality due to prematurity. Usually for pregnancies undergoing IUTs, the delivery is planned at about 34–35 weeks of pregnancy depending upon timing of last IUT. Pediatricians should be informed before planning induction of labor. They should be prepared for the need of frequent monitoring of infant Hb and bilirubin levels and need of neonatal blood transfusion or exchange transfusion.

Outcome

The overall outcome depends upon the cause and degree of fetal anemia. In case of Rh alloimmunization, it appears to be satisfactory in 90–95% of cases in case timely IUT is done. Survival is better in nonhydropic (90%) fetuses when compared with hydropic fetuses (70%). Neonate needs to be intensively monitored for development of neonatal anemia and bone marrow suppression. Iron and multivitamin supplementation should be advised to infants with 2–4 weekly measurement of Hb, total leukocyte count (TLC) and platelet count up to 3 months of age. The overall neurodevelopmental outcome seems to be satisfactory in more than 90% cases in babies who have received IUTs.[8]

In case of parvovirus B19 infection, outcome is expected to be satisfactory in 80–85% of cases. Fetal loss occurs in about 5–10% of the cases. Fetal anemia even if present gradually improves within 3–4 weeks and less than 1% of the cases develop hydrops and is amenable to be treated by IUT. Weekly monitoring by MCA-PSV should be done starting from 18 weeks of gestation to 12 weeks after the initial exposure. Exposed fetuses are not at increased risk of congenital malformations.[9]

Fetomaternal hemorrhage is usually self-limiting. If fetal hydrops develops, then it can be treated by IUT and carries a good prognosis.

For conditions like twin-to-twin transfusion syndrome, placental chorioangiomata, strategies such as fetoscopic laser ablation of communicating vessels are main modality of treatment and again outcome depends upon severity of fetal anemia and other complications.

Homozygous alpha thalassemia is a lethal disease and has no curative treatment as of now. Other genetic hemolytic anemia if diagnosed *in utero* can be helpful in preventing future recurrences in the family. Usually, these conditions are of varying severity resulting in chronic anemia which may be transfusion-dependent after birth.

CONCLUSION

Fetal anemia is a treatable cause of fetal hydrops. Rh isoimmunization and parvovirus B19 infection are the most common causes of fetal anemia. Clinical suspicion on basis of history, appropriate use of antenatal ultrasonography and Doppler measurement of MCA PSV, intrauterine transfusion, timely delivery and neonatal management are keys to success in most of the cases.

KEY POINTS

- Perform Rh-ABO in every pregnant lady in the first antenatal visit.
- Identify the potential cases (Rh-negative wife with Rh-positive husband) of Rh alloimmunization in first antenatal visit.
- Prophylactic Anti D immunoglobulin administration in Rh negative mother who are negative for Rh antibody, after any threatened abortion, at 28 weeks and within 24–48 hours of delivery.
- Review complete obstetric history and investigations records in the present pregnancy to identify the cases with high risk of developing fetal anemia.
- Perform ultrasonography for fetal growth, malformation, placental abnormalities, liquor amount, size of liver and spleen, presence of hydrops or evidence of twin-to-twin transfusion syndrome and peak systolic velocity of middle cerebral artery to diagnose fetal anemia.
- Investigations for mother include, Rh-ABO, indirect Coombs test, Rh antibody titer and polymerase chain reaction for parvovirus B19 if history is suggestive of exposure.
- In case of placental chorioangiomata or twin-to-twin transfusion, refer to fetal medicine specialist for fetoscopic laser coagulation of communicating vessel. If fetal hematological investigations suggest the hemolytic disease of the fetus other than maternal alloimmunization, refer

to a medical geneticist for work-up for genetic hemolytic anemia.

- Intrauterine infection by parvovirus B19 is usually self-limiting. Intrauterine transfusion, however, may be planned if fetus is diagnosed to have severe anemia, and/or shows signs of hydrops. In case USG shows signs of fetal anemia, plan for conservative management or intrauterine transfusion.
- In case of maternal Rh-alloimmunization, follow-up antenatally by repeated measurement of peak systolic velocity of middle cerebral artery should be done which is usually done at the interval of 3–4 weeks till fetal lung maturity.
- Plan for delivery at a center with good neonatal care facilities.
- In infants, 2–4 weekly measurement of Hb, TLC and platelet count up to 3 months of age and iron and multivitamin supplementation.

REFERENCES

1. Mari G, Norton ME, Stone J, Berghella V, Sciscione AC, Tate D, Schenone MH. Society for Maternal-Fetal Medicine (SMFM): Clinical Guideline #8: the fetus at risk for anemia—diagnosis and management. Electronic address: pubs@smfm.org. Am J Obstet Gynecol. 2015;212(6):697-710.
2. Bizzarro MJ, Colson E, Ehrenkranz RA. Differential diagnosis and management of anemia in the newborn, Pediatr Clin North Am. 2004;51:1087-1107.
3. Moise KJ Jr. Management of rhesus alloimmunization in pregnancy. Obstet Gynecol. 2002;100(3):600-11.
4. Mari G, Deter RL, Carpenter RL, Rahman F, Zimmerman R, et al. Noninvasive diagnosis by Doppler ultrasonography of fetal anemia due to maternal red-cell alloimmunization. Colloborative Group for Doppler Assessment of the Blood Velocity in Anemic Fetuses. N Engl J Med. 2000;342:9-14.
5. Oepkes D, Seaward PG, Vandenbussche FP, Windrim R, Kingdom J, Beyene J, Kanhai HH, Ohlsson A, Ryan G. DIAMOND Study Group. Doppler ultrasonography versus amniocentesis to predict fetal anemia. N Engl J Med. 2006;355(2):156-64.
6. Moise KJ. Fetal anemia due to non-Rhesus-D red-cell alloimmunization. Seminars in Fetal & Neonatal Medicine. 2008;13(4):207-14.
7. Papantoniou N, Sifakis S, Antsaklis A. Therapeutic management of fetal anemia: review of standard practice and alternative treatment options. J Perinat Med. 2013;41(1):71-82.
8. Lindenburg IT, van Klink JM, Smits-Wintjens VE, van Kamp IL, Oepkes D, Lopriore E. Long-term neurodevelopmental and cardiovascular outcome after intrauterine transfusions for fetal anaemia: a review. Prenat Diagn. 2013;33(9):815-22.
9. Cosmi E, Mari G, Delle Chiaie L, Detti L, Akiyama M, et al. Noninvasive diagnosis by Doppler ultrasonography of fetal anemia resulting from parvovirus infection. Am J Obstet Gynecol. 2002;187(5):1290-3.

CHAPTER

6

Thalassemia in the Fetus: Prenatal Diagnosis

Prajnya Ranganath

INTRODUCTION

The dictum "Prevention is better than cure" though applicable for all diseases in general, is particularly true for genetic disorders as most of the genetic disorders do not have any curative therapy or the treatment is costly, burdensome and many a times lifelong. The most effective way to reduce the burden of common genetic disorders in the population is to prevent the birth of affected children and the most widely practiced method to achieve this is prenatal diagnosis followed by termination of affected pregnancies within the medically and legally permissible gestational period.

Hemoglobinopathies are amongst the most common single gene disorders all over the world with around 300,000 affected individuals being born every year all over the world.[1,2] In India, beta-thalassemia is the most prevalent inherited hemoglobinopathy with an estimated 7,500–12,000 affected children being born per year and a country-wide carrier prevalence rate of 1.5–4% with some communities having a carrier rate as high as 4–17%.[1,3,4] Affected individuals with the thalassemia major or severe intermedia phenotype require lifelong blood transfusions along with iron chelation therapy and/or bone marrow transplantation for survival, which poses a huge financial and emotional burden on the family and a strain on the country's health resources. Though the life expectancy for thalassemia has improved significantly with regular treatment and improved management of associated complications, the quality of life remains poor for majority of the patients. Furthermore, it has been estimated that only 5–10% of the thalassemic children born in India receive optimal treatment and majority do not reach the age of 20 years.[5,6] Therefore, prevention of the birth of thalassemia-affected children through prenatal diagnosis remains the most effective strategy of tackling this health burden.

PREVENTIVE STRATEGIES FOR BETA-THALASSEMIA

The usual preventive strategy followed for most genetic disorders including beta-thalassemia is a sort of secondary prevention, wherein the birth of further affected children in the family is avoided, after the diagnosis of one or more affected children, through prenatal diagnostic testing in subsequent pregnancies. As beta-thalassemia is an autosomal recessive disorder, the risk of recurrence is 25% for each offspring of carrier parents. Identification of the exact disease-causing mutations in the family is the prerequisite for prenatal diagnostic testing. Ideally, the disease-causing mutations should be identified in the proband (index case) through a suitable molecular genetic test before the parents plan the next pregnancy. Appropriate preconception counseling can also be offered to such couples, so that after conception, invasive testing can be done at the correct gestational age in a planned manner. However, quite often, couples are referred to the geneticist or fetal medicine expert for the first time after conception of the next pregnancy. In such situations, mutation of the proband is done first, as quickly as possible and then prenatal testing is offered. However, if the gestational age is advanced, prenatal testing may not be feasible or useful, as the legally permissible limit for medical termination of pregnancies in India is 20 weeks. If genetic testing of the proband cannot be done either because he/she is not alive or for any other reason, mutations can be identified by testing both the parents.

Though the above strategy still remains the most common measure followed in India for preventing the birth of thalassemia-affected children, a primary preventive approach is a better tactic for tackling common genetic disorders like thalassemia. In view of the high carrier frequency in India, a population-based screening of all couples, irrespective of their family history, would help to identify their carrier status before conception or early in the 1st trimester in the very first pregnancy itself. This would help in taking appropriate prenatal diagnostic measures to prevent the birth of even one affected child. Screening for beta-thalassemia carriers can be done easily through estimation of mean corpuscular volume (MCV), mean corpuscular hemoglobin (MCH) and hemoglobin (Hb) A2 percentage [by Hb electrophoresis or-high performance liquid chromatography (HPLC)], which are readily available. Beta-thalassemia carriers usually have MCV less than 80 fL, MCH less than 27 pg and HbA2 more than 3.5%. Though carrier testing of couples should ideally be done preconceptionally, in the current Indian scenario, carrier testing in the 1st trimester at the time of the first antenatal visit is the most practical approach. Premarital carrier testing, though practiced in some countries, is not a good option for our country because of various sociocultural reasons. If both partners are found to be carriers of the beta-thalassemia trait, mutation detection has to be done in both to identify the exact pathogenic mutations, and only then can prenatal diagnostic testing be done.

National level programs of population-based carrier screening and genetic counseling for beta-thalassemia have been successfully implemented in several at-risk populations in Mediterranean countries such as Greece, Cyprus and Italy and have been very effective in reducing the burden of thalassemia in these countries.[7,8] Implementation of such population-based carrier testing programs is likely to significantly bring down the birth prevalence of this serious disorder in our country also.[5]

Cascade screening is another practically useful carrier testing approach, wherein the extended family members of an affected individual are counseled and screened for carrier status.

Mutation Testing for Beta-Thalassemia

Identification of the disease-causing mutations in beta-thalassemia can be done in two different ways: mutation-specific testing and whole gene sequencing of the *HBB* gene. Ethnic preponderance of specific mutations is a known feature of beta-thalassemia and some mutations are known to be common in specific populations. For instance, five mutations [IVS I-5 (G/C), 619-bp deletion, Codon 8/9 (+G), Codon 41/42(-TCTT) and IVS I-1 (G/T)] have been found to account for approximately 94% of beta-thalassemia alleles in Northern and Western India.[9] On the other hand, in Southern India, the most common alleles reported are the IVS I-5 (G/C), Codon 15 (G/A) and poly A (T/C) and there is also a higher frequency of homozygosity for rare mutations because of consanguinity.[9]

The most cost-effective strategy for mutation identification would be to first do mutation-specific testing for mutations known to be common in the community or region of origin of the individual and if these are found to be absent, whole gene sequencing of the *HBB* gene needs to be done. Mutation-specific testing can be done through various techniques such as ARMS-PCR (amplification-refractory mutation system-polymerase chain reaction), reverse dot blot or PCR-RFLP (restriction fragment length polymorphism).

Prenatal Diagnostic Testing for Beta-Thalassemia

As mentioned above, identification of the disease-causing mutations in the family is essential for prenatal diagnostic testing. Once the mutations are identified, targeted mutation analysis, i.e. testing for those specific mutations is done in the fetal DNA. Fetal DNA is obtained either through chorionic villus sampling (CVS) at around 11–13 weeks of gestation or through amniocentesis after 16 weeks of gestation. Both procedures are done under ultrasound guidance and between the two, CVS is preferred for antenatal testing of single gene disorders including beta-thalassemia because it can be done at an earlier gestational age and gives a higher DNA yield, but it has a slightly higher risk of pregnancy loss of 0.2–0.5%.[10] Amniocentesis is usually done when the pregnant lady presents at a later gestation or when CVS fails or is difficult to do, because of reasons such as a posteriorly positioned placenta; the risk of pregnancy loss after amniocentesis has been reported to vary between 0.1 and 0.3%.[10] DNA is extracted from the CVS or amniocytes and then subjected to mutation-specific testing. If the fetal DNA is found to have mutations on both copies (alleles) of the *HBB* gene (i.e. homozygous or compound heterozygous state), the fetus is considered to be affected, whereas in case of absence of both mutations or presence of a mutation in only copy of the gene (heterozygous state) the fetus is considered to be unaffected **(Figs 6.1A and B)**.

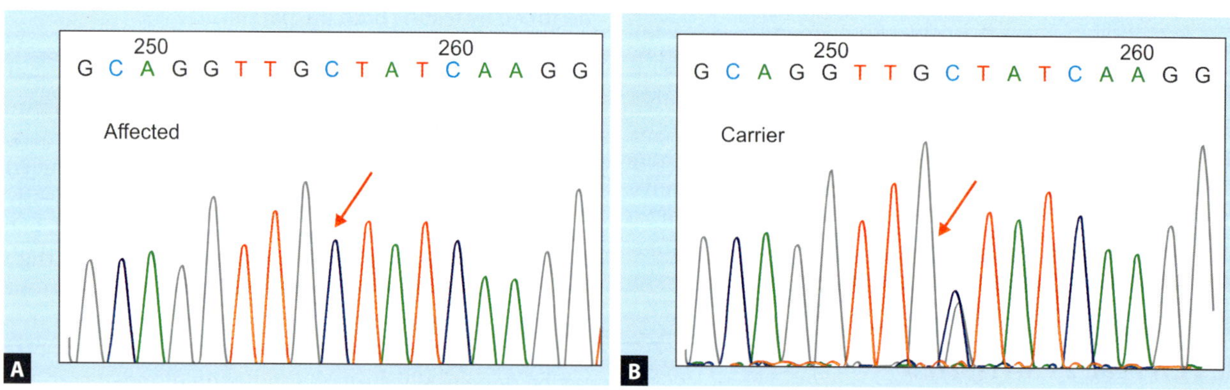

Figures 6.1A and B (A) Sequence chromatogram of a child affected with beta-thalassemia major showing homozygosity for the common mutation IVS 1–5 (G > C); (B) Sequence chromatogram of the fetus (chorionic villus sample) showing heterozygosity for the IVS 1–5 (G > C) mutation indicating that the fetus is only a carrier and not affected with beta-thalassemia disease

Sometimes, there may be some amount of admixture of maternal tissue in the fetal sample (CVS or amniocytes), which may give a wrong result and, therefore, it is important to rule out maternal DNA contamination in the fetal DNA sample in every case. Ruling out of maternal contamination is particularly essential if the fetal DNA is found to be a heterozygous carrier of the same mutation that is present in the mother.

Pretest and Post-test Genetic Counseling

Genetic counseling of the couple is essential both before and after the prenatal diagnostic procedure. Pretest counseling includes a detailed explanation about the autosomal recessive pattern of inheritance of beta-thalassemia, the 25% risk of recurrence in each offspring and the importance of prenatal diagnostic testing in preventing this recurrence. Many couples have a mistaken notion that prenatal detection of disease in the fetus would be followed by some form of curative fetal therapy. Though some fetal therapeutic strategies such as in utero hematopoietic stem cell transplantation and fetal gene therapy are being explored, as of now, there are no fetal curative modalities available and the couple has to be clearly counseled about this. The risk of pregnancy loss associated with the invasive procedure being done is also discussed. It is also important at this stage to clarify the fact that genetic testing of the *HBB* gene is informative for only beta-thalassemia disease status in the fetus and does not provide information about any other genetic disorder. Most often, either karyotyping or testing for at least the common chromosomal aneuploidies (i.e. trisomies 21, 13 and 18) is offered alongside the *HBB* testing for the collected fetal sample. Though an uncommon scenario, sometimes the fetus may be at risk for some other known genetic condition (especially in consanguineous families) and testing of these other relevant mutation(s) would have to be additionally done in the fetal sample.

Post-test counseling involves explanation about the implications of the negative or positive test results and about the error rate of the test. Every DNA-based test has an error rate, though very minimal (usually mentioned as about 1%). As genetic counseling is a nondirective process, the couple is not advised to terminate an affected pregnancy; rather, they are told about the postnatal prognosis for an affected fetus, so that they can autonomously take an informed decision about termination or continuation of the pregnancy. In case the fetus is found to be unaffected, they are advised to continue regular antenatal care and undergo fetal anomaly scans and follow-up scans as for any other normal pregnancy.

Role of Hemoglobin Electrophoresis or HPLC in Prenatal Diagnosis

Hemoglobin electrophoresis or HPLC in the fetal blood is another prenatal diagnostic modality which was being used commonly before the widespread availability of genetic testing. Due to its numerous limitations, it is no longer preferred. It requires fetal blood sampling or cordocentesis, which is a more invasive procedure with a pregnancy loss rate of around 1–2% and can be done only after 18 weeks of gestation. The fetal HbA levels are used to differentiate between fetuses affected with thalassemia major and carrier and normal fetuses with the HbA being in the range of 0–0.5% in thalassemia major-affected fetuses and more than 1.3% in carrier and normal fetuses. However, a significant amount of overlap has been found to be present between the HbA values of thalassemia intermedia affected and carrier fetuses.[11,12]

Newer Modalities for Fetal Testing

Preimplantation genetic diagnosis allows for the selection of disease-free embryos for transfer into the uterus in assisted reproduction (*in vitro* fertilization). Genetic analysis is carried out on one or two blastomeres that are microsurgically removed from the embryo on day-3 of culture. Single cell PCR amplification and molecular testing is done for testing of single gene disorders like beta-thalassemia. The disease-free embryos are then selected and transferred to the uterus for implantation. Preimplantation genetic diagnosis is becoming increasingly available in developed countries such as the United States and many European nations, for beta-thalassemia and other common monogenic disorders such as sickle cell disease, cystic fibrosis, spinal muscular atrophy, Duchenne muscular dystrophy, fragile X syndrome, etc.[13,14] While prenatal diagnosis entails the termination of affected pregnancies, preimplantation genetic diagnosis obviates the need for such a termination, which makes it a more attractive option. However, the high costs, the need for assisted reproduction, the high failure rate of successful implantation after *in vitro* fertilization and limited availability are the deterrents to a more widespread use of this testing modality.

Noninvasive prenatal diagnostic methods, which are being extensively studied, include cell-based and cell-free methods of which the most popular technique involves study of cell-free fetal DNA (cffDNA) in maternal plasma. Cell-free fetal DNA represents 3–6% of the circulating cell-free DNA in the maternal plasma, is present in smaller fragments and has a different methylation pattern compared to the maternal cell-free DNA. These small fragments of cffDNA can be sequenced through next-generation sequencing technology which works on the principle of shotgun sequencing. Though this approach is more commonly being used for the detection of fetal chromosomal aneuploidies and the fetal (rhesus) D (RhD) status in an RhD-negative woman, its utility in the detection of single gene disorders such as beta-thalassemia is being increasingly explored. Presence of the paternal mutation in the cffDNA can be unequivocally ascertained; however, if the maternal mutation is detected, it is difficult to determine if the identified mutation is in the maternal DNA or the cffDNA.[13,15]

Alpha-Thalassemia

Alpha-thalassemia is not common in our country. The severe form of alpha-thalassemia, Hb Bart syndrome, which

Table 6.1 Common structural hemoglobin variants found in India[1,17,18]

Hemoglobin variant	*Genetic basis*	*Prevalence in India*	*Phenotype in homozygote*	*Phenotype in compound heterozygotes*
HbS	Substitution of glutamic acid to valine at the sixth amino acid position in the beta-globin chain	Prevalent in Central India and tribal belts of Western, Eastern and Southern India	*HbS/HbS:* Sickle cell disease	*HbS/Beta-thalassemia:* Moderate-to-severe thalassemia intermedia phenotype
HbE	Substitution of glutamic acid to lysine at the 26th amino acid position in the beta globin chain	Prevalent in West Bengal and the North-Eastern states	*HbE/HbE:* Asymptomatic	*HbE/Beta-thalassemia:* Moderate-to-severe thalassemia intermedia phenotype. Many are transfusion dependent
HbD-Punjab	Substitution of glutamic acid to glutamine at the 121st amino acid position in the beta-globin chain	Prevalent in North-Western India	*HbD/HbD:* Asymptomatic or mild anemia	*HbD/Beta-thalassemia:* Mild-to-moderate anemia

Abbreviations: Hb, hemoglobin

presents with fetal hydrops, is rarely seen in India and is prevalent in Africa and South-East Asia.[16] This condition presents with nonimmune fetal hydrops and has to be considered as a possible differential diagnosis when the fetal scan and Doppler studies show evidence of hydropic changes and severe anemia in the fetus, in the absence of Rh isoimmunization, the other important possibility being fetal parvovirus infection. Prenatal testing in such a scenario should include fetal sampling through cordocentesis and fetal Hb HPLC to document Hb Bart (which is made up of four gamma globin chains) and molecular genetic testing of the alpha globin (*HBA*) gene; amniocentesis and mutation analysis of the *HBA* gene in the amniocyte DNA can also be done. Majority of the alpha-thalassemia-causing *HBA* gene mutations are deletions, which can be tested for through techniques such as Gap-PCR and multiplex ligation-dependent probe amplification (MLPA).

Other Inherited Hemoglobinopathies

Apart from alpha-thalassemia and beta-thalassemia, other important inherited hemoglobinopathies include the abnormal structural Hb variants, which are caused by mutations within the coding, i.e. exonic regions of the globin genes. The structural Hb variants, which are prevalent in India (HbS, HbE and HbD-Punjab), are listed in **Table 6.1** with their underlying genetic defect, regional prevalence and phenotypic manifestations.[1,17,18] As is evident from the table, compound heterozygosity of these variants (especially HbS and HbE) with a beta-thalassemia mutant allele produces a severe disease phenotype and, therefore, it is important to screen the partner of a beta-thalassemia carrier for these variants through Hb HPLC. Following carrier screening of the parents or mutation testing of a previous affected sibling, if the fetus is identified to be at risk for homozygous sickle cell disease (HbS/HbS), compound heterozygous HbS-beta-thalassemia or compound heterozygous HbE-beta-thalassemia, prenatal diagnosis through mutation-specific testing is offered for the pregnancy.

Delta beta-thalassemia is caused by deletion of the entire delta and beta gene sequences with production of only gamma-globin. Heterozygotes for δβ-thalassemia are asymptomatic and homozygotes have a mild phenotype, but compound heterozygotes for beta-thalassemia and δβ-thalassemia can have a thalassemia major or severe thalassemia intermedia-like disease phenotype, which requires prenatal testing.[1] δβ-thalassemia carriers have a normal or reduced HbA2 and an elevated HbF (5–20%) due to which they may be mistaken to have hereditary persistence of fetal hemoglobin.[1] Therefore, it is recommended that exact genetic characterization be done to identify and confirm this entity in individuals showing elevated HbF on carrier testing. The most common δβ-thalassemia-associated mutation in India is the Asian Indian inversion-deletion GγAγ (δβ) mutation.[19]

CONCLUSION

Beta-thalassemia is a significant health problem in our country and coordinated national level programs for population-based carrier screening and prenatal diagnostic testing of at-risk pregnancies are the need of the hour, to bring down the prevalence of this severe and chronic disease.

KEY POINTS

- Beta-thalassemia is the most common monogenic disorder in India with a high carrier prevalence rate.
- The most effective way to reduce the burden of thalassemia in the population is through prenatal diagnosis and termination of affected pregnancies.
- Beta-thalassemia, being an autosomal recessive genetic disorder, has a 25% risk of recurrence in each offspring of a carrier couple.
- After the birth of one or more affected children, recurrence can be prevented in the family by prenatal diagnosis of subsequent pregnancies.
- The preferred modality of prenatal diagnosis for beta-thalassemia is mutation-specific testing of fetal DNA

obtained through chorionic villus sampling at 11–13 weeks of gestation or through amniocentesis after 16 weeks of gestation.

- Identification of the exact disease-causing mutations, either in the proband or in the carrier parents, is a prerequisite for prenatal diagnostic testing.
- Population-based carrier screening of all couples in the preconception period or early in the 1st trimester irrespective of the family history and prenatal testing to prevent the birth of even one affected child is a more ideal and effective preventive measure.
- Newer modalities for fetal testing such as preimplantation genetic diagnosis and noninvasive prenatal testing have also become available for clinical use.

REFERENCES

1. Colah RB, Gorakshakar AC, Nadkarni AH. Invasive and non-invasive approaches for prenatal diagnosis of haemoglobinopathies: experiences from India. Indian J Med Res. 2011;134:552-60.
2. Weatherall DJ. The inherited disorders of hemoglobin are an emerging global health burden. Blood. 2010;115(22):4331-6.
3. Madan N, Sharma S, Sood SK, Colah R, Bhatia HM. Frequency of β-thalassemia trait and other hemoglobinopathies in northern and western India. Indian J Hum Genet. 2010;16(1):16-25.
4. Modell B, Petrou M. The problem of hemoglobinopathies in India. Indian J Haematol. 1983;1:1-5.
5. Petrou M. Screening for beta thalassaemia. Indian J Hum Genet. 2010;16(1):1-5.
6. Mallik S, Chatterjee C, Mandal PK, Sardar JC, Ghosh P, Manna N. Expenditure to treat thalassaemia: an experience at a tertiary care hospital in India. Iran J Public Health. 2010;39(1);78-84.
7. Angastiniotis MA, Hadjiminas MG. Prevention of thalassemia in Cyprus. Lancet. 1991;1:369-70.
8. Petrou M, Modell B. Prenatal screening for hemoglobin disorders. Prenat Diagn. 1995;15(13):1275-95.
9. Edison ES, Shaji RV, Devi SG, Moses A, Viswabandhya A, Mathews V, et al. Analysis of beta globin mutations in the Indian population: presence of rare and novel mutations and region-wise heterogeneity. Clin Genet. 2008;73(4):331-7.
10. Akolekar R, Beta J, Picciarelli G, Ogilvie C, D'Antonio F. Procedure-related risk of miscarriage following amniocentesis and chorionic villus sampling: a systematic review and meta-analysis. Ultrasound Obstet Gynecol. 2015;45(1):16-26.
11. Wadia MR, Phanasgaokar SP, Nadkarni AH, Surve RR, Gorakshakar AC, Colah RB, et al. Usefulness of automated chromatography for rapid fetal blood analysis for second trimester prenatal diagnosis of beta-thalassemia. Prenat Diagn. 2002;22(2):153-7.
12. Rao S, Saxena R, Deka D, Kabra M. Use of HbA estimation by CE-HPLC for prenatal diagnosis of beta-thalassemia; experience from a tertiary care centre in north India: a brief report. Hematology. 2009;14(2):122-4.
13. Bodurtha J, Strauss JF 3rd. Genomics and perinatal care. N Engl J Med. 2012;366(1):64-73.
14. Ranganath P, Phadke SR. Genetics in Perinatal Care: An Overview. Perinatology. 2013;14:1-6.
15. Papageorgiou EA, Patsalis PC. Non-invasive prenatal diagnosis of aneuploidies: new technologies and clinical applications. Genome Med. 2012;4(5):46.
16. Bernini LF. Geographic distribution of alpha thalassemia. In: Steinberg MH, Forget PG, Higgs DR, Nagel RL (Eds). Disorders of Hemoglobin: Genetics, Pathophysiology and Clinical Management. Cambridge, UK: Cambridge University Press; 2001. pp. 878-94.
17. Balgir RS. Genetic epidemiology of the three predominant abnormal hemoglobins in India. J Assoc Physicians India. 1996;44(1):25-8.
18. Verma IC, Bijarnia S. The burden of genetic disorders in India and a framework for community control. Community Genet. 2002;5(3):192-6.
19. Nadkarni A, Wadia M, Gorakshakar A, Kiyama R, Colah RB, Mohanty D. Molecular characterization of delta beta-thalassemia and hereditary persistence of fetal hemoglobin in the Indian population. Hemoglobin. 2008;32(5):425-33.

CHAPTER 7

Genetic Counseling for Hematological Disorders

Roshan Colah, Khushnooma Italia

INTRODUCTION

Monogenic or single gene disorders are the disorders where a variation (known as a mutation) in a gene gives rise to a clinical phenotype. More than 5,000 single gene disorders are known and are catalogued in the Online Mendelian Inheritance in Man (OMIM). The causative genes for most of them are known. This is especially true for hematological disorders. They are most often inherited from the parents but can also be caused due to *de novo* mutations occurring during gametogenesis. Many of these disorders are usually difficult to cure and expensive to manage. However, by identification of the causative genes and molecular genetic technologies; prevention of genetic disorders is possible by carrier detection and prenatal diagnosis. Genetic counseling plays a central role in the process and needs to be a part of the management of genetic disorders.

BURDEN OF THE INHERITED HEMATOLOGICAL DISORDERS

The inherited hematological disorders, mainly the hemoglobinopathies and the hemophilias pose a significant burden on the health of the population in India. It has been estimated that there would be around 100,000 children with the β-thalassemias, as many or more with sickle cell disorders and around 65,000 cases of hemophilia in India. Although there are no national registries, estimates show that around 10,000 new cases of the β-thalassemias, 7,000–8,000 of sickle cell anemia and around 5,000 cases of hemophilia are added each year.[1-3] Though these disorders are treatable and the patients can lead a fruitful and relatively long life; the severe clinical course, costly and many a times lifelong treatment justify the control of these disorders by prevention programs. At the same time, the existing patients need optimum management to lead a good quality and productive life. Genetic counselors would play a major role in both these endeavors.

GENETIC TESTING VERSUS GENETIC SCREENING

Genetic testing is a process where a family with an affected child or those who are aware of their risk seek help to arrive at an accurate diagnosis. Genetic screening, on the other hand, involves screening individuals who are asymptomatic and totally unaware of the possibility of being a carrier of a genetic disorder. The counseling process in both these situations would be very different. Screening is usually a population-based program and needs a system in place, awareness amongst clinicians and laypersons and laboratory capabilities to take up the heavy load of tests in addition to technical and counseling expertise.

INDIAN SCENARIO

Health insurance cover to bear the expenses of management of patients with the inherited hematological disorders is not available for the vast majority of families with an affected child. Many a times, affected children particularly with a severe thalassemia syndrome are not treated and die both due to lack of awareness and nonaffordability by the family. Many of these families do not get information about the risk of recurrence and an option of prevention of recurrence as they are not referred or not able to reach genetic centers. Also, there are inadequate medical facilities to manage these diseases. Government hospitals in major cities bear a huge burden on their services as well as bear a part of the cost of managing few of these patients. The limited facilities also have to cope with the patient load referred from peripheral hospitals at peripheral small towns and villages. Most district places do not have facilities for management of thalassemia and hemophilia. Prevention by genetic counseling and prenatal diagnosis will bring a great relief not only to the families but will also reduce the burden of health economics of the country.

An effort was made to collect information from different centers in India working in the area of Human Genetics and put together all this data for the benefit of patients and parents of children with genetic disorders.[4] Only 50 of the more than 1,000 members of Indian Society of Human Genetics were involved in providing diagnostic and counseling services for genetic disorders. Molecular and prenatal diagnosis was done at 26 centers and genetic counseling at 40 centers. The Department of Biotechnology and Indian Council of Medical Research have provided financial support to establish genetic clinics for diagnosis of genetic disorders.[4]

Awareness and Screening: The Need for Population-based Programs

Awareness about the β-thalassemias and sickle cell disorders is lacking in the population. This needs to be generated in all sections of society starting from school going children to young adults of marriageable age, married couples and pregnant women. Awareness generation is also required among professionals particularly pediatricians, obstetricians and family physicians. It is the key to a successful community-based thalassemia/sickle cell disease control program. This can be done by personal communication, posters, booklets and mass media in different local languages not only in urban areas but also to reach the remotest of rural areas.[5-7] Awareness on the hemophilias is considerably better as there are 76 chapters of the Hemophilia Society of India spread all over the country and they are all very active.

Screening programs are conducted for the hemoglobinopathies by many National Institutes, Anthropological Survey of India, different non-government organizations (NGOs) and Thalassemia and Sickle Cell Societies. Based on these initiatives, the prevalence of β-thalassemia carriers is 3–4% in the country, being much higher (5–17%) in certain communities like *Sindhis, Kutchi, Bhanushalis, Lohanas, Punjabi Aroras* and *Khatris*, some Muslim groups and even some tribal populations. The prevalence of sickle cell trait varies from 5% to 35% in some scheduled castes and scheduled tribes and some other backward classes.[8] Also due to migration of people from different regions to metropolitan cities for employment and education and due to the recent trend of mixed marriages between different communities, there is a need to be extremely cautious in identifying individuals who are carriers or couples at risk even in a nonendemic area or among those individuals not belonging to a high-risk community. The carriers of hemophilia are generally identified after the birth of a hemophilia patient is identified in a family or during carrier screening of extended family members.

GENETIC COUNSELING

When a family first discovers that their child is affected by a genetic disorder, they have the following questions:

- What is the problem?
- Why did it happen?
- Is there any treatment or cure?
- Will it happen again?
- How can it be prevented?

Principles of Genetic Counseling: Definition and Process

Genetic counseling is a process of communication involving both pretesting and post-testing counseling to help individuals and families at-risk of a hereditary genetic disorder to come to terms with the situation and consequences of the disorder and take the right decision which may guide future reproductive choices to avoid the birth of another child with the disease, keeping ethical issues in mind.[9,10]

Steps of Genetic Counseling

The main elements of genetic counseling have been outlined as given here:[11]

- Accurate diagnosis and explaining the clinical presentation, severity and consequences of the disorders
- Documenting family history, consanguinity and drawing a pedigree chart
- The inheritance pattern and the risk of recurrence
- Communication in simple language and in a sympathetic way
- Information on all available options and ethical issues
- Support to the family while making decisions
- Social and psychological support including religious and cultural issues
- The need for screening extended family members
- Reassurance of having a normal child.

Accurate Diagnosis

This is extremely important and with the availability of molecular technology should not be a major issue, e.g. the diagnosis of a β-thalassemia carrier should not be missed. This is particularly so in case of silent carriers who may have a normal HbA_2 level and/or near normal red cell indices. This is particularly important in a couple where one partner is a β-thalassemia carrier and the other has borderline/normal HbA_2 levels. Molecular analysis must be done in such cases to avoid a misdiagnosis. The counselor should be aware of this and advice accordingly. This may be due to inheritance of a silent β-thalassemia mutation like the cap site +1 (A>C) mutation, the poly A mutation or coinheritance of a δ gene defect.[6] Also, couples with α-gene triplication in one partner and a β-thalassemia carrier status with a coinherited α-gene triplication in the other partner should be made aware that a β-thalassemia carrier who inherits additional α-genes can also present as a thalassemia intermedia and may at times require blood transfusion support. Compound heterozygosity for hereditary persistence of fetal hemoglobin (HPFH) and HbD, β-thalassemia and HbD or homozygosity for HbE usually results in very mild clinical phenotypes and hence couples who are at risk of these disorders do not require prenatal diagnosis.

Special Issues in Genetic Counseling for Sickle Cell Disease

The severity of the disorder cannot always be predicted especially in sickle cell anemia where some homozygotes can have a mild clinical presentation and live well into adulthood without much disability and others can have repeated crisis, severe anemia and other sickle cell-related complications like stroke, avascular necrosis and acute chest syndrome.[8] In such a situation, it is difficult for the counselor to predict the clinical severity.

Pedigree

Marriage patterns contribute to the incidence of genetic disorders in the population. Consanguinity is very common in South India, particularly uncle niece marriages among Hindus and first cousin marriage among Muslims.[12] This consanguinity can occur in several generations making the pedigree drawing sometimes difficult.

Once the carrier or homozygous status is established, color-coded cards can be given which are particularly helpful in rural tribal areas to avoid marriage between two carriers.

The Inheritance Pattern

The β-thalassemias and sickle cell disorders have an autosomal recessive inheritance, and **Figures 7.1 and 7.2** show the risk of recurrence of the disease in different matings in every pregnancy.

Hemophilia has an X-linked inheritance where females are carriers and males are affected **(Figs 7.3 to 7. 5)**. For a female to be affected by the disease, she must receive two defective X-chromosomes, one from her mother and the other from her father (who must therefore be a hemophiliac himself). Hence, hemophilia primarily affects males and is very rare in females. However, it is possible for female carriers to become mild hemophiliacs due to lyonization (inactivation) of the X-chromosomes.

Prevention by Prenatal Diagnosis and Available Options for Reproduction

Molecular diagnosis has made prenatal diagnosis a reality. Prenatal diagnosis with the possibility of terminating an affected child is usually an acceptable option to most of the families. Another option is preimplantation diagnosis, which

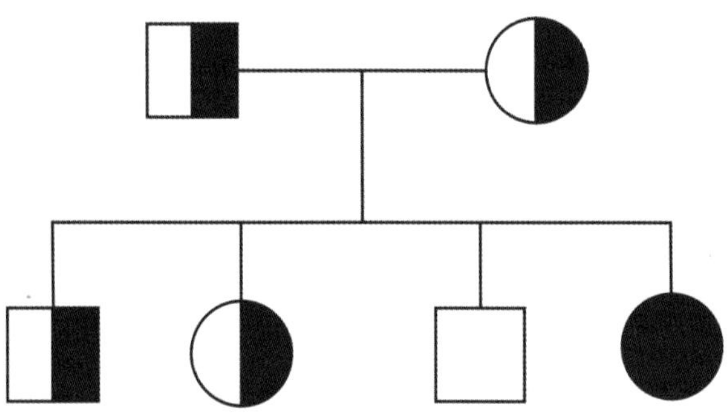

Figure 7.1 Both parents are β-thalassemia carriers
Note: When both parents are carriers, there is a 50% chance that the baby will be a carrier, 25% chance that the baby will be normal and 25% chance that the baby will be affected.

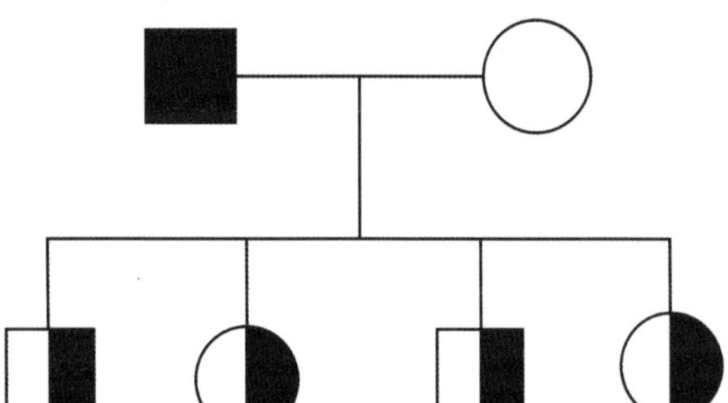

Figure 7.2 One parent is sickle homozygous and the other is normal
Note: If one parent is affected and the other is normal, all their children will be carriers.

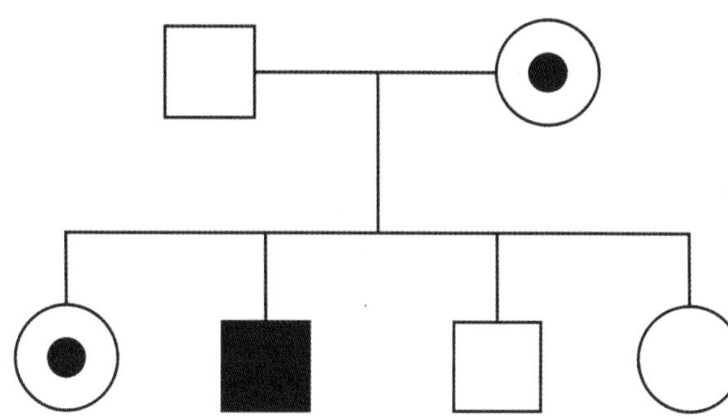

Figure 7.3 Mother is a carrier and father is normal
Note: Sons of a carrier woman have 50% chance of being affected with hemophilia; daughters have 50% chance of being a carrier.

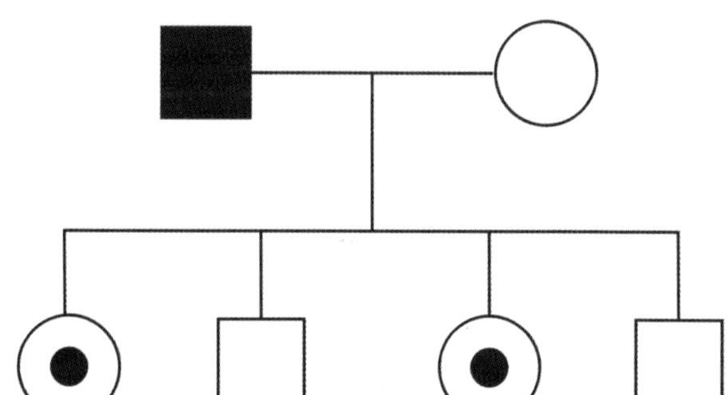

Figure 7.4 Father has hemophilia and mother is normal
Note: All daughters of a hemophilia male will be carriers and all sons will be normal.

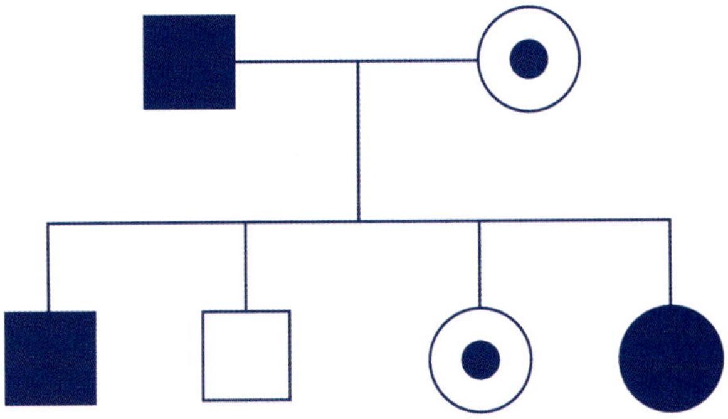

Figure 7.5 Father has hemophilia and mother is a carrier

Note: Sons have a 50% chance of having hemophilia and daughters have 50% chance of being a carrier and 50% chance of having hemophilia.

is of help to the families who do not accept termination of pregnancy for religious or other reasons. Other options, which may be discussed in relevant situations, are artificial insemination with a donor who is not a carrier of β-thalassemia or hemoglobinopathy or adoption.

Methodologies

After genetic counseling, most couples opt for prenatal diagnosis, which is ideally done in the first trimester of pregnancy by chorionic villus sampling and DNA analysis. Before undertaking fetal sampling for DNA analysis, the mutations in the family need to be identified by testing the affected member in the family (proband) or the carrier partners of the couple at risk. DNA-based prenatal diagnosis can also be done using amniotic fluid. The error rate of prenatal diagnosis is around 1% and this should be communicated during pre- and post-test counseling. If the couple at-risk is identified late and/or the mutations in the family are not identified; the genetic counselor can also suggest second trimester prenatal diagnosis in the case of hemoglobinopathies by high-performance liquid chromatography (HPLC) analysis of fetal blood obtained by cordocentesis at 18–19 weeks gestation and in the case of hemophilia by factor levels in fetal blood.[13,14] Fetal sexing can also tell whether the fetus is at risk of hemophilia or not.

Preimplantation genetic diagnosis is mainly for couples where termination of an affected pregnancy is not acceptable or when there is an unsuccessful reproductive history and the couple is undergoing assisted reproduction. It requires a collaboration between a competent *in vitro* fertilization center and a good molecular diagnostic laboratory.[15] It should be brought to the notice of the family opting for preimplantation diagnosis that as *in vitro* fertilization is necessary for preimplantation diagnosis the success rate of a liveborn child is around 40% and usually confirmation of fetal diagnosis by prenatal sampling is indicated to avoid errors. Recently, prenatal diagnosis by analyzing cell-free-fetal DNA in maternal plasma has also been shown to be technically possible.

Strategies of Prevention: Avoiding Recurrence in Sibs and Extended Family Members

Genetic counseling is an essential tool to educate a couple with a child with a genetic disorder. Through genetic counseling the parents can be made aware of the risk of having another child with a similar disorder in future pregnancies. They should also be advised to check the carrier status of all their first degree relatives who can be at high risk of being carriers and consequently capable of giving birth to a child with a genetic disorder.

Ethical Issues and the PCPNDT Act

Counseling has to be nondirective. Thus, facts have to be presented without influencing the decision which should be made by the couple. When couples are undergoing prenatal diagnosis, an informed consent must be taken. Often couples are accompanied by their parents and/or in-laws who influence decision making. The genetic counselor must also try to talk to the couple independently. Yet it is important for the genetic counselor to understand the family's beliefs and reasoning that lead to decision taking. An informed consent must be taken before a couple opts for genetic testing or prenatal diagnosis. According to the Preconception and Prenatal Diagnosis Technologies Act (PCPNDT Act), which was enacted to prevent female feticide, a written informed consent of the pregnant woman has to be taken by the counselor with prohibition of communicating the sex of the fetus. A genetic clinic, which undertakes screening, genetic counseling and prenatal diagnosis, must be registered with the respective State Governments and maintain detailed records as well as submit a monthly report of counseling and prenatal diagnosis done along with the results of the tests to the authorities. Any institution offering these procedures must have ethical clearance from their Institutional Ethics Committee.

Psychological, Social and Cultural Issues

Religious, social and emotional factors must be kept in mind while offering genetic counseling.[16] Abortion is not permissible in some religions; however, abortion up to 120 days is permitted in most countries, if a fetus is affected with a severe genetic disease.[17] There is often social stigmatization, and hence confidentiality must be maintained. It is always better to talk to both the husband and wife together and test them simultaneously. The woman is most often blamed and there is a feeling of guilt. This may lead to abandonment by the husband and the woman is often left to care for the affected child. This is mainly due to ignorance and lack of awareness. Long-term follow-up and support from the counselor is needed particularly when there is death of an affected child or termination of an affected pregnancy.

Who should Undergo Training in Genetic Counseling?

Pediatricians, obstetricians and primary physicians should undergo training in genetic counseling as they are the first to be approached by a family with a genetic disorder. Individuals from other specialties like nursing and those who have undertaken a Masters Degree in Social Science or Medical Social Work also most often serve as genetic counselors. There is only one course at present for human resource development in genetic counseling conducted at the Sanjay Gandhi Postgraduate Institute of Medical Sciences (SGPGIMS), Lucknow and more such courses are required to train genetic counselors in the country. Master of Science (MSc) in genetic counseling has also been started in some medical genetics departments.

CONCLUSION

Genetic counseling should be a part of management of genetic disorders and all clinicians need to know the concept of basic genetics and principles of genetic counseling and take up the responsibility of genetic testing and counseling. With increasing availability of genetic testing, there is a great need of medical geneticists and nonmedical genetic counselors. β-thalassemia being the most common genetic disorder, there is a need for a nationwide control program. The experience of pilot programs on thalassemia screening and prenatal diagnosis sponsored by Indian Council of Medical Research have proved the feasibility and brought some awareness amongst laypersons and policy makers. However, for a large country like India prevention by population screening and genetic counseling is a challenging task, which needs to be initiated.

KEY MESSAGE

Genetic counseling, genetic testing and prenatal diagnosis play a crucial role in providing information and support to families affected by or at risk of having a child with a severe inherited hemoglobin disorder or a bleeding disorder such as hemophilia. This makes training of healthcare professionals, clinicians and genetic counselors involved in genetic testing an important aspect of a control program. With advancement in genetic testing for many genetic disorders, a need for more medical geneticists and genetic counselors arises as this will not only help in bringing about awareness in the society but also help in reducing the burden of genetic disorders such as thalassemia and hemophilia in the country.

REFERENCES

1. Mohanty D, Colah RB, Gorakshakar AC, Patel RZ, Master DC, Mahanta J, et al. Prevalence of β-thalassemia and other haemoglobinopathies in six cities in India: a multicentre study. J Community Genet. 2013;4:33-42.
2. Verma IC, Saxena R, Kohli S. Past, present and future scenario of thalassaemia care and control in India. Indian J Med Res. 2011;134:507-21.
3. Shetty S, Ghosh K, Bhide A, Mohanty D. Carrier detection and prenatal diagnosis in families with haemophilia. Natl Med J India. 2001;14:81-3.
4. Singh JR, Singh AR, Singh AR. Directory of Human Genetic Services in India. Indian J Hum Genet. 2010;10:187-92.
5. Mohanty D, Das K. Genetic counselling in tribals in India. Indian J Med Res. 2011;134:561-71.
6. Colah RB, Gorakshakar AC. Control of thalassemia in India. Thal Rep. 2014;4:1955.
7. Puri RD, Verma IC. Screening, genetic counselling, prenatal diagnosis and pre-implantation diagnosis for thalassemia. In: Sachdeva A (Ed). Thalassemia: National guidelines for management of transfusion dependent and non-transfusion dependent thalassemia, New Delhi. 2014. pp. 272-84.
8. Colah RB, Mukherjee MB, Ghosh K. Sickle cell disease in India. Current Opin Hematol. 2014;21:215-23.
9. Muthuswamy V. Ethical issues in genetic counselling with special reference to haemoglobinopathies. Indian J Med Res. 2011;134:547-51.
10. Miller R. Genetic counselling for hemophilia. In Treatment of Hemophilia. May 2002 No. 25. World Federation Hemophilia.
11. Deka D, Malhotra N. Genetic counselling for obstetricians. Donald School J Ultrasound Obstet Gynecol. 2010;4:447-53.
12. Bittles AH, Devi AR, Rao NA. Consanguinity, twining and secondary sex ratio in the population of Karnataka, south India. Ann Hum Biol. 1998;15:455-60.
13. Colah RB, Gorakshakar AC, Nadkarni AH. Invasive and non-invasive approaches for prenatal diagnosis of haemoglobinopathies: experiences from India. Indian J Med Res. 2011;134:552-60.
14. Shetty S, Ghosh K. Robustness of factor assays following cordocentesis in the prenatal diagnosis of haemophilia and other bleeding disorders. Haemophilia. 2007;13:172-7.
15. Vrettou C, Traeger-Synodinos J, Tzetis M, Palmer G, Sofocleous C, Kanavakis E. Real-time PCR for single-cell genotyping in sickle cell and thalassemia syndromes as a rapid, accurate, reliable, and widely applicable protocol for preimplantation genetic diagnosis. Hum Mutat. 2004;23:513-21.
16. Bhat M. Social and cultural issues in genetic counselling. J Biosci. 2015;40:217-20.
17. Giordano PC. The Genetic Counselor. In: Carrier diagnostics and prevention of hemoglobinopathies using high-performance liquid chromatography. Companion handbood for the physician, the laboratory doctor and the genetic counselor. Hercules, CA: Bio-Rad Laboratories Inc; 2006. pp. 81-93.

CHAPTER

8

Fetal Hematological Disorders: Future Ahead

Shubha R Phadke

INTRODUCTION

There have been tremendous developments in the diagnosis and treatment of genetic disorders in the past few decades. Many of these disorders are congenital in nature or manifest during infancy or early childhood. In addition to these advancements, better understanding of fetal physiology, pathology and ability to access the fetus by invasive and noninvasive methods have led to the establishment of fetal medicine as a specialty. Though successful fetal interventions in the form of intrauterine fetal blood transfusions as well as surgical interventions for malformations such as meningocele and diaphragmatic hernia are now possible, the major component of fetal medicine still continues to be prenatal diagnosis. Prenatal diagnosis by ultrasonographic fetal imaging is possible for a number of structural malformations and has achieved a very high level of specificity and sensitivity due to the amazing resolution of current ultrasonographic equipment. Obtaining fetal DNA by chorionic villus sampling and amniocentesis is quite easy and prenatal diagnosis of chromosomal and single gene disorders in fetus is routinely done worldwide for the past more than two decades. This provides an option of avoiding the birth of a child with a serious, handicapping or untreatable disorder by terminating the pregnancy, if the fetus is found to be affected with the disorder. Availability of prenatal diagnosis provides families at risk of a genetic disorder an option of having a disease-free child without taking the risk of occurrence or recurrence of the disorder. Though prenatal diagnosis and associated termination of pregnancy are legal in most countries and acceptable for majority of families, termination of pregnancy will always remain an ethically debatable issue and an extremely emotionally traumatic situation for the family. Diagnosis of fetus should lead to the development of fetal therapies. The newer developments in fetal diagnosis and research in the direction of development of new fetal therapies are discussed in this chapter.

DIAGNOSIS OF FETUS

Preimplantation Diagnosis and Noninvasive Genetic Diagnosis

Preimplantation genetic diagnosis (PGD) allows individuals who are carriers or who are affected by genetic diseases to select unaffected embryos for transfer before becoming pregnant. This involves *in vitro* fertilization and screening of embryos by molecular techniques and selecting embryos without mutation. The main advantage of PGD is avoiding termination of pregnancy which is needed sometimes with the option of prenatal diagnosis. The embryo biopsy (blastomere or blastomere stage) is the preferred option over polar body testing for PGD. It involves molecular diagnosis on a single cell which is technically challenging. The success rates of continued pregnancies are usually up to 35%; however, PGD resulting in successful unaffected babies in up to 68.4% of the pregnancies have been reported.[1]

Beta thalassemia is probably the most common indication for PGD other than screening for common chromosomal aneuploidies.[2] PGD for other monogenic disorders of blood-like alpha thalassemia, Wiskott-Aldrich syndrome, Fanconi anemia, sickle cell anemia, Glanzmann's thrombasthenia, Diamond-Blackfan anemia, hemophilia and nonhematological monogenic disorders such as X-linked adrenoleukodystrophy, cystic fibrosis, fragile X syndrome, Duchenne muscular dystrophy and mucopolysaccharidosis type I, etc. are being done. In addition to preimplantation diagnosis for the genetic disorder in concern, a choice of human leukocyte antigen (HLA) matched embryo for implantation is also available in PGD by doing simultaneous HLA typing of the embryo. This helps in choosing not only an unaffected child but also a HLA-matched stem cell donor for the affected sib.[3] PGD for selection of HLA-matched donor sib for patients with leukemias are also being done, though this continues to remain an area of ethical debate. After PGD, confirmation by prenatal diagnosis is suggested.

Although PGD avoids the option of termination of pregnancy, there are ethical issues surrounding life in fetus, views about prospective parents and society toward the individuals with genetic disorders and level of severity of phenotype justifying such preventive actions. The scientific and other social, family-related issues are complex. Detailed and appropriate counseling about the PGD versus prenatal diagnosis and other options is an essential part of the PGD process. However, as will be seen in the next few paragraphs, the newer upcoming options of fetal treatment may make preimplantation diagnosis the first step toward fetal therapy.

Noninvasive Prenatal Diagnosis from Free Fetal DNA from Maternal Plasma

For a long time, fetal diagnosis by isolating fetal cells from maternal blood was being tried and shown to be possible. But soon it became obvious that this technique also detects fetal cells from previous pregnancies. Hence, now the thrust is on using cell-free fetal DNA (cffDNA) in maternal plasma for prenatal diagnosis. Fetal DNA accounts for about 10% of cell-free DNA in the maternal plasma. The life of cffDNA is only for few hours. Fetal diagnosis using cffDNA can be done as early as 9 weeks. Fetal Rh typing using cffDNA has become the standard of care in the management of pregnancies with Rh-isoimmunization.[4] Prenatal diagnosis for alpha- and beta-thalassemia and sickle cell disease using cffDNA has also been shown to be possible.[5,6] One of the initial strategies used was to demonstrate the paternal unmutated allele in the maternal plasma, thus excluding homozygous thalassemia in the fetus. Quantitative polymerase chain reaction (PCR) is another option used for detecting copies of normal gene for prenatal diagnosis of hemoglobin Hb Bart's disease (homozygous alpha (0)-thalassemia).[7] Correct fetal diagnosis of sickle cell genotype was achieved in 80% of cases using digital PCR on cffDNA.[8] Prenatal testing using noninvasive methods for autosomal recessive disorders still continues in research mode and confirmation by invasive sampling of fetus is considered necessary even for unaffected results.

The advent of next generation sequencing (NGS) technique, which is a high throughput sequencing technique, brought a revolution in noninvasive prenatal diagnosis of aneuploidies. Use of NGS for detection of aneuploidies has achieved a very high sensitivity of 99% or more. However, occasional false results and failure rate of about 3% still make it a screening test and is being used on a large scale for high- and low-risk pregnant women.[9] NGS-based testing has been shown to be successful for detection of the fetal Kell blood group (KEL1)[10] and beta-thalassemia.[11] Noninvasive prenatal diagnosis has been successfully used for other monogenic disorders as well.[12] NGS technology has opened up many more options for noninvasive prenatal diagnosis of monogenic disorders and may also be used for screening for many disorders in the future.

FETAL THERAPY

Fetal Stem Cell Therapy

The diagnosis should lead to cure with treatment and that is always the expectation of the patient and family and the will of the treating clinician. Fetal diagnosis of a wide variety of disorders is available in clinical practice for decades and has achieved a great degree of accuracy. However, cure of fetal disorders still appears a distant dream for most of the genetic disorders and termination of the fetus affected with a serious untreatable disorder or a disorder with poor outcome is the only option most of the times. Successful surgical interventions for some malformations, medical therapies for arrhythmias, fetal goiter, congenital adrenal hyperplasia and intrauterine blood transfusions for fetal anemia are some of the fetal treatments in practice, to a variable extent. Success of a great magnitude as is seen in fetal transfusions in Rh isoimmunized patients is not seen in most other fetal therapies. Postnatal treatments for genetic disorders are also limited. Hematopoietic stem cell therapy is one modality that offers complete cure for hematological disorders such as sickle cell disease, thalassemia, Fanconi anemia, dyserythropoietic anemia and immunodeficiency disorders. This modality is also successful in nonhematological disorders like osteopetrosis, lysosomal storage disorders, adrenoleukodystrophy, etc. *In utero* hematopoietic stem cell transplantation (IUHCT) is an attractive approach and a potentially curative modality for several congenital hematopoietic diseases. Over the past two decades, several attempts at IUHCT have been made to cure numerous underlying congenital diseases with limited success. It has been successful only in immunodeficiency disorders. It is thought that IUHCT has promise due to the naïve immunological status of the fetus, as a result of which immunological hurdles associated with postnatal hematopoietic stem cell therapy will not have to be tackled. This can help in avoiding cytotoxic host myeloablative conditioning. It has been long known that exposure to foreign antigens is well accepted in fetal life. The IUHCT has proven to be successful in mice[13] and other mammals including nonhuman primates.[14]

The first successful IUHCT was performed for bare lymphocyte syndrome by Touraine et al. (1989).[15] Successful transplantation of fetuses with severe combined immunodeficiency (SCID) was also achieved by several groups.[16] However, IUHCT for other hematological disorders including hemoglobinopathies was not effective. Over the years, the understanding of immune function has been improving.[17] Maternal immune system is also found to be a factor to be taken care of for the success of IUHCT. For this, maternal stem cells have been tried. The other issue is that of lack of space in the fetus for transplanted cells.[18] It is showed in mice model that by conditioning fetal mice using a monoclonal antibody against the c-kit receptor (ACK2) found on hematopoietic stem cells (HSCs), space can be made for donor stem cells.[19] It used IUHCT for creating tolerance and then successfully did nonmyeloablative stem cell transplantation postnatally from the same donor. Success of some degrees are also observed in nonhematological disorders as well.[20] Research studies in animal models are many more fold numerous than studies in humans. One hopes that the promise shown in animal models would hold true in humans as well.

Fetal therapy for alpha-thalassemia (Hemoglobin Bart's disease) needs special mention not only for the reason that it is the most common genetic disease worldwide but also because the only option to treat it is fetal therapy as the fetus develops hydrops fetalis and survival is impossible. Nearly 20 documented cases of Hb Bart's disease have been treated with *in utero* transfusions and outcomes have been generally favorable.[21] These children need lifelong blood transfusions postnatally and develop iron overload and related complications, if untreated. In addition, cognitive deficits and limb reduction defects are reported. Though Hb Bart's disease is the model disease for IUHCT, all three efforts at IUHCT till date have failed. In only one of the three fetuses, chimerism was detected at autopsy.[21]

Fetal Gene Therapy

Gene therapy has been considered the ultimate goal of research in molecular medicine. With the advent of recombinant DNA technology, gene therapy appeared to be the feasible goal. However, the journey in this direction had been arduous and the success is still limited. Germline gene therapy is not permitted for ethical reasons and the possibility of unknown adverse effects on future generations. Successful gene therapy has been possible for immunodeficiency disorders. Hematological disorders including hemophilia B and Griscelli syndrome are amongst the few monogenic disorders for which somatic gene therapy trials are going on. Though trials for gene therapy for beta-thalassemia started 2 decades ago, success in a single case has been reported recently.[22] Advent of new gene editing techniques has opened up options of foolproof corrections of genetic mutations and successes have been reported in experiments on cell lines.[23]

The option of fetal gene therapy opened up long ago.[24] The reasons to consider fetal gene therapy are similar to fetal stem cell therapy and include naïve immune system and acceptance of foreign proteins better than in postnatal life. In addition, it can provide a better outcome for disorders with prenatal onset of organ involvement. This is specific for alpha-thalassemia-Hb Bart's disease and some neurodevelopmental and neurodegenerative disorders. Fetal gene therapy has another advantage of the immature blood-brain barrier allowing access to the nervous system. Practically, fetal gene therapy may provide an option of cure for disorders such as cystic fibrosis, metachromatic leukodystrophy, hemophilia, etc. before birth. Major proof of principle for fetal gene therapy has been demonstrated in rodent and large animal systems as a method to prevent the onset of inherited genetic disease; however, safety and ethical issues still need to be addressed prior to human application.[25] Fetal application of gene therapy in mouse models of monogenic disease such as hemophilia A, hemophilia B, congenital blindness, Crigler-Najjar type 1 syndrome and Pompe disease (glycogen storage disease type II) have shown phenotypic correction of the condition.[26] In addition to the possible adverse effects due to the integration of a gene in another gene leading to cancer, fetal gene therapy poses a risk of integration of the recombinant gene in the germline. The procedure involves risk to the mother which may not be justified or acceptable. Though the option of fetal gene therapy appears feasible and attractive, many hurdles need to be negotiated and social, psychological and ethical issues addressed.

CONCLUSION

Fetal therapies have opened up new therapeutic strategies and the option of cure for many congenital serious disorders, especially with onset of organ involvement during fetal life. Fetal diagnostics have been advancing at a greater speed and have become a part of clinical practice. Progress in fetal therapy shows a hope of treatment as a second option after prenatal diagnosis. The advantage of lack of immune competence in fetuses as well as better access to the nervous system due to the immature blood-brain barrier and possibility of immune tolerance due to exposure of deficient protein during fetal life are points supporting the need and efficacy of fetal therapies. NGS can sequence the whole genome of an individual before or after birth and diagnosis of many monogenic disorders in all fetuses, even without a family history of a genetic disorder, has become possible. Targeted repair of mutated genes by genome editing tools during embryogenesis may not only offer cure for hematological and metabolic disorders but has now led us dream about normal brain development in zygotes with mutation for even serious intracranial malformations like holoprosencephaly. After decades of research in the area and marginal successes, a consensus has been reached that *in utero* transplantation is a viable strategy to treat fetuses with selective congenital disorders[27] and a society for fetal stem cell transplantation and gene therapy is being formed Fetal Transplantation and Immunology Society (FeTIS). The future of fetal therapies will depend on the safety and efficacy of these strategies.[28]

REFERENCES

1. Rechitsky S, Pakhalchuk T, San Ramos G, Goodman A, Zlatopolsky Z, Kuliev A. First systematic experience of preimplantation genetic diagnosis for single-gene disorders, and/or preimplantation human leukocyte antigen typing, combined with 24-chromosome aneuploidy testing. Fertil Steril. 2015;103(2):503-12.
2. Chow JF, Yeung WS, Lee VC, Lau EY, Ho PC, Ng EH. Experience of more than 100 preimplantation genetic diagnosis cycles for monogenetic diseases using whole genome amplification

and linkage analysis in a single centre. Hong Kong Med J. 2015;21(4):299-303.
3. Kahraman S, Beyazyurek C, Yesilipek MA, Ozturk G, Ertem M, Anak S, et al. Successful haematopoietic stem cell transplantation in 44 children from healthy siblings conceived after preimplantation HLA matching. Reprod Biomed Online. 2014;29(3):340-51.
4. Finning K, Martin P, Daniels G. The use of maternal plasma for prenatal RhD blood group genotyping. Methods Mol Biol. 2009;496:143-57.
5. Ho SS, Chong SS, Koay ES, Ponnusamy S, Chiu L, Chan YH, et al. Noninvasive prenatal exclusion of haemoglobin. Bart's using foetal DNA from maternal plasma. Prenat Diagn. 2010;30(1):65-73.
6. Phylipsen M, Yamsri S, Treffers EE, Jansen DT, Kanhai WA, Boon EM, et al. Non-invasive prenatal diagnosis of beta-thalassemia and sickle-cell disease using pyrophosphorolysis-activated polymerization and melting curve analysis. Prenat Diagn. 2012;32(6):578-87.
7. Sirichotiyakul S, Charoenkwan P, Sanguansermsri T. Prenatal diagnosis of homozygous alpha-thalassemia-1 by cell-free fetal DNA in maternal plasma. Prenat Diagn. 2012;32(1):45-9.
8. Barrett AN, McDonnell TC, Chan KC, Chitty LS. Digital PCR analysis of maternal plasma for noninvasive detection of sickle cell anemia. Clin Chem. 2012;58(6):1026-32.
9. Quezada MS, Gil MM, Francisco C, Oròsz G, Nicolaides KH. Screening for trisomies 21, 18 and 13 by cell-free DNA analysis of maternal blood at 10-11 weeks' gestation and the combined test at 11-13 weeks. Ultrasound Obstet Gynecol. 2015;45(1):36-41.
10. Rieneck K, Clausen FB, Dziegiel MH. Next-Generation Sequencing for Antenatal Prediction of KEL1 Blood Group Status. Methods Mol Biol. 2015;1310:115-21.
11. Xiong L, Barrett AN, Hua R, Tan TZ, Ho SS, Chan JK, et al. Non-invasive prenatal diagnostic testing for β-thalassaemia using cell-free fetal DNA and next generation sequencing. Prenat Diagn. 2015;35(3):258-65.
12. Chitty LS, Mason S, Barrett AN, McKay F, Lench N, Daley R, et al. Non-invasive prenatal diagnosis of achondroplasia and thanatophoric dysplasia: next-generation sequencing allows for a safer, more accurate, and comprehensive approach. Prenat Diagn. 2015;35(7):656-62.
13. Carrier E, Lee TH, Busch MP, Cowan MJ. Induction of tolerance in nondefective mice after *in utero* transplantation of major histocompatibility complex-mismatched fetal hematopoietic stem cells. Blood. 1995;86(12):4681-90.
14. Tarantal AF, Goldstein O, Barley F, Cowan MJ. Transplantation of human peripheral blood stem cells into fetal rhesus monkeys (Macaca mulatta). Transplantation. 2000;69(9):1818-23.
15. Touraine JL, Raudrant D, Royo C, Rebaud A, Roncarolo MG, Souillet G, et al. *In utero* transplantation of stem cells in bare lymphocyte syndrome. Lancet. 1989;1(8651):1382.
16. Wengler GS, Lanfranchi A, Frusca T, Verardi R, Neva A, Brugnoni D, et al. *In utero* transplantation of parental CD34 haematopoietic progenitor cells in a patient with X-linked severe combined immunodeficiency (SCIDXI). Lancet. 1996;348(9040):1484-7.
17. Loewendorf AI, Csete M, Flake A. Immunological considerations in *in utero* hematopoietic stem cell transplantation (IUHCT). Front Pharmacol. 2015;5:282.
18. Derderian SC, Moradi PW, MacKenzie TC. Placental drug delivery for treatment of congenital hematopoietic disorders. J Pediatr Surg. 2015;50(9):1517-20.
19. Peranteau WH, Hayashi S, Abdulmalik O, Chen Q, Merchant A, Asakura T, et al. Correction of murine hemoglobinopathies by prenatal tolerance induction and postnatal nonmyeloablative allogeneic BM transplants. Blood. 2015;126(10):1245-54.
20. Ihara N, Akihiro U, Onami N, Tsumura H, Inoue E, Hayashi S, et al. Partial rescue of mucopolysaccharidosis type VII mice with a lifelong engraftment of allogeneic stem cells *in utero*. Congenit Anom (Kyoto). 2015;55(1):55-64.
21. Derderian SC, Jeanty C, Walters MC, Vichinsky E, MacKenzie TC. *In utero* hematopoietic cell transplantation for hemoglobinopathies. Front Pharmacol. 2015;5:278.
22. Cavazzana-Calvo M, Payen E, Negre O, Wang G, Hehir K, Fusil F, et al. Transfusion independence and HMGA2 activation after gene therapy of human β-thalassaemia. Nature. 2010;467(7313):318-22.
23. Xie F, Ye L, Chang JC, Beyer AI, Wang J, Muench MO, et al. Seamless gene correction of β-thalassemia mutations in patient-specific iPSCs using CRISPR/Cas9 and piggy. Bac Genome Res. 2014;24(9):1526-33.
24. Couzin J. RAC confronts *in utero* gene therapy proposals. Science. 1998;282(5386):27.
25. Themis M, Schneider H, Kiserud T, Cook T, Adebakin S, Jezzard S, et al. Successful expression of beta-galactosidase and factor IX transgenes in fetal and neonatal sheep after ultrasound-guided percutaneous adenovirus vector administration into the umbilical vein. Gene Ther. 1999;6(7):1239-48.
26. David AL, Peebles D. Gene therapy for the fetus: is there a future? Best Pract Res Clin Obstet Gynaecol. 2008;22(1):203-18.
27. MacKenzie TC, David AL, Flake AW, Almeida-Porada G. Consensus statement from the first international conference for *in utero* stem cell transplantation and gene therapy. Front Pharmacol. 2015;6:15.
28. Mehta V, Abi-Nader KN, Carr D, Wallace J, Coutelle C, Waddington SN, et al. Monitoring for potential adverse effects of prenatal gene therapy: use of large animal models with relevance to human application. Methods Mol Biol. 2012;891:291-328.

SECTION 2

RBC Disorders and Anemia in Newborn

Section Editors

MR Lokeshwar, Ratna Sharma

CHAPTER

9

Developmental Erythropoiesis

Nimish Kulkarni, Ratna Sharma

INTRODUCTION

The 19th century was a witness to the discovery that the newborns hemoglobin is alkali-resistant, whereas adult hemoglobin (HbA) is alkali-sensitive. This triggered the curiosity of various researchers to figure out the differences in hemoglobin at various stages of life. In 1930, the first physical evidence of the difference between and adult and fetal hemoglobin (HbF) was obtained. By the beginning of the 20th century, the differences in oxygen affinity between embryonic and adult blood were discovered.[1]

In this chapter, we will discuss the various stages in the development of erythropoiesis and the factors that influence these changes.

BASICS OF ERYTHROPOIESIS

Erythropoiesis is a complex multistep process. The circulating enucleated red blood cells are the end result of differentiation process starting with the early erythroid progenitors. The cell differentiation starts from the pluripotent hematopoietic stem cells (HSCs) and early multipotent progenitors (MPPs), which generate committed erythroid precursors (erythroblasts). These further differentiate into mature erythrocytes red blood cells (RBCs).

Cell-to-cell interactions and soluble macromolecules, which act as extrinsic factors stimulate the HSCs in the bone marrow and initiate signaling pathways to prime the hematopoietic progenitors. These cells undergo several transition steps of differentiation and form the common myeloid progenitor (CMP) and the common lymphoid progenitor (CLP). T- and B-lymphocytes, natural killer (NK) cells, and mostly dendritic cells (DCs) are generated from CLP. CMP differentiates into megakaryocytic/erythroid progenitors (MEPs) and granulocyte-myeloid progenitors (GMPs). Growth factors act upon the MEP cells to differentiate them into colony forming unit-erythroid (CFU-E) and erythropoietin (EPO) responsive erythroid burst forming unit-erythroid (BFU-E). The CFU-Es are further differentiated into orthochromatic normoblasts. These normoblasts undergo enucleation to form reticulocytes, which further transform into mature RBCs[2] **(Fig. 9.1)**.

GLOBIN LOCI

The human β-globin locus has been located on chromosome 11. A corresponding set of elements that work as strong enhancers, termed as the "β locus control region" (βLCR), located upstream (5′) of the β locus structural genes has been identified.[3-8] The ε-globin gene is active in early fetal life. The γ-globin genes (Gγ and Aγ) are similar to the β-genes and are expressed in most of fetal life. As the fetus develops, δ and β-globin genes are activated late in fetal life. After birth and in the adult life, the β-globin gene is the most highly expressed gene in the erythroid cells.

The other major globin locus is the α-globin locus on chromosome 16. Unlike the β-globin gene, the α-globin gene is expressed early in fetal life and persists throughout fetal and adult life.[3,9]

The mRNA precursors are generated in the nucleus by human globin gene transcription, which subsequently form mature globin mRNAs in the cytoplasm.[10,11] This translational machinery of the cell along with enzymes and ribosomes result in the production of globins, which further combine with heme to form the normal human hemoglobins.[3]

As the hematopoietic process progresses erythroid cell mature and gradually lose their potential for cell proliferation finally form the mature enucleated cells. Mature RBCs are biconcave disks without mitochondria and other organelles.[2]

EMBRYONIC DEVELOPMENT OF ERYTHROPOIESIS

Hematopoiesis originates in the yolk sac/blood islands, then shifts to the aorta-gonad mesonephros region, then to the chorioallantoic placenta, then the fetal liver and eventually

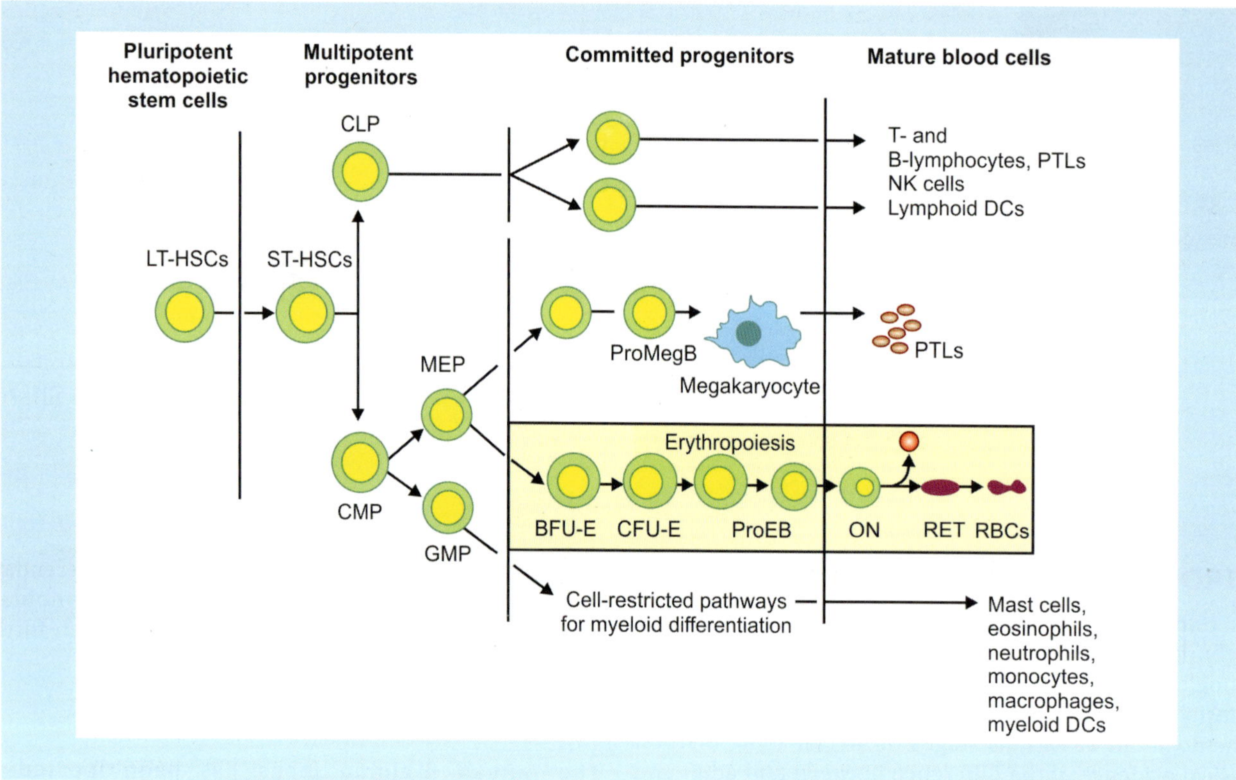

Figure 9.1 Maturation of the cell lines originating from the hematopoietic stem cells (HSCs)[2]
Abbreviations: CMP, common myeloid progenitor; GMP, granulocyte-myeloid progenitor; MEP, megakaryocytic/erythroid progenitor; CLP, common lymphoid progenitor; DC, dendritic cell; PTLs, platelets; BFU-E, burst forming unit-erythroid; CFU-E, colony forming unit-erythroid; LT, long-term; ST, short-term.

the bone marrow during adult life. The hemogenic blasts and the hemogenic endothelium of embryonic vasculature are the direct precursors of the hematopoietic cells in early embryonic life.

Hematopoiesis occurs in two stages during development:

Primitive Hematopoiesis or Embryonic Hematopoiesis

It occurs in blood islands in yolk sac and generate enucleated RBCs that express embryonic hemoglobins (Gower-1, Gower-2 and Portland hemoglobin).[2]

Definitive Hematopoiesis

It occurs in fetal liver and in the fetal bone marrow after the third trimester and gives rise to be enucleated RBCs that express HbF.[2,4]

The yolk sac, which is a transient extraembryonic tissue, is the site of origin of hematopoiesis. The early erythroid lineage production starts here. These erythroid cells are nucleated and short-lived. The epiblast cells that ingress through the primitive streak give rise to the mesodermal cells, which in turn form the erythroid cells.[12,13] These mesodermal cells migrate posteriorly and come in close contact with endoderm cells after entering the yolk sac. Initiation of erythropoiesis is dependent on this interaction between the two cell layers.[5,14] What is noteworthy here is that the mesodermal cells that migrate to the yolk sac from the blood islands not only have erythroid lineage cells but also have endothelial cells. This common ontogeny suggests a common mesodermal precursor. That precursor is the hemangioblast, which is said to have bilineage potential.[5,15]

The genetic basis for these two lineages show an overlap of characteristics, further supporting the common origin. For instance, the expression of Flk-1 kinase insert domain receptor (KDR), stem cell leukemia/T-cell acute lymphoblastic leukemia-1 (SCL/Tal-1), and CD34 genes in genetic programs for both and the lack of both lineages in embryos deficient for some of these genes.[16-18] *In vivo*, however, the hemangioblasts are not located in the yolk sac. They are found to be in the posterior primitive streak.[19] They then migrate to the yolk sac, and it is during this migration, they get committed to the endothelial and hematopoietic lineage progenitor cells. Each blood island is formed by several such cells.[20]

By 16–20 days of gestation, the yolk sac islands are easily detectable.[21]

Definitive fetal hematopoiesis eventually shifts to the bone marrow from the fetal liver and enucleated RBCs produce HbA.[22,23] Erythropoiesis in bone marrow occurs in erythroblastic islands, which are made up of a central macrophage and surrounding erythroblasts. The nuclei derived from enucleated orthochromatic normoblasts undergo phagocytosis by the central macrophage. The macrophage also provides the iron needed for erythropoiesis. Cell adhesive macromolecules including integrins support the communication between the central macrophage and the erythroblasts and also the interactions among the erythroblasts. The mechanism of stress hematopoiesis is thought to be due to increase in the number of the erythroblasts surrounding the central macrophage.[2]

During the third trimester, the fetus grows rapidly and the production of red cells is approximately 3–5 times that of adult steady state levels.[4]

Regulation of the Erythroblastic Islands

Erythropoiesis is regulated by the positive and negative feedback regulatory mechanisms operating within the erythroblastic islands. Soluble factors, such as stem cell factor (SCF), EPO, the ligand for the SCF receptor (c-kit), vascular endothelial growth factor (VEGF), etc. and cell-to-cell interactions are responsible for this regulation. SCF, EPO, and VEGF have a positive feedback mechanisms whereas interleukin-6 (IL-6), transforming growth factor-beta (TGF-β), tumor necrosis factor-alpha (TNF-α), etc. appear to have a negative inhibitory effect on erythropoiesis and promote cell death. IL-6 predominantly reduces iron release from the central macrophage thus reduces erythropoiesis. Finally, extracellular matrix components (EMCs), such as fibronectin and laminin, influence the terminal differentiation and migration of erythroid cells via fibronectin receptors, integrins and some other molecules.[2,24]

Beyond the Fetal Life

Birth and thereafter, origin of erythropoiesis shifts to a different line of cells. The HSCs become the founder cells for erythropoiesis after birth. HSCs anchor in the bone marrow and thereafter replenish the circulating cells all throughout adult life. HSCs undergo a distinct and long process of proliferation and differentiation to form the adult red cells along with cells of other lineages like lymphocytes, macrophages, granulocytes and megakaryocytes.

These adult erythrocytes are smaller than the primitive erythrocytes of the fetal life.[5]

Hemoglobin Switch

Hemoglobin tetramers composed of α-globin and β-globin ($\alpha_2\ \beta_2$, HbA_1) account for 97% of all hemoglobin in adult erythrocytes. HbF ($\alpha_2\gamma_2$) and HbA2 ($\alpha_2\delta_2$) account, respectively, for 1% and 2% of total hemoglobin in most adults. High HbF is restricted to a few cells, termed F cells, in normal adults.[5,25] Clonal analysis has shown that F cells are derived from the same progenitor cells as the adult red blood cells containing adult globin, ruling out the possibility that fetal and adult stem cell lineages coexist.[5,26]

Two globin gene switches occur during the development:

- *The embryonic to fetal globin switch*: Coincides with the transition from embryonic hematopoiesis (yolk sac) to definitive hematopoiesis (fetal liver).
- *The fetal to adult globin switch*: Occurs in the perinatal period.

The switches from ε to γ and from γ- to β-globin gene expression are controlled primarily at the transcriptional level. The transcriptional mechanism predominantly controls the ζ to α switch; however, the post-transcriptional mechanisms also play some role.[1]

Transcriptional Regulation of Erythropoiesis

Various transcription factors are involved in forming the hematopoietic cell lineages. For instance, TAL1, a basic helix–loop–helix transcription factor, and Lim domain only 2 (LMO2), a LIM-domain transcription factor, are of utmost importance for the onset of hematopoiesis. Null embryos in regard to these show complete absence of primitive and definitive hematopoiesis.[5,27-29]

GATA-1 binds to the promoters of many erythroid cell-specific genes and to β-LCR sequences, and is necessary for the normal erythroid cell differentiation.[3]

GATA-2 transcription factor is essential for the early stages of hematopoiesis. If *GATA-2* gene is deleted, both primitive and definitive hematopoieses get defected. It is also important for the proliferation of the early precursors rather than just their differentiation.[5,30,31]

Runt-related transcription factor 1 (RUNX1) is also very important for the early stages of definitive hematopoiesis. In RUNX1- null embryos, yolk sac hematopoiesis is normal but fetal liver hematopoiesis is absent.[5,32]

The HSCs are MPP cells and once these arise and proliferate, the process of lineage restriction begins. Restriction to either the myeloid or the lymphoid lineage is the first step. Some transcription factors are preferentially expressed in cells destined to one of these fates. For instance, PU.1 from the E26 transformation-specific (ETS) family of transcription factors is known to be involved in lineage restriction at this stage. The effect of PU.1 on lineage commitment is dependent on its expression level. A high level leads to commitment to the myeloid lineage, whereas lower levels of expression lead to commitment to the lymphoid lineage.[33-35] Inactivation of these factors thus affects erythropoiesis.

One of the important transcription factors is KLF1. It is required for terminal erythroid differentiation and is one of the best-studied examples of an erythroid transcriptional regulator. Expression of the KLF1 is largely restricted to the erythroid cell lineage. KLF1 specifically binds the sequence 50—CCACACCCT-30. KLF1 was formerly known as erythroid Krüppel-like factor (EKLF).[5,36]

The absence of KLF1 does not influence the embryonic globin gene expression, even though KLF1 normally binds these genes *in vivo*.[37] When the embryos switch to definitive erythropoiesis in the fetal liver, KLF1-null mutants rapidly develop anemia because of a deficit in β-globin expression. Remarkably, the number of CFU-E in the KLF1-null fetal livers is similar to those found in wild-type fetal livers, showing that KLF1 deficiency causes a very late erythroid defect.[38,39] Furthermore, fetal liver-derived erythroid cells of KLF12/2 fetuses have an abnormal morphology, and most of the cells remain nucleated, thus indicating that the adult β-globin genes are not the only target genes of KLF1. The analyses of genome-wide expression of KLF12/2 erythroid cells depicted that KLF1 activates many other genes specific to the erythroid lineage, including genes encoding proteins, like band 4.9/dematin, which are associated with the erythroid cell membrane. The function and stability of the erythrocytes depend on these proteins. Also, KLF1 plays an important role in regulating the cell cycle to facilitate proliferation arrest required for terminal differentiation.[40] Thus, KLF1 is crucial for activation of essential erythroid genes, which when up-regulated, help in terminal erythroid differentiation.

Importance of Hemoglobin Switch

The observation that HbF reduces the severity of sickle cell disease was appreciated in the late 1940s and the 1950s. Thus, the importance of the hemoglobin switch was understood long before the specific research had begun. Patients with severe β-thalassemia have alkaline-resistant, i.e. HbF, were first discovered by Italian hematologists in 1943. Thereafter, various genetic and biochemical studies have been conducted, which have concluded that the reason patients with severe β-chain deficiency remain alive is production of HbF. It was thus clear that substantial production of HbF can be very helpful to ameliorate symptoms of β-thalassemia and sickle cell disease. The research and efforts taken to understand the hemoglobin switch in the last 3 decades have been based on the understanding of this benefit in these patients.

In the early 1970s, immunochemical staining was introduced to visualize red cells containing HbF. It was then found that the low amounts of HbF present in all adult individuals were restricted to a few red cells called F cells.[41,42] Various researchers since then have tried to study their significance and their relationship to hemoglobin switching.

It was hypothesized that fetal to HbA switching in humans is because of two successive stem cell lineages that have discrete globin gene expression.[43] A fetal stem cell lineage committed to fetal globin formation is replaced around the perinatal period by an adult stem cell lineage committed to adult globin formation was the theory. According to this theory, F cells in adults were from the remnants of the fetal lineage that persisted in the adult bone marrow. This hypothesis was influenced by the presence of two successive cell lineages found in frogs and chicken.[44]

In the early 1970s, clonal erythroid cultures were introduced to study hematopoiesis.[45] Colonies grown from a single erythroid progenitor could be analyzed for their hemoglobin phenotype using fluorescent anti-γ and anti-β antibodies within each erythroid BFU-E colony. According the prior clonal model hypothesis, the BFU-E colonies should have been segregating into two categories, i.e. one containing HbF (derived from the fetal stem cell lineage) and the other containing HbA (derived from the adult stem cell lineage). However, it was found that majority of the colonies contained both types of cells,[46] thus giving evidence that fetal and adult hemoglobins are produced by cells of the same lineage. Such studies on cultures suggested that hemoglobin switching does not happen due to a change in stem cell populations representing fixed globin gene transcription programs. Instead, a change in transcription programs occurs in the cells of the same stem cell lineage.[46]

This was further supported by the findings in patients with clonal hematopoietic cell disorders, like polycythemia vera, chronic myeloid leukemia (CML), etc. where the cells should have belonged to either of the clones depending on the clone carrying the mutation, i.e. either 100% F cells or 100% non-F cells. Instead, both fetal and adult globin producing cells were found.[47,48]

ERYTHROID CELL MATURATION

Erythroid cells are derived from HSCs, but the differentiation path, they follow is still a matter of debate.[49] Immature progenitors are capable of giving rise to multilineage colonies, but it still remains unclear whether a cells fate is fixed, i.e. at each stage a cell has only limited options of differentiation or whether the potential of the cell to differentiate into different forms is variable. Weissman and group put forth the classical model where a decision is made between two fates at each step of differentiation, and thus gradually diminishing lineage potential. Adolfsson et al.[50] proposed an alternative scheme recently. They identified a highly-proliferative lymphoid primed multipotent progenitor (LMPP). This progenitor has a granulocyte/monocyte potential but is completely unable to adopt the erythroid or megakaryocytic lineage fates (dotted arrows, **Fig. 9.2**). Cell surface markers help purify the cell populations corresponding to the progenitors by using flow-cytometry. The mature differentiated cells emerging in colony assays in response to growth factors determine the lineage output. Immature erythroid-restricted progenitors are identified as the BFU-E, so-called because its earliest progeny are motile, giving rise to a multisubunit colony (or burst).

As the age progresses, there may be a change occurring in the globin gene transcription programs from a program allowing γ-globin expression to one that supports only β-globin expression. The erythroid cells mature normally and produce erythroblasts that synthesize only HbA in a normal adult. Few progenitor cells become terminal prematurely before any change in programs takes place. On stimulation,

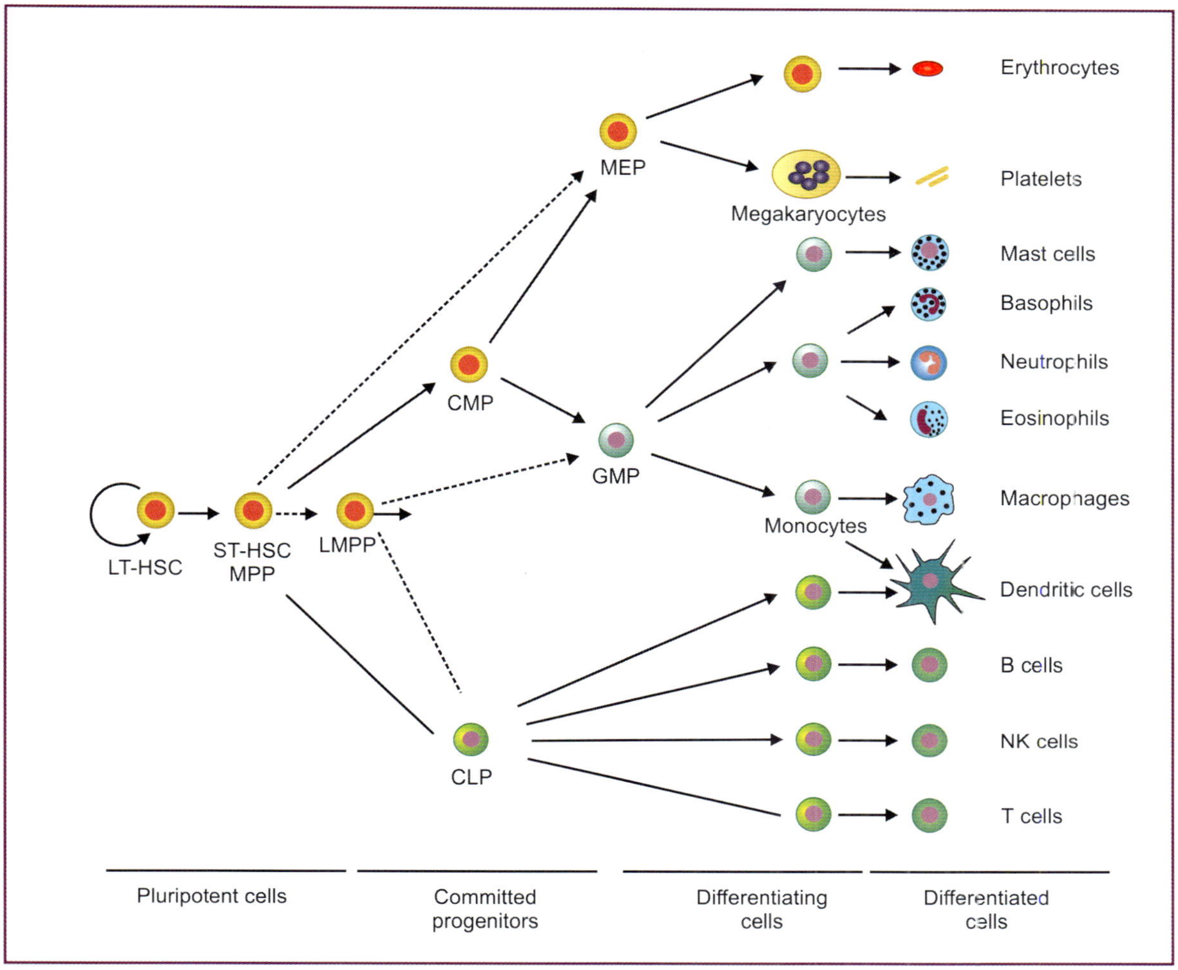

Figure 9.2 Proposed models for the hematopoietic hierarchy. In the model proposed by the Weissman group[51-53] (solid arrows), multipotential progenitors (MPPs) or short-term HSCs (ST-HSCs) give rise to either a common lymphocyte progenitor (CLP) or a common myeloid progenitor (CMP), which, in turn gives rise to either a granulocyte-macrophage progenitor (GMP) equivalent to CFU-GM or a megakaryocyte-erythroid progenitor (MEP). The alternate model suggested by the Jacobson group[50] (dotted arrows) involves the generation of MEPs directly from the MPPs/STHSCs, whereas a lymphoid-primed multipotential progenitor (LMPP) has the potential to generate both CLPs and GMPs

Abbreviations: LT-HSC, long-term hematopoietic stem cell; NK cell, natural killer cell

these cells produce HbF. Based on this hypothesis, the production of HbF during stress erythropoiesis could thus be explained.[54-57] The rapid erythroid regeneration during stress stimulates the terminal cells also, as there is acceleration of downstream differentiation and thus inducing the production from terminal cells that still possess the primitive fetal globin program.[57]

Several laboratories were attempting to identify the proteins involved in regulation of globin gene expression by around 1980. The study of chromatin finally proved to be useful. In the early 1980s, Groudine et al.[58] observed that the switch from fetal to adult globin gene expression is accompanied by a switch in the DNAse I hypersensitive sites (HSs) located in the γ- and β-promoters. These observations were a result of applying DNAse I sensitivity assays to assess the status of the chromatin of the human β-globin locus during development. Subsequently, Tuan et al.[59] and Groudine's group[60] found that upstream of the ε-globin gene, a series of DNAse I HSs are located. Two experiments published in 1987 showed that this upstream region has regulatory relevance to the β-locus. It was observed that the activation of the genes of the locus was preceded by formation of the upstream DNAse I hypersensitive region. It was proposed that the upstream region containing these HSs is responsible for activation of the locus. Therefore, this region was named locus activation region. Grosveld et al. conducted experiments on transgenic mice to identify and describe the same loci.[60,61] They attributed this effect to the upstream region that they called dominant control region. Both terminologies were used in the past, until the term LCR was adapted in 1990 at the 7th conference on hemoglobin switching.

Now it is clear that the hemoglobin switch occurs predominantly at the transcriptional level, one needs to understand how the β-gene expression takes over the γ expression. Gene competition and autonomous gene silencing are the two mechanisms responsible for turning off the γ-genes during development.

Gene Competition

Behringer et al. and Enver et al. provided proof of the competitive mechanism of γ- to β-globin gene switching by their experiments on transgenic mice.[62,63] When the LCR was linked either to the γ-gene alone or to the β-globin gene alone, these genes failed to display proper developmental regulation. The β-gene was active at all stages of development. Even in the embryonic cells, β-gene expression was as abundant as in adult cells. The γ-gene were also expressed in the adult life apart from being predominant in the fetal life. However, in the adult life, they were expressed at a much lower level. But, when these genes were linked to the LCR sequence, the developmental regulation was as *in vivo*. That is, β-gene expression was restricted to the adult erythropoiesis whereas the γ-gene expression was restricted only to the fetal erythropoiesis. Thus, originated the conclusion that the γ- and β-genes compete for interaction with the LCR.[63] There is a preferential interaction between the LCR and the γ-genes during the fetal life and the β-globin genes are turned off competitively. Whereas, the LCR interacts preferentially with the β-gene during the adult stage of development, thus silencing γ-globin genes expression. Experimental data points toward the observation that competition by the upstream ε and γ-genes silences the β-gene in embryonic erythropoiesis. And the γ-gene is turned off in adult erythropoiesis predominantly due to autonomous silencing but also to some extent due to competition by the β-gene **(Fig. 9.3)**.

AUTONOMOUS SILENCING

The concept of autonomous silencing states that all the elements responsible for turning off gene expression are contained within the same gene or in the adjacent sequences.[64] This was supported by the experiments on transgenic mice carrying the embryonic human ε-gene. A failure to express the gene at any stage of development was noted. However, when the ε-gene was linked to the LCR, the ε-expression was abundant. Thus, indicating that transcription of this gene is dependent on the presence of the LCR. However, this expression was totally restricted to yolk sac erythropoiesis. Many experiments have attempted to describe the ε gene promoting elements that contain these

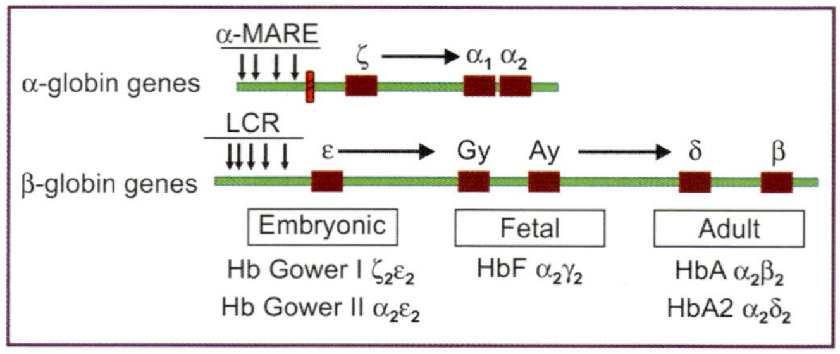

Figure 9.3 Structure and organization of human α- and β-globin gene family loci. The black boxes depict the corresponding globin genes, whereas the horizontal arrows above represent a switching event leading to expression of the next downstream gene in the locus. The vertical arrows denote the position of upstream DNAse I hypersensitive sites identified as the locus control region (LCR) in β-globin and as the α-major regulatory element (MARE) in α-globin gene family. The composition of embryonic, fetal, and adult hemoglobins produced at each developmental stage during erythropoiesis is also indicated[2]

silencing sequences. Sequences participating in the silencing process were identified in both the proximal and the distal ε gene promoter.[65,66] Also, mutation of GATA-1, YY1, or SP1 sites in the upstream ε-promoter abolish ε-gene silencing.[67] Hence, the possibility that globin gene silencing is the combined effect of several transcription factors participating in the formation of a silencing complex. The autonomous silencing of the ε-globin gene is a complex phenomenon that involves sequences in the proximal and distal promoter and participation of several DNA binding proteins. It is now believed that the ε gene expression is turned off by the silencing sequence by inhibiting the interaction between the ε gene and the LCR.[1,65,67,68]

PYR Complex: A Possible Switch Complex

Some studies have also found a chromatin remodeling complex called PYR complex. This complex is an intergenic complex on the γ-δ-globin sequence found only in adult hematopoietic cells. Thus, suggesting their additional role in the hemoglobin switch.[69] PYR complex binds to a 250-bp polypyrimidine (PYR)-rich DNA sequence 1 kb upstream of the human δ-globin gene.[69] Experiments on mice transgenic for human β-globin locus-containing cosmid have led to the observation that deletion of 511 bp of DNA including the PYR binding site upstream of the human δ-globin gene delays human γ to β-switching.[63,70]

Data combined from various studies suggest that PYR complex has a role in normal human γ- to β-switching. Inhibition of the PYR complex action may be an additional therapeutic approach to reactivation of γ-globin in adult erythroid cells. For instance, Ikaros activity inhibition by siRNA.[70,71]

Butyrate compounds, known inhibitors of histone deacetylases (HDAC) action,[72,73] increase HbF in patients with SS disease and β-thalassemia.[74,75] HDAC inhibitors are said to increase HbF production in humans by preventing the HDACs in the PYR complex from repressing γ-globin gene expression.

It was initially unclear whether competition[63] or autonomous silencing[68] account for turning off the γ globin gene. Current consideration is that both these mechanisms are involved in a variable degree. Autonomous silencing is the principal mechanism that turns off the γ-gene but evidence from human mutants suggests that competition by the β-gene also contributes.

SEQUENCE OF ACTIVATION OF GLOBIN GENES

The order of position of the genes determines the order of their activation. The sequential activation of ε, $^{G}\gamma$, $^{A}\gamma$, δ, and β-globin genes during development reflects the order of their arrangement in the chromosome. The gene located next to the LCR is expressed first during development, and the genes beyond that are expressed thereafter. Thus, proximity to the LCR is important as it increases the probability of interaction with that dominant regulatory element.[1]

FUTURE POSSIBILITIES

Further studies of developmental erythropoiesis will help us understand better the mechanisms of hemoglobin switching and will have a place for practical implementation in cases that increase survival with induction of HbF.

REFERENCES

1. Stamatoyannopoulos G. Control of globin gene expression during development and erythroid differentiation. Exp Hematol. 2005;33(3):259-71.
2. Tsiftsoglou AS, Vizirianakis IS, Strouboulis J. Erythropoiesis: model systems, molecular regulators, and developmental programs. IUBMB Life. 2009;61(8):800-30.
3. Bank A. Regulation of human fetal hemoglobin: new players, new complexities. Blood. 2006;107(2):435-43.
4. Palis J, Segel GB. Developmental biology of erythropoiesis. Blood Rev. 1998;12(2):106-14.
5. Dzierzak E, Philipsen S. Erythropoiesis: development and differentiation. Cold Spring Harb Perspect Med. 2013;3(4):a011601.
6. Tuan D, Solomon W, Li O, London IM. The "beta-like-globin" gene domain in human erythroid cells. Proc Natl Acad Sci USA. 1985;82(19):6384-8.
7. Grosveld F, van Assendelft GB, Greaves DR, Kollias G. Position-independent, high-level expression of the human beta-globin gene in transgenic mice. Cell. 1987;51(6):975-85.
8. Tuan DY, Solomon WB, London IM, Lee DP. An erythroid-specific, developmental-stage-independent enhancer far upstream of the human "beta-like globin" genes. Proc Natl Acad Sci USA. 1989;86(8):2554-8.
9. Weatherall DJ, Clegg JB. The Thalassemia Syndromes, 4th edition. Oxford, United Kingdom: Blackwell Science; 2001.
10. Bank A, Mears JG, Ramirez F. Disorders of human hemoglobin. Science. 1980;207(4430):486-93.
11. Stamatoyannopoulos G, Grosveld F. Hemoglobin switching. In: Stamatoyannopoulos G, Majerus PW, Perlmutter RM, Varmus H (Eds). The Molecular Basis of Blood Disease, 3rd edition. Philadelphia, PA, USA: WB Saunders; 2001: pp. 135-83.
12. Lawson KA, Meneses JJ, Pedersen RA. Clonal analysis of epiblast fate during germ layer formation in the mouse embryo. Development. 1991;113(3):891-911.
13. Kinder SJ, Tsang TE, Quinlan GA, Hadjantonakis AK, Nagy A, Tam PP. The orderly allocation of mesodermal cells to the extraembryonic structures and the anteroposterior axis during gastrulation of the mouse embryo. Development. 1999;126(21):4691-701.
14. Belaoussoff M, Farrington SM, Baron MH. Hematopoietic induction and respecification of A-P identity by visceral endoderm signaling in the mouse embryo. Development. 1998;125(24):5009-18.
15. Sabin FR. Studies on the origin of blood vessels and of red blood corpuscles as seen in the living blastoderm of chicks during the second day of incubation. Contrib Embryol Carnegie Inst Publ Wash. 1920;36:213-59.
16. Tavian M, Hallais MF, Péault B. Emergence of intraembryonic hematopoietic precursors in the pre-liver human embryo. Development. 1999;126(4):793-803.
17. Park C, Ma YD, Choi K. Evidence for the hemangioblast. Exp Hematol. 2005;33(9):965-70.
18. Shalaby F, Rossant J, Yamaguchi TP, Gertsenstein M, Wu XF, Breitman ML, et al. Failure of blood-island formation and vasculogenesis in Flk-1-deficient mice. Nature. 1995;376(6535): 62-6.
19. Huber TL, Kouskoff V, Fehling HJ, Palis J, Keller G. Haemangioblast commitment is initiated in the primitive streak of the mouse embryo. Nature. 2004; 432(7017):625-30.
20. Ueno H, Weissman IL. Clonal analysis of mouse development reveals a polyclonal origin for yolk sac blood islands. Dev Cell. 2006;11(4):519-33.
21. Tavian M, Péault B. Embryonic development of the human hematopoietic system. Int J Dev Biol. 2005;49(2-3):243-50.
22. Orkin SH, Zon LI. Hematopoiesis: an evolving paradigm for stem cell biology. Cell. 2008;132(4):631-64.
23. Palis J. Ontogeny of erythropoiesis. Curr Opin Hematol. 2008;15(3):155-61.
24. Eshghi S, Vogelezang MG, Hynes RO, Griffith LG, Lodish HF. Alpha-4-beta-1 integrin and erythropoietin mediate temporally distinct steps in erythropoiesis: integrins in red cell development. J Cell Biol. 2007;177(5):871-80.
25. Boyer SH, Belding TK, Margolet L, Noyes AN. Fetal hemoglobin restriction to a few erythrocytes (F cells) in normal human adults. Science. 1975;188(4186):361-3.
26. Papayannopoulou T, Brice M, Stamatoyannopoulos G. Hemoglobin F synthesis *in vitro*: evidence for control at the level of primitive erythroid stem cells. Proc Natl Acad Sci U S A. 1977;74(7):2923-7.
27. Robb L, Lyons I, Li R, Hartley L, Köntgen F, Harvey RP, et al. Absence of yolk sac hematopoiesis from mice with a targeted disruption of the scl gene. Proc Natl Acad Sci USA. 1995;92(15):7075-9.
28. Shivdasani RA, Mayer EL, Orkin SH. Absence of blood formation in mice lacking the T-cell leukaemia oncoprotein tal-1/SCL. Nature. 1995;373(6513):432-4.

29. Porcher C, Swat W, Rockwell K, Fujiwara Y, Alt FW, Orkin SH. The T cell leukemia oncoprotein SCL/tal-1 is essential for development of all hematopoietic lineages. Cell. 1996;86(1):47-57.
30. Tsai FY, Orkin SH. Transcription factor GATA-2 is required for proliferation/survival of early hematopoietic cells and mast cell formation, but not for erythroid and myeloid terminal differentiation. Blood. 1997;89(10):3636-43.
31. Tsai FY, Keller G, Kuo FC, Weiss M, Chen J, Rosenblatt M, et al. An early haematopoietic defect in mice lacking the transcription factor GATA-2. Nature. 1994;371(6494):221-6.
32. Okuda T, van Deursen J, Hiebert SW, Grosveld G, Downing JR. AML1, the target of multiple chromosomal translocations in human leukemia, is essential for normal fetal liver hematopoiesis. Cell. 1996;84(2):321-30.
33. Nerlov C, Graf T. PU.1 induces myeloid lineage commitment in multipotent hematopoietic progenitors. Genes Dev. 1998;12(15):2403-12.
34. Scott EW, Simon MC, Anastasi J, Singh H. Requirement of transcription factor PU.1 in the development of multiple hematopoietic lineages. Science. 1994;265(5178):1573-7.
35. Huang G, Zhang P, Hirai H, Elf S, Yan X, Chen Z, et al. PU.1 is a major downstream target of AML1 (RUNX1) in adult mouse hematopoiesis. Nat Genet. 2008;40(1):51-60.
36. Miller IJ, Bieker JJ. A novel, erythroid cell-specific murine transcription factor that binds to the CACCC element and is related to the Krüppel family of nuclear proteins. Mol Cell Biol. 1993;13(5):2776-86.
37. Zhou D, Pawlik KM, Ren J, Sun CW, Townes TM. Differential binding of erythroid Krupple-like factor to embryonic/fetal globin gene promoters during development. J Biol Chem. 2006;281(23):16052-7.
38. Nuez B, Michalovich D, Bygrave A, Ploemacher R, Grosveld F. Defective haematopoiesis in fetal liver resulting from inactivation of the EKLF gene. Nature. 1995;375(6529):316-18.
39. Perkins AC, Sharpe AH, Orkin SH. Lethal beta-thalassaemia in mice lacking the erythroid CACCC-transcription factor EKLF. Nature. 1995;375(6529):318-22.
40. Tallack MR, Keys JR, Perkins AC. Erythroid Kruppel-like factor regulates the G1 cyclin dependent kinase inhibitor p18INK4c. J Mol Biol. 2007;369(2):313-21.
41. Boyer SH, Belding TK, Margolet L, Noyes AN. Fetal hemoglobin restriction to a few erythrocytes (F cells) in normal human adults. Science. 1975;188(4186):361-3.
42. Wood WG, Stamatoyannopoulos G, Lim G, Nute PE. F-cells in the adult: normal values and levels in individuals with hereditary and acquired elevations of Hb F. Blood. 1975;46(5):671-82.
43. Weatherall DJ, Clegg JB, Wood WG. A model for the persistence or reactivation of fetal haemoglobin production. Lancet. 1976;2(7987):660-3.
44. Ingram VM. Embryonic red cell formation. Nature. 1972;235(5337):338-9.
45. Papayannopoulou TH, Brice M, Stamatoyannopoulos G. Stimulation of fetal hemoglobin synthesis in bone marrow cultures from adult individuals. Proc Natl Acad Sci USA. 1976;73(6):2033-37.
46. Papayannopoulou T, Brice M, Stamatoyannopoulos G. Hemoglobin F synthesis in vitro: evidence for control at the level of primitive erythroid stem cells. Proc Natl Acad Sci USA. 1977;74(7):2923-7.
47. Papayannopoulou T, Bunn HF, Stamatoyannopoulos G. Cellular distribution of hemoglobin F in a clonal hemopoietic stem-cell disorder. N Engl J Med. 1978;298(2):72-5.
48. Hoffman R, Papayannopoulou T, Landaw S, Wasserman LR, DeMarsh QB, Chen P, et al. Fetal hemoglobin in polycythemia vera. cellular distribution in 50 unselected patients. Blood. 1979;53(6):1148-55.
49. Buza-Vidas N, Luc S, Jacobsen SE. Delineation of the earliest lineage commitment steps of haematopoietic stem cells: new developments, controversies and major challenges. Curr Opin Hematol. 2007;14(4):315-21.
50. Adolfsson J, Månsson R, Buza-Vidas N, Hultquist A, Liuba K, Jensen CT, et al. Identification of Flt3+ lymphomyeloid stem cells lacking erythro-megakaryocytic potential a revised road map for adult blood lineage commitment. Cell. 2005;121(2):295-306.
51. Kondo M, Weissman IL, Akashi K. Identification of clonogenic common lymphoid progenitors in mouse bone marrow. Cell. 1997;91(5):661-72.
52. Akashi K, Traver D, Miyamoto T, Weissman IL. A clonogenic common myeloid progenitor that gives rise to all myeloid lineages. Nature. 2000;404(6774):193-7.
53. Manz MG, Miyamoto T, Akashi K, Weissman IL. Prospective isolation of human clonogenic common myeloid progenitors. Proc Natl Acad Sci USA. 2002;99(18):11872-7.
54. Dover GJ, Boyer SH, Zinkham WH. Production of erythrocytes that contain fetal hemoglobin in anemia. Transient in vivo changes. J Clin Invest. 1979;63(2):173-6.
55. Papayannopoulou T, Vichinsky E, Stamatoyannopoulos G. Fetal Hb production during acute erythroid expansion. I. Observations in patients with transient erythroblastopenia and post-phlebotomy. Br J Haematol. 1980;44(4):535-46.
56. DeSimone J, Biel SI, Heller P. Stimulation of fetal hemoglobin synthesis in baboons by hemolysis and hypoxia. Proc Natl Acad Sci USA. 1978;75(6):2937-40.
57. Stamatoyannopoulos G, Veith R, Galanello R, Papayannopoulou T. HbF production in stressed erythropoiesis: observations and kinetic models. Ann NY Acad Sci. 1985;445:188-97.
58. Groudine M, Kohwi-Shigematsu T, Gelinas R, Stamatoyannopoulos G, Papayannopoulou T. Human fetal to adult hemoglobin switching: changes in chromatin structure of the β-globin gene locus. Proc Natl Acad Sci USA. 1983;80(24):7551-5.
59. Tuan D, Solomon W, Li Q, London IM. The "beta-like-globin" gene domain in human erythroid cells. Proc Natl Acad Sci USA. 1985;82(19):6384-8.
60. Forrester WC, Thompson C, Elder JT, Groudine M. A developmentally stable chromatin structure in the human beta-globin gene cluster. Proc Natl Acad Sci USA. 1986;83(5):1359-63.
61. Grosveld F, van Assendelft GB, Greaves DR, Kollias G. Position-independent, high-level expression of the human beta-globin gene in transgenic mice. Cell. 1987;51(6):975-85.
62. Behringer RR, Ryan TM, Palmiter RD, Brinster RL, Townes TM. Human gamma- to beta-globin gene switching in transgenic mice. Genes Dev. 1990;4(3):380-9.
63. Enver T, Raich N, Ebens AJ, Costantini F, Papayannopoulou T, Stamatoyannopoulos G. Developmental regulation of human fetal-to-adult globin gene switching in transgenic mice. Nature. 1990;344(6264):309-13.
64. Raich N, Enver T, Nakamoto B, Josephson B, Papayannopoulou T, Stamatoyannopoulos G. Autonomous developmental control of human embryonic globin gene switching in transgenic mice. Science. 1990;250(4984):1147-9.
65. Raich N, Papayannopoulou T, Stamatoyannopoulos G, Enver T. Demonstration of a human epsilon-globin gene silencer with studies in transgenic mice. Blood. 1992;79(4):861-4.

66. Li Q, Blau CA, Clegg CH, Rohde A, Stamatoyannopoulos G. Multiple epsilon-promoter elements participate in the developmental control of epsilon-globin genes in transgenic mice. J Biol Chem. 1998;273(28):17361-7.
67. Raich N, Clegg CH, Grofti J, Roméo PH, Stamatoyannopoulos G. GATA1 and YY1 are developmental repressors of the human ε-globin gene. EMBO J. 1995;14(4):801-9.
68. Dillon N, Grosveld F. Human gamma-globin genes silenced independently of other genes in the beta-globin locus. Nature. 1991;350(6315):252-4.
69. O'Neill D, Bornschlegel K, Flamm M, Castle M, Bank A. A DNA-binding factor in adult hematopoietic cells interacts with a pyrimidine-rich domain upstream from the human delta-globin gene. Proc Natl Acad Sci USA. 1991;88(20):8953-7.
70. O'Neill D, Yang J, Erdjument-Bromage H, Bornschlegel K, Tempst P, Bank A. Tissue-specific and developmental stage-specific DNA binding of a mammalion SWI/SNF complex associated with human fetal-to-adult globin switching. Proc Natl Acad Sci USA. 1999;96(2):349-54.
71. O'Neill DW, Schoetz SS, Lopez RA, Castle M, Rabinowitz L, Shor E, et al. An ikaros-containing chromatin-remodeling complex in adult-type erythroid cells. Mol Cell Biol. 2000;20(20):7572-82.
72. Rodgers GP, Saunthararajah Y. Advances in experimental treatment of beta-thalassaemia. Expert Opin Investig Drugs. 2001;10(5):925-34.
73. Witt O, Monkemeyer S, Rönndahl G, Erdlenbruch B, Reinhardt D, Kanbach K, et al. Induction of fetal hemoglobin expression by the histone deacetylase inhibitor apicidin. Blood. 2003;101(5):2001-7.
74. Perrine SP, Miller BA, Faller DV, Cohen RA, Vichinsky EP, Hurst D, et al. Sodium butyrate enhances fetal globin gene expression in erythroid progenitors of patients with Hb SS and beta thalassemia. Blood. 1989;74(1):454-9.
75. Atweh GF, Schechter AN. Pharmacologic induction of fetal hemoglobin: raising the therapeutic bar in sickle cell disease. Curr Opin Hematol. 2001;8(2):123-30.

CHAPTER 10

Normal Hematological Values and Variation in Newborn Period with Special Reference to Hb and RBC Parameters

MR Lokeshwar, Sheikh Minhaj Ahmed, Ratna Sharma

INTRODUCTION

Neonatal period is the most dynamic period in human life. During this period, there occur profound alterations and adjustments especially during transit of a fetus from hypoxic intrauterine life to totally independent extrauterine existence. Although the fetus is nourished and protected by the mother during this period, fetus may suffer adverse effects related to maternal malnutrition, illnesses, infections, drug ingestions, etc. The proximity of two circulatory systems (mother and the baby) also permits the free passage of formed blood elements between mother and fetus as seen in fetomaternal hemorrhage leading to anemia and sensitization to red blood cell (RBC) antigens and also leads to maternofetal hemorrhage leading to hyperviscosity. Erythrocyte system undergoes serial adaptation to meet progressively changing demand to oxygen in embryo and numerous physiological changes occur in succession and rapidity in fetus and neonates to adapt to a new pattern of life. This leads to rapid changes in normal hematological parameters from fetal period, which continues throughout neonatal period. A switch finally occurs mainly after delivery wherein, fetal hemoglobin (HbF) is replaced by adult hemoglobin (HbA) because the breathing neonate starts to extract oxygen from lungs rather than from its mother's blood.

Pediatricians or neonatologists caring for sick or normal newborn and premature infants are often confronted with a variety of life-threatening and/or routine hematological problems particularly anemia. These problems are most often reactive, secondary or even iatrogenic. Anemia in neonatal period remains a cause for concern due to likelihood of rapid decompensation in this vulnerable group. Numerous physiological changes occur in succession and rapidity in fetus and neonate, as the erythrocyte system adapts to the progressively changing demand for oxygen from embryo stage to term.

An understanding about the basic physiology of hematopoiesis and appreciation of normal hematologic and laboratory values at birth is important because they form the basis for the diagnosis, treatment and prevention of many diseases that afflict these neonates. Interpretation of laboratory findings and institution of appropriate therapy require understanding of maturational process and normal physiological variations that takes place during this period.[1-3]

ANTENATAL ERYTHROPOIESIS

Embryonic erythropoiesis begins by the 20th day of gestation and is evidenced as blood islands in the yolk sac. During mid-gestation, the site of erythropoiesis migrates from the yolk sac to the liver to the spleen and eventually to the bone marrow in the third trimester. All RBCs originate from a pluripotent stem cell, which is capable of differentiation into erythroid lineage.

The primitive progenitors are designated as erythroid burst-forming units and the more differentiated group called colony-forming units, which under the stimulus of erythropoietin and other humoral factors give rise to identifiable erythroblasts, which proliferate, begin to synthesize hemoglobin and mature into differentiated nucleated RBCs. During the subsequent stage of maturation, the nucleus is extruded and the cell enters the circulation as a mature RBC.

By the mid-trimester, HbF composed of two alpha and two gamma chains is the predominant hemoglobin and remains so throughout the remaining gestation and early infancy. At birth 55–65% of total hemoglobin synthesis consists of HbF and decrease to less than 5% by 4 months of age. Immediately prior to term, the infant begins to synthesize beta-hemoglobin chains; thus the term infant has some HbA (two alpha chains and two beta chains).[2,3] HbF has a higher oxygen affinity than HbA.

Fetal and neonatal erythrocytes differ greatly from adult red cells. They have larger mean cell volumes and mean cell hemoglobin and vary in their surface antigens and metabolic patterns.

Fetal hemoglobin is resistant to both alkali and dilute acid forming the basis for two tests for its measurement (the Kleihauer-Betke stain for HbF in individual cells and quantitative measurement of HbF in a hemolysate). By the end of the 1st year of life, erythropoiesis in the infant is similar to that of the adult.

NORMAL HEMATOLOGICAL VALUES AND VARIATION IN NEWBORN PERIOD

Hemoglobin Values

Hemoglobin values vary at different gestational age and reported 10 g/dL at 12 weeks of gestation to 13.7-20.1 g/dL (mean of 16.8) at term. In 100 full-term normal infants studied at Lokmanya Tilak Municipal General (LTMG) Hospital, Mumbai only 2% of neonates in this study had hemoglobin value less than 13 g% in the cord blood.[4] Approximately 95% of all values for term babies fall between 13.7 g/dL and 20.1 g/dL.[1,4,5,7-10,12-16] Most authorities, Naiman and Oskin, Mollison et al.[6] Sisson,[17] Lokeshwar et al.[12] and others have suggested that aHb concentration of 13.5 g/dL or less in cord blood should be considered as the lower limit of normal hemoglobin. Value for umbilical artery blood tends to be about 0.5 g/dL higher than sample obtained from umbilical vein.[18]

Mean cord blood hemoglobin of term neonates ranges from 14 g% to 20 g%, which increases in the first few hours due to reduction in plasma volume and placental transfusion. Hemoglobin increases by 17-20% of the initial value in the first 24 hours of life but then falls slightly during the next 24 hours decreasing thereafter. At the end of 1st week of life, hemoglobin concentration is as high as it was in the cord blood. Preterm infants have lower baseline values. In the case of preterm neonates, the hemoglobin levels start decreasing earlier in the 1st week of life. Cord blood hemoglobin can be calculated in premature infants as 7+ gestational age in lunar months g/dL as found by Burmann and Morris in female neonates infants. Capillary specimens obtained by heel stick have higher hemoglobin and hematocrit values than samples obtained from the umbilical vein or peripheral blood. A hemoglobin value less than 13 g/dL in first 2 weeks of life is labeled as anemia and warrants evaluation. Beyond the 1st week of life many factors influence what is considered as normal hematological parameters in newborn period **(Box 10.1)**.

Box 10.1 Factors affecting hematological parameters in newborn

- Site of sampling
- Time of sampling
- Treatment of umbilical vessels
- Fetomaternal transfusion
- Erythropoietin in newborn period
- Variation in blood volume
- Erythrocyte life span
- Red cell—osmotic and mechanical fragility

The postnatal drop in hemoglobin is universal in newborns. It is typically asymptomatic requiring no intervention. Immediately after birth, there is successful transition from fetal to neonatal circulation-there is increase in blood oxygen content and tissue oxygen leading to down regulation of erythropoietin production so that erythropoiesis is suppressed. In the absence of erythropoiesis, hemoglobin levels decrease as there is no replacement of aged RBC's. As a result of this, the hemoglobin concentration in healthy full-term and premature infants undergoes typical changes during the 1st week of life leading to a decrease in hemoglobin and hematocrit concentrations after birth. The postnatal drop in hemoglobin is universal in newborns. It is typically asymptomatic requiring no intervention. The hemoglobin levels in both term and preterm infants fall after the 1st week of life to reach a plateau and after 1 year of age, there is no difference between the hemoglobin values of term and preterm infants **(Tables 10.1 and 10.2)**.

Table 10.1 Normal cord blood hemoglobin by various authors

	Mean (g/dL)	Hemoglobin (Hb) range (g/dL)
Mollison (1951)[6]	16.6	–
Dochain et al. (1952)[7]	17.9	14.4–21.6
Walker et al. (1953)[8]	16.5	
Marks et al.(1955)[9]	16.9	12.3–22
Guest et al.(1957)[10]	17.1	13.6–25
Sturgeon (1956)[11]	15.7	
Dalal and Lokeshwar[12]	16.2	13.2–22
Rama Rao[13]	15.13	14.16 to ± 3.26

Table 10.2 Hemoglobin, hematocrit, red blood cell (RBC) at different age in neonatal period studied at Lokmanya Tilak Municipal General Hospital (LTMGH), Mumbai

	Hb (g%)	Hematocrit	RBC (million/mm)
Cord blood	16.2 ± 3.6	46.66 ± 5.1	4.9 ± 1.2
12–18 hours	18.79 ± 2.8	49 ± 4.8	5.3 ± 0.8
72 hours	17.38 ± 3.0	46.9 ± 5.3	5.2 ± 0.6
15 days	16.36 ± 2.2	43.4 ± 4.1	5.01 ± 0.9
28 days	14.17 ± 2.4	42.1 ± 3.8	4.7 ± 1.0

Hematocrit

Capillary hematocrit on 1st day of life is reported to be 62.9 ± 3.2% reaching 56.6 ± 2.6 by day 7, and 53.7 ± 2.5% by day 10 mean capillary hematocrit value is 2% points higher than the mean venous hematocrit values at 1 week of age. Capillary specimens obtained by heel stick have higher hemoglobin and hematocrit values than samples obtained from the

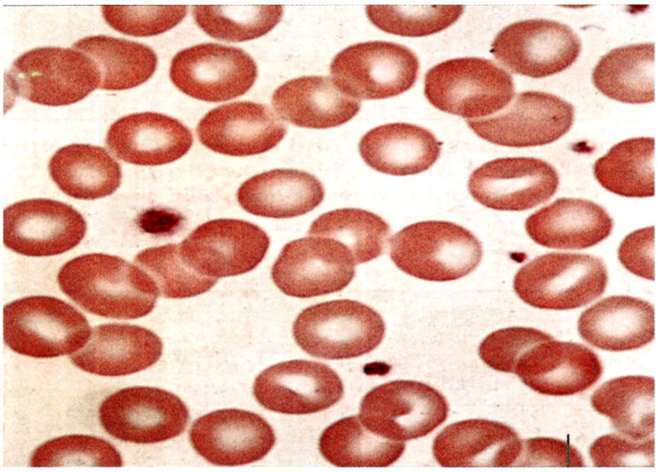

Figure 10.1 Normal red blood cell (RBC) in newborn

umbilical vein or peripheral blood. Just as hemoglobin value, hematocrit value also increases during the first few hours of life and reaches the original value of cord blood by 1 week **(Table 10.2)**.

Normal RBC Values (Fig. 10.1)

Red Cell Count and Red Cell Indices

Red cell count also shows a great variability at the time of birth and ranges from 4.6 million/mm^3 to 5.2 million/mm^3. Red cell count rises rapidly during first few hours of life reaching approximately 5 million/mm^3 stabling to 5.2 million/mm^3 attend of 1 week and remains the same during neonatal period.[19-21] In the case of preterm neonates the hemoglobin levels start decreasing earlier in the 1st week of life.

Of note, in the term infant, the normal mean corpuscular volume (MCV) is high. The MCV and mean corpuscular hemoglobin (MCH) decrease with increasing gestational age and postnatal age.

Mean Corpuscular Volume

Average MCV is 107 fL. The MCV and MCH decrease with increasing gestational age and postnatal age. The MCV at 24–25 weeks of gestation is markedly elevated at 135 ± 0.2, but decreases to 119 ± 9.4 at term. Of note, in the term infant, the normal MCV is high. An MCV less than or equal to 95, which is normal for an adult, would be defined as microcytic in the newborn period and may indicate an alpha thalassemia syndrome. MCV at birth ranges from 105 fL to 125 fL compared to normal adult value of 82–92 fL. MCV rapidly decreases in 1st week of life and at the age of 2 months, cell size is comparable to those in adult cells. MCV less than or equal to 95, which is normal for an adult, would be defined as microcytic in the newborn period and may indicate thalassemia syndrome or iron deficiency.

Newborn red cells are generally much larger than adults; average diameter of RBC is 8.5–9.3 *μ at birth* reaching the adult diameter of 7.5 *μ around 6 months of age* **(Table 10.3)**.

Mean Corpuscular Hemoglobin

Hemoglobin content of the RBC in neonatal cells is 35–38 pg/cell, which is greater than that of adult cells and hypochromia is defined as MCH less than 34 pg/cell.[19-21] MCH is also increased at birth ranging from 33.5 pg to 41.4 pg as compared to 27–37 pg in adults.

However, the mean corpuscular hemoglobin concentration (MCHC) is fairly constant throughout life.

MCHC in newborn period is quite similar to that in adults ranging from 30% to 35% in newborn and 30–36% in adults. It is higher in preterm infants. High MCHC should lead to suspicion of spherocytosis or sickle cell anemia.

Average value for central venous hemoglobin at birth for more than 34 weeks gestational age is 17 g/dL. Anemia in newborn defined as central venous hemoglobin 13 g/dL or capillary hemoglobin less than 14.5 g/dL in infant more than 34 weeks gestation and 0–28 days old. Hemoglobin values rise from 8 g/dL to 10 g/dL at 12 weeks of gestation to 13.7–20.1 g/dL (mean of 16.8) at term; preterm infants have lower base line values.

Reticulocyte Count

The reticulocyte count declines continuously during the course of gestation.

Average reticulocyte count in cord blood is 3–7%. Normal values for the first 3 days range from 4.1% to 6.3%,

Table 10.3 Mean corpuscular volume (MCV), mean corpuscular hemoglobin (MCH), mean corpuscular hemoglobin concentration (MCHC) and normoblast counts studied at Lokmanya Tilak Municipal General Hospital (LTMGH)

	MCV (fl)	*MCH (Pg)*	*MCHC (%)*	*Normoblasts (cells/mm^3)*
Cord blood	113.04 ± 5.3	34.33 ± 1.4	33.9 ± 0.8	600 ± 186
12–18 hours	108.96 ± 5	35.1 ± 1.9	34.4 ± 0.6	283 ± 122
72 hours	98.54 ± 2.9	35.82 ± 0.8	34.9 ± 0.5	36 ± 48
7 days	96.0 ± 3.4	34.0 ± 1.0	34.6 ± 0.8	—
15 days	95.5 ± 4.0	33.2 ± 9.0	34.54 ± 0.5	—
28 days	96.1 ± 3.2	31.6 ± 0.93	34.2 ± 0.7	—

Table 10.4A Red blood cell (RBC) values in preterm neonates during the 1st week of life

	Hb-g/dL	Hematocrit (HCT)	Reticulocyte %	Nucleated RBC (cells/1,000 RBC)
Preterm cord blood	16.0 (13–18.5)	49	<10	<3.00
Day 7	14.8	45	<3	<0.01

Table 10.4B Red blood cell (RBC) values in term neonates during the first week of life

	Hb (g/dL)	Hematocrit (HCT)	Reticulocytes (%)	Nucleated RBC (cells/1,000 RBC)
Term				
Cord blood	17 (14–20)	53	<7	<1
Day 1	18.4	58	<7	<0.01
Day 3	17.8	55	<3	0
Day 7	17.0	54	<1	0

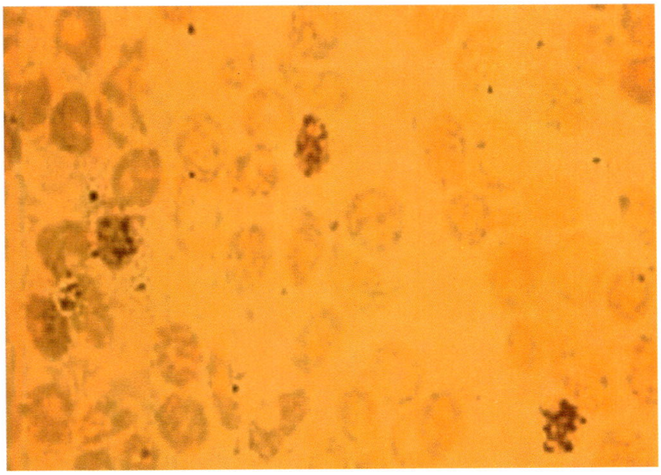

Figure 10.2 Reticulocyte on peripheral smear

approximately 300,000 reticulocytes per cubic millimeter. Although elevated at birth, it is normal by the 3rd day. Approximately 500 nucleated RBC per cubic millimeter of blood may be seen at birth in the term infant; however, by the 4th day of life, these cells should not be detected in the peripheral blood of normal infants.[22,23] Capillary specimens obtained by heel stick have higher hemoglobin and hematocrit values than samples obtained from the umbilical vein or peripheral blood. Reticulocytes and nucleated RBCs decrease in number with increasing postgestational age as shown in **Tables 10.4A and B**. Persistence of reticulocytosis and nucleated RBCs suggests the possibility of hemorrhage and hemolysis. Hypoxia in the absence of anemia also can be associated with increased release of reticulocytes and nucleated RBCs **(Fig. 10.2)**.

CONCLUSION

It is essential to know changing pattern of normal variation of hematological parameters in relation to gestational age, weight and other factors that affects pregnancy and its outcome. An understanding about the basic physiology of hematopoiesis and an appreciation of normal hematologic laboratory values at birth is important because they form the basis for the prevention, diagnosis and treatment of many causes that afflict these neonates.

KEY MESSAGE

Failure to recognize the importance of physiologic process of hematological parameters, particularly anemia, may lead to inappropriate investigations and treatment of apparent anemia and avoid subjecting these infants to unnecessary investigations, blood transfusions as it needs no therapy unless symptomatic.

REFERENCES

1. Oski FA, Nathan JL. Normal blood values in newborn period – hematological problems of the newborn. Vol IV in the series. Major Problems in Clinical Pediatrics. WB Saunders Company, 1982. pp. 1-31.
2. Christensen RD. Hematopoiesis in the fetus and neonate. Pediatr Res. 1989;26:531-5.
3. Brown MS. Fetal and neonatal erythropoiesis. In: Stockman JA, Pochedly C (Eds). Developmental and neonatal hematology. New York: Raven Press, 1988. p. 39.
4. Dalal Raksha. Hematological parameters in the newborn period. Thesis submitted for MD (Ped) Exam, University of Bombay, under the guidance of Dr MR Lokeshwar.
5. Wegelius R on changes in the peripheral blood picture of newborn infant immediately after birth. Acta Pediatr. 1948;35: 1 Nov. 1986. p. 12.
6. Mollison PL. Blood transfusion in clinical medicine. 1st Edn, Oxford Blackwell, 1951.
7. Dochain J, Lemage L, Lambrechts A. Cited in Oski & Naiman. Normal blood values in newborn period. Hematologic problems in the newborn. WB Saunders Co, Philadelphia; 1982. pp. 1-31.

8. Walker JL, Turnbull EPN. Hemoglobin and red cells in human foetus and their relation to the oxygen content of the blood in the vessels of umbilical cord. Lancet. 1953;2:312.
9. Marks J, Gairdner D, Rescoe JD. Blood formation in infancy III cord blood. Arch Dis Child. 1955;30:117.
10. Guest GM, Brown EW. Erythropoiesis and hemoglobin of blood in infancy and childhood. Am J Dis. 1957;93:486.
11. Sturgeon P. Iron metabolism—a review with special consideration of iron requirement during normal infancy. Pediatrics. 1956;18:267.
12. Lokeshwar MR, Dalal Raksha, Manglani Mamta, Shah N. Anemia in newborn. Ind J Pediatr. 1998;65:651-61.
13. Rama Rao BR, Krishnamurthy PN, et al. Study of neonatal hematological values in relation to maternal and foetal factors and incidence of transplacental passage of foetal erythrocytes. Ind Pediatr. 1979;16:591-5.
14. Krisnamurthy PN. Physiological variation in hematological parameter in fetus an neonates. Problems in pediatric Hematology and oncology. Hematology and oncology chapter of IAP Publication. 1988. pp. 10-17.
15. Manroe BL, Weinberg AG, Rosenfeld CR, Browne R. The neonatal blood count in health and disease. I. Reference values for neutrophilic cells. J Pediatr. 1979;95:89-98
16. Aneja S, Mandranda R, Patwari A, Sagreiya K, Bhargava SK. Normal Hematological values in Newborns. Indian Pediatr. 1979;16:781-6.
17. Sisson TRC, Lund CJ, Whalen LE, Telek A. The blood volume of infant. 1. The full-term infant in the first year of life. J Paediatr. 1959;55:163-79.
18. Lanzkowosky P. Effect of early and late clamping of umbilical cord on infants hemoglobin level. Br Med J. 1980;2:1777.
19. Mitchell SL. Reference ranges and normal values. Dacie Lewis Pract Haematol. 2006;10:13-20.
20. Qaiser DH, Ahmed ST, Sandila MP, Kazmi T. Haematological reference intervals in Indian population. Indian J Clin Biochem. 2005;20:110-8.
21. Keramati MR, Zadeh MA, Farhat AS. The determination of haematological reference values in neonates in Mashard J Ofoghe Danesh J. 2010;16(1):64-71.
22. Kato. Physiological variations in reticulocyte in newborn study of 219 cases. Cited Oski FA & Naiman JL. Normal blood value in newborn period - hematological problems in newborn Vol.1 in the series; Major problems in clinical pediatrics. WB Saunders Co, 1982. pp. 1-31.
23. Seip M. The reticulocyte level and erythrocyte production judged from reticulocyte studies in the newborn infants during first week of life. Acta Pediatr. 1955;44:355.

CHAPTER 11

Effect of Nutritional Deficiency Anemia during Pregnancy on Fetus and Newborn

BD Bhatia, Shweta Singh, Nagendra Chaudhary

INTRODUCTION

Among nutritional disorder in pregnancy, anemia constitutes most common micronutrient deficiency predominantly in developing countries. The origin of word "anemia" is from Greek literature, which denotes lack of blood. The World Health Organization has defined anemia as "condition in which the number of red blood cells (RBCs) or their oxygen carrying capacity is inadequate to meet physiologic demands of the body, which vary by sex, age, altitude, smoking and pregnancy status".

EPIDEMIOLOGY

Nutritional anemia in pregnancy is a grave issue owning to the fact that it has deleterious effect on mother as well as fetus. This is the cause of high maternal and perinatal mortality in developing countries.[1] The highest proportions of individuals affected with anemia are in Africa and in Southeast Asia[2] with highest prevalence in India. Two billion people constituting over 30% of the world's population are anemic. Prevalence of anemia in pregnant women in India is 49.7% (up to more than 80% in certain states) against the global prevalence of 41.8%.[2] Sri Lanka and Thailand have low prevalence (22.3–29.3%) as against 74.6% in Nepal. Studies done in India clearly show that prevalence as well as severity of anemia during pregnancy and lactation is grave. In spite of affordable technology and decades of National Anemia Prophylaxis Programme (since 1968), no sizeable impact has been evident on prevalence, except in state of Kerala.

According to the WHO scientific group, anemia in pregnant women should be considered when hemoglobin values are lower than 11 g/dL, and diet must be supplemented with medical iron **(Table 11.1)**.[3]

Table 11.1 The Indian Council of Medical Research (ICMR)[4] categories of anemia

Category	*Type*	*Hemoglobin level*
1	Mild	10.0–10.9 g%
2	Moderate	7–10 g%
3	Severe	<7 g%
4	Very severe (decompensated)	<4 g%

ETIOLOGY

Determining the etiology of anemia is challenging because hematological parameters (e.g. hematocrit, reticulocyte, ferritin, unsaturated iron binding capacity) are altered by usual physiological mechanism. The most common causes of anemia seen during pregnancy are iron-deficiency anemia and megaloblastic anemia due to folate deficiency. Vitamin B12 deficiency less commonly causes megaloblastic anemia in pregnancy. The main causes for this anemia are inadequate diet lacking these micronutrients and anemic women not taking iron and folate supplementation in prenatal period; the other contributing factors are poor absorption, increased losses and incomplete utilization of hemopoietic nutrients. Malaria, human immunodeficiency virus (HIV) infection and hemolytic anemia are less commonly encountered during pregnancy, still can have significant adverse influence on mother and fetus health.

The major contributory factors are incomplete absorption, increased daily requirements, poor utilization and increased losses.

PHYSIOLOGICAL ANEMIA

The estimated increase in maternal red cell mass varies from 17% to 25% and for plasma volume is approximately 43%.

The cause for physiological anemia is hemodilution as a result of larger increase in plasma volume as compared to red cell mass.[5]

However, the RBC morphology remains normocytic normochromic. In normal pregnancy, iron requirements

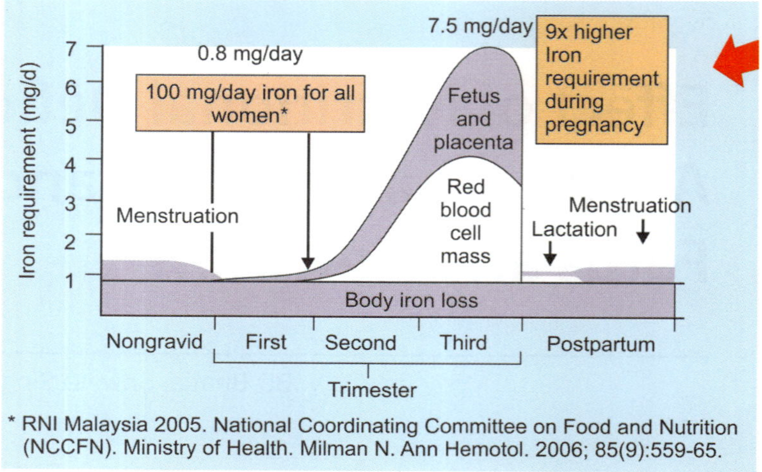

Figure 11.1 Iron requirement during pregnancy, postpartum and nonpregnant female[9]

are increased by two- to threefold and folate requirements by ten- to twentyfolds. The initial decrease in hemoglobin and hematocrit starts in first trimester, continue to decrease in second trimester and finally reaches their nadir in late second to early third trimester. At term, once again, there is upsurge of hemoglobin and hematocrit. The differentiation of physiological anemia from iron-deficiency anemia becomes tough in late pregnancy.[6] Therefore, early pregnancy is the right time for detection of risk related with maternal anemia.[7]

Megaloblastic anemia caused by folic acid deficiency is as a result of lesser intake, poor absorption and increased demands owning to fetal development and maternal erythropoiesis. Furthermore, there is an inhibitory effect of increased levels of estrogen and progesterone on folate absorption during pregnancy.[8]

Iron requirement during pregnancy is 9 times more than prepregnancy state. **Figure 11.1** depicting iron requirement during prepregnancy stage, pregnancy and postpartum phase.[9]

MATERNAL EFFECTS OF ANEMIA

Maternal Risks during Pregnancy

Poor pregnancy outcome like increased duration of hospitalization, infectious diseases and general health issues too are associated with mild-to-moderate anemia. Complications of pregnancy like postpartum abruptio placentae, placenta previa, cesarean delivery and postpartum hemorrhage have been found to be associated with severe anemia (hemoglobin less than 6 g/dL). It can also lead to serious life-threatening complications as a consequence of congestive heart failure. Anemia has been attributed to be the single main cause of 20–40% of maternal deaths in developing countries. The risk increases dramatically in severe anemia.

There are increased chances of preeclampsia, recurrent infection, puerperal sepsis and preterm delivery.

Lactation

Iron-deficient anemic mothers are equally competent as nonanemic mothers for lactation. Furthermore, milk composition with regards to macro and micronutrients has not been found to be altered. The physiological trapping leads to increased iron content in breast milk of hypoferremic mothers.[10] Nevertheless, after 4–6 months of age breast milk has been demonstrated inadequate to sustain sufficient iron metabolism.

Risk of Infections

Anemia depresses the immune status and increases the morbidity from infections. Evidence has showed lower levels of lymphocyte stimulation indices in severe iron-deficient pregnant women and with iron therapy lymphocyte stimulation increases.[11]

FETAL EFFECTS

Fetal complications like premature birth, LBW and also fetal demises have been reported in anemic mothers.

Preterm Delivery

Preterm delivery has been reported to be increased by 20% in pregnant women with hemoglobin levels between 10 g/dL and 11 g/dL while 60% with hemoglobin levels between 9 g/dL and 10 g/dL. Hemoglobin levels lower than 9 g/dL in pregnancies have further increased risk and for every 1 g fall in hemoglobin below 9 g/dL, risk doubles, triples and so forth.[12]

Preterm delivery in iron-deficient pregnant women is initiated essentially by three mechanisms namely hypoxia, oxidative stress and lastly infections.[13]

Stress response generated by chronic hypoxia from anemia liberates CRH (corticotropin-releasing hormone) by placenta, which further accelerates production of fetal cortisol leading to preterm delivery. Also, CRH can increase the maternal and fetal stress and lead to early rupture of membrane, pregnancy-induced hypertension and premature labor. Linear growth of fetus is also reduced by high levels of cortisol.

A different way of inducing CRH could be through oxidative damage to fetoplacental red cells by iron deficiency. Risk of infections increases due to decreased immune response in iron-deficient pregnant women, which finally leads to higher levels of cytokines, CRH and prostaglandins finally increasing the chances of preterm delivery.

Apgar Score

Low Apgar score has been found to be associated with maternal anemia. In one Indian study, higher maternal hemoglobin during first stage of labor had been correlated with better Apgar score and with decreased risk of birth asphyxia.[14]

Birth Weight

Studies have established that LBW is correlated with low maternal hemoglobin levels. Perinatal mortality has been reported to increase by 3 times with maternal hemoglobin level below 8 g/dL in contrast to mother with hemoglobin level more than 11 g/dL.[15]

Varanasi study revealed that proportion of LBW babies increased with fall in maternal hemoglobin levels and maternal hemoglobin levels exerted independent significant influence on birth weight even after controlling maternal weight, height, serum albumin status. Maternal hemoglobin alone explained 16% variation in birth weight in a multivariate analysis.

Growth and Neurological Development

Poor neurological development (decreased vision, deafness, autism, cerebral palsy and lower education attainment) along with increased morbidity has been found in LBW babies born to anemic mother. With decreasing birth weight, damage to central nervous system increases.[16]

Prenatal iron deficiency induced in fetal rats had shown alterations mainly in neurometabolic, electrophysiological and behavioral functions.[17]

However, there are two schools of thought regarding the level of maternal hemoglobin and effects on the fetus. Even a mild reduction in maternal hemoglobin during pregnancy can have deleterious effects on the fetus while others believe that those effects only manifest when maternal hemoglobin falls below 6 g/dL.[18]

Fetal Iron Stores

Liver iron stores are decreased in fetus of mother with low ferritin levels. With advancing gestational age and increasing birth weight, the fetal iron store in liver, spleen and kidney rises. There is sharp rise in tissue iron content in last 8 weeks of pregnancy. Hepatic iron reserve is half for infants born before 36 weeks of gestation as compared to those born after 36 weeks.[10]

Neurotransmission

Iron content of fetal brain is decreased. Neurotransmitters are also reduced along with alterations in receptors.[19] Enzymes of carboxylic acid cycle were reduced in fetal brain. Fetal latent iron deficiency had been associated with decrease in brain neurotransmitters. Among the neurotransmitters of central nervous system, most irreparable depletion was noticed for brain gamma-aminobutyric acid (GABA) levels, enzymes involved in the biosynthesis of GABA and L-glutamic acid

Reduction was found in whole brain catecholamine, dopamine, norepinephrine, tyrosine and monoamine oxidase. Increased tyrosine aminotransferase in corpus striatum despite reduced whole brain content has been reported.[10]

Study done of the iron content in different parts of fetal rat brain born to mother with latent iron deficiency anemia in mother showed:

- Iron content in cerebral cortex: 17%
- Cerebellum: 18%
- Hypothalamus: 19%
- Midbrain: 21%
- Corpus striatum: 32%

Iron content remains constant in pons and medulla oblongata.[20] Fetal brain iron content did not change after maternal iron supplementation. Low brain iron content was associated significant alteration in brain Cu, Zn, Ca, Mn, Pb and Cd levels.

Effect on Fetoplacental Unit

Initially, fetus gets its iron from maternal transferring entrapped in placenta regardless of maternal iron stores. At last progressively, though, fetal iron reserve decreases with diminished maternal store and also hemoglobin mass is insufficient than normal counter parts. The phenomenon of reduced fetal iron store as a consequence of iron-deficiency anemia in pregnant mother is known as hidden iron deficit.

Babies born to mother with decreased ferritin, cord blood hemoglobin was found to be decreased in both preterm as well as full-term babies. In maternal iron deficiency, gradient for iron transport from mother to fetus is increased. Mother and fetus do not regulate iron transport as it is an exclusively placental function. This has been confirmed by findings of trapping of iron despite removal of placenta in animal. However, in severe maternal hypoferremia, iron content of placenta decreases despite this maternal protective process.

In maternal hypoferremia, placenta undergoes morphological (weight, volume, number of cotyledons are reduced, cotyledons have poor septation and are ill-defined), pathophysiological (decreased vascularity, endarteritis obliterans), biochemical (compensatory changes to impaired

Flow chart 11.1 Algorithm for managing nutritional anemia in pregnancy

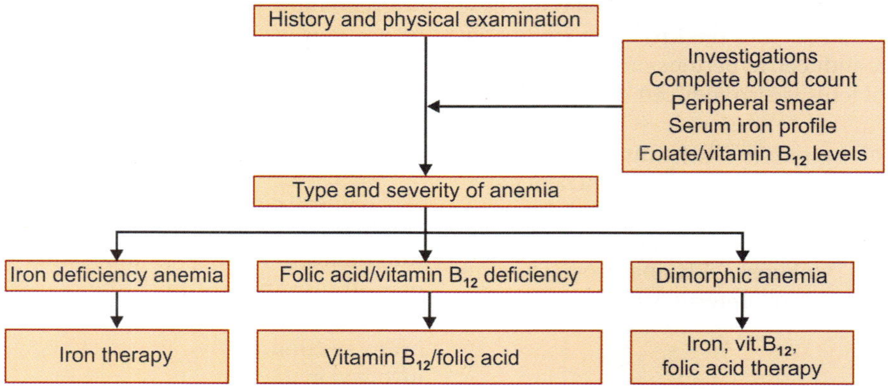

Note: In severe anemia, consider blood transfusion

citric acid cycle), reduced cell number with hypertrophy. Some of these changes are purely to improve functioning parenchyma in placenta.

Studies done in past reported that babies born to anemic and nonanemic mothers do not have significant differences in cord blood hemoglobin, iron and ferritin regardless of maternal hypoferremia. Still, these findings might be applicable for mothers having mild-to-moderate anemia but not in severely anemic mothers where most workers have reported that in maternal hypoferremia, cord blood hemoglobin and iron levels are decreased. There is direct relationship of cord serum iron levels with maternal and fetus iron levels. Moreover, studies done using serum ferritin as a measure of iron status showed poor iron store at birth in babies born to mother not on iron supplementation during pregnancy. Perinatal outcome improved, mean weight, Apgar score and hemoglobin level at 3 months of age have been found to increase considerably with supplementation of iron during pregnancy as compared with control (placebo) group.

Maternal iron levels improve and iron depletion during third trimester decreases with iron supplementation during pregnancy.

Pregnant women, who have poor iron store prepregnancy state, do not respond to iron supplementation despite iron deficiency.[20,21]

Placental transferrin receptors increase for better utilization of iron in pregnant woman with low iron store. Still, the magnitude of iron utilization by this process is insufficient to transfer iron to fetus from iron-deficient mother.

There is direct correlation of maternal hemoglobin with cord blood hemoglobin, hematocrit and red cell count. At 32–34 weeks of pregnancy with maternal hemoglobin level lower than 11 g, these parameters have lower values **(Flow chart 11.1)**.[20]

An altered temperament has been reported in first 7 days of life in newborn with low cord blood hemoglobin and iron.[22]

Criteria for diagnosis of iron-deficiency anemia during pregnancy:

- Serum iron levels: Less than 30 mg/dL
- Low serum ferritin levels: Less than 55 µg/L
- Serum transferring saturation: Less than 15%
- Unsaturated iron binding capacity (UIBC): More than 400 µg/dL.

TREATMENT OF IRON DEFICIENCY ANEMIA

Iron supplementation in pregnancy is universally advised. There is also another school of thought that advocates hemoglobin level at or above 10 g/dL; iron supplementation has no role because hemodilution during pregnancy is a physiological mechanism required for adequate placental circulation.[23]

While iron supplementation increases maternal iron status and stores, maternal complications like gestational diabetes and increased oxidative stress have also been reported.

Therefore, iron therapy in pregnancy is a double-edged sword. On the one hand, in iron-deficient pregnant women, iron uptake improves outcome of pregnancy. At the other end, iron uptake in pregnant women without iron deficiency increases the risk of complications.

Iron therapy in iron-deficiency anemia should be followed to detect iron refractory or unresponsive anemia **(Table 11.2)**.

Oral iron therapy (60 mg) with folic acid (5 mg) daily must be started early in pregnant woman and continued till 6 months postpartum.

Erythropoietin

It is the new agent used in treatment of anemia. Erythropoietin is gaining popularity as at therapeutic option during pregnancy and the postpartum period.

Table 11.2 Iron content of different salts[24]

Salt	*Dose of salt*	*Elemental iron in milligram*
Ferrous fumarate	200	65
Ferrous gluconate	300	35
Ferrous glycine sulfate	225	45
Ferrous succinate	100	35
Ferrous sulfate	300	60

FOLIC ACID DEFICIENCY ANEMIA

Megaloblastic anemia due to folic acid deficiency has predominantly gastrointestinal symptoms like anorexia, nausea, vomiting, diarrhea and glossitis.

Skin and oral pigmentation, hepatosplenomegaly and petechiae can be found. However, alternative diagnosis like leukemia and aplastic anemia must be considered and ruled out before considering folic acid deficiency.

The two important functions of folates and its metabolite are DNA synthesis and production of amino acid. Vitamin B_{12} is required for folate metabolism via active tetrahydrofolate.

Deceased serum levels of vitamin B_{12} in pregnancy lead to megaloblastic anemia, which commonly exists with folic acid deficiency anemia.

Diagnostic Criteria for Megaloblastic Anemia

Minimum two of the criteria are required for diagnosis of megaloblastic anemia:

- Hypersegmented neutrophils (contain six or more lobes) more than 4%
- Macrocytes with diameter more than 12 mm
- Presence of Howell-Jolly bodies [basophilic nuclear remnants (clusters of DNA) in circulating erythrocytes]
- Nucleated erythrocytes
- Presence of macropolycyte (unusually large neutrophilic leukocyte with multisegmented nucleus).

Red cell indices usually seen in megaloblastic anemia are mean corpuscular volume (MCV) more than 96 fL and mean corpuscular hemoglobin (MCH) more than 33 pg. Folic acid deficiency is diagnosed by decreased serum folate (<3 mg/mL) along with red cell folate level (<150 ng/mL).

DIMORPHIC ANEMIA

It refers to dual deficiency of iron and folic acid with predominance features of one.

Additional causes of micronutrient deficient anemia encountered in pregnancy:

- *Deficiency of phosphorus*: Severe deficiency leads to depletion of adenosine triphosphate (ATP) inside red cells resulting in osmotic rupture causing hemolytic anemia.
- *Deficiency of zinc*: In thalassemia and sickle cell anemia, zinc deficiency has been reported. But, there is no clue that zinc deficiency aggravates anemia.
- *Deficiency of pyridoxine*: This is rarely found during the course of pregnancy, levels of pyridoxine have been reported to decrease to 25% of normal. It leads to microcytic hypochromic anemia.
- *Deficiency of vitamin C*: Deficiency of vitamin C leads to microcytic hypochromic anemia.
- *Deficiency of vitamin A*: Anemia is a common consequence of vitamin A deficiency. In cases of deficiency, iron is trapped in the liver and spleen and is not effectively released for erythropoiesis by bone marrow.

Prevention of anemia in fertile age women:

- Countrywide awareness about anemia and its effect on fetus
- Universal supply of iron and folic acid to girls until age of 19 years
- Liasioning with and strengthening of school health schemes and adolescent friendly health services for nutrition counseling, and yearly deworming of adolescents
- Improvements in legislative and other support for woman's nutrition
- The delivery of micronutrient and food supplements to female adolescents through the school system can also be considered
- In pregnant women without iron deficiency, dose of iron may be reduced to 30 mg. All the women of childbearing age especially teenage girls should be screened and given iron supplementation.

Prevention of anemia in pregnancy:

- *Prepregnancy counseling*: Dietary advice and treatment is very important for ensuring best pregnancy outcomes.
- *Screening during pregnancy*: All pregnant ladies should get full blood count done during booking of pregnancy and should be repeated at 28 weeks to screen for anemia. In high-risk mothers and multiple pregnancies, an additional hemoglobin check should be performed near term.
- Dietary advice:
  - *Iron-rich food*: Dark green leafy vegetables (spinach, beans, legumes and lentils), meat, poultry, fish, egg yolk, dry fruits and iron-fortified cereals
  - Cast iron utensils for cooking
  - Taking iron with vitamin (orange juice) can improve its intake and absorption
  - *Iron inhibitors*: The common iron inhibitors present in diet include phytic acid (grains and legumes), egg protein (from both the white and the yolk), minerals competing with iron for absorption: calcium, zinc, magnesium, copper and tannic acid. These food items should not be taken concomitantly with iron or iron rich diet

- *Weekly iron therapy*: At places where iron deficiency is more common, weekly iron along with folic acid may be attempted to all vulnerable females
- *Deworming*: Increased intake of iron, treatment of underlying conditions like deworming (antihelminthic therapy) are important preventive measures
- *Vitamin B_{12} and folate deficiencies*: Both of these vitamins help in embryogenesis. Folate deficiency is known to cause neural tube defect. From neonatal point of view, a delay in cord clamping by 1-3 minutes is an inactive toward prophylaxis for neonatal anemia.

FUTURE PERSPECTIVE

- In poor resource area, there are many problems in assessment of iron deficiency. Limited resources again poses hurdle in prevention as well as treatment of iron-deficiency anemia
- The standard levels of biochemical markers of iron status are easily influenced by inflammation. The diagnosis can be difficult in diseases in which there is an acute-phase response like ferritin is an acute-phase reactant. A newer alternative laboratory measurement is the soluble transferrin receptor. Further studies are needed to evaluate their response to inflammations
- Newer studies must be performed for evaluating the response of iron supplementation on immune function in pregnant women
- *Transferrin receptor (TfR), transferring receptor saturation*: Serum ferritin ratio, total iron binding capacity (TIBC), zinc protoporphyrin (ZPP), reticulocyte hemoglobin (CHr) and stainable bone marrow are important biomarkers of iron exposure that might be useful in pregnancy
- Role of neuroimaging in infants of anemic mother and their neurodevelopment must be evaluated
- Measures should be taken to increase drug compliance and bioavailability
- Food-based approach should be tried like fortification of staple food and food variety. Agricultural production should be boosted and prices lowered. Targeted agricultural programs can complement these investments by supporting livelihoods, enhancing access to diverse diets in poor populations and fostering women's empowerment
- Advantages of staple food fortification and promotion of dietary diversity, that is, food-based approach rather than food supplementation must be searched.

KEY POINTS

- Among nutritional disorder in pregnancy, anemia constitutes most common micronutrient deficiency predominantly in developing countries
- Full blood counts must be assessed at booking and 28 weeks
- In pregnancy, iron-deficiency anemia and folate-deficiency megaloblastic anemia constitute the most common causes of anemia
- Serum ferritin levels less than 15 µg/mL are diagnostic of iron deficiency and levels below 30 µg/mL should prompt treatment. ZPP and saturated transferring receptors may be helpful adjuncts
- Nutritional anemia increases maternal morbidity and mortality and leads to pregnancy complications
- Maternal anemia can lead to prematurity, LBW and even fetal deaths
- Daily oral iron (60 mg) and folic acid (5 mg) should be started and continued till 6 months postpartum. In case of poor compliance, iron can be given by intramuscular or intravenous route. Parenteral iron should be considered from second trimester onward. Folic acid deficiency causing megaloblastic type of anemia should be treated with folic acid 5 mg daily
- *Prevention of anemia*: Prepregnancy counseling, screening during pregnancy, dietary advice, iron-rich food, cast iron utensils for cooking, avoidance of inhibitors of iron.

REFERENCES

1. UNICEF and Micronutrient Initiative. Vitamin and mineral deficiency: a global progress report. March, 2004.
2. McLean E, Cogswell M, Egli I, Wojdyla D, de Benoist B. Worldwide prevalence of anaemia, WHO Vitamin and Mineral Nutrition Information System, 1993-2005. Public Health Nutr. 2009;12(4):444-54.
3. Nutritional anaemias. Report of a WHO scientific group. World Health Organ Tech Rep Ser. 1968;405:5-37.
4. Indian Council of Medical Research. Evaluation of the National Nutritional Anemia Prophylaxis Programme. Task Force Study. New Delhi: ICMR, 1989.
5. Goodlin RC, Dobry CA, Anderson JC, Woods RE, Quaife M. Clinical signs of normal plasma volume expansion during pregnancy. Am J Obstet Gynecol. 1983;145(8):1001-9.
6. Scholl TO, Hediger ML. Anemia and iron-deficiency anemia: complication of anemia on pregnancy outcome. Am J Clin Nutr. 1994;59(2 Suppl):492S-500S.
7. Institute of Medicine. Nutrition during Pregnancy. Washington DC, USA: National Academy Press; 1990.
8. Pritchard JA, McDonald PC. Medical and surgical illnesses during pregnancy and the puerperium in Williams Obstetrics, 16th edn. New York, Appleton-Century-Crofts, 1980.
9. Milman N. Iron and pregnancy—a delicate balance. Ann Hematol. 2006;85(9):559-65.
10. Agarwal KN, Gupta V, Agarwal S. Effect of maternal iron status on placenta, fetus and newborn. J Med Med Sci. 2013;5(9):391-5.
11. Kandoi A, Bhatia BD, Pandey LK, Pandey S, Sen PC, Satya K. Cellular immunity status in anemia in pregnancy. Indian J Med Res. 1991;94:11-5.
12. Kaltreider DF, Kohl S. Epidemiology of preterm delivery. Clin Obstet Gynecol. 1980;23(1):17-31.
13. Allen LH. Biological mechanisms that might underlie iron's effects on fetal growth and preterm birth. J Nutr. 2001;131(2S-2):581S-589S.

14. Rusia U, Madan N, Agarwal N, Sikka M, Sood SK. Effect of maternal iron deficiency anaemia on foetal outcome. Indian J Pathol Microbiol. 1995;38(3):273-9.
15. Meyer MB, Tonascia JA, Buck C. The interrelationship of maternal smoking and increased perinatal mortality with other risk factors. Further analysis of the Ontario Perinatal Mortality Study, 1960-1961. Am J Epidemiol. 1974;100(6):443-52.
16. Williams MD, Wheby MS. Anemia in pregnancy. Med Clin North Am. 1992;76(3):631-47.
17. Rao R, Tkac I, Townsend EL, Gruetter R, Georgieff MK. Perinatal iron defieciency alters the neurochemical profile of the developing rat hippocampus. J Nutr. 2003;133(10):3215-21.
18. Pryor JA, Morrison JC. Nutritional anemias. In: Bern MM, Frigoletto FD (Eds). Hematologic Disorders in Maternal-Fetal Medicine. New York, USA: Wiley-Liss; 1990. pp. 93-111.
19. Agarwal KN. Iron and the brain: neurotransmitter receptors and magnetic resonance spectroscopy. Br J Nutr. 2001;85 Suppl 2:S147-50.
20. Allen LH. Pregnancy and iron deficiency: unresolved issues. Nutr Rev. 1997;55(4):91-101.
21. Svanberg B, Arvidsson B, Norrby A, Rybo G, Sölvell L. Absorption of supplemental iron during pregnancy - a longitudinal study with repeated bone-marrow studies and absorption measurements. Acta Obstet Gynecol Scand Suppl. 1975;48:87-108.
22. SWachs TD, Pollitt E, Cueto S, Jacoby E, Creed-Kanashiro H. Relation of neonatal iron status to individual variability in neonatal temperament. Dev Psychobiol. 2005; 46(2):141-53.
23. Koller O. The clinical significance of hemodilution during pregnancy. Obstet Gynecol Surv. 1982;37(11):649-52.
24. Stoltzfus RJ, Dreyfuss ML. Guidelines for use of iron supplement to prevent and treat iron deficiency anaemia. Geneva: INACG, WHO, UNICEF, 1998.

CHAPTER 12

Anemia of Prematurity

Jayashree Mondkar

INTRODUCTION

Anemia of prematurity (AOP) is characterized by a decline in the hemoglobin concentration after birth in prematurely born babies. The anemia generally becomes manifested by 3–4 weeks of age and is often associated with manifestations that can be attributed to anemia.

ETIOPATHOGENESIS

Due to the relative hypoxic state *in utero*, the erythropoietin (EPO) levels in the fetus are high resulting in a larger RBC mass and hemoglobin at birth. After birth, due to improved blood and tissue oxygenation, the hypoxic stimulus for EPO ceases, as a result, the RBC mass and hemoglobin gradually decrease resulting in a state of relatively low hemoglobin. This state is termed as "physiological anemia" and is characteristically seen in the term baby by 8–12 weeks of life and is asymptomatic.[1] The hemoglobin generally drops from 17 g/dL to 19 g/dL at birth to 10–11.5 g/dL at the nadir of the anemia. Thereafter as tissue oxygenation reaches a critical point, EPO production starts and hemoglobin starts to rise again.

In preterm babies, the pathophysiology of the anemia is similar. However, the drop in hemoglobin starts earlier and the nadir is lower; hemoglobin often drops to 6–8 g/dL and occurs earlier by 4–6 weeks, especially in the more premature, extremely low-birth-weight (ELBW) babies. Babies are often symptomatic; hence, AOP is considered "nonphysiologic".[2] The principal cause of AOP is failure of the EPO levels to rise in response to anemia.[3] *In utero*, EPO is produced by the liver. In term babies with physiological anemia of infancy, switch to the renal production of EPO occurs, which is a far more sensitive mechanism for detecting low-tissue oxygenation than the hepatic mechanism that persists till 40 weeks gestational age. The blunted hepatic response in preterm babies results in a lower nadir of hemoglobin.[4] Increased metabolism of EPO in preterm babies has also been shown to be a mechanism causing AOP.[5]

Several additional factors contribute to the severity of AOP. The life span of RBCs in preterms is shorter 35–50 days in preterm babies compared to 60–70 days in term babies contributing to the anemia.[6] Additionally, repeated phlebotomy losses during the neonatal period contribute in a large way to early onset of anemia; deficiency of vitamin E, folic acid and iron are additional contributory factors.

CLINICAL FEATURES

Anemia of prematurity is associated with various manifestations, none of which are specific for this condition. Among the most common presenting features are pallor manifesting by the 3rd–4th weeks of life. Some preterms may present with failure to gain weight despite optimizing nutritional intake. Lethargy and poor activity may also be manifested due to anemia.

Cardiorespiratory manifestations in the form of tachypnea, tachycardia, and occasionally systolic murmurs may also occur. Late onset of apneas in the 3rd week or later is often manifestations of AOP and responds to packed cell transfusion.

INVESTIGATIONS

Complete Blood Count

Hemoglobin is low often as low as 6–8 g/dL.[7] The platelet and WBC counts are normal. Peripheral blood smear reveals a normochromic, normocytic anemia and the red cell indices are normal for age. The reticulocyte count is disproportionately low in relation to the degree of anemia due to the low EPO levels.[7]

DIFFERENTIAL DIAGNOSIS

Anemia mimicking AOP may occur in the following conditions:

- *Anemia due to intrauterine infections*: Parvovirus, syphilis and cytomegalovirus (CMV)

- Substrate deficiencies (e.g. iron, vitamin E and folic acid)
- Diamond-Blackfan anemia
- Disseminated intravascular coagulation with bleeding
- Hereditary spherocytosis, elliptocytosis
- G6PD deficiency, pyruvate kinase and isomerase deficiency
- Iatrogenic (e.g. excessive phlebotomy losses)
- Hemorrhage [e.g. gastrointestinal (GI), central nervous system, subcutaneous tissues].

MANAGEMENT

Red blood cell transfusions are the mainstay of management of AOP. Recombinant human erythropoietin (rHuEPO) has been tried but has not been successful in significantly reducing the need for RBC transfusions. Almost 95% of ELBW infants and 80% sick VLBW infants will need at least one transfusion.[5] RBC transfusion practices vary widely, though over the years more conservative approach toward RBC transfusion is practiced. Bell et al. studied 100 infants randomized to receive small-volume RBC transfusions as per either restricted (RES) or liberal (LIB) guidelines.[8] The guidelines were based on a combination of the pretransfusion hematocrit or hemoglobin level, age of the neonate, and clinical condition (i.e. need for ventilation, oxygen, etc.) at the time each transfusion was given. Infants in the liberal-transfusion group received more RBC transfusions [5.2 ± 4.5 (mean ± SD) versus 3.3 ± 2.9 in the restrictive-transfusion group]. However, the number of donors to whom the infants were exposed was not significantly different (2.8 ± 2.5 vs 2.2 ± 2.0) in the LIB versus the RES groups. There was also no difference between the groups in the percentage of infants who avoided transfusions altogether (12% in the liberal-transfusion group versus 10% in the restrictive-transfusion group). However, they observed that infants in the restrictive-transfusion group were more likely to have frequent episodes of mild-to-severe apnea, intraparenchymal hemorrhage or periventricular leukomalacia.

Kripalani et al. in a randomized study of 451 babies found fewer infants received one or more transfusions in the low-threshold group (89% low versus 95% high, *P=.037*); however, there was no significant difference between the groups for the composite primary outcome of death before home discharge or survival with any of either severe retinopathy, bronchopulmonary dysplasia, or brain injury on cranial ultrasound [74.0% in the low-hemoglobin threshold group and 69.7% in the high (*P = 0.25*; risk difference, 2.7%; 95% CI -3.7% to 9.2%)].[9]

Although there are no clear guidelines, some common indications for transfusion include the following:

Liberal Transfusion Guidelines[10]

- Replacing blood after more than 10% of the infant's blood volume has been removed
- Maintaining a hematocrit more than 35–40% in patients with severe respiratory distress or symptomatic heart disease
- Maintaining hematocrit more than 30% in neonates with mild-to-moderate cardiopulmonary problems, growth failure, or significant apnea, and/or
- Transfusing any asymptomatic infant with a hematocrit less than 21% and reticulocytes less than 3%.

Restrictive Transfusion Guidelines[11]

Transfusion should be considered:
- If acute blood loss of more than or equal to 10% associated with symptoms or if significant hemorrhage of more than or equal to 20% of total blood volume occurs.
- For infants requiring mechanical ventilation with mean airway pressure (MAP) more than 8 cm H_2O and fraction of inspired oxygen (FiO_2) more than 0.40 on a conventional ventilator, or MAP more than 14 and FiO_2 more than 0.40 on high-frequency ventilator, consider transfusion if hematocrit is less than or equal to 30% (hemoglobin ≤10 g/dL).
- For infants requiring mechanical ventilation with MAP less than or equal to 8 cm H_2O and/or FiO_2 less than or equal to 0.40, or MAP less than 14 and/or FiO_2 less than 0.40 on high frequency, consider transfusions, if the hematocrit is less than or equal to 25% (hemoglobin ≤8 g/dL).
- For infants on supplemental oxygen, not requiring mechanical ventilation, consider transfusion if hematocrit is less than or equal to 20% (hemoglobin ≤7 g/dL), and one or more of the following is present:
  - More than or equal to 24 hours of tachycardia (heart rate >180 beats/minute) or tachypnea [risk ratio (RR) >60 breaths/minute]
  - Doubling of the oxygen requirement from the previous 48 hours
  - Lactate more than or equal to 2.5 mEq/L or an acute metabolic acidosis (pH <7.20)
    - Weight gain less than 10 g/kg/day over the previous 4 days while receiving more than or equal to 120 kcal/kg/day.
    - Infant needing major surgery within next 72 hours.
- Asymptomatic infants, consider transfusion if the hematocrit is less than or equal to 18% (hemoglobin ≤ 6 g/dL) associated with an absolute reticulocyte count less than 100,000 cells/μL (<2%).
- Small volume of compatible packed cell transfusions of 10–15 mL/kg is administered. In order to minimize donor exposure, it is preferable to use dedicated stored units (satellite packs) of packed cells from the same donor for the same baby as far as possible.

Role of Recombinant Human Erythropoietin for Treatment of Anemia of Prematurity

As low level of EPO is postulated as a primary cause of AOP, exogenous EPO has been used in an effort to reduce the need for blood transfusions and multiple donor exposure. Several studies in the 1990s were reported regarding the use of rHuEPO for treatment of AOP with varying results. Different doses ranging from 70 IU/kg/week to 2,100 IU/kg/week along with oral iron in doses ranging from 2 mg/kg/week to 10 mg/kg/week have been used.[12] In a meta-analysis of EPO studies to reduce need for blood transfusions in 2001 though EPO significantly reduced RBC transfusion needs during the first few weeks of hospitalization inconclusive results were obtained and were not found to be of clinical importance.[13] A meta-analysis in 2012 regarding early (<8 days) use of EPO to prevent use of red cell transfusion in preterm and low-birth-weight babies, the total volume of RBC transfusions in mL/kg, the number of RBC transfusions per baby were reduced and the number of donor exposure was significantly reduced.[12] However, a nonsignificant increase in risk of stage 3 retinopathy of prematurity (ROP) or more was noted. On posthoc analysis, this was found to be significantly increased. In the meta-analysis to study the effect of late use of EPO between 8 days and 30 days, the authors concluded that late EPO does not significantly reduce or increase any clinically important adverse outcomes except for a trend in increased risk for ROP. The authors have recommended focusing on limiting donor exposure during the first few days of life in sick neonates, when RBC requirements are most likely to be required and cannot be prevented by late EPO treatment.[14] In view of variable results, EPO therapy is currently not considered a standard of care in AOP.

Clinical Practices that can Help to Reduce the Need for Blood Transfusions

Minimizing Phlebotomy Losses

Extremely low-birth-weight babies have a small circulating blood volume, this coupled with severe cardiorespiratory illness results in repeated blood sampling with phlebotomy losses mandating blood transfusions in the 1st week of life. Minimizing these losses by micro sampling methods and performing several tests on the same sample may help reduce the number of transfusions required.

Delayed Cord Clamping

Several trials have demonstrated benefit of delayed cord clamping (DCC) in premature neonates. Benefits include stabilize transitional circulation, lessening needs for inotropic medications, reducing need for blood transfusions, necrotizing enterocolitis and intraventricular hemorrhage.[15,16] The timing of "late" clamping time has varied in different studies from 30 seconds to 180 seconds after birth and positioning of the infant relative to the placenta or uterus before clamping. On an average, a 39% reduction in the need for blood transfusion in preterm babies was observed in with delayed umbilical cord clamping.[16]

Katheria et al. performed the first trial comparing umbilical cord milking (UCM) (stripping 4 times) with DCC (45–60 seconds) and demonstrated higher systemic blood flow with UCM in preterm neonates compared with DCC. They concluded that UCM may be a more efficient technique to improve blood volume in premature infants delivered by cesarean section.[17]

OPTIMIZING NUTRITIONAL SUPPORT

Iron Therapy

Maximum transplacental transfer of iron occurs in the third trimester of pregnancy; iron stores in the baby thus vary inversely with the gestational age at birth. Hence, preterm babies less than 32 weeks gestational age are more likely to manifest iron-deficiency anemia in the first 6 months especially those babies showing a rapid catch-up growth due to rapid depletion of tissue stores. Besides anemia, iron deficiency can cause poor growth, altered immunity and GI disturbances. All preterm babies need iron supplementation. Controversy exists whether iron supplements should be started early or late. In a small meta-analysis of 246 patients, early supplementation (by 3 weeks after birth) group was associated with significantly smaller decreases in serum ferritin and hemoglobin levels [the rate of blood transfusions compared with late iron supplementation (at or after 4 weeks)].[18] In another small study, Joy R et al. showed better serum ferritin and hemoglobin in the early supplemented group.[19] However, a word of caution that multiple transfusions may lead to increased iron with a potential for causing oxidant injury to tissues of preterm infants.[20]

The dose of oral iron for preterm infants not receiving EPO is 2–4 mg/kg/day depending on the degree of prematurity.[21] The American Academy of Pediatrics (AAP) recommends that the breastfed preterm infant receive at least 2 mg/kg/day of elemental iron supplementation beginning at 1 month of age until 12 months of age.[22] Iron-deficiency anemia is treated with oral iron dose of 3–6 mg/kg/day for 4 weeks.[23] Supplementation of preterm babies with vitamin B_{12} and folic acid also helps increase in hemoglobin.

In summary, AOP is an exaggeration of physiological anemia due to a variety of factors important among which is phlebotomy losses in tiny preterm babies. Babies are often symptomatic and need packed cell transfusions for the same. Restricting phlebotomy losses along with early iron administration may help reduction in the number of transfusions required. EPO has been found useful to reduce the number of transfusions but is not accepted as a standard of care.

REFERENCES

1. O'Brien RT, Pearson HA. Physiologic anemia of the newborn infant. J Pediatr. 1971;79(1):132-38.
2. Wardrop CA, Holland BM, Veale KE, Jones JG, Gray OP. Nonphysiological anemia of prematurity. Arch Dis Child. 1978;53(11):855-60.
3. Stockman JA 3rd, Graeber JE, Clark DA, McClellan K, Garcia JF, Kavey RE. Anemia of prematurity: determinants of the erythropoietin response. J Pediatr. 1984;105(5):786-92.
4. Dame C, Fahnenstich H, Freitag P, Hofmann D, Abdul-Nour T, Bartmann P, et al. Erythropoietin mRNA expression in human fetal and neonatal tissue. Blood. 1998;92(9):3218-25.
5. Widness JA, Veng-Pedersen P, Peters C, Pereira LM, Schmidt RL, Lowe LS. Erythropoietin pharmacokinetics in premature infants: developmental, nonlinearity, and treatment effects. J Appl Physiol. 1996;80(1):140-8.

6. Brugnara CP, Orah S. The neonatal erythrocyte and its disorders. In: Nathan DG, Orkin SH, Ginsburg D (Eds). Hematology of Infancy and Childhood. Philadelphia, PA, USA: WB Saunders; 2003.
7. Luchtman-Jones L, Wilson DB. Hematologic Problems in the Fetus and Neonate. In: Martin RJ, Fanaroff AA, Walsh MC, (Eds). Fanaroff and Martin's Neonatal-Perinatal Medicine, 9th edition. United States: Elsevier Mosby; 2011.pp.1303-60.
8. Bell EF, Strauss RG, Widness JA, Mahoney LT, Mock DM, Seward VJ, et al. Randomized trial of liberal versus restrictive guidelines for red blood cell transfusions in preterm infants. Pediatrics. 2005;115(6):1685-91.
9. Kirpalani H, Whyte RK, Andersen C, Asztalos EV, Heddle N, Blajchman MA, et al. The Premature Infants in Need of Transfusion (PINT) study: a randomized, controlled trial of a restrictive (low) versus liberal (high) transfusion threshold for extremely low birth weight infants. J Pediatr. 2006;149(3):301-7.
10. Strauss RG. Anemia of prematurity: Pathophysiology and treatment. Blood Rev. 2010;24(6):221-5.
11. Bishara N, Ohis RK. Current controversies in the management of the anemia of prematurity. Semin Perinatol. 2009;33(1):29-34.
12. Ohlsson A, Aher SM. Early erythropoietin for preventing red blood cell transfusion in preterm and/or low birth weight infants. Cochrane Database Syst Rev. 2014;(4):CD004863.
13. Vamvakas EC, Strauss RG. Meta-analysis of controlled clinical trials studying the efficacy of rHuEPO in reducing blood transfusions in the anemia of prematurity. Transfusion. 2001;41(3):406-15.
14. Aher SM, Ohlsson A. Late erythropoietin for preventing red blood cell transfusion in preterm and/or low birth weight infants. Cochrane Database Syst Rev. 2014;(4):CD004868.
15. Jelin AC, Zlatnik MG, Kuppermann M, Gregorich SE, Nakagawa S, Clyman R. Clamp late and maintain perfusion (CLAMP) policy: delayed cord clamping in preterm infants. J Matern Fetal Neonatal Med. 2016;29(11):1705-9.
16. Rabe H, Diaz-Rossello JL, Duley L, Dowswell T. Effect of timing of umbilical cord clamping and other strategies to influence placental transfusion at preterm birth on maternal and infant outcomes. Cochrane Database Syst Rev. 2012;(8):CD003248.
17. Katheria AC, Truong G, Cousins L, Oshiro B, Finer NN. Umbilical cord milking versus delayed cord clamping in preterm infants. Pediatrics. 2015;136(1):61-9.
18. Joy R, Krishnamurthy S, Bethou A, Rajappa M, Ananthanarayanan PH, Bhat BV. Early versus late enteral prophylactic iron supplementation in preterm very low birth weight infants: a randomised controlled trial. Arch Dis Child Fetal Neonatal Ed. 2014;99(2):F105-9.
19. Jin HX, Wang RS, Chen SJ, Wang AP, Liu XY. Early and late iron supplementation for low birth weight infants: a meta-analysis. Ital J Pediatr. 2015;41:16.
20. Inder TE, Clemett RS, Austin NC, Graham P, Darlow BA. High iron status in very low birth weight infants is associated with an increased risk of retinopathy of prematurity. J Pediatr. 1997;131(4):541-4.
21. Iron fortification of infant formulas. American Academy of Pediatrics. Committee on Nutrition. Pediatrics. 1999;104(1 Pt 1):119-23.
22. Georgieff RR. Micro minerals. In: Tsang RC, Uauy R, Koletzko B (Eds). Nutrition of the Preterm Infant: Scientific Basis and Practical Guidelines, 3rd edition. Cincinnati, Ohio: Digital Educational Publishing, 2005.
23. American Academy of Pediatrics (AAP), Committee on Nutrition. Iron deficiency. In: Kleinman RE (Ed). Pediatric Nutrition Handbook, 5th edition. Elk Grove Village, Ill: American Academy of Pediatrics; 2004.

CHAPTER

13

Clinical Aspect of Immune Hemolytic Disease of Newborn

ATK Rau, Soundarya M, Aarathi R Rau

INTRODUCTION

Immune hemolytic disease of the newborn had initially been described in literature with the clinical features of only RhD isoimmunization, a common disease (especially in the West) occurring in Rh-positive infants born to Rh-negative mothers and resulting in high neonatal morbidity and mortality. As similar clinical diseases were later found even in Rh-positive mothers and infants, further research into blood group systems and isoimmunization progressed rapidly over the years resulting now in the identification and characterization of almost 35 incriminating blood group systems as reported by the International Society of Blood Transfusion in 2012.[1] This chapter deals with immune hemolytic disease of newborn (IHDN) with respect to each of the blood group systems beginning with the Rh system.

Rh BLOOD GROUP SYSTEM AND Rh ISOIMMUNIZATION

Historical Background

Immune hemolytic disease in the newborn (IHDN) was first described in Western literature as early as in 1609 but was studied in some detail and termed erythroblastosis fetalis in 1932 by Diamond and colleagues.[2] Levine and Stetson[3] described the process of RBC surface antigen sensitization in a woman following the birth of a stillborn infant in 1939 in which the earliest association of maternal sensitization due to fetal RBC's was made. The Rh system in its entirety was described by Landsteiner and Wiener[4] in 1940, a Nobel prize winning effort, following, which rapid strides in research has identified more than 30 RBC antigens, which can cause similar disease even in Rh-positive mothers **(Figs 13.1A and B)**. In 1954, Chown et al. reported that sensitization of the mother to fetal antigens occurred mainly during the delivery process due to transplacental hemorrhage[5] and many further studies showed that maternal sensitization to fetal antigens could be countered by antibodies given to the mother, leading to the use of RhD immunoglobulin to prevent isoimmunization in future pregnancies. Further research has led to other options like exchange transfusions and intrauterine transfusions in the management of the newborn with IHDN and have drastically changed the outcomes of such pregnancies over the last 4–5 decades.

Rh Blood Group System

The Rh blood group system includes almost 45 antigens, of which the most common encountered in clinical practice are the "D", "C", "c", "E" and "e". There is no Rh "d" antigen and Rh-negativity is defined as the absence of the RhD antigen. The proteins coded by the RhD and the Rh C and E genes are nonglycosylated palmitoylated integral membrane proteins on the surface of the RBC. These are responsible for maintaining the shape of the RBC along with the functional integrity of the RBC cell membrane. This identification explains the findings in some Rh-deficient (who do not possess any type of Rh antigens, i.e. Rh null) individuals in whom stomatocytosis, spherocytosis and chronic hemolysis

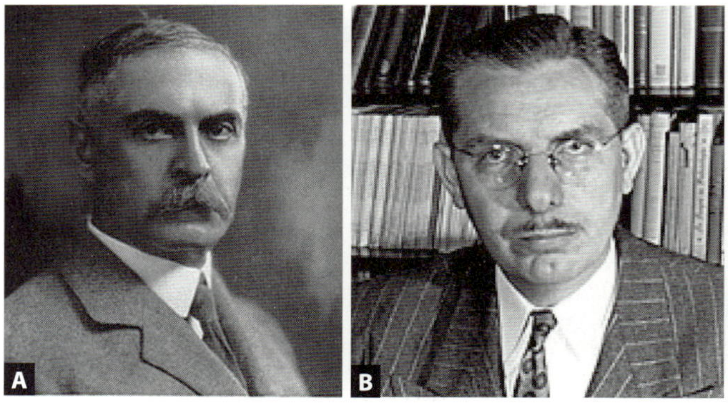

Figures 13.1A and B (A) K Landsteiner; (B) Alexander Wiener

of varying severity have been seen. This is because of the deficient linkage of the Rh complex with the spectrin-based RBC membrane skeleton causing significant membrane dysfunction, which highlights the significance of this protein.[6] In between these two groups of Rh-positive and Rh null individuals lie the "weak" and partial D phenotypes. Weak D and partial D type imply reduced number of antigenic sites on the RBCs and the failure of the RBCs to react with some of the monoclonal anti-D antibodies respectively. To encompass these two variants and their overlapping types the term aberrant "D" has been proposed.[5] These subgroups can also cause significant reactions in transfusion and during pregnancy.

Incidence

The incidence of Rh isoimmunization varies from 5% to 15% and depends upon the widely different prevalence of the Rh-negative antigen in the population among countries and among between different population groups in the same country.[7] The incidence of Rh sensitization also differs with the ABO status of the fetus. In ABO compatible Rh-positive pregnancies, the incidence of Rh sensitization is as high as 8% without anti-D prophylaxis[8] in contrast to ABO incompatible Rh-positive pregnancies where the incidence is only 1.5–2%,[9] suggesting that ABO incompatibility provides partial protection against Rh sensitization. This protection occurs only in the first pregnancy and has no influence on later gestations.[9] Estimated perinatal mortality without antenatal diagnosis and treatment is reported to be approximately 17.5% with 14% of the deaths being stillborn.[10] After the introduction of postnatal anti-D immune prophylaxis, this incidence has reduced to 1–2% and these benefits incur irrespective of the ABO status of the baby. Immune prophylaxis, if started antenatally and continued postnatally, has brought down the incidence even further to 0.1%.[11,12] However, Chávez and colleagues have reported that the anticipated massive reduction in the incidence of Rh isoimmunization worldwide has not occurred despite anti-D therapy being advocated universally for the last so many years[13] and poor compliance to the protocol and the nonavailability of anti-D in many countries may be the reasons. Safety issues of anti-D, being a blood product, have resulted in the accelerated search for monoclonal antibodies many of which are under trials today.[14]

ETIOPATHOGENESIS

The pathogenesis of Rh isoimmunization occurs in three phases:

- *1st phase*: Maternal alloimmunization.
- *2nd phase*: Antibody transfer to fetus.
- *3rd phase*: Fetal response.

Maternal Alloimmunization

This can occur as a result of spontaneous transplacental hemorrhage during any of the three trimesters of pregnancy. The Rh antigen is expressed by the fetal cells as early as 30–45 days postconception and being a very potent immunogen, very small quantities (0.1 to 1 mL) of fetal cells can stimulate maternal antibody production.[15] The risk of this sensitization increases when the volume of transplacental hemorrhage increases as in situations like antepartum-hemorrhage, toxemia of pregnancy, cesarean sections,[16] external version[17] and manual removal of placenta. The number of fetal cells entering the maternal blood at delivery and causing sensitization has traditionally been determined by the Kleihauer test on maternal blood. While most studies done on this topic have only focused upon how the maternal circulation and hematological system reacts to the exposure to fetal antigens, other maternal tissues may also show equally strong but different responses when exposed to fetal cells. Many of these are yet to be identified.

Antibody Transfer to the Fetus

This occurs maximally during delivery when there is significant maternofetal bleeding but can also occur at any time during the pregnancy. Though initially maternal antibodies of the immunoglobulin M (IgM) class are formed which do not cross the placenta, later immune response is antibodies of the IgG class which do. Here they bind to the RBC surface membrane resulting in the extravascular destruction of the RBC in the reticuloendothelial organs. Anti-D antibodies do not bind to complement unlike the anti-A and B antibodies but the significance of this is unknown. The other mechanisms of RBC destruction include antibody-dependent cellular cytotoxicity and lysis by natural killer (NK) cells. The severity of RBC destruction is dependent on the nature of the antigen and the antibody characteristics:

- Nature of the antigen:
  - The antigens, which are almost exclusively present on erythroid cells like the Rh antigens, have a greater potential of causing IHDN than those antigens, like the A and B antigens, which are distributed on other tissues as well.
  - The antigens must be present and expressed in the fetus and neonate. Hence, while the Rh and Kell antigens, which are expressed early in gestation, cause severe HDN, the Lewis antigen, which is expressed only postnatally almost never causes IHDN.
  - *Antigen density*: Higher the titers of the maternal anti-D antibody, the greater is the potential to cause hemolysis in the fetus, though this is not applicable if the fetus has an aberrant D phenotype.
  - *Antigen structure*: Some antigens promote the recognition by and presentation of the RBC to the phagocytic cells and hence hasten hemolysis.
- *Characteristics of antibody*:
  - The presence of particular subclasses of IgG antibodies plays a significant role in determining the severity of the isoimmunization and consequently the hemolysis. The anti-A and anti-B antibodies are of the IgG 2 subtype while anti-D antibodies are of the IgG1 and IgG3

Flow chart 13.1 Pathophysiology explaining the evolution of the clinical features in IHDN

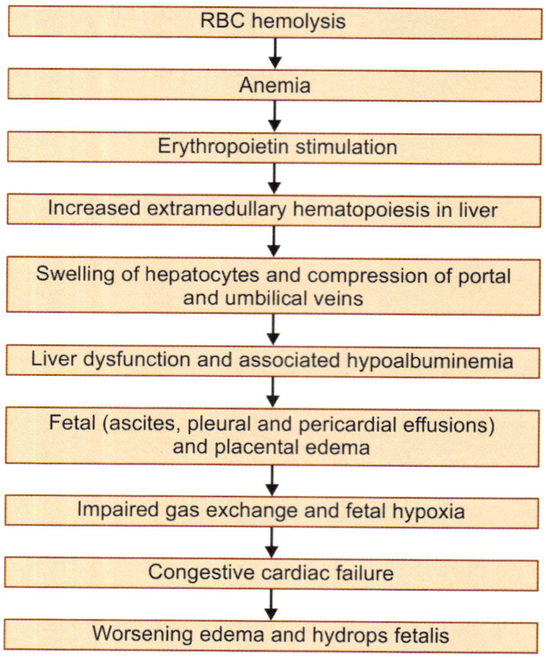

subtypes. The tenacity and binding capacity of the IgG3 subtype is much more than the others which causes more efficient and severe hemolysis.
  - Antibody structure and density too play a role in the severity of hemolysis.

Fetal Response

Erythropoiesis begins in the fetal yolk sac by the 3rd week of gestation and ends by the 7th–8th weeks when the liver takes over and continues till late into the third trimester after which it occurs almost entirely in the bone marrow. The first expression of the Rh antigens occurs by the 6th week of intrauterine life. Fetal RBCs are at risk of destruction from maternal antibodies at any time during pregnancy, which then leads to fetal anemia, which stimulates erythropoiesis via erythropoietin and other growth factors resulting in the enhanced presence of early immature nucleated RBCs, i.e. erythroblasts in the circulation, giving the name of erythroblastosis fetalis **(Flow chart 13.1)**.

Summary of the pathophysiology and the genesis of clinical features—(Details of the pathogenesis has been detailed in **Flow chart 13.1**).

CLINICAL FEATURES

The main triad of symptoms in infants with immune hemolytic disease is jaundice, pallor and enlargement of the liver and spleen. The degree of the anemia and jaundice decides the severity of the hemolysis and is classified as:

- *Mild HDN*: Where the infant is born with either minimal or no anemia, does not develop significant icterus and exchange transfusion is only rarely required.
- *Moderate HDN*: These fetuses usually have anemia *in utero*, which is reflected after birth but they do not show features of hydrops. They can develop significant icterus and hence are at risk of kernicterus and thus require frequent monitoring, intensive phototherapy and at times exchange transfusion.
- *Severe HDN*: These are infants who are born with hydrops. There is usually associated polyhydramnios, which is seen at the onset of hydrops. Over the ensuing weeks ascites, pleural and pericardial effusions also develop, which when massive can cause compressive hypoplasia of the lungs and result in deficient oxygenation at birth. It is in these infants that the term hydrops fetalis is used. The outcome without intensive supportive management is poor.

  There can also be late and chronic anemia due to continued erythrocyte destruction in some mild-to-moderately affected newborns manifesting as cardiac failure as late as 21 days of life. This is because of the presence of the anti-D Ig in the baby's blood. Petechiae and purpura with features of early disseminated intravascular coagulation (DIC) may also be seen at times in this disorder, due hepatic dysfunction and consequent clotting factor deficiency.[18]

DIAGNOSIS OF IMMUNE HEMOLYTIC DISEASE IN THE NEWBORN

Investigations are divided into:

- Those that identify fetuses at risk for IHDN
- Those that determine the severity of the IHDN.
- To identify fetuses at risk for IHDN:
  - *Maternal blood grouping and Rh typing*: It is done at the first antenatal visit. In those who are D negative or weakly D positive and if the father is D positive, antibody screening and titers at 24–28 weeks of gestation is required.
  - *Paternal blood typing*: This is done whenever the mother is Rh-negative. If the father if Rh-positive, fetal blood typing is essential.
  - *Fetal blood typing*: In cases where there is a high index of suspicion of incompatibility and the fetus is at a risk of developing HDN as mentioned above, fetal cells are tested either by performing amniocentesis or chorionic villus sampling. These procedures do carry an inherent risk of worsening maternal sensitization and are usually done by 18–20 weeks of gestation. However, when there is history of a previously affected fetus or ultrasound evidence of fetal hydrops, earlier intervention and diagnosis may be needed.
- To identify the severity of the disease by:
  - *Maternal history*: In Rh-negative mothers, history of a previously affected fetus or bad obstetric history should lower the threshold for monitoring fetal well-being. The first pregnancy is usually the least affected and subsequent pregnancies are likely to be increasingly affected, if the baby is incompatible.
  - *Maternal antibody testing and titers*: The indirect antiglobin or the indirect Coombs test is done using the Coombs serum (the test result is interpreted

as the maximum dilution of the maternal serum that causes fetal RBC agglutination and detects the antibodies circulating in the maternal blood). The higher the dilution of the maternal serum that causes agglutination, more significant is the fetomaternal hemorrhage and chances of subsequent sensitization. The titers of these antibodies can be estimated using an auto analyzer that has been standardized to identify a critical titer, above which the fetus is deemed at risk. Rising titers in a mother with a bad obstetric history requires urgent fetal assessment and monitoring.

- *Amniotic fluid analysis and spectrophotometry*: Amniocentesis is performed under ultrasound guidance and the fluid, normally clear, may be colored yellow because of the bile pigment released from hemolyzed RBCs. Fetal blood group and DNA from the fetal cells in the amniotic fluid are identified and analyzed. If the fetus types as Rh-positive and shows signs of hemolysis, the amniotic fluid optical density is measured in a spectrophotometer and the results are interpreted as per the Queenan and Liley[19] graph which reveals fetal outcomes based on amniotic fluid spectrophotometry identified as a deviation from the 450 nm line due to the adsorption spectrum of bilirubin (delta OD450). Further, based on severity, three zones are identified where in the risk of developing pathological jaundice and the requirement for exchange transfusion is plotted. The readings in zone 1 reflect an unaffected or mildly affected fetus with no anemia while zone 2 indicates a moderately affected fetus. The disease severity increases as the readings fall closer to zone 3 and readings falling in zone 3 indicate severe disease with hydrops either already present or at a risk of developing it over the next 10 days.
- *Ultrasound*: The use of the ultrasound with the incorporation of the ultrasound Doppler has emerged as a very useful tool for fetal assessment and therapy. Routine obstetric ultrasound is done to assess the fetal size, fetal liver, placenta and as a guide for procedures, both diagnostic and therapeutic. The ultrasound Doppler is used to measure the flow velocities in the major fetal vessels, which has been found to be a reliable indicator of fetal anemia. The middle cerebral artery flow velocimetry is currently the most extensively used parameter.[20]
- *Percutaneous fetal blood sampling*: The development of sophisticated ultrasound and skills have paved the way for percutaneous fetal blood sampling from the umbilical vein at its junction with the placenta from the 18th–21st weeks of gestation. This allows for direct diagnosis of fetal blood group, hemoglobin levels and other metabolic parameters. Despite the risks of being an invasive procedure, it is still the procedure of choice for fetal diagnosis.[21]
- *Neonatal analysis in an infant born with suspected IHDN*: At birth, hemoglobin and bilirubin levels from the cord blood are analyzed for determining the severity of hemolysis. The peripheral smear in these children will show increased number of nucleated RBCs, polychromasia and anisocytosis. The most important confirmatory test remains the direct antiglobin test or the direct Coombs test, which tests the sensitization of the fetal cells using the Coombs reagent. A positive result confirms fetal hemolysis but this must be interpreted along with clinical findings. Regular monitoring of the infant's hemoglobin and bilirubin levels are done subsequently to determine therapeutic interventions and transfusion needs.

MANAGEMENT OF Rh ISOIMMUNIZATION

Management of Maternal Alloimmunization

Prevention of alloimmunization is done by giving anti-D immunoglobulin antenatally between the 28th week and 34th week of gestation.[8,22] While this has been found to have significant benefits in reducing the antibody response in subsequent pregnancies, it may not be very useful in the current pregnancy[23] and is also not significantly cost effective.[24]

Treatment of the established alloimmunization wherein the risk to the fetus is high has few options—plasmapheresis may be used to remove the antibodies that have the potential to cross the placenta but due to the inherent risks of this procedure, its benefits still remain to be proven. High-dose intravenous immunoglobulin (IVIG) has been tried in severely alloimmunized mothers but as the treatment must begin by the end of the first trimester, its risk and cost benefit ratios are yet to be established.[25]

Fetal Therapy

Once the fetus has been proven to be affected, intrauterine transfusion is the management of choice. These begin at 20–22 weeks of gestation and continue as required till the fetus is mature enough for delivery. These can be given either as intraperitoneal transfusions (IPTs) wherein the blood is placed in the peritoneal cavity of the fetus or as intravascular transfusions (IVTs) wherein the blood is transfused into the fetus through a placental or umbilical blood vessel. IVT is preferred as it allows for diagnostic sampling and is very rapidly effective in treating fetal anemia and reversing hydrops. Recent reports suggest that almost 87% of patients with isoimmune anemia have been salvaged with this intervention.[26] Blood should be O negative packed RBCs, cytomegalovirus (CMV) negative, less than 7 days old, compatible with maternal serum, leukocyte depleted and irradiated. Fetal hemoglobin is measured before and after the transfusion till a target level is reached. Complications like premature labor, cord hematomas, infections and bleeding can occur and hence skilled personnel and tertiary care centers are needed to perform IVT.

Neonatal Management

At delivery, the newborn should be carefully examined for hemodynamic instability, pallor, jaundice, organomegaly and petechiae. Management of the hydropic infant may need surfactant therapy, mechanical ventilation, albumin infusions and treatment of the associated ascites, effusions and cardiac failure. Even the mildly affected infant needs careful monitoring and anticipatory management. Cord blood is sent for estimation of hemoglobin, hematocrit, bilirubin levels, direct Coombs (antiglobin) test and reticulocyte count. Any cord blood hemoglobin value less than 11 g/dL or a cord bilirubin level more than 4.5 mg/dL is an indicator for exchange transfusion.[27] In infants whose values do not initially reach the above levels, frequent serial estimation of serum bilirubin is done. Phototherapy is started early as it is very effective in preventing exchange transfusions in many of these infants and is stopped when the bilirubin values show a steady falling trend. Exchange transfusion is the mainstay in the management of rapidly rising serum bilirubin levels. Here the antibody-coated RBCs are replaced by donor RBCs uncoated by the sensitizing antigen, which then halts the hemolysis, corrects the anemia and prevents further hyperbilirubinemia. Exchange transfusions are carried out at birth in severely affected fetuses or in other high-risk infants when the serum bilirubin rises at the rate of more than 0.4–0.6 mg/dL/hour (8–13 μmol/L/hour) despite intensive phototherapy in full-term infants.[28] A double volume (130–170 mL/kg body weight) exchange transfusion is traditionally performed during, which approximately 90% of the affected RBCs are removed. However, the procedure removes only 30% of the total bilirubin, as bilirubin is sequestered in the extravascular spaces and tissues and hence a rebound rise of bilirubin may occur after 6–8 hours of the procedure warranting frequent monitoring and continued phototherapy. The main complications of exchange transfusion are the same as with any transfusion and additionally complications of the catheter and technique may also occur. Necrotizing enterocolitis (NEC) is a potentially dangerous complication related to the technique and avoidance of rapid and wide pulse pressure and volume changes during the procedure minimizes its risk. It is obvious that best results are obtained when the procedure is done in a tertiary care unit with a well-equipped blood bank.

Apart from management of the IHDN, all the infants must be breastfed and started on folic acid at the dose of 100–200 μg per day continued for several weeks, as folate reserves are less in the newborn and exchange transfusion replaces neonatal blood with adult blood that has less folate.[29]

Follow-up Care

Despite the initial presentation, follow-up care of the infant with hemolytic disease is important as late anemia can develop. Hemoglobin levels should be checked regularly at 2–3 weekly intervals till the infant is 3 months old. If anemic, a small volume transfusion of cross-matched, packed RBCs compatible with the infant's blood is given in the dose of 10–15 mL/kg. Folic acid and at times vitamin B_{12} supplementation are continued till 6 months of age.

ABO BLOOD GROUP SYSTEM AND ABO HEMOLYTIC DISEASE

ABO hemolytic disease results from the interaction between maternal anti-A or anti-B antibodies on fetal erythrocytes of the same blood group. The ABO IHDN is different from the Rh IHDN in that, unlike in adults, where ABO mismatched blood transfusions can cause violent life-threatening reactions, in the fetus, ABO IHDN is a relatively milder condition, rarely contributing to anemia and hydrops. The reasons for this are:

- The anti-A and anti-B antibodies are often of the IgA, IgM or IgG2 class, which either do not cross the placenta or play a minor role in the development of IHDN.
- There are fewer A or B antigenic sites on the RBC membrane as these antigens are not restricted to the erythrocyte and are distributed on many other tissues as well.
- The IgG antibodies that do cross the placenta bind not only to the RBC antigens but also to the tissue antigens and hence reduce the extent of hemolysis.
- There are also soluble blood group A and B substances in the fetal and newborn blood that neutralize the transplacentally transmitted antibodies.

The ABO IHDN is found to be more frequent in O Rh-positive mothers with A or B fetuses than with any other combination[30] and of these O-A incompatibility occurs more frequently than O-B incompatibility because the A antigen is the 7s fraction of the gamma globulin (lower molecular weight) while the B antigen is the 17s fraction of the gamma globulin (higher MW) and hence relatively poorly transmitted across the placenta. It is thus routine practice in some institutions to assess the newborn's blood group from the cord blood in all infants born to O Rh-positive mothers to identify "at risk" newborns, as is done in Rh-negative mothers.

Clinical Features and Investigations

Jaundice occurring on the 1st day of life in infants of Rh-positive mothers is usually the characteristic of ABO IHDN and is confirmed once other causes of hyperbilirubinemia are ruled out. Anemia is not as common as in Rh IHDN. Peripheral blood films show increased number of spherocytes and an elevated reticulocyte count. Coombs test may be negative or weakly positive but this is not specific for ABO IHDN as it may occur even in nonaffected infants.

Management

The principles of management are similar to Rh IHDN with phototherapy and frequent monitoring of serum bilirubin as the modalities. Exchange transfusion is only rarely needed and the risks of late anemia are much lesser than in Rh IHDN.

Hemolytic Disease due to Minor Blood Group Incompatibility

The prevalence of minor blood group incompatibility in pregnancy is reported to be around 0.15–1.1%.[31] This is usually due to anti-E, anti-c and anti-K (Kell) antibodies and cases have been reported of severe IHDN and hydrops due to these antibodies[32,33] as well as due to multiple maternal antibodies.[34] Other blood groups associated with hemolytic disease of the newborn include Duffy and Kidd. In contrast, some minor antigens like Lewis and others never cause IHDN because of the reduced number of these antigenic sites on the fetal cells or absorption of the antibodies by the fetal antigens on the placenta.[35] Nevertheless, ideally, it is recommended that screening of all pregnancies for all blood group antibodies be done once in pregnancy before the 34th week of gestation and fetal blood testing for evidence of hemolysis and blood typing be done in case the father is heterozygous for the offending antigen.

Immune Hemolytic Anemia Following Maternal Causes

In certain conditions, maternal autoimmune hemolytic anemia or lupus erythematosus during pregnancy may cause neonatal hemolytic disease due to passive transfer of antibodies to the fetus. This is suspected in the absence of blood group incompatibility and a positive direct Coombs (antiglobin) test in the clinical setting of IHDN. Treatment of the mother with prednisolone reduces the maternal hemolysis and therefore fetal and neonatal morbidity.[36] Rarely, drugs like penicillin, cephalosporin and alpha methyldopa (Aldomet) given to the mother have been implicated in causing drug-induced immune hemolysis in the newborn, which usually reverses when drug levels fall after delivery.

CONCLUSION

Immune hemolytic disease in the newborn is a significant contributor to neonatal morbidity and mortality. Though Rh incompatibility is the most widely prevalent and usually most severe disease of this group, other incompatibilities including those between minor blood groups also play a role in the etiopathogenesis of this disorder. While prevention is certainly better than cure, early detection of incompatibility status in pregnancy and subsequent intervention can greatly improve fetal outcomes. Fetal therapy is now a part of standard care in advanced countries while phototherapy and exchange transfusion remains the standard in ours. Latest research into this field offers exciting possibilities ahead.

REFERENCES

1. Table of blood group systems v 4.0 141125. International Society of Blood Transfusion, Oct 2012. http://www.genenames.org/
2. Diamond L, Blackfan K, Baty J. Erythroblastosis fetalis and its associations with universal edema of the fetus, icterus gravis neonatorum and anemia of the newborn. J Pediatr. 1932;1:269-309.
3. Levine P, Stetson RE. Landmark article July 8, 1939. An unusual case of intra-group agglutination. By Philip Levine and Rufus E Stetson. JAMA. 1984;251(10):1316-7.
4. Landsteiner K, Wiener A. An agglutinable factor in human blood recognized by immune sera for rhesus blood. Proc Soc Exp Biol Med. 1940;43:223-4.
5. Chown B. Anemia from bleeding of the fetus into the mother's circulation. Lancet. 1954;266(6824):1213-5.
6. Prasad MR, Krugh D, Rossi KQ, O'Shaughnessy RW. Anti-D in Rh positive pregnancies. Am J Obstet Gynecol. 2006;195(4):1158-62.
7. Daniels G, Green C, Smart E. Differences between RhD-negative Africans and RhD-negative Europeans. Lancet. 1997;350(9081):862-3.
8. Bowman J. Thirty-five years of Rh prophylaxis. Transfusion. 2003;43(12):1661-6.
9. Woodrow J. Rh immunization and its prevention. The immune response in the mother. In: Jensen K, Killman S (Eds). Series Haematologica, volume III. Copenhagen, Munksgaard; 1970. p. 3.
10. Zipursky A. Hemolytic anemia of the newborn. In: Nathan DG, Oski FA (Eds). Hematology of Infancy and Childhood. Philadelphia, PA, USA: WB Saunders; 1974. pp. 46-99.
11. Kinnock S, Liley AW. The epidemiology of severe hemolytic disease of newborn. N Z Med J 1970;71(453):76-83.
12. Liumbruno GM, D'Alessandro A, Rea F, Piccinini V, Catalano L, Calizzani G, et al. The role of antenatal immunoprophylaxis in the prevention of maternal-foetal anti-Rh(D) alloimmunisation. Blood Transfus. 2010;8(1):8-16.
13. Chávez GF, Mulinare J, Edmonds LD. Epidemiology of Rh hemolytic disease of the newborn in the United States. JAMA. 1991;265(24):3270-4.
14. Scott ML, Voak D. Monoclonal antibodies to Rh D-development and uses. Vox Sang. 2000;78 Suppl 2:79-82.
15. Carton JP. Rh blood group system and the molecular basis of Rh-deficiency. Baillieres Best Pract Res Clin Haematol. 1999;12(4):655-89.
16. Feldman N, Skoll A, Sibai B. The incidence of significant fetomaternal hemorrhage in patients undergoing cesarean section. Am J Obstet Gynaecol. 1990;163(3):855-8.
17. Lau TK, Lo KW, Chan LY, Leung TY, Lo YM. Cell-free fetal deoxyribonucleic acid in maternal circulation as a marker of fetal-maternal hemorrhage in patients undergoing external cephalic versions near term. Am J Obstet Gynaecol. 2000;183(3):712-6.
18. Chessells JM, Wigglesworth JS. Hemostatic failure in babies with rhesus isoimmunization. Arch Dis Child. 1971;46(245):38-45.
19. Queenan JT, Tomai TP, Ural SH, King JC. Deviation in the amniotic fluid optical density at a wavelength of 450 nm in Rh-immunized pregnancies from 14 to 40 weeks' gestation: a proposal for clinical management. Am J Obstet Gynecol. 1993;168(5):1370-6.
20. Whitecar PW, Moise KJ Jr. Sonographic methods to detect fetal anemia in red blood cell alloimmunization. Obstet Gynecol Surv. 2000;55(4):240-50.
21. Daffos F, Capella-Pavlovsky M, Forestier F. Fetal blood sampling during pregnancy. In: Nathan DG, Oski FA (Eds). Hematology of Infancy and Childhood. Philadelphia, PA, USA: WB Saunders; 2003. p. 72.
22. Fung Kee Fung K, Eason E, Crane J, Armson A, De La Ronde S, Farine D, et al. Prevention of Rh alloimmunisation. J Obstet Gynaecol. 2003;25(9):765-73.

23. de Silva M, Contreras M, Mollison PL. Failure of passively administered anti-Rh to prevent secondary Rh responses. Vox Sang. 1985;48(3):178-80.
24. Torrance GW, Zipursky A. Cost-effectiveness of antepartum prevention of Rh immunization. Clin Perinatol. 1984;11(2):267-81.
25. Porter TF, Silver RM, Jackson GM, Branch DW, Scott JR. Intravenous immune globulin in the management of severe Rh D hemolytic disease. Obstet Gynecol Surv. 1997;52(3):193-7.
26. Grannum PA, Copel JA, Moya FR, Scioscia AL, Robert JA, Winn HN. The reversal of hydrops fetalis by intravascular intrauterine transfusions in severe isoimmune fetal anemia. Am J Obstet Gynecol. 1988;158(4):914-9.
27. Zipursky A, Bowman JM. Isoimmune hemolytic diseases. In: Nathan DG, Oski FA (Eds). Hematology of Infancy and Childhood. Philadelphia, PA, USA: WB Saunders; 1993. pp. 44-73.
28. Wennberg RP, Depp R, Heinrichs WL. Indications for early exchange transfusion in patients with erythroblastosis fetalis. J Pediatr. 1978;92(5):789-92.
29. Purugganan G, Leikin S, Gautier G. Isoimmune hemolytic diseases. In: Nathan DG, Oski FA (Eds). Hematology of Infancy and Childhood. Philadelphia, PA, USA: WB Saunders; 2009. pp. 87-99.
30. Ozolek JA, Watchko JF, Mimouni F. Prevalence and lack of clinical significance of blood group incompatibility in mothers with blood type A or B. J Pediatr. 1994;125(1):87-91.
31. Judd WJ; Scientific Section Coordinating Committee of the AABB. Practice guidelines for prenatal and perinatal immunohematology, revisited. Transfusion. 2001;41(11): 1445-52.
32. Kornstad L. New cases of irregular blood group antibodies other than anti-D in pregnancy. Frequency and clinical significance. Acta Obstet Gynecol Scand. 1983;62(5):431-6.
33. Poole J, Daniels G. Blood group antibodies and their significance in transfusion medicine. Transfus Med Rev. 2007;21(1):58-71.
34. Markham KB, Rossi KQ, Nagaraja HN, O'Shaughnessy RW. Hemolytic disease of the fetus and newborn due to multiple maternal antibodies. Am J Obstet Gynecol. 2015;213(1):68.e1-5.
35. Reid ME, Chandrasekaran V, Sausais L, Pierre J, Bullock R. Disappearance of antibodies to Cromer blood group system antigens during mid-pregnancy. Vox Sang. 1996;71(1):48-50.
36. Schick P. Hemolytic anemia-immune hemolysis. In: Besa EC (Ed). Avery's Textbook of the Newborn, 8th edition; 2005. p. 1192.

CHAPTER 14

Laboratory Management of ABO and Rh Hemolytic Disease of the Fetus and Newborn

Snehalata C Gupte

INTRODUCTION

Hemolytic disease of the newborn (HDN) is the condition in which infant's red blood cell (RBC) life span is shortened. The shortened RBC life span could be due to immune or nonimmune-mediated hemolysis. Blood group antigens are expressed on the surface of erythrocyte membrane as proteins, glycoproteins or glycolipids. The Committee on Terminology of Red Cell Antigens of International Society of Blood Transfusion has recognized 36 blood group systems in the year 2015, consisting 346 antigens. Red cell antigens have potential to produce immune antibodies when a woman is exposed to foreign antigen. Maternal alloimmunization against the fetal blood group antigens of father's origin is responsible for immune hemolysis.

PATHOPHYSIOLOGY OF HEMOLYTIC DISEASE OF THE NEWBORN

ABO HDN shows a spectrum of severity but in majority of the cases it is mild because ABH antigens are not fully developed at birth. Rarely hydrops fetalis is reported,[1] therefore it is important to detect severe ABO HDN cases in the antenatal. Generally, Rh D antibodies cause severe most hemolytic disease of the fetus and newborn (HDFN). Women having partial or weak D antigen also have a potential to develop anti-D, hence determining correct Rh D status is important. Besides D antigen other antigens of Rh system like C, e, E, e and compound antigens like Ce, cE, ce can also produce antibodies and responsible for severe HDN. This article will deal with laboratory management of ABO and Rh HDFN.

ABO HEMOLYTIC DISEASE OF THE NEWBORN

Halbrecht described a concept "icterus precox" to designate jaundice arising during the first 24 hours of life unlike physiological jaundice. During the years after his report, HDN was reported in number of cases due to ABO incompatibility. ABO HDN occurs almost exclusively in the ABO incompatible infants born to O group women. Severity of the disease varies in different populations.[2]

Origin of ABO Antibodies

ABO blood group system significantly differs from other systems as all normal, healthy individuals have antibodies to ABO antigens they lack on their red cells. These naturally occurring IgM antibodies exist since birth, as a rule. Bacteria are chemically similar to human ABO antigens and serve as a continuous source of antigenic stimulus. Association between vaccination and increase in anti-A/anti-B levels is well established.[3,4] The ABH antigens are present in majority of living organisms and everybody is exposed to them. Therefore, IgG anti-A and/or anti-B antibodies are present in all individuals except AB group persons. Thus, mother already has IgG antibodies when she is pregnant and her first-born ABO incompatible infant has the risk of ABO HDN. However, it may not occur in subsequent pregnancies.[5]

INCIDENCE

About 25–30% pregnancies are usually ABO incompatible but all incompatible infants are not affected with HDN. The overall incidence of ABO HDN is about 1 in 150–200 pregnancies.[5,6] HDN more frequently occurs in A group infants of "O" mothers than B group infants of "O" mothers. Rare cases of ABO HDN in ABO incompatible infants born to A or B group mothers are reported.[5,6] Risk of ABO HDN increases twofold in mothers receiving tetanus toxoid injections during pregnancy.[7]

DIAGNOSIS

Serological Diagnosis

The laboratory diagnosis of ABO HDN is difficult as in majority of cases direct antiglobulin test (DAT) is negative or weakly positive. The reasons for negative or weakly positive DAT are given below:

- Weaker strength of fetal A and B antigens at birth
- Antihuman globulin reagent may not be sensitive enough to detect A/B antibody coating
- Antibody may be removed during washing of RBC in the centrifuge
- Complement action may be necessary.

Serological tests for estimation of IgG anti-A/-B are complicated because of the presence of naturally occurring IgM anti-A/-B in the maternal serum. Prenatal testing is required for a woman having severely affected child in previous pregnancy. The prenatal tests on mother include ABO grouping, maternal IgG anti-A/-B estimation and antibody-dependent cell-mediated cytotoxicity (ADCC) if previous fetus was hydrops.

Postnatal tests include ABO group, DAT on baby's RBC; if baby is ABO incompatible with mother and DAT is negative then elute antibody on baby's red cells and test for IgG anti-A or ant-B. Anti-A/-B positive result confirms ABO HDN diagnosis.

Several techniques like Witebsky's partial neutralization test, treatment of maternal serum with 2-mercaptoethanol (2-ME) or dithiothreitol (DTT) prior to IgG anti-A/-B titer and diethylaminoethyl (DEAE) cellulose column chromatography are available for estimation of IgG anti-A/-B levels.[8] Generally IgG anti-A/-B titer levels of more than or equal to 1:32 are considered diagnostic for ABO HDN.[9]

Brief procedures for estimation of IgG anti-A/anti-B are given below:

Witebsky's Partial Neutralization Test

- Determine saline (IgM) anti-A/anti-B titer levels
- Dilute secretor A and B saliva, adjusting the titer to 1:8
- Add appropriate amount of saliva to maternal serum till it is partially neutralized
- Titrate neutralized serum using IAT method or Andersen medium (Dextran-AB serum medium).

2-Mercaptoethanol or Dithiothreitol Method

2-ME or DTT treatment cleaves the IgM molecules and makes them nonreactive. Thus, it is possible to estimate IgG anti-A/anti-B levels using IAT or Andersen medium.

Diethylaminoethyl Column Chromatography

Diethylaminoethyl, an anion exchanger, separates IgG immunoglobulins.

- Pack DEAE suspended in 0.02 M phosphate buffer (pH 6–5) in a baby column or 10 mL syringe
- Equilibrate it with phosphate buffer
- Percolate 0.5 mL of maternal serum in the column
- Add 10 mL phosphate buffer and elute the fraction. Raise the molarity of this fraction by addition of a few grains of sodium chloride
- Determine IgG anti-A/anti-B of the fraction (starting dilution 1:20) using IAT or Adersen medium.

Hematological Changes

Hematological changes like microspherocytosis and increased osmotic fragility though diagnostic may not be associated with every case. Slight increase in reticulocyte count and presence of normoblasts in blood smear may be observed. Red cell acetylcholinesterase levels are reduced in some cases of ABO HDN.[10]

Rh HEMOLYTIC DISEASE OF THE FETUS AND NEWBORN

History

In the year 1939, Levine and Stetson[11] described a case of a woman delivering stillborn child. She had severe hemolytic transfusion reaction after receiving transfusion of her husband's blood for postpartum hemorrhage. An antibody was detected in her serum, which caused agglutination of her husband's red cells. They discussed the possibility of mother's immunization with red cell of fetus having father's antigen and antibody may also be responsible for fetal death in uterus. In the year 1940, Landsteiner and Wiener[12] discovered Rh blood group system by injecting red cells of Rhesus monkey into rabbits and guinea pigs and by testing resulting antibody with human red cells. The antibody detected by Levine and Stetson was termed as Rh antibody, which is synonymous to anti-D. The subsequent work on Rh system revealed that although it appeared that antibody produced in rabbits and guinea pigs with Rhesus monkey red cells by Landsteiner and Wiener was identical to human antibody, there is no similarity between Rhesus antigen and D antigen on human RBC. However, because of the universal acceptance of Rh blood group system, it was not possible to change the name of this system. But the system discovered with Rhesus monkey red cells and having resemblance to Rhesus red cell antigens was termed as LW system.[5]

Incidence

The incidence of Rh (D) negative group in Indian population is about 5%. When anti-D IgG prophylaxis was not available then about 5% Rh (D) negative pregnant women produced anti-D.[13] The incidence of Rh alloimmunization has declined significantly over the years because of the extensive use of anti-D IgG and family planning practices.[14] However, the complete eradication of Rh HDN is yet to be achieved. In small towns and villages in India, the blood group of pregnant women may not be determined. Moreover, many women having spontaneous abortion or medical termination of pregnancy are not receiving anti-D IgG and antenatal anti-D IgG prophylaxis is not administrated to majority of Rh (D) negative pregnant women.[15]

Rh Alloimmunization

Rh antibody is not naturally occurring and D antigen exists only on human red cells. Hence, exposure to Rh (D) positive red cells is essential for anti-D formation. Rh (D) positive pregnancy is the main source of D antigen stimulus. Majority of Rh (D) negative women in India will have Rh (D) positive husband and in 75% cases fetus will be Rh (D) positive. If antenatal and/or postnatal Rh prophylaxis is not administered then few of them may have the risk of producing anti-D. Passage of fetal Rh (D) positive red cells from fetus to mother is the prerequisite for Rh (D) immunization in pregnancy. Therefore, generally there is no immunization during first pregnancy. However, Rh (D) negative woman may get immunized in the next pregnancy with previous abortion. Majority of Rh (D) negative women get immunized during second pregnancy.

Rh (D) incompatible blood transfusion is another source of D antigen stimulus. Generally, Rh (D) negative patients receive Rh (D) negative red cell components but often Rh (D) positive platelet products, which always have slight red cell contamination, are given to Rh (D) negative patients. Thus, these patients have a risk of alloimmunization. All female patients should have priority for Rh (D) negative blood components until they cross the childbearing age.

Transplacental Hemorrhage

Transplacental hemorrhage (TPH) during first or second trimester of pregnancy is rare. During the third trimester, about 7% women have the risk.[16] About 20% women have TPH if delivery is normal but complicated or instrumental deliveries increase the risk of TPH.[17] Mollison compiled the data of three large studies and reported that approximately 99% women have less than 3 mL fetal cell leak (FCL), 0.7% have 3–10 mL and only 0.3% women will have more than 10 mL FCL.[18] A massive FCL occurs only in one in 1,000 deliveries.

The D antigen has many variants. Thus, currently there is a practice of using two potent anti-D reagents for D typing. Rh (D) antigen has more than 37 epitopes or antigenic determinants.[5] Monoclonal anti-D antibodies have been raised against each of them, which have helped in analyzing these epitopes. Partial D antigen individuals who lack some D epitopes have potential to produce anti-D.[19] Kulkarni et al.[20] have observed 0.15% frequency of partial D antigen in Western India with DFR as the predominant Rh variant.

Among Rh antibodies other than D, the most common antibodies are anti-c and anti-E.[5] Anti-E can occur naturally. Occurrence of anti-C without anti-D is rare. Anti-CE is the most common compound antibody while anti-CE is sometimes found with anti-D.[21]

Laboratory Tests for Prediction of Severity of Rh Hemolytic Disease of the Fetus and Newborn

Diagnosis of Rh HDFN is easy; i.e. Rh (D) negative mother has anti-D, husband/fetus is Rh (D) positive and DAT of the fetal RBC is positive. The antenatal investigations are carried out to prevent hydrops fetalis by predicting severity and treating the fetus.

Rh Genotype of Father

The knowledge of zygosity of father is helpful as anti-D found in maternal serum could be of previous pregnancy if he is heterozygous. Serological tests cannot determine the correct Rh genotype therefore most probable genotype is derived. However, several molecular methods are available for determination of true zygosity when the father is Rh (D) positive.[22]

MATERNAL LABORATORY INVESTIGATIONS

Routine antenatal investigations include ABO and Rh (D) typing of mother at her first antenatal visit. If she is Rh (D) negative then her serum is repeatedly tested for presence of anti-D. In-depth investigations are needed for Rh (D) alloimmunized mother.

Rh (D) Titer

Manual Rh (D) antibody titration is a universally accepted test because it is simple, cheap and could be easily repeated frequently. A rise in titer indicates Rh (D) positive fetus. Techniques like enzyme, bovine albumin and IAT are available.[5] Though IAT is preferred it is time-consuming and skilled technician is required to get the reliable results. Incorporation of positive and negative controls is also essential. A vast degree of correlation is not expected from anti-D titer but majority of stillbirth cases have maternal titer more than or equal to 1:32.[23] In general the titer of 1:16–1:32 at first antenatal visit is significant requiring repeated follow-up titer.

Anti-D Concentration

Quantification of maternal anti-D concentration is considered better parameter of assessment as Rh (D) titer is semiquantitative, visual test thus having limitations. Anti-D could be quantified on the autoanalyzer or by immunoradiometric assay using ^{125}I or enzyme-linked immunosorbent assay (ELISA).[24,25] Anti-D concentration of more than 4 µg/mL is significant when intrauterine transfusion (IUT) is considered.

Each laboratory should develop its own critical levels by reviewing outcome of Rh alloimmunized pregnancies.

Functional Tests

Anti-D being a noncomplement binding IgG antibody, destruction of anti-D-coated fetal red cells occurs extravascularly. The adherence of sensitized erythrocytes (target cells) to Fc receptors on monocytes or macrophages (effectors cells) is the initial event that leads to erythrophagocytosis or cytolysis of attached cells. Several bioassays are available for measurement of lytic potential of anti-D using peripheral lymphocytes, monocytes or cultured macrophages. ^{51}Cr antibody-dependent cell-mediated cytotoxicity (ADCC) assay using monocytes appears to have more predictive value than other assays.[26,27]

Immunoglobulin G (IgG) subtypes of anti-D are also important while determining severity. All IgG subclasses can transfer the placental barrier but the transfer ranks in the order IgG1 > IgG3 > IgG4 > IgG2. The most predominant subclasses of anti-D are IgG1 and IgG3. IgG1 anti-D mediates red cell destruction by phagocytosis while IgG3 by prolonged cytolysis. They exist as a single class or in combination with other classes.[28] The affinity of IgG3 to bind the Fc receptor is greater than IgG1 but IgG3 has only 7 days half-life while IgG1 has 21 days. Both the classes are clinically significant.

SPECTROPHOTOMETRIC ANALYSIS OF AMNIOTIC FLUID

Although placenta clears bilirubin of the affected fetus, a significant portion enters the amniotic fluid. In the year 1961, Liley[29] introduced a spectrophotometry method to measure bilirubin pigments in the amniotic fluid at 450 nm. It is a time-tested method of assessing severity of Rh HDN. The measurement on spectrophotometer needs a clear specimen of amniotic fluid. If there is a contamination of maternal or fetal blood then the optical density (OD) values are not reliable. The amniotic fluid is centrifuged and/or filtered prior to measurement to remove the floating particles. Information about an accurate gestational age at the time of amniotic fluid collection is essential. The serial OD values at different wave lengths of Rh alloimunized mother's sample and normal amniotic fluid collected at the same gestation are plotted as seen in **Figure 14.1**.[30] If the fetus is severely affected then at 450 nm a peak is observed; the delta OD value above 0.2 indicates that the fetus is in danger. **Figure 14.2** shows three zones of Liley's chart at 16–30 weeks. Zone III represents the highest risk, i.e. either hydrops fetalis or severely affected fetus. The utility of Liley's graph before 27 weeks is questionable as graph needs to be extrapolated to get the values at earlier gestations. The graph has been modified by Queenan[31] **(Fig. 14.3)** to get the accurate diagnosis at earlier gestations. The considerable number of OD values of the graph fall in zone II beginning or middle even when the fetus is Rh (D) negative. Hence, IUT is recommended only if the results indicate end of the zone II or zone III.[32]

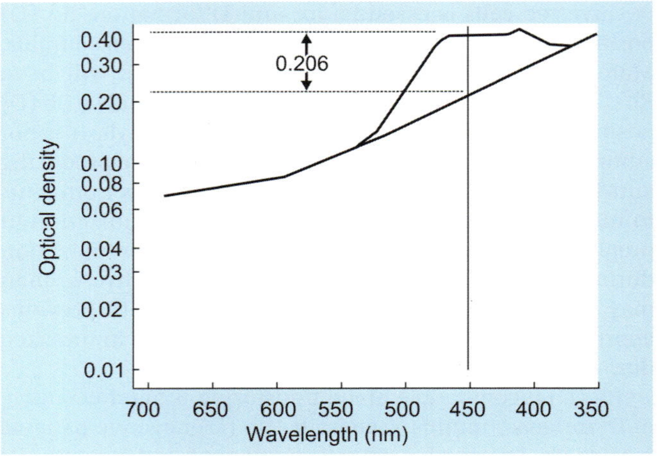

Figure 14.1 Liley curve. This graph illustrates an example of amniotic fluid spectrophotometric reading of 0.206, which when plotted at 35 weeks' gestation falls into zone 3, indicating severe hemolytic disease[30]

Source: *http://emedicine.medscape.com/article/974349-clinical*

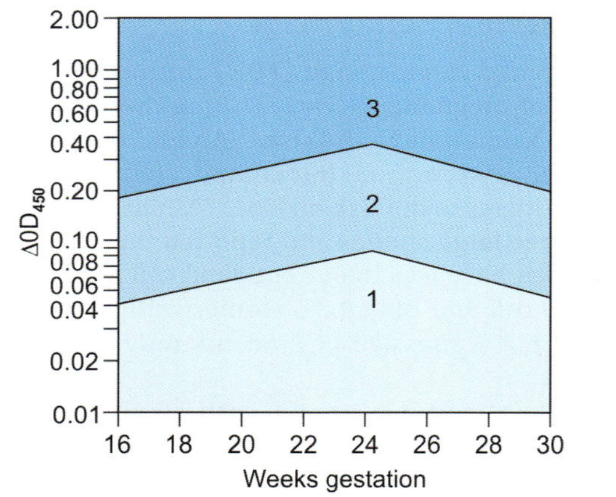

Figure 14.2 Modified Liley curve for gestation of less than 24 weeks showing that bilirubin levels in amniotic fluid peak at 23–24 weeks' gestation[30]

Source: *http://emedicine.medscape.com/article/974349-clinical*

INVESTIGATION OF FETUS

Prenatal Determination of Rh (D) Status of Fetus by DNA Analysis

The determination of the Rh type of a fetus early in pregnancy facilities the decision making for IUT of affected child due Rh disease, when the father is heterozygous or his zygosity is not known. If the fetus is Rh (D) negative parents are assured about the safety of fetus and invasive management is avoided. Information about Rh (D) status of fetus is also useful for administrating prophylaxis anti-D IgG after the sensitizing event in the early pregnancy, when fetus of Rh (D) negative nonimmunized mother is Rh (D) positive. Bennett et al.[33] reported a technique based on polymerase chain reaction (PCR) for detecting Rh status by analysis of DNA expected from amniotic fluid fibroblasts. The same method could be used for chorionic villus tissue also. The amniotic fluid is preferred because amniocentesis procedure is safer. Rh (D) typing can also be carried out by noninvasive method using cell-free fetal DNA in maternal plasma and real-time quantitative PCR.[34]

Fetal Blood Sampling

Fetal sample collected by ultrasonography (USG)-guided cordocentesis or percutaneous umbilical sampling allows examination of blood for Hb, hematocrit, blood group, DAT, etc.[35] This has revolutionized antenatal management as severity of HDN is directly known.

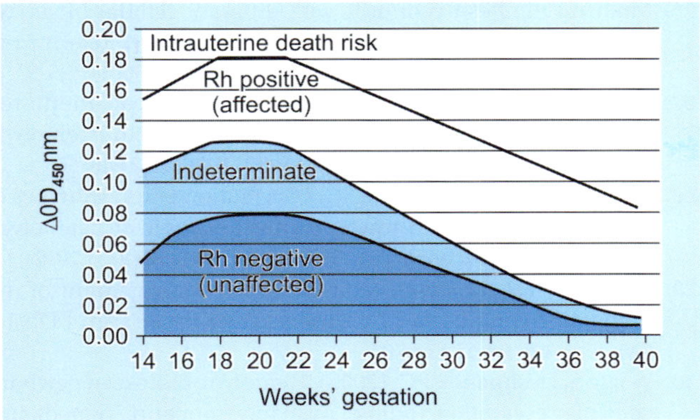

Figure 14.3 Queenan curve: Modified Liley curve that shows delta-OD 450 values at 14–40 weeks' gestation. Chart for predicting severity of rhesus isoimmunization[30]

Source: *http://emedicine.medscape.com/article/974349-clinical*

Postnatal Laboratory Investigations

Rh (D) positive group and positive DAT on cord blood sample confirm the diagnosis of Rh HDN. Sometimes in spite of strong positive DAT, Rh D typing of the infant shows negative result, because of the blocking of D antigen sites due to anti-D sensitization. In this situation, multiple washings of RBC with warm saline help in removal of coated antibody and test gives Rh (D) positive results. Reticulocyte count and blood smear examination for immature erythrocytes are carried out to assess degree of red cell destruction. At birth cord blood Hb is an important investigation to assess anemia and repeated bilirubin levels during the postnatal period can determine rise in bilirubin per hour. The goal is to perform timely exchange transfusion to prevent kernicterus. Serum albumin levels and the ability of albumin to bind bilirubin vary significantly between newborns. In sick, premature infants albumin binding capacity of bilirubin is diminished. Estimation of albumin and albumin binding levels helps in preventing kernicterus.

Thus, serological, hematological and biochemical investigations play a significant role in successful management of ABO HDN and Rh HDFN.

CONCLUSION

ABO HDN though assumed to be mild to moderate could be severe enough to cause kernicterus and death. Therefore it is important to distinguish it from physiological jaundice and establish diagnosis based on serology and hematological investigations.

In India Rh HDNF still exists. Antenatal laboratory investigations of Rh (D) negative mother are necessary to identify Rh (D) alloimmunized cases. Laboratory work-up is also essential for prediction of severity of HDNF to prevent hydrops fetalis.

Prevention of Rh (D) alloimmunization is the best approach to eradicate Rh HDNF. Administration of prophylaxis anti-D IgG is necessary for all Rh (D) negative non-immunized women having Rh (D) positive husband, in the antenatal and postnatal period as per the need.

Besides anti-D other Rh specific antibodies like anti-c, anti-e, anti-C, anti-E and compound Rh antibodies are capable of causing hyperbilirubinemia. Hence antenatal detection of atypical blood group antibodies is essential.

KEY MESSAGE

Investigate all ABO incompatible jaundice infants and their mothers to detect severe cases of ABO HDN.

Every maternity hospital should have antenatal serology clinic to identify non-immunized and immunized Rh (D) negative women and laboratory facility to predict severity of Rh HDNF. There should be facility to screen antenatal women for atypical blood group antibodies

REFERENCES

1. McDonnell M, Hannam S, Devane SP. Hydrops fetalis due to ABO incompatibility. Arch Dis Child Fetal Neonatal Ed. 1998;78(3):F220-1.
2. Toy PT, Reid ME, Papenfus L, Yeap HH, Black D. Prevalence of ABO Maternal-infant incompatibility in Asians, Blacks, Hispanics and Caucasians. Vox Sang. 1988;54(3):181-3.
3. Crawford H, Cutbush M, Falconer H, Mollison PL. Formation of immune A iso-antibodies, with special reference to heterogenetic stimuli. Lancet. 1952;2(6727):219-23.
4. Gupte SC, Bhatia HM. Anti-A and anti-B titre response after tetanus toxoid injections in normal adults and pregnant women. Indian J Med Res. 1979;70:221-8.
5. Klein HG, Anstee DJ. Mollison's blood transfusion in clinical medicine, 11th edition. Copenhagen, Denmark, UK: Blackwell Publishing; 2006. pp. 496-545.
6. Gupte SC, Bhatia HM. Factors influencing the seropathology and severity of ABO HDN. J Obstet Gynecol India. 1980;30:865-72.
7. Gupte SC, Bhatia HM. Increased incidence of haemolytic disease of the new-born caused by ABO-incompatibility when tetanus toxoid is given during pregnancy. Vox Sang. 1980;38(1):22-8.
8. Gupte SC, Bhatia HM. Comparison of Witebsky's partial neutralization, 2-mercaptoethanol and DEAE column chromatography techniques in detection of IgG anti-A/anti-B and their significance in neonatal jaundice. Proc Recent Trends in Immuno Haematology. BGRC (ICMR) Publication, Bombay. 1982. pp. 19-24.
9. Gupte SC, Bhatia HM. Studies on neonatal jaundice: a role of ABO incompatible pregnancy. Indian J Med Res. 1973;61(9):1335-45.
10. Gupte SC, Bhatia HM. Erythrocyte membrane enzyme acetyl cholinesterase in neonatal jaundice. Indian J Pediatr. 1980;47(387):267-71.
11. Levine R, Stetson RE. An unusual case of intra group agglutination. J Am Med Assoc. 1939;113:126-7.
12. Landsteiner K, Wiener AS. An agglutinable factor in human blood recognizable by immune sera of Rhesus blood. Proc Soc Exp Biol Med (NY). 1940;43:223-4.
13. Gupte SC, Bhatia HM. Changing pattern of Rh D immunization in Bombay. J Obestel Gynecol India. 1984;34:776-9.
14. Gupte SC, Kulkarni SS. Incidence of Rh immunization between 1981 and 1992. Natl Med J India. 1994;7(2):65-6.

15. Gupte SC, Dalal RM, Kulkarni RR, Satam SD, Bhatia HM. Follow up studies in Rh (D) negative women receiving and not receiving anti-D immunoglobulin injection. J Obstet Gynaecol India. 1983;33:579-84.
16. Mehta DM, Gupte SC, Bhatia HM. Transplacental haemorrhage and maternal iso-immunization. J Postgrad Med. 1979;25(2):75-80.
17. Gupte SC. Laboratory techniques in evaluating rhesus alloimmunized pregnancy. Chapter 4 in: The Rhesus factor current concepts. In: Shah D, Salvi V (Eds). New Delhi, India: FOGSI Publication, Jaypee Brothers Medical Publishers; 2002. pp. 41-57.
18. Mollison PL. Blood Transfusion in Clinical Medicine, 6th edition. Oxford, UK: ELBS and Blackwell Scientific Publication; 1979. pp. 292-352.
19. Mayne K, Bowell P, Woodward T, Sibley C, Lomas C, Tippett P. Rh immunization by partial D antigen category of DVa. Br J Haematol. 1990;76(4):537-9.
20. Kulkarni S, Colah R, Gorakshakar A, Gupte S, Vasantha K, Mohanty D, et al. Frequency of partial D in Western India. Transfus Med. 2008;18(2):91-6.
21. Gupte SC, Merchant RH, Joshi SR, Bhatia HM. Hemolytic disease of newborn in Rh(D) positive mothers. Indian Pediatr. 1983;20(8):577-81.
22. Simsek S, Faas BH, Bleeker PM, Overbeeke MA, Cuijpers HT, van der Schoot CE, et al. Rapid Rh D genotyping by polymerase chain reaction-based amplification of DNA. Blood. 1995;85(10):2975-80.
23. Gupte SC, Bhatia HM. Correlation of Rh (D) antibody titre and obstetric history with severity of Rh haemolytic disease of the newborn. Indian J Haematol. 1985;3:75-9.
24. Austin EB, McIntosh Y. Anti-D quantification by flow cytometry: a comparison of five methods. Transfusion. 2000;40(1):77-83.
25. Gupte SC, Dumasia AN, Kulkarni SS, Patil JS. Rhesus hemolytic diseases of the newborn: Comparison of four assays developed for anti-D quantitation. Lab Med Intl. 1994;11:12-5.
26. Mollison PL. Results of tests with different cellular bioassays in relation to severity of RhD haemolytic disease. Report from nine collaborating laboratories. Vox Sang. 1991;60(4):225-9.
27. Patil JS, Gupte SC. Antibody-dependent cell-mediated cytotoxicity and erythrophagocytosis assays in Rh haemolytic diseases of the newborn. Ceylon Med J. 1996;41(2):46-50.
28. Iyer YS, Kulkarni SV, Gupte SC. Distribution of IgG subtypes in maternal anti-D sera and their prognostic value in Rh haemolytic disease of the new born. Acta Haematol. 1992;88(2-3):78-81.
29. Liley AW. Liquor amnil analysis in the management of the pregnancy complicated by rhesus sensitization. Am J Obstet Gynecol. 1961;82:1359-70.
30. Wagle S, Deshpande PG. (2003). Hemolytic disease of newborn clinical presentation. [online] Available from http://emedicine.medscape.com/article/974349-clinical. [Accessed October, 2016].
31. Queenan JT, Tomai TP, Urak SH, King JC. Deviation of amniotic fluid density at a wave length of 450 nm in Rh immunized pregnancies from 14 to 40 weeks gestation. A proposal for clinical management. Am J Obstet Gynecol. 1993;168:1370-6.
32. Gupte SC, Lulla CP, Kulkarni SS, Korgaonkar SA, Walvekar VR, Merchant RH. Experience with intrauterine transfusions for severe Rh alloimmunization in a developing country. J Matern Fetal Med. 1998;7(6):287-91.
33. Bennett PR, Le Van Kim C, Colin Y, Warwick RM, Chérif-Zahar B, Fisk NM, et al. Prenatal determination of fetal RhD type by DNA amplification. N Engl J Med. 1993;329(9):607-10.
34. Grootkerk-Tax MG, Soussan AA, de Haas M, Maaskant-van Wijk PA, van der Schoot CE. Evaluation of prenatal RHD typing strategies on cell-free fetal DNA from maternal plasma. Transfusion. 2006;46(12):2142-8.
35. Gupte SC. Transfusion therapy for fetus and newborn. In: Gupte S, Desai PK (Eds). Recent Trends in Transfusion Medicine. Surat, India: SRKRC Publication; 2002. pp. 155-64.

CHAPTER 15

Nonimmune Hemolytic Anemia

Anirban Das, Deepak Bansal

INTRODUCTION

Hemolysis is a common cause of anemia in the neonate. The evaluation of hemolysis in the newborn must be considered in the context of normal neonatal physiology, which is different from older infants and children. Neonatal erythropoiesis, hemoglobin (Hb) synthesis and the metabolism of neonatal red blood cells (RBCs) have different characteristics as compared to older children **(Box 15.1)**.[1] Hence, while several of the common hemolytic disorders of childhood appear first in the neonatal period, other disorders do not present until the child is several months old. Similarly, selected rare hemolytic anemias occur only in the newborn period.[2]

Approach to a neonate with a suspected hemolytic disorder involves confirming the increased destruction of RBCs and their accelerated production. The next step is to identify the mechanism of destruction. As in adults, it is useful to classify hemolytic disorders as extrinsic or intrinsic **(Box 15.2)**.[1,2]

- *Extrinsic*: Extrinsic or extracellular factors are usually acquired. Acquired disorders include those that are associated with infection, immune-mediated, or are secondary to some other underlying pathology.
- *Intrinsic*: Intrinsic red cell defects are more likely to be genetic in origin. Inherited disorders are due to defects in RBC membrane, abnormalities in cell metabolism or a consequence of an Hb defect.

Box 15.1 Characteristics of neonatal RBCs with relevance to hemolytic disorders

- Larger erythrocyte size and higher mean corpuscular volume (MCV)
- Increased membrane phospholipid and cholesterol content, higher osmotic resistance
- Increased membrane rigidity and reduced membrane deformability
- Higher sialic acid content, more negative surface charge
- Reduced structural stability secondary to increased unbound 2, 3-diphosphoglycerate
- *Surface antigen expression:* Reduced A, B, Lewis, I antigens, I antigen present
- Increased glucose consumption and adenosine triphosphate (ATP) production
- Increased activity of several glycolytic enzymes
- Decreased membrane potassium influx
- Increased susceptibility to oxidant induced damage
- Presence of membrane surface pits secondary to splenic hypofunction
- Abundance of irregular shaped erythrocytes secondary to splenic hypofunction
- Reduced erythrocyte lifespan

Box 15.2 Causes of hemolysis in the neonate

Extrinsic causes of hemolysis

- Alloimmune hemolysis (Rh, ABO, rarer blood group incompatibilities)
- Immune hemolysis due to maternal autoimmune disease or drug intake
- *Infections*: Intrauterine infections, malaria, sepsis, T-activation
- *Microangiopathic anemias*: Kasabach-Merritt phenomenon, arteriovenous malformations, renal artery stenosis and thrombosis
- Oxidant exposure
- *Others*: Vitamin E deficiency, galactosemia, prolonged or recurrent acidosis

Intrinsic causes of hemolysis

- *Membrane defects*: Hereditary spherocytosis, hereditary elliptocytosis
- *Enzymopathies*: Disorders of the hexose monophosphate shunt (G6PD deficiency) and glycolytic pathways (pyruvate kinase deficiency)
- *Hemoglobinopathies*: α-thalassemias, γδ-thalassemia, unstable hemoglobinopathies

CONFOUNDING FACTORS IN THE EVALUATION OF NEONATAL HEMOLYSIS

Hemolytic anemia in older children typically presents with anemia, reticulocytosis and hyperbilirubinemia. In neonates, these must be interpreted in context of the values appropriate for gestational and postgestational age.

Hemoglobin

In neonates, a mean Hb of 17 g/dL decreases to 11 g/dL over the first 3–4 months of life as a result of physiological adaptation to the extra-uterine environment.[3] In mild hemolysis, the anemia may be masked by the physiological anemia of infancy. On the other hand, neonates have a limited capacity for compensatory erythropoiesis as a response to hemolysis; this may increase the severity of anemia in disorders with significant hemolysis. Hence, several of the hemolytic anemias may have more severe manifestations in the neonate.

Mean Corpuscular Volume

The mean corpuscular volume (MCV) reduces from birth (100–130 fL) over the 1st year of life (70–85 fL).[4] A relatively high MCV may mask microcytosis, characteristic of certain hemolytic disorders, including α-thalassemia. The reticulocyte count in term infants at birth (3–7%) decreases to 1–3% by 4 days and to less than 1% by day 7 of life.[4] In premature infants, reticulocyte values at birth are higher (6–10%). This may remain elevated for an increased period of time. In addition, the physiologic anemia of infancy is a normal response to the improved oxygen-carrying capacity of extra-uterine life. As a result, mild hemolysis might not be sensed as an oxygen-deficit in the newborn. As a result, compensatory erythropoiesis or reticulocytosis may be absent.

Nucleated RBCs

These are frequently observed in newborn infants. nRBCs typically disappear by the 3rd day of life in term infants and in 7–10 days in preterms. The persistence of nRBCs suggests the possibility of a hemolytic disorder.[2] On the other hand, hypoxia per se, even in the absence of anemia, can be associated with increased release of nRBCs. In such a scenario, the bone marrow examination will demonstrate an increased compensatory erythropoiesis in patients with hemolytic anemia; however, this is seldom required for diagnosis.[2]

Peripheral Blood Smear

The peripheral blood smear (PBS) is invaluable in diagnosing hemolytic anemias. However, several abnormalities in the peripheral smear are observed in a normal newborn as well. Howell-Jolly bodies, siderocytes, target cells, and other atypical RBCs are demonstrated due to relative hyposplenism.[5] Such changes are more profound in premature infants and disappear by 3–4 months of age.

Hyperbilirubinemia

Reduced RBC survival, increased enterohepatic circulation of bilirubin and reduced glucuronyl transferase activity are responsible for the physiological hyperbilirubinemia in the neonates. Levels up to 12 mg/dL (maximum on day 4) are observed in term neonates, and levels as high as 15 mg/dL (maximum on day 7) are observed in preterms.[6] Beyond the first few days, different metabolic problems and breastfeeding can result in hyperbilirubinemia. This further confounds the recognition of increased RBC destruction. However, in the presence of hemolysis, bilirubin levels exceed the physiological levels. Clinical jaundice may appear early at less than 36 hours of age.[6] In neonates, mild hemolysis can occur without anemia or significant reticulocytosis. Disproportionate hyperbilirubinemia may often be the only manifestation of an underlying hemolytic disorder.

Other Markers of Hemolysis

Serum haptoglobin is a marker of intravascular hemolysis. It is an α-2 glycoprotein that reacts with free Hb and forms a complex, which is removed by the reticuloendothelial system. In newborns, the serum haptoglobin levels are low. Values that are normal for a child or adult may not be achieved until the child is several months old.[7] Hence, serum haptoglobin is not a reliable parameter in diagnosing hemolysis in newborns.

Carboxyhemoglobin is the circulating form of carbon monoxide generated from breakdown of heme, and is useful as a marker of accelerated RBC destruction. In addition, noninvasive measurement of exhaled carbon monoxide can be used as a marker of increased breakdown of Hb to bilirubin.[8] Elevated serum lactic dehydrogenase (LDH) secondary to the release of LDH2 isozyme from RBCs is a marker of hemolysis. However, typically it is the hyperbilirubinemia that triggers the evaluation of hemolytic anemia in a neonate.[2]

EXTRINSIC CAUSES OF HEMOLYSIS IN NEONATES

Exposure to Drugs and Other Oxidants

Maternal drug intake can cause hemolysis in the fetus and neonate. Dapsone has been frequently incriminated including instances of hemolysis in the fetus during pregnancy, and in the neonate via exposure through breast milk.[9] Episodes are reversible with cessation of the drug. Maternal ingestion of valproic acid has resulted in hemolysis and thrombocytopenia in a breastfed infant.[10,11]

Hemolysis secondary to exposure to oxidants in the newborn is not infrequent. This may be associated with an inherited metabolic abnormality of the erythrocyte or with congenital Heinz body anemia. Neonatal RBCs may be more oxidant-sensitive. The presentation is with acute onset anemia and hyperbilirubinemia with "bite" and "blister" cells, spherocytes and irregularly shaped RBCs on a peripheral blood smear.[1] Often no recognizable source of the presumed oxidant stress is identified. The episode resolves in a few days and transfusions are rarely required.[1]

Infections

Intrauterine Infections

Transplacentally acquired infections including cytomegalic inclusion disease, disseminated toxoplasmosis, syphilis, rubella, herpes simplex and human immunodeficiency viral infections can present with anemia, hepatosplenomegaly and jaundice. Stigmata including cataracts, developmental delay and microcephaly often coexist.[1]

Neonatal Sepsis

Bacterial sepsis may be associated with conjugated as well as unconjugated hyperbilirubinemia. The hemolysis is postulated to be associated with macrophage activation and RBC sequestration secondary to infection. In addition, certain bacterial enzymes including phospholipases and neuraminidase may alter membrane lipids or affect the glycoprotein surface structure, reducing their survival. Disseminated intravascular coagulation (DIC) is frequently associated with anemia in neonates with sepsis. In addition, neutrophilic leukocytosis with left-shift in maturation and toxic granules are demonstrated in the peripheral smear along with evidence of hemolysis **(Fig. 15.1)**. Group B *Streptococcus*, *Escherichia coli* and *Pseudomonas aeruginosa* have been frequently incriminated.[1]

Postnatal Viral Infections

Neonatal enteroviral infection has been complicated by DIC and anemia.[11] Parvovirus B19 infection, which typically presents as hypoplastic anemia, may be associated with hemolysis as well.[12]

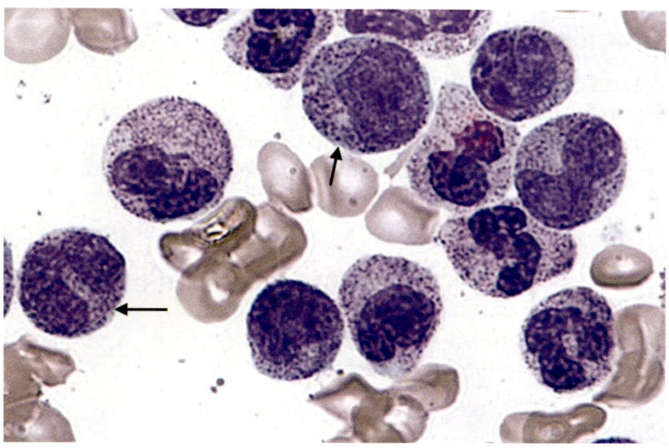

Figure 15.1 Peripheral blood film demonstrating toxic granulation and shift to left with myelocytes and metamyelocytes (arrows) in a case of neonatal sepsis (Oil immersion 100X)

Courtesy: Dr Prateek Bhatia, Department of Pediatrics, PGIMER, Chandigarh.

T-activation: Exposure of an occult galactosyl residue on the RBC surface membrane, the Thomsen-Friedenreich cryptoantigen or the T-antigen, is mediated via neuraminidase-mediated cleavage of sialic acid residues from sialoglycoproteins in the RBC membrane.[13] Neuraminidase-producing organisms including *Clostridium perfringens, Clostridium welchii* and *Streptococcus pneumonia* are frequently incriminated.[2,14] However, *Bacteroides, Escherichia coli,* and other gram-negative organisms have been incriminated as well.[2] The exposed T-antigen may then bind with anti-T-immunoglobulin M (IgM) antibodies resulting in destruction by immune-mediated intravascular hemolysis. An alternative mechanism involves rapid clearance from circulation because of reduced surface charge of the RBC membrane secondary to the reduced sialic acid content of the RBC membranes.[15]

Anti-T IgM antibodies are absent at birth. They are formed in later life following antigenic stimulation by intestinal bacteria that possess T-like antigens. However, neonates with necrotizing enterocolitis (NEC), particularly complicated cases requiring surgical interventions, have been demonstrated to have a higher frequency of T-activation. It is hypothesized that RBCs in newborns are exposed to bacterial neuraminidase locally released from devitalized bowel, resulting in T-activation. In addition, anti-T antibodies are present in adult plasma. The transfusion of adult blood to a neonate lacking T antibodies can lead to life-threatening hemolysis. T-activation should be suspected in a sick or septic infant with intravascular hemolysis following transfusion of blood products. Failure to achieve an expected post-transfusion increment of Hb should point toward this diagnosis as well.[16]

T-activation can be diagnosed by compatibility testing, where agglutination is demonstrated when the neonate's RBCs are added to the donor serum. Routine minor cross-match between the donor serum and the recipient RBCs is infrequently performed in infants less than 4 months of age because the formation of alloantibodies is extremely rare in this age. As a consequence, T-activation may not be recognized before the newborn is transfused. However, once identified, neonates with T-activated RBCs should be transfused with washed or plasma-reduced RBCs or platelets. The compatibility of donor plasma and the newborn RBCs needs to be assessed. Low-titer anti-T plasma should be considered if plasma products are clinically indicated in such circumstances. Screening of high-risk infants including those with NEC or sepsis could prevent T-activation-related hemolysis.[17]

Malaria: Neonatal malaria is rare. In endemic areas, it is reported in up to 10% of nonimmune and 0.1% of immune mothers. However, placental infection is described in as many as 30% of women who acquire infection during pregnancy. In endemic areas, the spontaneous clearance of infection in neonates may be as high as 93%.[18] This has been attributed to the protective effect of maternal antibodies that are passed on to the newborn. Fetal Hb plays a protective role in slowing the rate of development of the parasite as well.

Neonatal malaria is described as disease presenting within the first 28 days of life. Cases presenting later may be included once the possibilities of postpartum infection by either a mosquito bite or blood transfusion have been confidently excluded. However, this is difficult in endemic regions including India. Congenital malaria is defined as the presence of asexual stages of the parasite in cord blood at the time of delivery or in the peripheral smear of the infant in the first 7 days of life. While malaria caused by *Plasmodium falciparum* has been implicated in most studies from Africa, *Plasmodium vivax* associated disease has been described from the Indian subcontinent.[19,20]

The clinical features of malaria in newborns are nonspecific and are similar to those of sepsis. The infant has fever, irritability, excessive cry and refusal to suck along with anemia. The characteristic paroxysm is absent.[21] Anemia is documented in up to half the cases. It is caused by a combination of factors including hemolysis of parasitized erythrocytes and marrow suppression. Other manifestations include symmetric fetal growth retardation and low-birth-weight.[19-21]

Even though the demonstration of the malarial parasite remains the gold standard for diagnosis, it is prone to interobserver variation. Antigen capture dipstick assays are useful, especially in field settings. The therapy for the infecting plasmodium species is curative. As the infection is produced by the transmission of the infected erythrocytes rather than forms that invade the liver, the infant does not need treatment targeted toward the exoerythrocytic stages of *Plasmodium*.

Microangiopathic Anemias

Neonatal hemolytic anemia with microangiopathic changes including the presence of schistocytes (fragmented RBCs) in the peripheral blood suggests that hemolysis is secondary to altered RBC-vessel wall interactions. Causes include arteriovenous malformations, cavernous hemangiomas, renal artery stenosis, severe coarctation of aorta and large vessel thrombi.[2] Abnormalities of placental microcirculation or macrovascular anomalies including an umbilical-vein varix are infrequent causes.[22] The Kasabach-Merritt syndrome, a local consumptive coagulopathy with microangiopathic anemia, thrombocytopenia and hypofibrinogenemia occur in association with kaposiform hemangioendotheliomas and tufted angiomas and typically presents in the neonatal period **(Fig. 15.2)**.[23] Fibrin deposited in the vessel walls interacts with the RBCs. It results in breaking off of RBC fragments, producing fragile schistocytes, which are removed by the reticuloendothelial system. The coagulopathy and anemia, which may be persistent and severe, improve with regression or removal of the malformation.

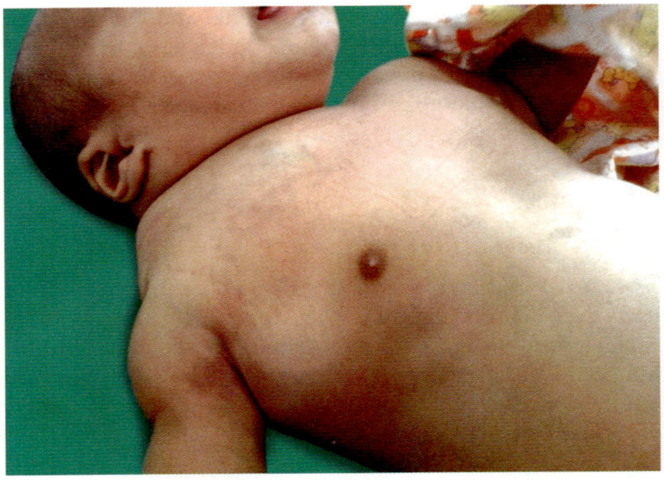

Figure 15.2 Kaposiform hemangioendothelioma presenting as a progressively enlarge swelling in the right upper chest in a neonate. The baby presented with thrombocytopenia, consumptive coagulopathy and microangiopathic hemolytic anemia, the components of the Kasabach-Merritt phenomenon

Vitamin E Deficiency

Premature infants are deficient in vitamin E. The deficiency persists for 2–3 months, unless supplemented. Vitamin E has antioxidant properties. This is vital to the integrity of the RBCs. Vitamin E deficiency makes RBCs susceptible to membrane injury due to lipid peroxidation. Hence, vitamin E deficiency in small premature babies (<1,500 g) can lead to hemolytic anemia at 6–10 weeks of age.[24] The hemolysis subsides following vitamin E administration. In addition, preterms administered prophylactic vitamin E (15 IU) daily have been demonstrated to have higher Hb levels and lower reticulocyte levels as compared to controls.[25] However, several subsequent studies failed to demonstrate such a benefit.

Infantile Pyknocytosis

Pyknocytes account for approximately 2% of RBCs in normal neonates and up to 6% in preterms. These are abnormal, densely staining RBCs with a distorted, irregular contracted appearance and few, short, irregular and projections.[2]

Epidemiology

Tuffy et al. first reported infantile pyknocytosis.[26] Recent reports have been scarce. Over a 3-year period, it was reported in 9% of neonatal hemolytic anemias from a specialty erythrocyte diagnostic center in France (n = 149).[27]

Etiopathogenesis

Exact pathophysiology of this disorder is unknown. An unidentified extrinsic factor is deemed responsible because of the following reasons: (1) the transfused RBCs develop a shortened survival as well, and appear to take on the appearance of pyknocytes and (2) examination of red cell Hb concentration suggests that it is the mature erythrocytes that take on the hyperdense state and not the reticulocytes.[2]

Clinical Features

Infantile pyknocytosis has been described as a hemolytic anemia affecting multiple siblings presenting with hemolysis, jaundice, pallor and sometimes hepatosplenomegaly.[27]

Investigations

Laboratory features include anemia, reticulocytosis and elevated aspartate aminotransferase. Increased pyknocytes and polychromasia are apparent on the peripheral blood smear.

Differential Diagnoses

Infantile pyknocytosis is a diagnosis of exclusion. Similar, findings are observed in other hemolytic disorders including Heinz body hemolytic anemia, glucose-6-phosphate dehydrogenase (G6PD) deficiency, pyruvate kinase (PK) deficiency and vitamin E deficiency. In addition, microangiopathic disorders, hereditary elliptocytosis and may produce a similar morphology.

Management

Treatment consists of transfusion for symptomatic disease. Erythropoietin (EPO) has been documented to be useful as well.[28]

Other Causes of Hemolysis Extrinsic to RBCs

Causes include galactosemia, prolonged or recurrent metabolic acidosis, lysosomal storage disease and a few aminoacidopathies.[1] Although typically associated with a hypoplastic anemia and thrombocytopenia, hemolysis may be found in neonates with osteopetrosis as well.[29]

Intrinsic Causes of Hemolysis in Neonates

Neonatal hemolysis caused by intrinsic disorders in RBCs is usually inherited and can be divided into three major groups of disorders, viz.

1. Disorders of RBC membrane
2. Disorders of enzymatic pathways
3. Hemoglobinopathies.

DISORDERS OF THE RBC MEMBRANE

Hereditary Spherocytosis

Epidemiology

Hereditary spherocytosis (HS) is a heterogeneous disorder in which abnormalities of RBC structural proteins lead to loss of erythrocyte membrane surface area, resulting in spherical-shaped, hyperdense, poorly deformable RBCs with a shortened lifespan. It is the most common cause of inherited chronic hemolysis in Northern Europe and North America, where it affects nearly one person in 2,000.[30] Although, the disease arises in all racial and ethnic groups, data suggest that it is less common in African-Americans and Southeast Asians. In the West, approximately 65% of neonates with HS have a parent with HS. However, in India, family history is present in approximately one-third of patients.[31]

Etiopathogenesis

The loss of membrane surface area in HS erythrocytes is due to defects in various erythrocyte membrane proteins including ankyrin-1, band 3, β-spectrin, α-spectrin and protein 4.2. Numerous mutations in the genes encoding these membrane proteins have been described. Destruction of poorly deformable HS erythrocytes in the spleen is the primary cause of hemolysis in patients with HS.[31] The wide spectrum of manifestations are related to the various genes and specific mutations involved as well as to the presence or absence of coinherited conditions including mutations or polymorphisms of genes involved in bilirubin uptake into hepatocytes (SLC01B1) or intrahepatic bilirubin conjugation (UGT1A1), which increase the risk of hyperbilirubinemia and kernicterus in neonates with HS.[30,32]

Clinical Features

Hereditary spherocytosis in the neonate has several unique manifestations and complications, which make establishing the diagnosis, a priority. The triad of anemia, splenomegaly and jaundice, which is found in older children and adults with HS, is infrequent in neonates. More than one-half of neonates with HS are not anemic in the 1st week of life, and splenomegaly is rarely detected. Jaundice is the most frequent presenting feature of HS in the newborn.[30]

Delhommeau et al. reported 34 infants with HS during their 1st year of life.[33] Thirty-one of the 34 infants had pallor and dyspnea during the 1st month. Twenty-six (76%) required more than or equal to one RBC transfusion during the 1st year; 12 had a single transfusion and 14 had more than or equal to two transfusions. Transfusions were rarely needed in the 1st week of life; however, were commonly administered in the 2nd month of life. Merely eight (24%) infants with HS continued to receive transfusions after 6 months of age. Six underwent splenectomy at 2–5 years of age.[33] HS during the 1st week of life can present with hyperbilirubinemia, which is sometimes severe, leading to bilirubin-induced neurologic dysfunction. In the USA Kernicterus Registry, 23 of the 125 patients with kernicterus had a hemolytic condition, of whom three had HS and severe icteric sequelae.[34] In the study by Delhommeau et al. neonatal jaundice (NNJ) was present in virtually all the infants. Twenty-seven infants were treated with phototherapy, and three received exchange transfusion in the 1st week due to hyperbilirubinemia.[33] In a study of 82 children with HS by the authors, the earliest age at diagnosis was 1 month; merely seven (8.5%) were diagnosed in infancy. However, a history of NNJ was present in 25 (30.5%); one had received an exchange transfusion.[31] It is likely that a diagnosis of HS is often missed in neonates presenting with hyperbilirubinemia.

Investigations

In neonates with HS, the typically sluggish physiological erythropoietic response often renders the reticulocyte count low relative to the degree of anemia. The presence of spherocytes is helpful when considering the diagnosis of HS **(Fig. 15. 3)**. However, up to one-third of neonates with HS do not have spherocytes identified prominently on their blood smear.[30] A few neonates with band 3 deficiency have pincered RBCs. One way to suspect HS in a jaundiced neonate is to obtain a complete blood cell count for interpretation of the RBC indices, in particular the mean corpuscular hemoglobin concentration (MCHC) and the MCV. Typically, a neonate with HS will have an elevated MCHC. In neonates, an MCHC more than 36 g/dL is a useful indicator for HS (specificity 98%, sensitivity 82%). In majority of neonates with HS, the MCV is low. The "neonatal HS ratio" can be calculated by dividing MCHC by MCV. With this ratio, little overlap is observed between normal neonates and those later proven to have HS. In fact a neonatal HS ratio more than 0.36 indicated that HS is present with 97% sensitivity, more than 99% specificity and more than 99% negative predictive value.[32]

When the diagnosis of HS is uncertain, eosin-5-maleimide (EMA) binding can be helpful **(Figs 15.4A and B)**.[32] EMA binding is a flow cytometry-based test that measures the relative amount of fluorescently labeled EMA dye bound to band 3 and Rh-related proteins in the erythrocyte membranes. In HS, the reduction in band 3 and other membrane proteins

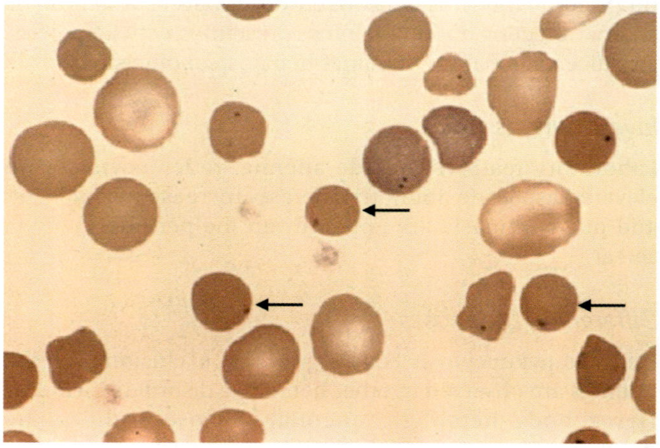

Figure 15.3 Peripheral blood film showing spherocytes in a case of hereditary spherocytosis (arrows). Oil immersion (100 X)
Courtesy: Dr Prateek Bhatia, Department of Pediatrics, PGIMER, Chandigarh.

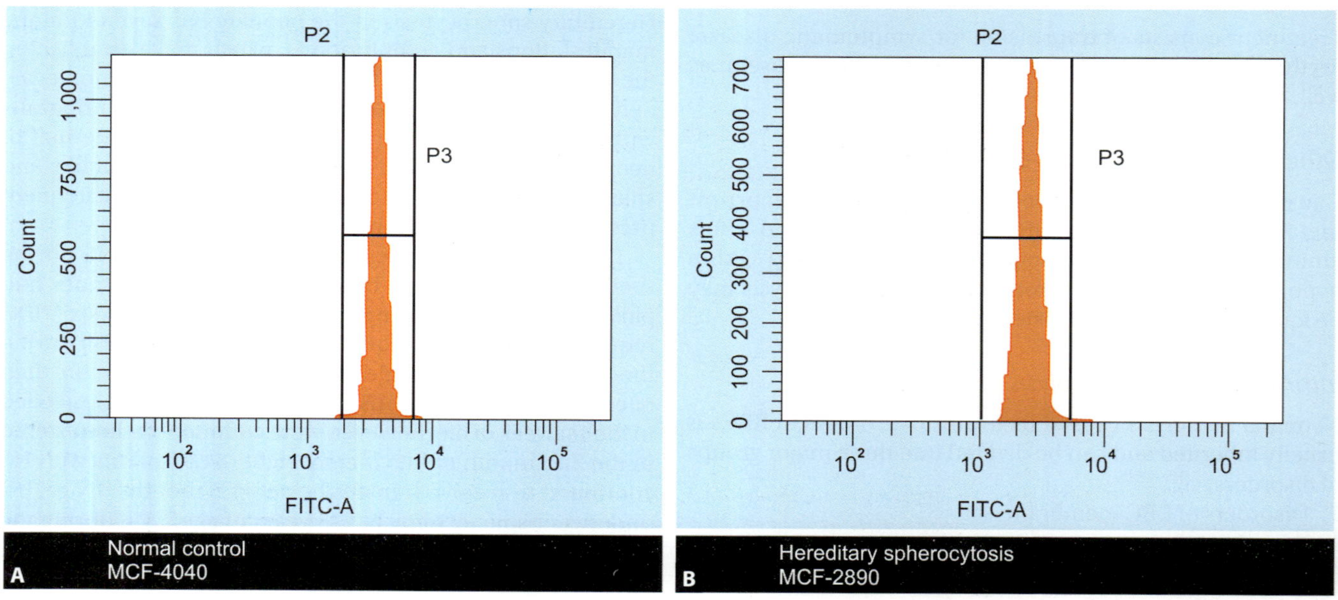

$$\text{MCF ratio} = \frac{\text{MCF of patient}}{\text{Mean MCF of normal controls}} = \frac{2890}{4040} = 0.71$$

Figures 15.4A and B (A) Fluorescence intensity (median channel fluorescence or MCF) recorded in histogram plot in a patient with hereditary spherocytosis, and, (B) in a normal control subject, showing population of RBC, stained with EMA. The MCF ratio is calculated by dividing the MCF of the patient with that of the control. An MCF ratio less than 0.8 is consistent with a diagnosis of HS in an appropriate clinical setting
Abbreviations: EMA, eosin-5-maleimide; MCF, median channel fluorescence
Courtesy: Prof Reena Das, Department of Hematology, PGIMER, Chandigarh.

leads to decreased fluorescence intensity. The EMA test is useful irrespective of the morphology and age of the newborn.

The erythrocytes in HS are more susceptible to osmotic lysis than normal erythrocytes due to decreased membrane surface area. Incubation overnight stresses the already fragile erythrocytes, accentuating the defect. Spherocytes from any cause, including ABO incompatibility, will yield a positive result on osmotic fragility test (OFT). Sodium dodecyl sulfate polyacrylamide gel electrophoresis (SDS-PAGE) of RBC membrane can detect the abnormal proteins. DNA sequencing is not needed in diagnosis of most cases of HS. However, it can establish the diagnosis in difficult cases. Sequencing of relevant genes is considered when family history is negative and severe Coombs-negative hemolysis is idiopathic.[30,32]

When HS is suspected in an otherwise well neonate, testing can be postponed till 6 months of age when the morphology may be less confusing.[32]

Differential Diagnoses

Spherocytes from any cause, including ABO incompatibility, will yield a positive result on OFT. Some neonates with ABO incompatibility have a negative direct antiglobin test; however, the hemolysis may be severe enough to produce spherocytes on peripheral smear. In most cases, the differentiation from HS is clear (e.g. family history, maternal or infant blood group analysis). Additional testing such as elution of anti-A or anti-B from neonatal erythrocytes or detection of free anti-A or anti-B IgG antibody in neonatal serum (indirect Coombs test) can clarify the diagnosis.[30] Other membrane disorders must be considered if the morphology is atypical.[35] Occasionally spherocytes may be demonstrated in other conditions unrelated to membranopathy including PK deficiency, pyrimidine-5′-nucleotidase deficiency (demonstrates basophilic stippling), glucose-6-phosphate deficiency in crisis and unstable hemoglobinopathies.[35] Decreased EMA binding may be observed in other disorders, such as hereditary pyropoikilocytosis and congenital dyserythropoietic anemia II (CDA II). The reticulocyte count is elevated in HS and helps differentiate it from in CDA II. SDS-PAGE of red cell membrane proteins demonstrates abnormality of the band 3 protein in the CDA II.

Management

Folate supplementation is recommended in severe and moderate HS. Phototherapy is the mainstay of treatment of jaundiced neonates with HS in the 1st day after birth. Severe jaundice may require exchange transfusion. However, this is not clearly related to the subsequent disease severity.[30]

When signs of anemia appear, packed erythrocyte transfusions are helpful. Some neonates with HS may be transfusion-dependent in the 1st year of life. This is due to their inability to mount an adequate erythropoietic response.[32] Treatment with EPO may reduce or avoid transfusions; this can usually be stopped by 9 months of age.[30] The rationale for EPO treatment relates to the relative hypoplastic phase of erythropoiesis during the 1st week to months after birth. This phase might be associated with the abrupt decrease after birth from the highly stimulated erythropoiesis during fetal life, the switch of EPO production from the liver to the kidney, the switch from fetal to adult Hb, or a lower serum level of EPO in infants compared with older children. Children requiring 1–2 transfusions early in life often become transfusion independent. Splenectomy is rarely undertaken in the 1st year of life because of the risk of sepsis. In addition, there remains the long-term possibility of development of thromboembolic disorders.[36] Partial splenectomy may be an option in those with persistent symptoms.

Hereditary Elliptocytosis and Related Disorders

Epidemiology: Hereditary elliptocytosis including its multiple variants occurs with an estimated frequency of 1:5,000 Caucasians. Higher prevalence is reported in countries endemic for malaria; it may be as high as 1:100 in some African countries. It has been described across all racial and ethnic groups including the Mediterranean countries the Middle East, the Far East and the Indian subcontinent.[35]

Etiopathogenesis: It is a clinically diverse group of disorders. All are caused by mutations of the cytoskeletal proteins in the RBC membrane (spectrin/protein 4.1). The abnormal proteins disrupt the horizontal integrity of the membrane by weakening interactions. This increases RBC mechanical fragility. It has an autosomal dominant mode of inheritance. However, heterogeneity of presentation among the members of the same family point to the presence of as yet undiscovered modifiers of disease phenotypes.

Clinical features: Most individuals are clinically asymptomatic. Anemia is infrequent. However, the peripheral blood smear can demonstrate up to 15–100% elliptocytes. In 5–20% of cases, hemolysis is evident. However, the hemolysis is frequently compensated with mild anemia (Hb 9–12 g/dL) and reticulocytosis (20–25%). In some cases, poikilocytes are demonstrated in the peripheral smear in addition to elliptocytes. Homozygous and compound heterozygous states may present with severe hemolytic anemia in the neonatal period.[2,35]

Hereditary pyropoikilocytosis is biochemically related to hereditary elliptocytosis. Both have been described in the same family. Many but not all patients are of African heritage.[2] It is recessively inherited and presents as a severe hemolytic anemia. The peripheral smear demonstrates budding of the RBC membrane, red cell fragments, poikilocytes and microspherocytes. The MCV is low (30–50 fL) and the MCHC is normal. Osmotic fragility is increased. Hemolysis, anemia, and jaundice may be severe in the neonatal period, requiring treatment with phototherapy and blood transfusion. Exchange transfusion may be required as well.

The peripheral blood smears of some neonates demonstrate both poikilocytes and elliptocytes. In these babies, the hemolysis often decreases with time. Clinical features convert to those of mild disease by 6–12 months of age. It has been hypothesized that the RBC membrane may be more fragile in the newborn due to the presence of elevated levels of free intraerythrocytic 2, 3-diphosphoglycerate (2, 3-DPG). This is a byproduct of fetal Hb. As fetal Hb levels decline after birth, the fragility of the RBC membrane improves, hemolysis decreases, and the morphology undergoes a transition from poikilocytosis to elliptocytosis. The term "infantile poikilocytosis" is often used, because it is difficult to distinguish this variant of hereditary elliptocytosis from hereditary pyropoikilocytosis. However, in most infants with both the hemolytic variant of hereditary elliptocytosis, as well as hereditary pyropoikilocytosis, the hemolysis, in general, wanes over the 1st year of life.[1,2]

Southeast Asian ovalocytosis, a common hereditary elliptocytosis syndrome in Southeast Asia and the South Pacific, usually presents with neonatal anemia and hyperbilirubinemia.[1]

Investigations: Anemia, reticulocytosis and the peripheral smear aid in diagnosis. The OFT is increased in the hemolytic variants with fragmentation and poikilocytosis. However, it is usually normal in the nonhemolytic forms of the common hereditary elliptocytosis.

Differential diagnoses: Individuals with the rare blood group Leach phenotype in the Gerbich blood group system (null phenotype) have elliptocytic RBCs; however, they are hematologically well and healthy. Patients with burns and blood specimens inadvertently stored at high temperatures may demonstrate elliptocytes.[35]

Management: No treatment is needed for the majority. Transfusions may be required in the newborn period. Hyperbilirubinemia might warrant phototherapy; in addition, exchange transfusions may be needed in severe cases. Splenectomy is beneficial for older children with chronic hemolysis.

Hereditary Stomatocytosis and Related Disorders

These include heterogeneous disorders characterized by variable numbers of stomatocytes on a peripheral blood film. Abnormal permeability of erythrocytes to sodium and potassium leads to modification of intracellular water content. The dehydrated variant, also known as hereditary xerocytosis, has been linked to mutations in the mammalian mechanosensory transduction protein PIEZO1. Hereditary stomatocytosis can present in the newborn with severe hemolysis, anemia, hyperbilirubinemia and hydrops fetalis. Hereditary xerocytosis may present in utero with nonimmune hydrops fetalis unrelated to the degree of fetal anemia.[35]

ENZYME DEFICIENCIES

Glucose-6-phosphate Dehydrogenase Deficiency

Epidemiology

Prevalence of G6PD deficiency is correlated with geographic distribution of malaria. It has been hypothesized that carriers of G6PD deficiency may incur partial protection against malarial infection.[37] It occurs with increased frequency throughout Africa, Asia, the Mediterranean and the Middle East. However, cases of sporadic gene mutation occur in all populations. In hospital-based studies from New Delhi and Kolkata, India, the incidence of G6PD deficiency in neonates was found to vary between 2% and 15%.[38,39]

Etiopathogenesis

Disorders of the hexose monophosphate shunt or the glutathione metabolic pathways impair the ability of the erythrocyte to adequately respond to oxidant stress. Reduced glutathione detoxifies intracellular oxidants. In G6PD deficiency, the inability to generate reduced nicotinamide adenine dinucleotide phosphate (NADPH) leads to inadequate levels of reduced glutathione. Reduced levels of glutathione lead to elevated levels of oxidants, which damage erythrocyte proteins. Oxidation of the sulfhydryl groups of Hb produces methemoglobin and intracellular precipitates of Hb called Heinz bodies.[2]

Clinical Features

All three clinical syndromes described in G6PD deficiency have been reported in neonates. These include NNJ, congenital nonspherocytic hemolytic anemia, and acute hemolysis following an oxidative stress.[1,37] The presentation is related to the severity of defect **(Table 15.1)**.

Table 15.1 Classes of glucose-6-phosphate dehydrogenase (G6PD) enzyme variants

Class	*Degree of deficiency*	*Presentation*	*Prevalence*
I	Very severe	Chronic nonspherocytic hemolytic anemia, severe neonatal jaundice	Uncommon; sporadic across populations
II	Severe (<10% of normal)	Intermittent hemolysis with oxidants (fava beans), predisposition to neonatal jaundice	Variable; frequent in Asian and Mediterranean population (e.g. G6PD-Mediterranean)
III	Moderate (10–60% of normal)	Intermittent hemolysis, typically with infections or drugs	10% of Afro-American population in the United States (e.g. G6PD)
IV	Mild-to-none (60–150% of normal)	Usually none	G6PD is the "wild" type variant

Jaundice is rarely present at birth. Levels peak between the 2nd and 3rd day of life. The severity of hyperbilirubinemia is variable; however, kernicterus has been reported. The pathogenesis of jaundice in G6PD deficiency is not known. It may result from reduced hepatic excretion of bilirubin or from low-grade hemolysis. Polymorphism of the uridine diphosphoglucuronosyl transferase gene (*UGT1A*) associated with Gilbert syndrome has been linked to the variable severity of jaundice.[40]

Anemia is rarely severe.[1] However, severe hemolytic anemia including nonimmune hydrops fetalis has been described in G6PD-deficient fetus or neonate following maternal ingestion of oxidants including sulfonamides, ascorbic acid or fava beans. Hemolysis has been reported in breastfed infants with G6PD deficiency following maternal ingestion of fava beans (*favism by proxy*).[41] In addition, hemolysis after transfusion or exchange transfusion with G6PD-deficient erythrocytes has been reported in neonates.[42] Screening of donors for G6PD deficiency before transfusing neonates can therefore be considered in endemic regions.[1]

Diagnosis

Acute hemolysis is characterized by marked morphologic abnormalities of RBCs with polychromasia, anisocytosis, bizarre poikilocytes, "bite cells" and "hemighost cells" **(Fig. 15.5)**. Supravital stain with methyl violet may demonstrate Heinz bodies. In patients presenting with chronic nonspherocytic hemolytic anemia, the morphologic abnormalities may be less pronounced; however, several poikilocytes and occasional bite cells are observed. Severity of NNJ often prompts screening for G6PD deficiency in neonates. A spectrophotometric method is utilized to directly measure the formation of NADPH via its characteristic absorption peak at 340 nm.[1] Activity is expressed in international units (micromoles of NADPH produced per minute) per gram of Hb. Leukocyte depletion is necessary as they are often rich in G6PD and their presence confounds results. In addition, increased G6PD levels in reticulocytes produced after an acute episode of hemolysis may falsely elevate enzyme levels warranting repeat measurement after a few weeks or using molecular methods to confirm the diagnosis in the acute phase.

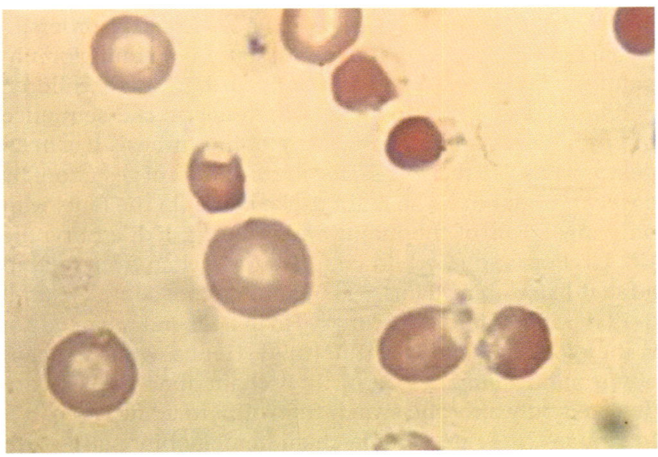

Figure 15.5 Blood smear demonstrating partially dehemoglobinized or "hemighost" cells in a case of G6PD deficiency. Oil immersion (100 X)

Courtesy: Dr Prateek Bhatia, Department of Pediatrics, PGIMER, Chandigarh.

Treatment

Hyperbilirubinemia is usually managed with phototherapy. An exchange transfusion may be indicated occasionally. Blood transfusion may be needed in the rare case presenting with hemolysis alone following exposure to oxidizing agents.[1,2] Advice to avoid potential oxidant triggers to hemolysis should be advised to all parents with babies with G6PD deficiency **(Box 15.3)**.

Pyruvate Kinase Deficiency

Epidemiology: Pyruvate kinase deficiency is an autosomal recessive disorder. It is the most common disorder of the Embden-Meyerhof glycolytic pathway. Heterozygotes are clinically as well as hematologically normal, even though they have roughly 50% of normal enzyme activity. It has been described in all ethnic groups. It has frequently been described in Northern Europeans (prevalence ~ 1:20,000).[2] In a study from Mumbai, India, the prevalence of PK deficiency among neonates with jaundice was 3.2%.[43]

Etiopathogenesis

Pyruvate kinase is involved in one of the two pathways that generate adenosine triphosphate (ATP) in RBCs. Nonerythroid tissues can utilize alternative pathways. Hence, clinical abnormalities in PK deficiency are manifested only in erythrocytes. It is a genetically diverse disorder with more than 180 mutations described in literature.

Box 15.3 List of selected agents to be avoided in patients with G6PD deficiency

- Furazolidone
- Methylene blue
- Nalidixic acid
- Naphthalene
- Nitrofurantoin
- Phenazopyridine
- Phenylhydrazine
- Primaquine
- Sulfacetamide
- Sulfamethoxazole
- Sulfanilamide
- Sulfapyridine
- Thiazolesulfone
- Toluidine blue
- Trinitrotoluene

Clinical Features

The phenotypic manifestations of the disorder reflect its genetic heterogeneity. History of neonatal hyperbilirubinemia is found in 33% of patients.[2] Jaundice frequently appears on the 1st day of life. Mortality and morbidity secondary to kernicterus have been described. Severe intrauterine anemia and hydrops fetalis have been reported as well.

Investigations

The diagnosis is considered in a jaundiced neonate with nonimmune hemolysis, especially in the absence of infections or definite exposure to hemolytic agents. Erythrocyte morphology is usually normal. Occasional dense cells with irregular margins (echinocytes) are seen. The peripheral smear helps to exclude hemoglobinopathies and membrane disorders. Assay for red cell PK activity is confirmatory.

Treatment

Exchange transfusion may be required in cases with severe NNJ. Splenectomy may reduce disease severity in cases with severe anemia; however, this is usually considered beyond 5 years of age.

Other Enzyme Deficiencies Presenting in the Newborn

Less frequent causes of enzyme deficiencies are usually considered if, (A) the level of PK is normal in a neonate with nonimmune hemolysis and (B) the peripheral smear is normal.[1,2]

Glucose phosphate isomerase (GPI) deficiency: It is the second most common enzymopathy of the glycolytic pathway that presents with hemolysis. Clinical manifestations are similar to PK deficiency. Severity of hemolysis is variable. Anemia and hyperbilirubinemia may be present. Hydrops fetalis has been reported.

Phosphoglycerate kinase (PGK) deficiency: It is an X-linked disorder. In addition to hemolysis, the newborn may present with neurologic abnormalities including seizures and movement disorders. Aphasia and mental retardation may be present in older children.

Phosphofructokinase (PFK) deficiency: It presents as severe myopathy due to profound enzyme deficiency in muscles, along with mild hemolysis secondary to partial enzyme deficiency in RBCs.

Triose phosphate isomerase (TPI) deficiency: It is characterized by severe neurologic abnormalities, including spasticity, motor retardation and hypotonia. It presents early in life. Most die before 5 years of age. Hemolysis is associated.

Hexokinase deficiency: It is a rare cause of hemolytic anemia. Splenectomy ameliorates however does not cure the disease.

Pyrimidine 5′-nucleotidase deficiency: It is the fourth common enzyme abnormality presenting with hemolytic anemia. It is inherited as an autosomal recessive disease. Though it has been described from geographically diverse regions, Mediterranean, Jewish, and African families often demonstrate a predisposition. Pyrimidine 5′-nucleotidase catalyzes the degradation of pyrimidine nucleotides to inorganic phosphate and the corresponding pyrimidine nucleoside. Deficiency leads to aggregation of ribosomes that produce membrane injury. The disorder is characterized by mild-to-moderate anemia, reticulocytosis and hyperbilirubinemia. RBCs demonstrate marked basophilic stippling due to the presence of partially degraded ribosomes. Spectrophotometric enzyme assay confirms the diagnosis.

Disorders of Glutathione Metabolism

Enzymes involved in glutathione metabolism include γ-glutamylcysteine synthetase and glutathione synthetase. Deficiency of these two enzymes has been associated with anemia in the neonatal period.[1]

HEMOGLOBINOPATHIES IN THE NEONATE

The basic pathophysiology of this autosomal group of disorders relates to the genetically determined abnormality of any of the multiple globin chains. The genes for these globin proteins are located on chromosome 16 for the α-like chains, and on chromosome 11 for the β-like chains. Deficient or mutated proteins promote chain imbalance compromising Hb stability. Hypoxia and hemolysis with or without ineffective erythropoiesis ensue leading to multiple complications. Phenotypic diversity ranges from an asymptomatic state to transfusion dependence in utero because of the multiple possible mutations in the different globin chains. In general, reduced production of normal Hb leads to the thalassemia syndromes, while the production of qualitatively abnormal Hb leads to disorders including the unstable hemoglobinopathies and the sickle cell disorders.

Salient differences in the manifestation of hemoglobinopathies in the neonatal age with respect to that in older children is related to the physiological difference in the sequence of synthesis of globin genes.[1,2] α-globin synthesis has been demonstrated in the yolk sac by the 3rd week of gestation. By 9 weeks, α-globin is the main α-like globin in the fetus with only low levels of the major embryonic α-like embryonic Hb, Hb Portland ($\zeta_2\gamma_2$). In contrast, the switch from fetal to adult β-like globin chains, γ to β-globin, is not complete until 6–12 months of life. The primary Hb in fetal and neonatal life is therefore the fetal Hb, HbF ($\alpha_2\gamma_2$). Hence, while α-chain abnormalities manifest at birth, β-chain abnormalities are detected only after the switch from HbF to adult Hb ($\alpha_2\beta_2$). In contrast, the rare gamma chain hemoglobinopathies are symptomatic in the fetus and neonate and disappear by 3–4 months of age. The carrier frequency of hemoglobinopathies in India varies from 3 to 17% in different populations.[44]

Gamma-thalassemia

In the presence of large deletions within the β-globin gene cluster, γ-globin genes ($^{A}\gamma$ and $^{G}\gamma$) may be removed along with δ and β-globin genes. About eight different γδβ-deletions have been reported mostly in families of European origin. This results in γδβ-thalassemia, which is lethal in the homozygous state. In the heterozygous state, this disorder produces a moderately severe albeit transient microcytic anemia in the neonate. The anemia improves over the next 3–4 months without any specific treatment. In older children, the hematological picture mimics β-thalassemia trait.[1,2]

Alpha Thalassemia

Epidemiology

Frequency of α-thalassemia in different populations of India vary from 0.05% to 0.2%.[44]

Etiopathogenesis

There are four genes coding for α-globin chains and these are located on chromosome 16. The clinical spectrum ranges from an asymptomatic state to hydrops fetalis depending on the number of genes involved as well as the mutation leading to either absence of the protein or a protein that is abnormal. Either way, chain imbalance leads to RBC destruction, resulting in ineffective erythropoiesis and hemolysis.

Clinical Phenotypes

A neonate can inherit deletions in one, two, three or all four of the α genes leading to four distinct clinical syndromes, viz. a silent carrier state, α-thalassemia trait, HbH disease and homozygous α-thalassemia presenting as hydrops fetalis.

Silent Carrier State

It occurs in individuals lacking one functional α-globin gene (–α/αα). Such individuals are clinically as well as hematologically normal. However, at birth, mildly elevated levels of Hb Barts (γ_4) (1–3%) can be demonstrated as compared to normal newborns (<1%). Beyond the newborn period, there is neither microcytosis nor anemia. Both HbF as well as HbA_2 are within normal limits.

Alpha-thalassemia Trait

It is due to deletion or nonfunctional status of two α-globin genes. In Southeast Asia, the deletions are frequently in *CIS*, i.e. located on the same chromosome (– –/αα). On the other hand, those of African inheritance have their deletions predominately in *trans*, i.e. on different chromosomes (–α/–α). This has the clinical implication that severe α-thalassemia disorders including HbH disease and homozygous α-thalassemia occur more frequently in Southeast Asians.

Alpha-thalassemia trait is associated with mild microcytic anemia. The MCV in neonates is less than 100 fL. Usually frank hemolysis and reticulocytosis are absent. The cord blood contains 3–10% Hb Barts. Significant clinical abnormalities are absent. Beyond the newborn period, the mild microcytic anemia often mimics that caused due to iron deficiency. HbA2 levels are in the low-to-low-normal range (1.5–2.5%) **(Fig. 15.6A)**.

Hemoglobin H Disease

It occurs in the presence of one functional α-globin gene and is more frequent in Southeast Asia. It occurs due to deletion of three genes (– –/–α). One parent is usually a trait (– –/αα),

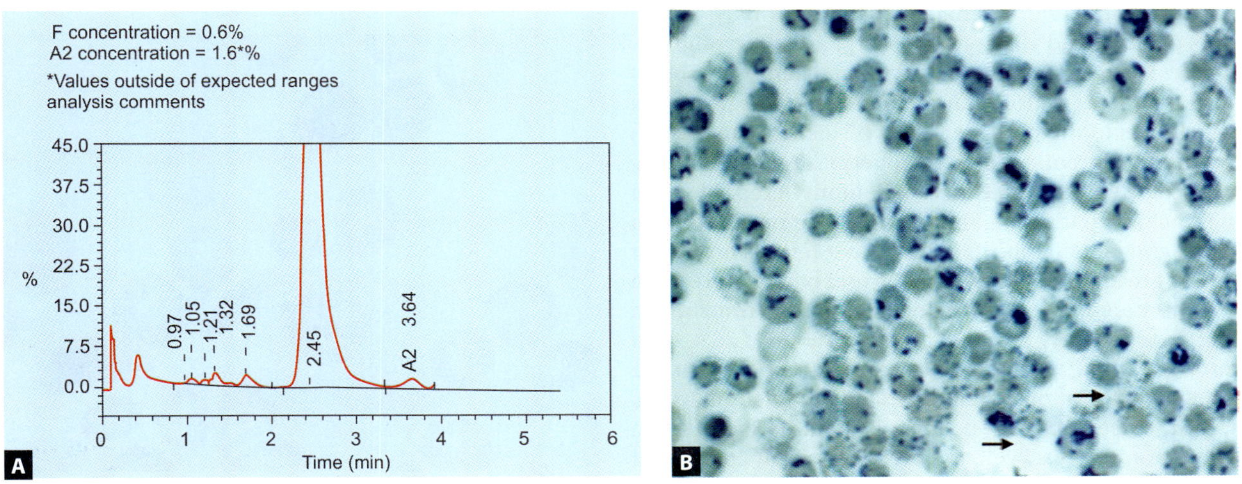

Figures 15.6A and B (A) HPLC of father demonstrating a low HbA2 (1.6%) suggestive of α-thalassemia trait; (B) "Golf ball" inclusions in a case of HbH disease

Abbreviations: HbH, hemoglobin H; HPLC, high-performance liquid chromatography

Courtesy: Prof Reena Das, Department of Hematology and Dr Prateek Bhatia, Department of Pediatrics, PGIMER, Chandigarh.

while the other is a silent carrier ($\alpha\alpha/\alpha$-). One of the two existing α-globin chains in an individual being abnormal often leads to a similar phenotype. Hb constant spring is the most well-known disorder in this group (- -/αcsα).

In the neonate, HbH disease is characterized by marked hypochromia and microcytosis. The cord blood demonstrates elevated levels of Hb Barts (20–30%). Beyond infancy, there is excess of β-globin chains and these form tetramers known as HbH. Brilliant cresyl blue demonstrates intra-erythrocytic HbH inclusions in a nonsplenectomized patient **(Fig. 15.6B)**. However, HbH is best demonstrated as rapidly migrating Hb on electrophoresis of a fresh blood sample on cellulose acetate at alkaline pH. In such cases, it comprises 5–40% of the total Hb.

Hemoglobin constant spring (HbCS) is due to a mutation that alters the translation codon for terminating α-globin synthesis. This leads to an elongated α-globin variant whose output is less than 1% of normal. The allele is observed only in the presence of another normal α-allele ($\alpha^{cs}\alpha$). Heterozygous HbCS ($\alpha^{cs}\alpha/\alpha\alpha$) presents similar to the α-thalassemia silent carrier and infrequently like the α-thalassemia trait. Findings are unremarkable other than the presence of 1–2% HbCS, demonstrated as a slow-migrating Hb on electrophoresis.[2]

The inheritance of an α^{cs} allele with an α-thalassemia trait ($\alpha^{cs}\alpha$/- -) results in a phenotype that is similar to HbH disease. The patient has 10–15% HbH and 2–3% HbCS. This hemolytic variant is more frequent in Southeast Asia. Homozygous HbCS ($\alpha^{cs}\alpha/\alpha^{cs}\alpha$) has a clinical phenotype akin to HbH disease. Despite the presence of two normal α-alleles, an unstable α^{cs} mRNA leads to membrane damage and basophilic stippling, secondary to precipitation. Splenomegaly is present. A mild hemolytic anemia with normocytic RBCs demonstrating basophilic stippling is described.

Homozygous α-thalassemia: Deletion of all four α-globin genes is incompatible to postnatal life. The cord blood demonstrates tetramers of non-α-globin chains: 70–80% Hb Barts, small amounts of HbH, and Hb Portland ($\xi_2\gamma_2$), an embryonic Hb. Intrauterine survival is related to the persistent function of Hb Portland. The predominance of Hb Barts in postnatal life contributes to the pathogenesis. This is because its high oxygen affinity impairs oxygen delivery. Anemia is severe (Hb 3–10 g/dL); erythroblastosis is demonstrated. Physical findings include marked pallor, hepatosplenomegaly, edema and other congenital abnormalities. Most fetuses are either aborted or are stillborn. However, several babies were born alive, resuscitated, and placed on chronic RBC transfusion programs. In a study from Thailand (n = 65), 25% died in utero, 18% died during delivery and 54% died within 1 hour of delivery.[2] Autopsy demonstrated enlarged placenta, heart, liver, spleen and adrenal glands. Retardation of brain growth was reported as well. Majority had a reduced weight for gestational age.[2]

Most live-borns receive a chronic transfusion regimen from birth.[45] Bone marrow transplantation is a viable option if a suitable donor is available.[46] In utero hematopoietic stem cell transplantation is under evaluation.

In families with homozygous α-thalassemia, both parents have α-thalassemia trait (- -/$\alpha\alpha$). Significant maternal complications during gestation and delivery have been reported. For reasons unknown, majority develop toxemia of pregnancy. Delivery is complicated by significant postpartum hemorrhage because of the retention of a bulky placenta. In the absence of appropriate obstetrical care, up to 50% of mothers might suffer lethal complications.

Sickle Cell Disease

Sickle cell disease (SCD) results from a single amino acid substitution in the β-globin gene. The abnormal Hb (HbS) undergoes intracellular polymerization in the deoxygenated state. This distorts the red blood cell (RBC) morphology leading to lysis of the cells **(Fig. 15.7)**. Individuals homozygous for the sickle mutation have the most severe form of the disease. They are susceptible to both acute and chronic sequelae, and are said to have sickle cell anemia (SCA). The mutation involves substitution of valine for glutamic acid at the 6th amino acid on the β-globin.[2]

Although no clinical abnormalities associated with SCD are present at birth, early diagnosis is important. Universal screening identifies babies with all forms of SCD including those with SCA, who are most at risk for invasive pneumococcal infection.[47] This provides opportunity to initiate the following three-pronged preventive strategy to prevent morbidity and mortality: (1) vaccination against encapsulated organisms; (2) twice-daily prophylactic penicillin beginning in early infancy and continuing till at least 5 years of age and (3) education of caregivers regarding the need to seek immediate medical attention in the event of fever.[47]

Infants who are born to mothers with SCD may develop several complications. There is an increased risk of stillbirth, intrauterine growth restriction and preterm delivery.[47] Fetal

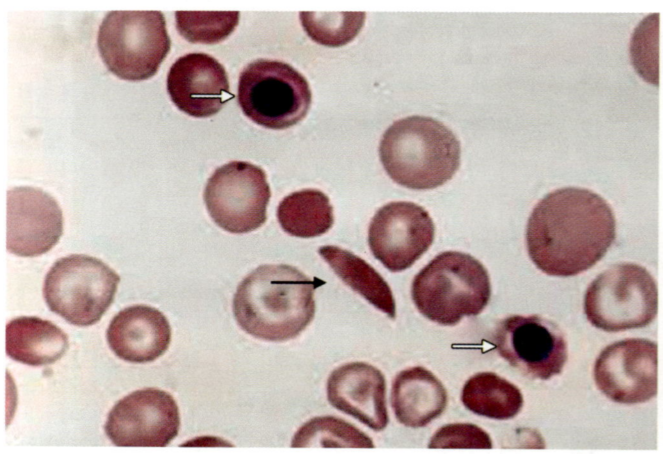

Figure 15.7 Peripheral blood film showing a sickle cell (black arrow) and nRBCs (white arrows) in a case of sickle cell anemia. (Oil immersion 100 X)

Courtesy: Dr Prateek Bhatia, Department of Pediatrics, PGIMER, Chandigarh.

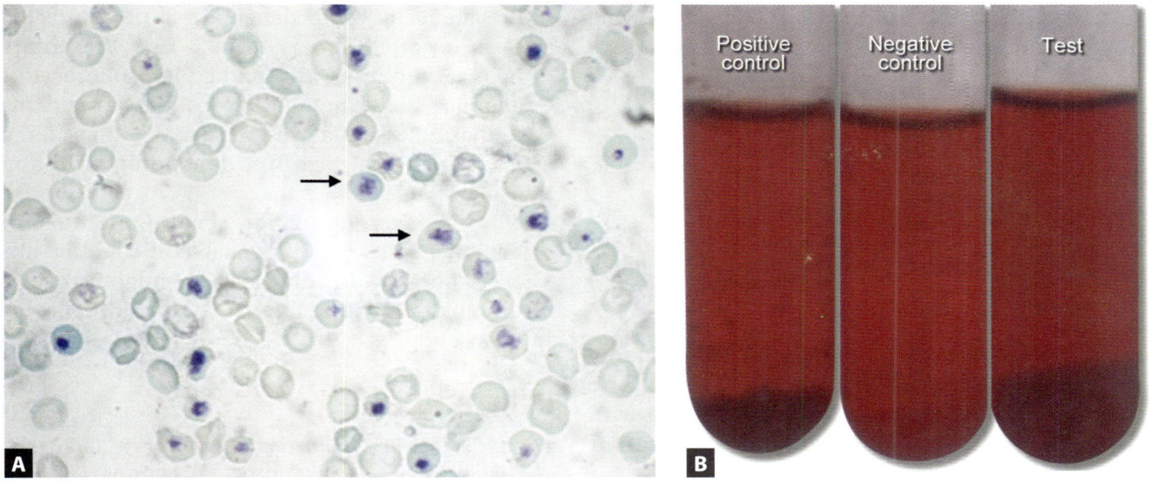

Figures 15.8A and B (A) Heinz bodies (black arrows) in a case of unstable hemoglobinopathy; (B) Heat instability test demonstrates precipitation reaction in the "test" and "positive control" samples
Courtesy: Prof Reena Das, Department of Hematology, PGIMER, Chandigarh.

surveillance is required during pregnancy. In addition, blood from an adult donor who has sickle trait should not be utilized for exchange transfusion in the newborn, particularly if hypoxemia is present, because this result in an adverse outcome.[2]

Unstable Hemoglobinopathies

Unstable Hbs have lower solubility than normal Hb. This leads to chronic nonspherocytic hemolytic anemia.[1] Both α and β-chains may be involved. Several unstable Hbs have been described. Many patients present with mild or moderate hemolysis. However, severe hemolysis can lead to hyperbilirubinemia in the newborn. Precipitation of the insoluble globin leads to the formation of Heinz bodies **(Fig. 15.8A)**. These can be difficult to detect in the young as well as in those with a functioning spleen. Hence, their absence in the perinatal period does not rule out the presence of an unstable hemoglobinopathy. Specific diagnosis is made by detecting Hb instability at 50°C or in the presence of isopropanol **(Fig. 15.8B)**. Diagnosis can be made with Hb electrophoresis in several cases. However, approximately 30% of unstable Hbs remain undetectable. Such cases are plausibly responsible for several of the undiagnosed transient hemolytic anemias of infancy.[1,2]

Two variants deserve attention in neonatal period. In both these disorders, the hemolysis abates after the first few months of life once fetal Hb ($\alpha_2\gamma_2$) is replaced by adult Hb ($\alpha_2\beta_2$). Hb F-Poole is a mutant fetal Hb in which the 130th residue of the γ-globin chain contains glycine instead of tryptophan. This leads to instability of fetal Hb and hemolysis.[48] Hb Hasharon results from a substitution of histidine for aspartate at position 47 of the α-globin gene. When coupled with γ-globin, this results in decreased stability, leading to hemolysis. When paired with the β-globin gene, Hb Hasharon is stable and the hemolysis subsides.[49]

Neonatal Screening for Hemoglobinopathies

Newborn screening for hemoglobinopathies is primarily for early diagnosis and treatment of an affected newborn with the aim of prevention of morbidity, rather than prospective primary prevention. In addition, it allows primary prevention for the parents who have had an affected or carrier child, and thereby at risk. An added advantage would be prevention of morbidities including those during anesthesia for HbS carriers. In the long-term, it provides information for healthy carriers to opt for testing of partners.

The first step in newborn screening is the direct separation and measurement of the Hb fractions present.[44] Those present at birth include HbF (~80%) with some HbA (~20%). Measurement of HbA, HbF and any abnormal fractions (HbS, C, E, D, Barts, etc.) if present assists in the diagnosis. Frequently used methods in newborn screening include high-performance liquid chromatography, capillary electrophoresis and isoelectric focusing. HbCS is measured via capillary electrophoresis because it is not detected on high-performance liquid chromatography. The sample used is either dry blood or fresh cord blood. Dry blood samples are reliable for up to 3 weeks after collection. The analysis takes only a few minutes.[44]

Newborn screening for α-thalassemia has importance in endemic regions. Early diagnosis might prevent unnecessary treatment with iron. Moreover, couples at risk of having babies with severe disease may be identified and informed regarding their reproductive choices. Hb-Barts is easily detected and its amount correlates with the number of defective α-globin genes. A single gene defect (-α/αα) presents with 1–4% Hb-Barts with two defective genes it will rise to 5–15%, reaching more than 25% in HbH disease with three defective genes (-/-α). Affected children should undergo a confirmatory DNA test. Genotype analysis is essential to exclude false positives including variants mimicking HbS, C, E or D. It also predicts the risk for subsequent children allowing informed reproductive choices for future pregnancies.

Potential drawbacks of neonatal screening for hemoglobinopathies include:[44]

- Hereditary persistence of fetal Hb (HPFH) may be mistaken as thalassemia major.
- Carriers of β-thalassemia cannot be diagnosed by measuring their elevated HbA_2 expression at birth. HbA_2 is not sufficiently expressed before 1 year of age to be a reliable diagnostic parameter. However, carriers can often be diagnosed at birth by measuring HbA expression.
- Physiologically reduced amounts of HbA confounding interpretation of homozygous states of HbS and HbE versus respective compound heterozygous state with β-thalassemia trait. Distinction requires molecular analysis.
- Small amounts of HbA (<2–3%) can be present in β^+-thalassemia major (or β^+-thalassemia/HPFH). Samples with 3–5% HbA should be evaluated for possible β-thalassemia intermedia or β-thalassemia carrier state.
- Unstable β-gene variants may not be detected with newborn screening and can manifest after 6 months of age with hemolysis of variable severity.

CONCLUSION

Disorders causing non-immune hemolysis in the neonate need to be diagnosed keeping in mind the unique physiology at this age. A few diseases may be missed at this age, others might have distinct features, while select disorders are exclusive to newborns. A systemic approach to diagnosis, including screening for disorders like hemoglobinopathies, will aid in limiting morbidity in later life.

KEY POINTS

- Diagnosis of hemolysis in the newborn has to be considered in the backdrop of physiological changes. These include decrease in Hb and MCV, reticulocytosis, increased nucleated RBCs, predominance of atypical cells, secondary to relative hyposplenism and hyperbilirubinemia.
- Nonimmune causes of hemolysis may be secondary to defects that may be extrinsic or intrinsic to RBCs.
- Maternal drug intake is a frequent cause of oxidant-related hemolysis in the neonate.
- Several infections can result in hemolysis—viral, bacterial or parasitic.
- HS is an important cause of nonimmune hemolysis among intrinsic disorders of the RBC membrane. Neonates may present with severe jaundice. Anemia could be transfusion-dependent during the 1st year of life. A lack of family history (common in India) may delay diagnosis. RBC indices are useful in screening. An EMA binding assay excludes majority of the confounding differential diagnoses in the neonatal period.
- Hereditary elliptocytosis and hereditary pyropoikilocytosis may demonstrate overlapping features in the neonate.
- Prevalence of G6PD deficiency in newborns in India has been reported to vary from 2–15%. Presentation in the neonate could be with jaundice, nonspherocytic hemolytic anemia or acute hemolysis secondary to oxidant exposure.
- Alpha-thalassemia presents as a silent carrier, trait, HbH disease or fetal hydrops, depending on the number of α-genes deleted.
- Newborn screening for several of the nonimmune hemolytic disorders is available. It could be utilized for a cost-effective early diagnosis in endemic regions of India, thereby preventing late morbidity and allowing genetic counseling.

REFERENCES

1. Gallagher PG. The neonatal erythrocyte and its disorders. In: Orkin SH, Fisher DE, Ginsberg D, Look AT, Lux SE, Nathan DG (Eds). Nathan and Oski's Hematology and Oncology of Infancy and Childhood, 8th editon. Philadelphia, PA, USA: Elsevier Saunders; 2015. pp. 52-4.
2. Glader B, Allen GA. Neonatal hemolysis. In: de Alarcon PA, Werner EJ, Christensen RD (Eds). Neonatal Hematology, 2nd edition. Cambridge, UK: Cambridge University Press; 2015. p.91.
3. Geaghan SM. Hematologic values and appearances in the healthy fetus, neonate, and child. Clin Lab Med. 1999;19(1):1-37.
4. Oski FA, Naiman JL. Hematologic problems in the newborn. 3rd edition. Major Probl Clin Pediatr. 1982;4:1-360.
5. Padmanabhan J, Risemberg HM, Rowe RD. Howell-Jolly bodies in the peripheral blood of full-term and premature neonates. Johns Hopkins Med J. 1973;132(3):146-50.
6. Martin CR, Cloherty JP. Neonatal hyperbilirubinemia. In: Cloherty JP, Eichenwald EC, Stark AR (Eds). Manual of Neonatal Care, 6th edition. Philadelphia, PA, USA: Lippincott Williams and Wilkins; 2008. pp. 181-92.
7. Landaas S, Skrede S, Steen JA. The levels of serum enzymes, plasma proteins and lipids in normal infants and small children. J Clin Chem Clin Biochem. 1981;19(10):1075-80.
8. Tidmarsh GF, Wong RJ, Stevenson DK. End-tidal carbon monoxide and hemolysis. J Perinatol. 2014;34(8):577-81.
9. Hocking DR. Neonatal haemolytic disease due to dapsone. Med J Aust. 1968;1(26):1130-1.
10. Stahl MM, Neiderud J, Vinge E. Thrombocytopenic purpura and anemia in a breast-fed infant whose mother was treated with valproic acid. J Pediatr. 1997;130(6):1001-3.
11. Pruekprasert P, Stout C, Patamasucon P. Neonatal enterovirus infection. J Assoc Acad Minor Phys. 1995;6(4):134-8.
12. Nobili V, Vento S, Comparcola D, Sartorelli MR, Luciani M, Marcellini M. Autoimmune hemolytic anemia and autoimmune hepatitis associated with parvovirus B19 infection. Pediatr Infect Dis J. 2004;23(2):184-5.
13. Klein RL, Novak RW, Novak PE. T-cryptantigen exposure in neonatal necrotizing enterocolitis. J Pediatr Surg. 1986;21(12):1155-8.
14. Mupanemunda RH, Kenyon CF, Inwood MJ, Leigh K. Bacterial-induced activation of erythrocyte T-antigen complicating necrotising enterocolitis: a case report. Eur J Pediatr. 1993;152(4):325-6.
15. Piagnerelli M, Boudjeltia KZ, Brohee D, Piro P, Carlier E, Vincent JL, et al. Alterations of red blood cell shape and sialic acid membrane content in septic patients. Crit Care Med. 2003;31(8):2156-62.

16. Osborn DA, Lui K, Pussell P, Jana AK, Desai AS, Cole M. T and Tk antigen activation in necrotising enterocolitis: manifestations, severity of illness, and effectiveness of testing. Arch Dis Child Fetal Neonatal Ed. 1999;80(3):F192-7.
17. Rodwell R, Tudehope DI. Screening for cryptantigen exposure and polyagglutination in neonates with suspected necrotizing enterocolitis. J Paediatr Child Health. 1993;29(1):16-8.
18. Barnett ED. Malaria. In: Feigin RD, Cherry JD, Demmler GJ, Kaplan S (Eds). Textbook of Pediatric Infectious Diseases, 6th edition. Philadelphia, PA, USA: WB Saunders; 2004. pp. 2714-29.
19. Rai P, Majumdar K, Sharma S, Chauhan R, Chandra J. Congenital malaria in a neonate: case report with a comprehensive review on differential diagnosis, treatment and prevention in Indian perspective. J Parasit Dis. 2015;39(2):345-8.
20. Gandhi A, Garg K, Wadhwa N. Neonatal Plasmodium vivax malaria: an overlooked entity. J Infect Dev Ctries. 2011;5(6):489-92.
21. Ekanem AD, Anah MU, Udo JJ. The prevalence of congenital malaria among neonates with suspected sepsis in Calabar, Nigeria. Trop Doct. 2008;38:(2):73-6.
22. Batton DG, Amanullah A, Comstock C. Fetal schistocytic hemolytic anemia and umbilical vein varix. J Pediatr Hematol Oncol. 2000;22(3):259-61.
23. Anai T, Miyakawa I, Ohki H, Ogawa T. Hydrops fetalis caused by fetal Kasabach-Merritt syndrome. Acta Paediatr Jpn. 1992;34(3):324-7.
24. Ritchie JH, Fish MB, McMasters V, Grossman M. Edema and hemolytic anemia in premature infants. A vitamin E deficiency syndrome. N Engl J Med. 1968;279(22):1185-90.
25. Zipursky A, Brown EJ, Watts J, Milner R, Rand C, Blanchette VS, et al. Oral vitamin E supplementation for the prevention of anemia in premature infants: a controlled trial. Pediatrics. 1987;79(1):61-8.
26. Tuffy P, Brown AK, Zuelzer WW. Infantile pyknocytosis; a common erythrocyte abnormality of the first trimester. AMA J Dis Child. 1959;98(2):227-41.
27. Eyssette-Guerreau S, Bader-Meunier B, Garcon L, Guitton C, Cynober T. Infantile pyknocytosis: a cause of haemolytic anaemia of the newborn. Br J Haematol. 2006;133(4):439-42.
28. Amendola G, Di Concilio R, D'Urzo G, Danise P, Parisi G, della Ragione F, et al. Erythropoietin treatment can prevent blood transfusion in infantile pyknocytosis. Br J Haematol. 2008;143(4):593-5.
29. Gamsu H, Lorber J, Rendle-Short J. Haemolytic anaemia in osteopetrosis. A report of two cases. Arch Dis Child. 1961;36:494-9.
30. Christensen RD, Yaish HM, Gallagher PG. A pediatrician's practical guide to diagnosing and treating hereditary spherocytosis in neonates. Pediatrics. 2015;135(6):1107-14.
31. Das A, Bansal D, Das R, Trehan A, Marwaha RK. Hereditary spherocytosis in children: profile and post-splenectomy outcome. Indian Pediatr. 2014;51(2):139-41.
32. Bolton-Maggs PH, Langer JC, Iolascon A, Tittensor P, King MJ. General Haematology Task Force of the British Committee for Standards in Haematology. Guidelines for the diagnosis and management of hereditary spherocytosis—2011 update. Br J Haematol. 2012;156(1):37-49.
33. Delhommeau F, Cynober T, Schischmanoff PO, Rohrlich P, Delaunay J, Mohandas N, et al. Natural history of hereditary spherocytosis during the first year of life. Blood. 2000;95(2):393-7.
34. Bhutani VK, Johnson L. Synopsis report from the pilot USA Kernicterus Registry. J Perinatol. 2009;29(Suppl 1):S4-7.
35. King MJ, Garçon L, Hoyer JD, Iolascon A, Picard V, Stewart G, et al. ICSH guidelines for the laboratory diagnosis of nonimmune hereditary red cell membrane disorders. Int J Lab Hematol. 2015;37(3):304-25.
36. Das A, Bansal D, Ahluwalia J, Das R, Rohit MK, Attri SV, et al. Risk factors for thromboembolism and pulmonary artery hypertension following splenectomy in children with hereditary spherocytosis. Pediatr Blood Cancer. 2014;61(1):29-33.
37. Frank JE. Diagnosis and management of G6PD deficiency. Am Fam Physician. 2005;72(7):1277-82.
38. Pao M, Kulkarni A, Gupta V, Kaul S, Balan S. Neonatal screening for glucose-6-phosphate dehydrogenase deficiency. Indian J Pediatr. 2005;72:835-7.
39. Bisoi S, Chakraborty S, Chattopadhyay D, Biswas B, Ray S. Glucose-6-phosphate dehydrogenase screening of babies born in a tertiary care hospital in West Bengal. Indian J Public Health. 2012;56(2):146-8.
40. Kaplan M, Renbaum P, Levy-Lahad E, Hammerman C, Lahad A, Beutler E. Gilbert syndrome and glucose-6-phosphate dehydrogenase deficiency: a dose-dependent genetic interaction crucial to neonatal hyperbilirubinemia. Proc Natl Acad Sci USA. 1997;94(22):12128-32.
41. Kaplan M, Vreman HJ, Hammerman C, Schimmel MS, Abrahamov A, Stevenson DK. Favism by proxy in nursing glucose-6-phosphate dehydrogenase-deficient neonates. J Perinatol. 1998;18(6 Pt 1):477-9.
42. Kumar P, Sarkar S, Narang A. Acute intravascular haemolysis following exchange transfusion with G-6-PD deficient blood. Eur J Pediatr. 1994;153(2):98-9.
43. Kedar PS, Warang P, Colah RB, Mohanty D. Red cell pyruvate kinase deficiency in neonatal jaundice cases in India. Indian J Pediatr. 2006;73(11):985-8.
44. Old J, Angastiniotis M, Eleftheriou A, Harteveld CL, Petrou M, Synodinos JT. Prevention of Thalassemias and Other Haemoglobin Disorders, 2nd edition. Volume 2: Laboratory Protocols. Nicosia, Cyprus: Thalassemia International Federation; 2012.
45. Singer ST, Styles L, Bojanowski J, Quirolo K, Foote D, Vichinsky EP. Changing outcome of homozygous alpha-thalassemia: cautious optimism. J Pediatr Hematol Oncol. 2000;22(6):539-42.
46. Chik KW, Shing MM, Li CK, Leung TF, Tsang KS, Yuen HL, et al. Treatment of hemoglobin Bart's hydrops with bone marrow transplantation. J Pediatr. 1998;132(6):1039-42.
47. Yawn BP, Buchanan GR, Afenyi-Annan AN, Ballas SK, Hassell KL, James AH, et al. Management of sickle cell disease: summary of the 2014 evidence-based report by expert panel members. JAMA. 2014;312(10):1033-48.
48. Lee-Potter JP, Deacon-Smith RA, Simpkiss MJ, Kamuzora H, Lehmann H. A new cause of haemolytic anaemia in the newborn. A description of an unstable fetal haemoglobin: F Poole, alpha2-G-gamma2 130 tryptophan yeilds glycine. J Clin Pathol. 1975;28(4):317-20.
49. Charache S, Mondzac AM, Gessner U. Hemoglobin Hasharon (alpha-2-47 his(CD5)beta-2): a hemoglobin found in low concentration. J Clin Invest. 1969;48(5):834-47.

CHAPTER 16

Inherited Bone Marrow Failure Syndromes

Tathagata Chatterjee, Ujjwal Dimri, VP Choudhry

INTRODUCTION

The inherited bone marrow failure syndrome (IBMFS) consists of various inherited disorders, which present as bone marrow failure (all or a single cell lineage) with first presentation in childhood but occasionally in adulthood and generally in association with one or more somatic abnormality. More than 33 genes have been identified till dates, which have been implicated in these syndromes. Genetic studies have provided fresh knowledge of various molecular pathways implicated in the pathogenesis of these disorders such as the DNA repair-FA/BRCA pathway; Telomere maintenance—Dyskeratosis congenita (DC) pathway; Ribosomes biogenesis—Shwachman-Diamond syndrome (SDS) as well as Diamond-Blackfan anemia (DBA) genetic pathway. In a way these disorders also provide insights into genesis of cancer since they have been associated with increased risk of development of cancer.

It is well documented that one-fourth of pediatric and one-tenth of adult patients who present with features of hypoplastic and aplastic anemia have some form of an inherited etiology; hence IBFMS must be considered in young patients presenting with specific types of cancers as well as in patients of aplastic anemia with characteristic somatic findings. International Registries have compiled data that help us in defining and categorizing the various IBFMS. These include the United Kingdom Dyskeratosis Congenita Registry (DCR), the Severe Chronic Neutropenia International Registry (SCNIR), the International Fanconi Anemia Registry (IFAR) and the Diamond-Blackfan Anemia Registry (DBAR). These registries help to define the clinical and laboratory features of the recognized patients. In all such cases the main presenting features are due to the various cytopenias. Fanconi anemia (FA) and DC patients generally present with pancytopenia whereas anemia is the usual presentation in DBA.

Isolated neutropenia is the most common presentation in patients of both SCN and SDS, whereas thrombocytopenia is the most prominent feature in patients with thrombo-cytopenia absent radii (TAR) and in amegakaryocytic thrombocytopenia (Amega). DBA, SCN and TAR are three categories of IBFMS, which generally present with monocytopenias unlike FA, DC and SDS. Most of these IBFMS may evolve to either MDS or AML with either of them as the first presenting sign. FA, DC and DBA are associated with characteristic solid tumors. Most of these syndromes are associated with mutated genes except possibly TAR. However, there are exceptions to the rule and some of them having the classical features may lack a mutated gene.

Among the various entities under IBFMS only TAR and Amega are predominantly diagnosed in childhood whereas FA and DC may be diagnosed in adults. On the other hand DBA, SCN and SCD may initially be diagnosed much later in adults. In fact more than half of the patients reported in the various above-mentioned registries were actually diagnosed in adulthood (at least > 16 years) and the median survival ranged from 16 years to 72 years. The possibility of IBMFS should be considered by adult hematologists or oncologists also, as cases of IBMFS may present to them.

FANCONI ANEMIA

Fanconi anemia is generally inherited as an autosomal inherited disorder though very rarely it can be inherited as an X-linked recessive disorder **(Fig. 16.1)** with usual presentation 1st decade in life's; however, there are patients who have presented at a much later age and few cases have been diagnosed even in the 4th decade of life.

Approximately 9% of cases are diagnosed in the adult age group. Patients usually present with characteristic birth defects, which are helpful in the diagnosis; however, their absence does not, for example exclude FA as more than one-fourth of such cases have no obvious physical anomalies **(Table 16.1)**. Classical features include café-au-lait spots, short stature, microphthalmia, hyper- and hypo-pigmentation, microcephaly and abnormal thumbs with or without hypoplastic radii **(Figs 16.2A and B)**. Hypogonadism

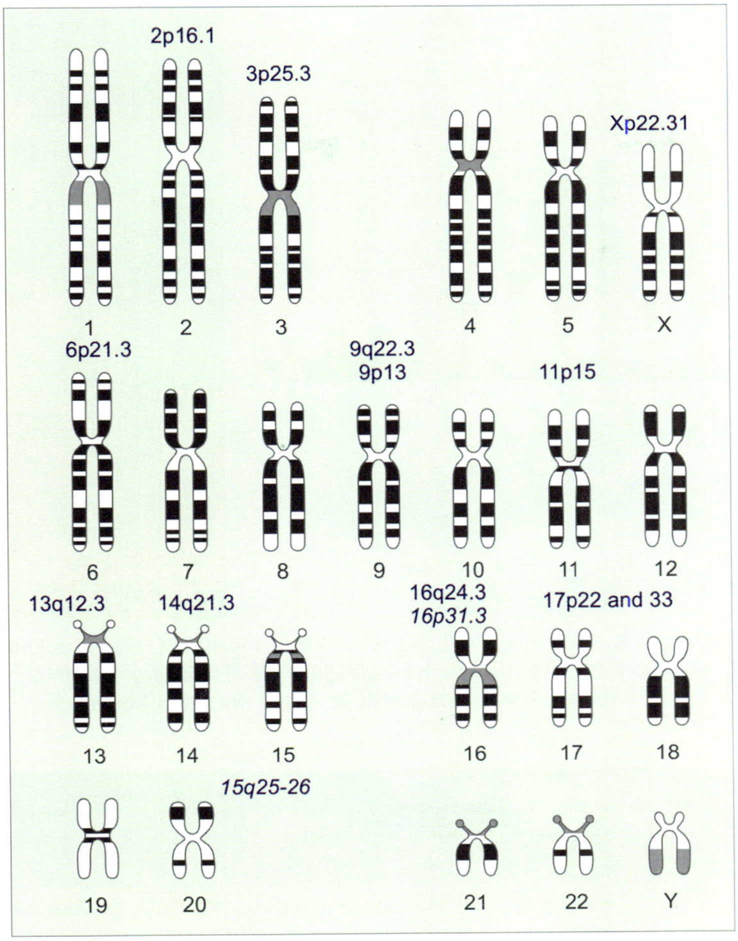

Figure 16.1 Fanconi anemia (FA) is genetically heterogeneous, there are 15 complementation groups
Courtesy: Dr Revathi Raj, Apollo Specialty Hospital, Chennai.

Table 16.1 Somatic abnormalities in Fanconi anemia

Abnormality	*Percentage of patients*
Skeletal (radial ray, hip, vertebral, scoliosis and rib)	71
Skin pigmentation (café-au-lait, hyper and hypopigmentation)	64
Short stature	63
Eyes (microphthalmia)	38
Renal and urinary tract	34
Male genitalia	20
Mental retardation	16
Gastrointestinal (e.g. anorectal, duodenal atresia)	14
Heart	13
Hearing	11
Central nervous system (e.g. hydrocephalous, septum pellucidum)	8
No abnormalities	30

Source: Auerbach AD, Buchwald M, Joenje H. In: Scriver CR (Ed). The Metabolic and Molecular Basis of Inherited Disease. New York, USA: McGraw-Hill Publisher; 2001. pp. 753-68.

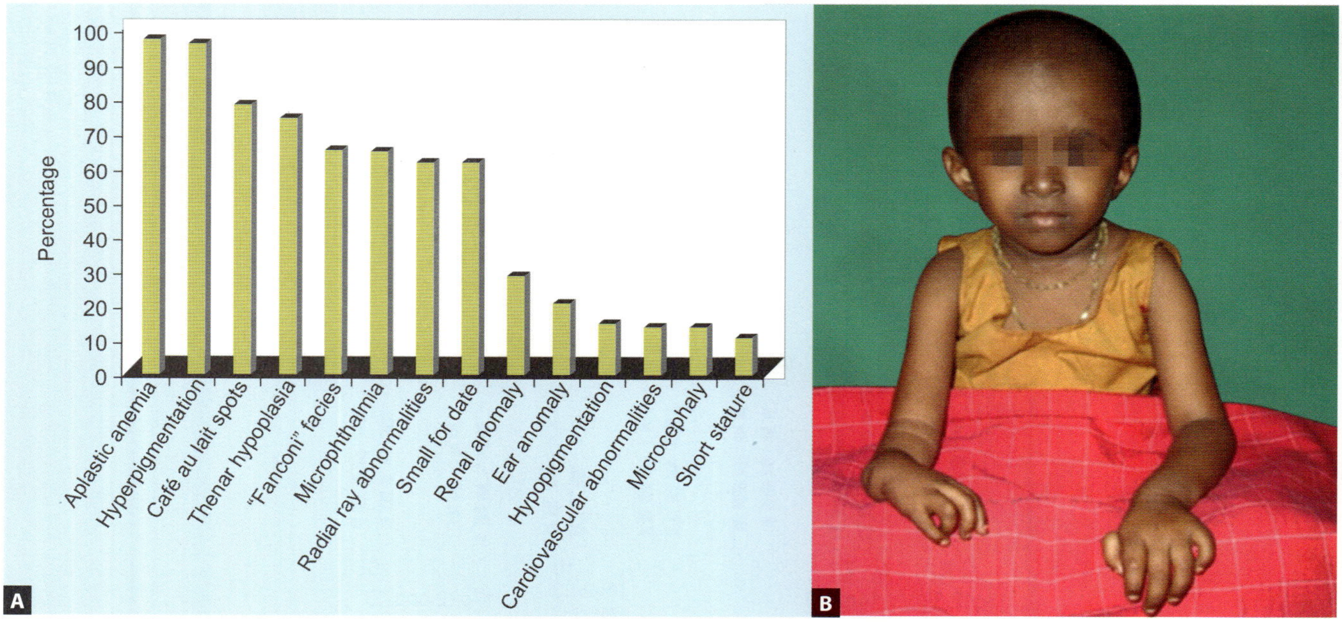

Figures 16.2A and B Spectrum of anomalies in FA from registry of Fanconi anemia in India. Also a 3-year-old patient with FA showing typical radial ray deformity
Courtesy: Dr Revathi Raj, Apollo Specialty Hospital, Chennai.

Table 16.2 Incidence of malignancies in Fanconi's anemia

Malignancy	*NAS study*	*IFAR*	*Registry of Fanconi anemia in India*	*Cumulative incidence from literature*
Leukemia (mainly AML M4 and M%)	10% by age of 48 years	40% by age of 50 years	For AML—median age 13 years (0.1–50) For ALL—median age 5 years (1–10)	33% by age of 40 years
Solid tumors (mainly hepatic tumors and squamous cell carcinoma affecting vulva, esophagus, head and neck)	29% by age of 48 years	35% by age of 50 years	Median age of occurrence—26 years (1–45)	28% by age of 40 years

Abbreviations: ALL, acute lymphoblastic leukemia; AML, acute myeloid leukemia; IFAR, International Fanconi Anemia Registry; NAS, North American Survey

Source: Alter BP. Diagnosis, genetics, and management of inherited bone marrow failure syndromes. Hematology Am Soc Hematol Educ Program. 2007. pp. 29-39.

and infertility may be the presentation in males presenting during adulthood, while women may have late onset of menarche and early onset menopause. Patients presenting with progressive failure of bone marrow and an increased predisposition to malignancy in very young age may lead to a high level of suspicion for diagnosis of underlying FA **(Table 16.2)**.

Diagnosis in such patients of aplastic anemia, acute myeloid leukemia (AML) or MDS and head and neck cancers as well as vaginal or vulvar cancers is facilitated by the occurrence of the same in much younger age groups usually less than 50 years. A North American Survey (NAS) study has also confirmed the high risk of development of aplastic anemia, solid tumors and leukemia in FA patients. Odds ratio of up to 800 for AML and 50 for all cancers may be seen. For head and neck squamous cell carcinoma (HNSCC) and liver tumors, relative risk may be to the tune of hundreds while for esophageal and vulvar cancers, the relative risk may run in thousands.

According to NAS study involving 145 participants, severe bone marrow failure leading to death or transplantation developed in 55%, solid tumor developed in 29% and leukemia developed in 10% (excluding MDS) of the participants by 48 years of age when subjected to a competing risk analysis (first adverse outcome is bone marrow failure, solid tumor or leukemia). Data from IFAR has revealed the cumulative incidence as highest for marrow failure followed by development of hematological malignancy and solid tumors in that order.

Similar observations were made by IFAR where by the age of 30 years the probability of leukemia was approximately 30%, and by the age of 45 years, the probability of a solid tumor was 75%. According to the literature, there is 85% probability of a malignancy by the age of 45 years with 15 years as the median age. It may be seen that with respect to occurrence of malignancy, there is consensus among data of IFAR and NAS. Stem cell transplant (SCT) has offered cure for bone marrow failure but has also been found to increase the risk of development of solid tumors by four folds.

According to the literature, SCT also lead to an early occurrence of tumor development, to the tune of median 16 years earlier than those individuals where SCT was not undertaken. In 30% of FA cases, the diagnosis of malignancy was made before the diagnosis of FA.

As per data maintained in registry for FA in India, similar figures for early development of leukemia and solid tumors among Indian FA patients have emerged **(Table 16.2)**, particularly for acute lymphoblastic leukemia (ALL) and renal Wilm's tumor with a median age of occurrence of 5 years and 1 year, respectively.

The hallmark in the diagnosis of FA is the chromosomal breakage test in the presence of DNA cross-linking substances like diepoxybutane **(Fig. 16.3)**. Diagnostic tests were developed targeting this genomic instability more than 2 decades ago. These tests have led to several advances in understanding of disease including elucidating the genetics of FA. The T lymphocytes in the blood are exposed to a mitogen by which they divide. This is followed by another exposure, this time to a DNA cross-linking agent like diepoxybutane (DEB) or mitomycin C (MMC). The cells, which have divided at the metaphase phase, have increased numbers of chromosomal breaks per cell and an increased fraction of cells with breaks. There is also an increase in quadriradial forms seen on exposure with MMC.

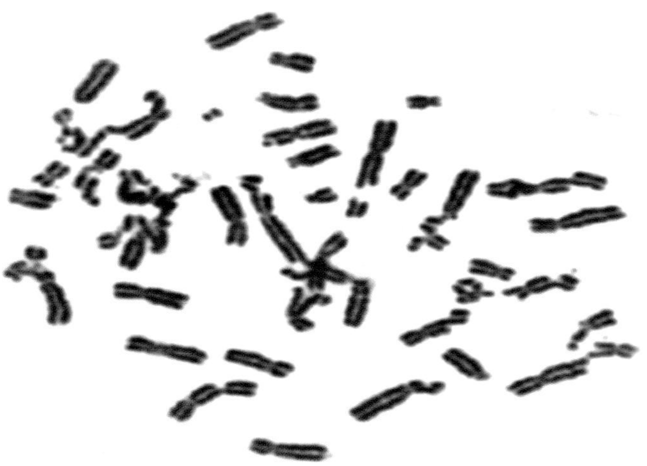

Figure 16.3 Karyotype in patients diagnosed with Fanconi anemia showing chromosome breakage

Some patients with FA may show normal results with this test where a hematopoietic stem cell has undergone gene correction leading to somatic mosaicism. Lymphocytes derived from corrected stem cell have a growth advantage and thus may show a normal chromosomal stability response. It is advisable to use skin fibroblasts for the breakage assay if mosaicism is suspected. Diagnosis of FA is clinched by identification of the gene complementation group, followed by demonstration of the disease-causing mutation.

Till date both alleles of at least 13 FA genes (exception being Fanconi anemia complementation group B (FANCB) responsible for X-linked recessive form of FA) affecting the FA patients have been cloned. There may still be some FA genes that have not been unidentified, as even after checking for the aforementioned 13 genes still some patients remain unclassifiable.

The known genes are *FANCA, FANCB, FANCC, FANCD1/BRCA2, FANCD2, FANCE, FANCF, FANCG, FANCI, FANCJ/BACH1/BRIP1, FANCL, FANCM,* and *FANCN/PALB2* **(Fig. 16.1)**. A multimeric nuclear complex is formed following DNA damage by the products of *FANCA, FANCB, FANCC, FANCE, FANCF, FANCG, FANCI, FANCL,* and *FANCM*. Monoubiquitination of *FANCD2* either in S phase or in response to DNA damage is caused by this multimeric nuclear complex. Monoubiquitination further leads to complex formation with other FA proteins including *FANCD1* and with non-FA proteins including BRCA1, RAD51, MRE11, ATM, BLM, RAD50, NBS and others. All these complex formations ultimately lead to formation of DNA damage repair foci. It leads to much increased rate of apoptosis of progenitor stem cells and is the main cause of failure of hematopoiesis in FA. Defective FA complex may not be contributing to hematopoietic failure in such cases of FA. Non-FA proteins are important in the sense that by their binding to FA proteins, they participate in preventing oxidative stress and programmed cell death.

Double stranded RNA, tumor necrosis factor-α, interferon-γ, fas ligand and macrophage inflammatory protein-1α (MIP-1α) are some other notable non-FA proteins that interact with FA proteins. FA cells contain defects in intra-S phase cell-cycle checkpoints. Inactivation of these checkpoints may be present in up to 25% of "sporadic" cancers associated with FA and includes breast, ovarian, cervical, nonsmall cell lung, pancreatic cancer (mutation of *FANCC* or *FANCG*), HNSCC and adult AML (deletion or mutation of *FANCA*). Management protocol for FA patients starts with a meticulous history and detailed physical examination, laboratory tests and cancer screening.

Fanconi anemia being a multisystem disease, involvement of every organ needs to be assessed clinically. Nonhematologic subspecialties like head and neck oncology, endocrinology, cardiology, neurology, gynecology, plastic surgery, hand surgery, otolaryngology, ophthalmology, radiology and dentistry should also be involved. Gynecologists, head and neck oncology teams, and dentists provide the best surveillance of solid tumors.

There is also interest about the type of impact that human papilloma virus (HPV) vaccine will have on gynecologic cancers and HNSCC. According to consensus guidelines developed by a panel of experts, treatment of bone marrow failure should be initiated when the hemoglobin (Hb) is less than 8 g/dL, platelets less than 30,000/μL, and absolute neutrophil count less than 500/μL (or there are symptoms from anemia, bleeding or infection). SCT is recommended provided a human leukocyte antigen (HLA)-matched sibling donor is available. Matched unrelated donor may also be considered if the earlier condition is not fulfilled. It is also very important to prove that FA is not present in sibling donor. Symptoms of aplastic anemia may also improve with androgen therapy, but it is not a definite cure for aplastic anemia.

Granulocyte colony-stimulating factor (G-CSF) alone or combined with erythropoietin and/or androgens may be helpful. As every cell in the case of FA has a chromosomal abnormality, preparative regimens need to be tailor-made for SCT in FA in comparison to SCT for acquired aplastic anemia. Along the same lines the chemotherapy for cancer treatment requires modification in sense that only those agents are used that do not cause DNA damage.

DYSKERATOSIS CONGENITA

In many patients of DC, diagnosis is delayed and they may present in their adulthood. Thus, there are high chances that the pediatric hematologists may under-recognize the classical DC. As a result most of these DC patients come directly under the care of adult hematologists. It is characterized by the classical triad of mucosal leukoplakia, nail dystrophy and abnormal skin pigmentation **(Figs 16.4A to F)**. Median age of diagnosis of DC is 15 years. More than 50% cases are diagnosed beyond 15 years of age.

The diagnostic triad of dysplastic nails, lacy reticulated pigmentation and oral leukoplakia may be absent, and the diagnosis of DC includes those with at least one triad feature plus at least two other somatic features, like hypogonadism, urethral strictures, lacrimal duct stenosis, rarely deafness, pulmonary fibrosis, liver fibrosis, esophageal strictures and osteoporosis.

Hoyeraal-Hreidarsson syndrome is the early childhood variant of DC (characterized by cerebellar hypoplasia, microcephaly, intrauterine growth retardation, immunodeficiency, developmental delay and bone marrow failure). Revesz syndrome is another early childhood variant of DC (identified by similar features plus exudative retinopathy).

Principle cause of mortality in these cases is bone marrow failure followed by malignancy and pulmonary complications. Based on inheritance pattern both autosomal dominant, autosomal recessive and X-linked recessive forms of DC have been identified. Till date the number of DC genes identified is six and includes *NOP10, TERC, DKC1, TINF2* and *TERT*. In X-linked DC, *DKC1* is the mutated gene that encodes for dykerin, which is a highly conserved nucleolar protein. Dyskerin is very important for the maturation of ribosomal RNA. This function of dyskerin is essentially linked to conversion of uracil to pseudouracil, which is affected by nucleolar ribonucleoprotein particles (snoRNPs) and guided by dyskerin in association with H/ACA class of small nucleolar RNA. Dyskerin also mediates another critical component of telomeres maintenance wherein it stabilizes the telomerase complex, brought about by association of dykerin with the RNA component of telomerase (TERC). Autosomal dominant DC has been found to share heterozygous mutations in TERC and TERT (telomerase reverse transblockdase) with some patients with pulmonary fibrosis, aplastic anemia and myelodysplastic syndrome. Mutations of DKC1 have also been found in some patients of Hoyeraal-Hreidarsson syndrome, a rare multisystem disorder.

Genetic heterogeneity has also been established for autosomal recessive DC wherein three subtypes have been described on the basis of biallelic mutations in NHP2, NOP10 and TERT. One subtype of autosomal dominant DC was recently found to be due to mutations in *TINF2*, which encodes a component of the shelterin complex that protects telomeres and controls access to the telomere.

Thus, these findings have shown that a defect in telomere maintenance is the culprit for the classical DC, Hoyeraal-Hreidarsson syndrome, and a subset of acute myeloid leukemia/myelodysplastic syndrome and aplastic anemia. This finding is further supported by the presence of very short telomeres in patients afflicted by above-mentioned conditions. The critical role of telomeres and telomerase in humans is especially highlighted by the multisystem abnormalities seen in these patients, including the increased incidence of malignancy. Occurrence rates of up to 9–10% of malignancy have been reported in DC patients and in the DCR; the majority of the cancers are carcinomas, particularly head and neck and esophageal in 60% of the patients and colon and anus in 15%. Three patients were reported who had MDS and one AML, but MDS may be underreported. DC has more frequency of solid tumors in comparison to FA.

According to the literature, 28 years is the median age for cancer; and the cumulative incidence of 35% has been reported for all malignancies by the age of 50 years. The diagnosis of DC can easily be made even in absence any hematologic signs, provided patient has the diagnostic triad. The converse is the problem to diagnose DC in a patient with thrombocytopenia or pancytopenia with minimal or no physical findings.

To substantiate these observations and the diagnosis, examination of the length of telomeres in leukocyte subsets using flow cytometry with fluorescence in situ hybridization (flow-FISH) had been attempted. Results showed that individuals with telomeres less than the first percentile of age matched control cells had DC with mutations in known genes where available. This also included silent carriers, who did not have physical or hematologic abnormalities. It was noted

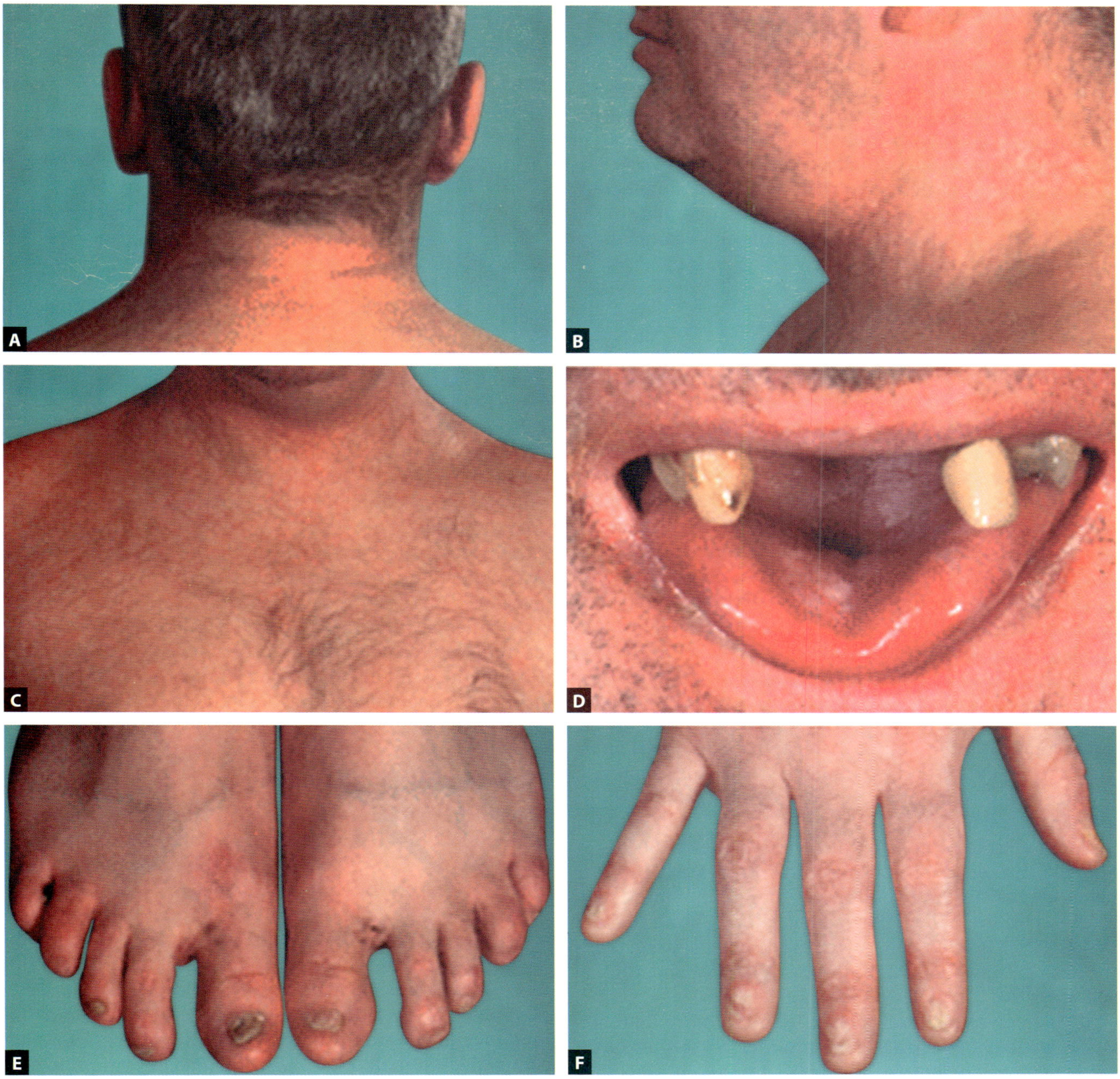

Figures 16.4A to F A selection of these features are shown in this 32-year-old X-linked recessive DC patient: abnormal skin pigmentation (A, B, C), premature greying of hair (A); leukoplakia and premature loss of teeth (D) and nail dystrophy (E, F)

that granulocytes of acquired aplastic anemia patients may also have short telomeres. However, DC patients had findings of short telomeres in all subsets of leukocytes.

Sensitivity and specificity values of above 90% in diagnosing DC from unaffected relatives as a separate entity from SDS, FA or DBA can be achieved from lymphocytes alone, or by B cells or naïve T cells in combination with lymphocytes. This test is somewhat analogous to the chromosome breakage test for FA. Guidelines for treatment of DC are similar to those for FA as to how and when to treat. If an unaffected HLA-matched sibling donor is present then SCT should always be given a preference. Due to the possibilities of silent carriers among siblings, it is suggested that examination of telomeres in leukocyte subsets is done. It is recommended to avoid a graft failure due to inadvertent selection of defective donor stem cells with low engraftment potential. The immunosuppression used to treat acquired aplastic anemia is unlikely to be successful. Patient with

DC respond favorably to androgens, similar to patients with FA. However, androgens plus G-CSF is fraught with risk of splenic rupture or peliosis and thus this combination is not recommended in DC. SCT for DC requires modified protocols on the same lines of SCT in FA, particularly since patients with DC are at risk of pulmonary and liver fibrosis as part of their underlying genetic disorder.

Monitoring of patients with DC and their "unaffected" family members with very short telomeres is similar to the protocol for FA, i.e. blood counts, bone marrow examinations and cancer surveillance.

Shwachman-Diamond Syndrome

Shwachman-Diamond syndrome primarily presents with the major symptom of malabsorption with excessive fatty stools and failure to thrive in childhood. Malabsorption is due to exocrine pancreatic insufficiency. Features of pancreatic insufficiency are apparent in infancy. It is an autosomal-recessive disorder. The spectrum of hematologic abnormalities includes neutropenia, pancytopenia, myelodysplastic syndrome and leukemia. The median age for leukemia is 18 years according to the literature reports.

Short stature is the usual physical findings and may also include metaphyseal dysostosis particularly at the hips and femurs in about half the patients. Learning disabilities may also be present in some patients. There are no reports of solid tumors in SDS unlike FA or DC. Exocrine pancreatic insufficiency can currently be demonstrated by reduced levels of serum trypsinogen (which may improve with age) and isoamylase (which fails to increase in the normal manner after age 3 years), and/or detection of a fatty pancreas by ultrasound, computerized tomography, or magnetic resonance imaging.

Documenting of neutrophil counts below 1,500/μL on more than one occasion is also required. Several patients with history of diarrhea and neutropenia do not fulfil these strict criteria, and are called "Shwachman-like". Bone marrow of SDS patients often show cytogenetic clones, particularly involving chromosome 7 [monosomy 7, der (7), and i(7q)] as well as del(20q).

SBDS gene mutation has been found in more than 90% of SDS patients. The *SBDS* gene product (SBDS) affect the biogenesis of ribosomes as it plays an important role in the maturation of the 60S ribosomal subunit. Supplements of pancreatic enzyme are given with food to treat malabsorption. Fat soluble vitamins (A, D, E and K) are also added to the diet. As functioning of pancreas often improves with age, thus adult patients may require fewer or no supplements.

Neutropenia rarely assumes clinical significance and responds well to low doses of G-CSF. SDS patients have responded excellently to SCT (stem cell transplant); however, cyclophosphamide-based preparative regime has been shown to have cardiac toxicity.

Congenital Amegakaryocytic Thrombocytopenia (Amega)

Apart from the thrombocytopenia induced bruises, no characteristic physical appearance has been associated with Amega unlike most of the other IBMFS. Isolated thrombocytopenia along with reduction or absence of megakaryocytes in the bone marrow albeit without somatic abnormalities is characteristically the first presentation of this condition.

Aplastic anemia may develop in up to 50% of patients (usually by the age of 5 years). Development of myelodysplastic syndrome or leukemia in patients with Amega has also been observed. Among the spectrum of IBMFSs, Amega has perhaps the easiest understandable genetic basis. Amega has been found to be associated with the recessive mutations in *MPL* gene in all the cases examined till date. This gene codes for the receptor for thrombopoietin. Thrombopoietin is the hematopoietic growth factor that drives the megakaryopoiesis. Treatment with androgens has shown improved blood counts in patients with Amega and pancytopenia.

However, the current recommendation is to consider SCT as first line treatment provided HLA matched donor is available. There are no published large series, but it appears that patients with Amega do well with the SCT protocols in current use for acquired aplastic anemia. SCT-associated toxicity does not appear to be as much relevant in Amega as that has been seen with DC and FA (and cardiotoxicity in SDS).

Diamond-Blackfan Anemia

Diamond-Blackfan anemia patients usually present in infancy with up to 90% patients reporting before their first birthday. Prognosis is relatively better and many patients eventually reach level of care by adult hematologists.

Subtle physical abnormalities in form of flattened thenar muscles may be present. Short stature is common, while rarer presentations include triphalangeal thumbs, microtia and cleft palates. The hallmark of classical DBA is a selective decrease in erythroid precursors and normochromic macrocytic anemia associated with a variable number of somatic abnormalities such as craniofacial, thumb, cardiac and urogenital malformations. AML and myelodysplastic syndrome have been reported in a few patients. There are also cases in which the disease has evolved into aplastic anemia.

A handful of solid tumors including half dozen cases of osteogenic sarcoma have also been reported. According to published reports, the median age for cancer is 23 years. DBA does not have a "chromosome breakage" or "telomere length" test. A specific but not entirely sensitive test is to analyze the level of red cell adenosine deaminase (ADA). It is elevated in majority of patients. However, it may also be noted that ADA levels may be normal in approximately 10% of patients with classical DBA.

Nonspecific findings common to most of IBMFS like macrocytic red cells with increased fetal hemoglobin (HbF) may be found in most of the DBA patients. Autosomal dominant inheritance pattern is associated with most cases of DBA (including new mutation sporadic cases). Nearly 25% of patients are represented by mutation of two genes coding for ribosomal proteins, RPS19 and RPS24. Heterozygous mutations in other genes encoding for ribosomal proteins of the small (RPS24, RPS17, RPS7, RPS10, RPS26) and large (RPL5, RPL11 and RPL35A) ribosomal subunits have also been reported; collectively the genetic basis of approximately 50–60% of cases of DBA can now be established.

These reports point to the fact that DBA essentially is a disorder of ribosomes. Response to corticosteroids is good in most of the patients with DBA. Hemoglobin level can be maintained adequately (usually > 8–10 g/dL) with corticosteroids. Corticosteroids, which are used initially at a higher dose, are then subsequently tapered to the minimum possible dose. An alternate day regime is always preferred.

Transfusions of packed red cells may also be required in those who are steroid resistant, or who require unacceptably high doses of steroids. These patients will eventually need iron chelation, however. The so called "spontaneous remission" may occur in 25% of DBA patients leading to remarkable improvement and no requirement of further treatment. However, as their age progress, they may relapse during late adulthood. Among some quarters of hematologist, there are concerns of steroids-induced impairment of growth especially during 1st year and prepubertal growth spurt. Thus, transfusion of red blood cells is advocated by some. The flip side of these transfusions is overload of iron and transfusion transmitted viruses. Despite widespread discussions and attempts, there is still no consensus to rational steroid doses for these children.

Stem cell transplant from both related and unrelated donors have reports of successful outcome.

SEVERE CONGENITAL NEUTROPENIA

Severe congenital neutropenia (SCN) is the term for a group of disorders characterized by early onset neutropenia (<500/µL), pyogenic infections and a marrow maturation arrest. This disease also has its first presentation in infancy like most of other IBMFS. Patients with the congenital disorder usually present with recurrent, life-threatening infections in infancy.

Features of maturation arrest in the myeloid lineage are usually revealed in bone marrow examination. Progression to myelodysplasia and leukemia has also been associated with SCN. It is the acquisition of secondary mutations including mutations in the G-CSF receptor that lead to malignant transformation in SCN. Dominant heterozygous mutations in the neutrophil elastase gene (ELA2) have been demonstrated in the majority of patients. Maturation arrest is thought to be due to an unfolded protein response triggered by the nonfunctional protein's accumulation brought on by these mutations. Among all patients of SCN, GFI1 mutation has been reported in up to 2%.

Wiskott-Aldrich syndrome (WAS) gene mutation leading to X-linked disease has also been reported in a small proportion of cases. Autosomal recessive SCN associated with biallelic mutations in the HAX1 gene was first described in the original family by Kostmann. This mutation has been predicted to lead to defects in cell death. Mutations in other genes (*GFI1, WASP*) are also known to be associated with SCN, demonstrating genetic heterogeneity. Patients with SCN respond to standard treatment protocols with G-CSF in form of improved neutrophil counts. Dose of G-CSF is usually 5–10 µg/kg/day or every other day with an aim of neutrophils count above 1,500/µL.

There have been suggestions to categorize SCN as a preleukemic disorder with report of three SCN patients developing AML in the pre-G-CSF era. Following more than 20 years of use of GCSF, it is clear that MDS or AML is a part of the syndrome. As to how G-CSF leads to malignancy, its role is still unclear. There is evidence from analysis of 374 patients in the SCNIR that demonstrate a time-dependent increase in cumulative incidence (reaching 21% after 10 years) of MDS or AML with G-CSF treatment. Sepsis accounted for 8% of total deaths. There are no reports of occurrence of solid tumors.

Stem cell transplant may be considered for unresponsive patients who have a matched sibling donor.

THROMBOCYTOPENIA ABSENT RADII

Diagnosis of TAR is relatively easier and is suspected when a child at birth presents with absence of radii but with presence of thumbs (may be a bit malformed). Diagnosis is clinched with the presence of a concomitant low platelet count. Adult hematologist may also encounter these cases as the 5 years survival rate may reach up to 78% and up to 16% of them reported to have reached age of 16 years. Additional physical malformations that may afflict these patients are—cardiac defects, short or absent ulnae, dislocated hips, absent humeri or abnormal knees.

Till date, 300 cases have been reported with four leukemia cases (age ranging from 1 month to 41 years). There are suggestions to classify TAR along with preleukemic IBMFS, based on three AML reports. Decreased and/or abnormal megakaryocytes as the sole abnormality was found in bone marrow examination. In TAR, 10–20% infants require transfusions during orthopedic surgery. However, even though platelets count do not come to normal, still the orthopedic surgery may not require platelet cover after 1 year of age when the counts start to rise. SCT is rarely required as a treatment modality.

BIBLIOGRAPHY

1. Alter BP. Diagnosis, genetics, and management of inherited bone marrow failure syndromes. Hematology Am Soc Hematol Educ Program. 2007. pp. 29-39.
2. Auerbach AD, Buchwald M, Joenje H. In: Scriver CR (Ed). The Metabolic and Molecular Basis of Inherited Disease. New York, USA: McGraw-Hill Publisher; 2001. pp. 753-68.
3. Bagby GC, Alter BP. Fanconi anemia. Semin Hematol. 2006;43(3):147-56.
4. Dokal I, Vulliamy T. Inherited bone marrow failure syndromes. Haematologica. 2010;95(8):1236-40.
5. Dokal I. Dyskeratosis congenita in all its forms. Br J Haematol. 2000;110(4):768-79.
6. Howlett NG, Taniguchi T, Olson S, Cox B, Waisfisz Q, De Die-Smulders C, et al. Biallelic inactivation of BRCA2 in Fanconi anemia. Science. 2002;297(5581):606-9.
7. Kutler DI, Singh B, Satagopan J, Batish SD, Berwick M, Giampietro PF, et al. A 20-year perspective on the International Fanconi Anemia Registry (IFAR). Blood. 2003;101(4):1249-56.
8. Registry for Fanconi Anaemia in India. 2015.
9. Rosenberg PS, Alter BP, Bolyard AA, Bonilla MA, Boxer LA, Cham B, et al. The incidence of leukemia and mortality from sepsis in patients with severe congenital neutropenia receiving long-term G-CSF therapy. Blood. 2006;107(12):4628-35.
10. Rothbaum R, Perrault J, Vlachos A, Cipolli M, Alter BP, Burroughs S, et al. Shwachman-Diamond syndrome: report from an international conference. J Pediatr. 2002;141(2):266-70.
11. Taniguchi T, D'Andrea AD. The molecular pathogenesis of Fanconi anemia: recent progress. Blood. 2006;107(11):4223-33.
12. Walne AJ, Dokal I. Advances in the understanding of dyskeratosis congenita. Br J Haematol. 2009;145(2):164-72.
13. Wang W. Emergence of a DNA-damage response network consisting of Fanconi anaemia and BRCA proteins. Nat Rev Genet. 2007;8(10):735-48.
14. Paulo Ricardo G Zen, Felipe Nora de Moraes, Rafael Fabiano M Rosa, Carla Graziadio, Giorgio Adriano Paskulin. Clinical characteristics of patients with Fanconi anemia. Rev Paul Pediatr. 2011;29(3):392-9.

CHAPTER

17 Polycythemia and Hyperviscosity Syndrome in Newborn

MR Lokeshwar, Sheikh Minhal Ahmed, Swati Kanakia

INTRODUCTION

Polycythemia is a relatively common disorder seen during early newborn period. It is also called as "thick blood syndrome" characterized by central venous hematocrit (HCT) level of more than 65%.[1-13] The most widely accepted definition of neonatal polycythemia is a venous HCT greater than 65% (capillary HCT > 70%) and/or a venous hemoglobin concentration in excess of 22.0 g/dL.[1-21] Polycythemia includes a venous HCT of 64% or more at 2 hours of age or an umbilical venous or arterial HCT of 63% or more.[8-10]

The terms polycythemia and hyperviscosity are often used interchangeably but are not synonymous. Polycythemia is significant only because it increases the risk of hyperviscosity syndrome. Although polycythemia may be associated with hyperviscosity of the blood, all infants with hyperviscosity are not polycythemic nor all polycythemic neonates are associated with hyperviscosity. Blood viscosity increases linearly with rising HCT up to 65% but subsequently viscosity rises exponentially.[1,3,4,7-9,14,18,20,21]

Among the many factors that determine blood viscosity, the primary factor in the newborn is the HCT. In neonates, the HCT rises soon after birth, peaks at around 2 hours of age and falls to about 57% in next 12–18 hours. It then declines until the infant is aged 24 hours[8] at which time it equals the HCT level of the cord blood. Fewer than 40% of infants with a HCT level greater than 64% at 2 hours still have a high value at 12 hours or later.[4,22] The mean venous HCT in term infants is 52% at 12–18 hours of age.[10,16,18,23] The mean cord blood HCT is 45 ± 5% and 50 + 5% in preterm and term infants, respectively, if they are born at sea level. Values are somewhat higher in infants born in locations at higher altitudes.[18] The incidence of polycythemia was found to be highest among the infants who were born either small or large for gestational age.[15,16]

The viscosity of a fluid is defined as the ratio of shear stress to shear rate. Hyperviscosity refers to any state in which there is increased viscosity of the blood.[3,9,11-21] Polycythemia must be distinguished from hyperviscosity, which is defined as a blood viscosity greater than 12 centipoise, measured at a shear rate of 11.5 per second or greater than 6 centipoise, measured at a shear rate of 10.6 per second. The normal blood viscosity (mean ± SD) in the neonate is 1.18 ± 0.17 centipoise at a shear rate of 11.5 seconds.[4,15]

Shearing occurs as the result of internal friction of the fluid layers moving over one another during flow. It can be measured with a cone plate viscometer (such as Wells-Brookfield microviscometer) over a range of shear rates. Two commonly used shear rates for blood are 11 and 10.6 seconds. These shear rates presumably approximate those in small venules and large arteries, respectively.

INCIDENCE[1-4,7,11-18,20]

The true incidence of polycythemia and hyperviscosity is not known since majority of the infants are likely to be asymptomatic and normal. Also, HCT is not routinely recommended or performed in this population. Polycythemia (venous HCT > 65%) occurs in approximately 4% of newborn infants.[1,2,4,7] Symptomatic polycythemia occurs in 0.4–0.6% of the screened infants. Hyperviscosity syndrome (>2 SD above population mean) occurs in 5% of infants.[1] However, reported incidence of polycythemia is about 3–4% (range 0.4–12%) and about half of the infants with polycythemia have hyperviscosity.[1,3,5,7,9-12]

PATHOPHYSIOLOGY[3,8,9-21]

Neonatal polycythemia is an abnormal increase in RBC mass causing hyperviscosity with sludging of blood within vessels with a tendency to form microthrombi leading to impairment of tissue oxygenation **(Flow chart 17.1)**. The hyperviscosity syndrome is a symptom complex associated with decreased blood fluidity, tardy flow and sludging of blood within the blood vessels especially in small arteries and capillaries.

Hyperviscosity is influenced not only by the red cell mass but also by other factors such as increased RBC volume and decreased deformability of the erythrocyte, plasma proteins, plasma fibrinogen, increased circulating serum

Flow chart 17.1 Pathophysiology of polycythemia hyperviscosity

↑Hematocrit >65%(Hyperviscosity)
↓
Intravascular blood sludging
↓
Impairment of tissue oxygenation and perfusion
↓
Microthrombi
↓
Tissue hypoxia, metabolic acidosis, hypoglycemia
↓
Damage in the cerebral cortex, kidneys, intestine, adrenal glands
↓
Multiple organ dysfunctions

immunoglobulins (e.g. macroglobulinemia, multiple myeloma), clotting factors, platelets, WBCs, increased cellular blood components in hyperproliferative states, e.g. leukemia.[1,2,6,9,10] As the central HCT level increases, viscosity increases.[1-3,5,9-12]

Hyperviscosity syndrome can lead to thrombosis and infarcts in the territory supplied by the vessels. In neonates, the focus is generally on red cell excess.[8-10] Significant damage may occur, if these events occur in the cerebral cortex, kidneys and adrenal glands leading to multiple organ dysfunction. Thrombosis may result in cerebral infarction, renal venous thrombosis, necrotizing enterocolitis (NEC) and adrenal insufficiency. These clinical conditions require early identification and effective prompt interventions.

ETIOLOGY[1,2-4,7-9,17-21]

Placental Insufficiency

Increased fetal erythropoiesis secondary to intrauterine hypoxia may occur in association with placental insufficiency, growth restriction, hypertension or maternal-smoking causing neonatal polycythemia.[1,2,24]

Placental Red Cell Transfusion

Hyperviscosity occurs in 6.7% of infants with delayed cord clamping, which may increase blood volume and red cell mass by as much as 55%. A study of 242 newborns by Rincon et al.[8,25,26] demonstrated changes in blood values in newborns based on the period of time between birth and clamping of the umbilical cord. HCT levels were found to have risen in accordance with the amount of time to clamping with values at 48 hours of 53.4%, 58%, and 59%, respectively when clamped after 1 minute, between 1 minute and 2 minutes and more than 3 minutes. In addition, the number of infants with symptomatic polycythemia was significantly higher in the group that was clamped at 2–3 minutes. When cord clamping is delayed more than 3 minutes after birth, blood volume increased 30%. In the event of delayed cord clamping, blood flow to the infant is enhanced by oxytocin and milking of umbilical cord.[27-29]

Twin-to-twin Transfusion Syndrome

Vascular communication occurs in approximately 10% of monozygotic twin pregnancies (feto-fetal transfusion) causing neonatal polycythemia.

Maternofetal Transfusion

Secondary to pre-eclampsia, small for gestational age infants, postmature infants, chronic or recurrent abruptio placentae, maternal cyanotic congenital heart disease,[30-35] infants of hypertensive mothers or those on propranolol, postdate pregnancy and maternal smoking[3,24,36-52] cause neonatal polycythemia.

Intrauterine Growth Retarded, Small for Gestational Age Neonates

Infants who are intrauterine growth retarded (IUGR), small for their gestational age (SGA), large for gestational age infant (LGA) are prone for polycythemia. However, many infants with appropriate size or weight for their gestational age (AGA) are reported with polycythemia.[51]

Infants of a Diabetic Mother

With poor glycemic control reported incidence of polycythemia is more than 40% and those born to mothers with gestational diabetes reported incidence is more than 30%.[7-9]

Endocrine Abnormalities

Adrenogenital syndrome, hypothyroidism, congenital thyrotoxicosis, congenital adrenal hyperplasia and Beckwith-Wiedemann syndrome are associated with polycythemia.[7-9]

Genetics Disorders

Chromosomal abnormality (trisomy13, 18 and 21) are associated with polycythemia.[33,34]

High Altitudes

Neonatal polycythemia is increased at high altitude.[7,14,15,17,18]

CLINICAL FEATURES

Many cases of polycythemia are seen in normal healthy neonates. The clinical features depend on organs involved. Polycythemia in newborn babies may manifest with serious, sometimes life-threatening insults to brain, heart, kidneys, lungs and intestines with multiple organ dysfunction, which may affect present and long-term outcome.[1-3] The most obvious finding is plethora and other symptoms include lethargy, feeding problems, irritability, jitteriness, tremors, hypoglycemia, hypocalcemia, jaundice and thrombocytopenia.[37-39]

Central Nervous System

Central nervous system (CNS) manifestations are the most serious problems observed with polycythemia, presenting in the form of tremors, drowsiness, seizures, irritability, jitteriness and cerebrovascular accidents.[3,42]

Cardiopulmonary

In those with a HCT level of 65% or more, the decrease in pulmonary blood flow may be associated with respiratory distress and cyanosis, tachypnea, apnea and congestive heart failure.[32,40,43]

Gastrointestinal

Loss of appetite and poor feeding are reported in more than one-half of all infants with polycythemia. Studies have shown that polycythemia is a known risk factor in the development of NEC.[37-39]

Renal Manifestations

Polycythemia is known to be associated with decreased glomerular filtration rates, oliguria, hematuria, proteinuria and renal vein thrombosis.

Metabolic

Hypoglycemia and hypocalcemia are the most common metabolic derangements observed in 12–40% and 1–11% of neonates with polycythemia.[40]

Coagulation Abnormalities

Thrombocytopenia and coagulation cascade abnormalities including disseminated intravascular coagulation (DIC) have been noted with polycythemia.[40]

INVESTIGATIONS

Diagnosis of hyperviscosity syndrome is largely clinical.[44-46] Many babies with polycythemia and hyperviscosity may be asymptomatic. High index of suspicion is important and follow up of the child with HCT measurement particularly in high-risk baby is essential. Infants with symptoms consistent with hyperviscosity should be tested immediately. As blood viscosity measurements are not easily available, perform HCT on cord blood (if suspected early) or on a central venous sample (venipuncture) or heel prick.

Central venous HCT measurement is used for diagnosis of hyperviscosity in newborns with polycythemia because it is readily available. Due to variability in measurements obtained from capillary samples, the diagnosis of polycythemia is based upon peripheral venous sample. In neonates, initial screening tests are often obtained via capillary sampling (heelstick). Either microcentrifuge 3,000 rpm for 4 minutes [available in neonatal intensive care unit (NICU)] or the laboratory analyzer measurement (counter—which is usually slightly lower due to trapped plasma) is used. High-risk infants who are asymptomatic for hyperviscosity should have a screening capillary HCT (heel prick) obtained at 4–6 hours of age. The mean HCT and hemoglobin concentrations from these capillary samples in normal term infants at birth are 61 ± 7.4 (SD) percent and 19.3 ± 2 2 g/dL (SD), respectively.[1] Capillary samples often overestimate HCT and may not be reliable, and hence a venous or arterial HCT and hemoglobin should be obtained before confirming the diagnosis.

Capillary HCT more than 60% drawn before 4 hours of life should be repeated with a second capillary HCT at 4–6 hours of life, which should be followed up immediately with a peripheral venous (or arterial) HCT. Venous HCT may be as much as 15% lower than those of capillary HCT whereas Coulter counter results are lower than HCT values determined by microcentrifugation.

Blood viscosity is difficult to measure and is not readily available in majority of the laboratories.

It is measured by Wells-Brookfield cone-plate microviscometer and is not available in most neonatal intensive care units.

Other Investigations

- Complete hemogram
- Blood peripheral smear examination
- Reticulocyte count
- Bleeding profile
- Hyperbilirubinemia
- Blood sugar and Ca^{++} levels
- Arterial blood gases (ABGs)
- X-ray chest for cardiomegaly, increased vascularity, hyperaeration, if any
- Maternal blood sugar levels to rule out maternal diabetes and gestational diabetes.

MEDICAL MANAGEMENT OF POLYCYTHEMIA

Therapy in newborns with polycythemia is based on both the presence or absence of symptoms and the central venous HCT level.

Asymptomatic Patient with Hematocrit Level of 65–75%

Monitor cardiorespiratory symptom, HCT and glucose levels every 6–12 hours and observe the patient for symptoms until the HCT level declines. Continue monitoring in asymptomatic patients with HCT level of more than 75% with additional fluid intake. An extra fluid intake of 20 mL/kg may be added to the daily basal fluid requirement.[4,7] Hemodilution decreases the viscosity, however, fluid therapy should be titrated and reserved for hemodynamically stable babies with asymptomatic polycythemia.[4,45,52]

Treatment for Symptomatic Patients

In patients with a HCT level more than 65% and symptoms attributable to polycythemia and hyperviscosity, partial exchange transfusion (PET) should be considered though treatment of polycythemia with PET remains debatable.[45-55]

Partial Volume Exchange Transfusion

Partial exchange transfusion corrects the polycythemia and hyperviscosity; however, improvements in clinical signs have not been unequivocally documented in randomized trials of PET compared to no exchange. Though PET improves symptoms by improving capillary perfusion, cerebral blood flow and cardiac functions, there is little data to suggest improvement in the long-term outcome, like neurodevelopmental behavioral problems, etc.[45-55]

Using an umbilical venous catheter PET is performed to reduce the HCT to 50–55%.Umbilical venous catheter may be used for both withdrawal of the blood and replacement of saline. Umbilical venous cannulation can also be used for withdrawal of the blood from the catheter and replacing same volume of the saline through the peripheral vein. PET done via peripheral or central route, which avoids umbilical vessels cannulation and is done by using peripheral arterial and venous line, blood is withdrawn from arterial line and replaced simultaneously through the venous line. No major complications are reported in babies undergoing PET.

The volume of partial exchange required is calculated as follows:

$$\text{Volume to be exchanged} = \frac{\text{Observed HCT} - \text{Desired HCT}}{\text{Observed HCT}} \times \text{Blood volume}$$

The blood volume was calculated by weight in kg × 85 mL.

In majority of NICUs, it is a routine practice to use plasma for correcting polycythemia. In view of the fact that adult plasma has higher viscosity as compared to newborn blood, PET with plasma may lower the HCT to the desired level but viscosity may remain unaltered. Normal saline has been shown to be a promising alternative to plasma.[49-57] Normal saline is the replacement fluid of choice (crystalloids) for exchange transfusions because it is effective, economical and easily available.[53] Other solution used for PET includes 5% albumin. The colloid products have been associated with complications such as NEC. In addition, both 5% albumin and fresh-frozen plasma are blood products and are associated with risks of transfusion-transmitted illnesses of variable severity.[46,48-54,56-59]

However, none of these are more effective than normal saline. Aliquots should not exceed 5 mL/kg delivered or removed over 2–3 minutes.

KEY POINTS

- Good antenatal care to prevent growth retardation during the antenatal period
- To avoid polycythemia, early cord clamping is desirable
- Hold the baby at the level of introitus at the time of delivery to minimize hypertransfusion
- Avoid and treat dehydration. HCT should be measured after correction of dehydration
- Treat promptly metabolic problems, like hypoglycemia, hypocalcemia, hyperbilirubinemia and acidosis
- Though PET improves symptoms of polycythemia and hyperviscosity; however, long-term outcomes are uncertain despite this modality of management
- High index of suspicion is required for diagnosing polycythemia and its complications in high-risk newborns.

REFERENCES

1. Oski FA, Naiman JA, Pearson JA. Polycythemia and hyperviscosity in the neonatal period. In: Marcovitz M (Ed). Hematological Problems in Newborn. Major Problems in Clinical Pediatrics, 3rd edition. Volume IV. Philadelphia, PA, USA: WB Sunders; 1982. pp. 87-96.
2. Phibbs RH. Neonatal polycythemia. In: Rudolph AM (Ed). Pediatrics, 20th edition. New York, USA: Appleton Century Crofts; 1997. p. 179.
3. Gross GP, Hathaway WE, McGaughey HR. Hyperviscosity in the neonate. J Pediatrics. 1973;82(6):1004-12.
4. Humbert JR, Abelson H, Hathaway WE, Battaglia FC. Polycythemia in small for gestational age infants. J Pediatr. 1969;75(5):812-9.
5. Kontras SB. Polycythemia and hyperviscosity syndrome in infants and children. Pediatr Clin North Am. 1972;19(4):919-33.
6. Gomella TL, Cunningham MD, Eyal FG. Polycythemia-Neonatology, 7th edition. Philadelphia, PA, USA: McGraw Hill Medical Publisher; 2013. pp. 484-9.
7. Faridi MMA, Krishnamurthy Sriram. Polycythemia and hyperviscosity syndrome. Textbook of Pediatric Hematology and Hemato-Oncology, 1st edition. New Delhi, India: Jaypee Brothers Medical Publishers (Pvt.) Ltd; 2016. pp. 57-63.
8. Werner EJ. Neonatal polycythemia and hyperviscosity. Clin Perinatol. 1995;22(3):693-710.
9. Krishnan L, Rahim A. Neonatal polycythemia. Indian J Pediatr. 1997;64(4):541-6.
10. Mentzer WC, Glader BE. Erythrocyte disorders in infancy. In: Ballard RA, Taeusch HW (Eds). Avery's Diseases of the Newborn, 7th edition. Philadelphia, PA, USA: WB Saunders; 1998. p. 1080.
11. Jeevasankar M, Agarwal R, Chawla D, Paul VK, Deorari AK. Polycythemia in the newborn. Indian J Pediatr. 2008;75(1):68-72.
12. Mimouni FB, Merlob P, Dollberg S, Mendel D; Israeli Neonatology Association. Neonantal polycythemia: critical review and a consensus statement of the Israeli Neonatology Association. Acta Paediatr. 2011;100(10):1290-6.
13. Gupta G, Wilson CG. Polycythemia in neonate. Textbook of Neonatal Hematology-Oncology, 1st edition. New Delhi, India: Jaypee Brothers Medical Publishers (Pvt) Ltd; 2003. pp. 118-25.
14. Oh W. Neonatal polycythemia and hyperviscosity. Pediatr Clin North Am. 1986;33(3):523-32.
15. Brooks GI, Backes CR. Hyperviscosity secondary to polycythemia in the appropriate for gestational age neonate. J Am Osteopath Assoc. 1981;80(6):415-8.
16. Ramamurthy RS, Berlanga M. Postnatal alteration in hematocrit and viscosity in normal and polycythemic infants. J Pediatr.1987;110(6):929-34.
17. Drew JH, Guaran RL, Grauer S, Hobbs JB. Cord whole blood hyper viscosity: measurement, definition, incidence and clinical features. J Paediatr Child Health. 1991;27(6):363-5.
18. Stevens K, Wirth FH. Incidence of neonatal hyperviscosity at sea level. J Pediatr.1980;97(1):118-9.

19. Mackintosh TF, Walker CH. Blood viscosity in the newborn. Arch Dis Child. 1973;48(7):547-53.
20. Wirth FH, Goldberg KE, Lubchenco LO. Neonatal hyperviscosity: I. Incidence. Pediatrics. 1979;63(6):833-6.
21. Riopel L, Fouron JC, Bard H. Blood viscosity during the neonatal period: the role of plasma and red blood cell type. J Pediatr. 1982;100(3):449-53.
22. Gordon EA. Polycythemia and hyperviscosity of the newborn. J Perinat Neonatal Nurs. 2003;17(3):209-19.
23. American Academy of Pediatrics Committee on Fetus and Newborn: Routine evaluation of blood pressure, hematocrit and glucose in newborns. Pediatrics. 1993;92(3):474-6.
24. Bada HS, Korones SB, Pourcyrous M, Wong SP, Wilson WM 3rd, Kolni HW, et al. Asymptomatic syndrome of polycythemic hyperviscocity: effect of partial plasma exchange transfusion. J Pediatr. 1992;120(4 Pt 1):579-85.
25. Linderkamp O, Nelle M, Kraus M, Zilow EP. The effect of early and late cord-clamping on blood viscosity and other hemorheological parameters in full-term neonates. Acta Paediatr. 1992;81(10):745-50.
26. Rincon D, Foguet A, Rojas M, Segarra E, Sacristán E, Teixidor R, et al. Time of cord clamping and neonatal complications, a prospective study. An Pediatr (Barc). 2014;81(3):142-8.
27. Rabe H, Reynolds G, Diaz-Roselllo J. Early versus delayed umbilical cord clamping in preterm infants. Cochrane Database Syst Rev. 2004;(4):CD 003248.
28. McDonald SJ, Middleton P, Dowswell T, Morris PS. Effect of timing of umbilical cord clamping of term infants on maternal and neonatal outcomes. Cochrane Database Syst Rev. 2013;(7):CD004074.
29. Upadhyay A, Gothwal S, Parihar R, Garg A, Gupta A, Chawla D, et al. Effect of umbilical cord milking in term and near term infants: randomized control trial. Am J Obstet Gynecol. 2013;208(2):120.
30. Brossard Y, Pons JC, Jrad I, van Nifterik J, Gillot R, Saure C, et al. Maternal-fetal hemorrhage: a reappraisal. Vox Sang. 1996;71(2):103-7.
31. Jennings ER, Clauss B. Maternal-fetal hemorrhage: its incidence and sensitizing effects. Am J Obstet Gynecol. 1978;131(7):725-7.
32. Michael AF Jr, Mauer AM. Maternal-fetal transfusion as a cause of plethora in the neonatal period. Pediatrics. 1961;28:458-61.
33. Widness JA, Pueschel SM, Pezzullo JC, Clemons GK. Elevated erythropoietin levels in cord blood of newborns with Down's syndrome. Biol Neonate. 1994;66(1):50-5.
34. Lappalainen J, Kouvalainen K. High hematocrits in newborns with Down's syndrome: a hitherto undescribed finding. Clin Pediatr (Phila). 1972;11(8):472-4.
35. Mukhtar AI, Halliday HL. Eisenmenger syndrome in pregnancy: a possible cause of neonatal polycythemia and persistent fetal circulation. Obst Gynecol. 1982;60(5):651-2.
36. Awonusonu FO, Pauly TH, Hutchison AA. Maternal smoking and partial exchange transfusion for neonatal polycythemia. Am J Perinatol. 2002;19(7):349-54.
37. Hakanson DO, Oh W. Necrotizing enterocolitis and hyperviscosity in the newborn infant. J Pediatr. 1977;90(3):458-61.
38. Wilson R, del Portillo M, Schmidt E, Feldman RA, Kanto WP Jr. Risk factors for necrotizing enterocolitis in infants weighing more than 2,000 grams at birth: a case-control study. Pediatrics. 1983;71(1):19-22.
39. Martinez-Tallo E, Claure N, Bancalari E. Necrotizing enterocolitis in full-term or near-term infants: risk factors. Biol Neonate. 1997;71(5):292-8.
40. Wiswell TE, Cornish JD, Northam RS. Neonatal polycythemia: frequency of clinical manifestations and other associated findings. Pediatrics. 1986;78(1):26-30.
41. Ozek E, Soll R, Scimmel MS. Partial exchange transfusion to prevent neurodevelopmental disability in infants with polycythemia. Cochrane Database Syst Rev. 2010;(1):CD005089.
42. Black VD, Lubchenco LO, Lucky DW, Koops BL, McGuinness GA, Powell DP, et al. Development and neurological sequelae of neonatal hyperviscosity syndrome. Pediatrics. 1982;69(4):426-31.
43. Murphy DJ Jr, Reller MD, Meyer AR, Kaplan S. Effects of neonatal polycythemia and partial exchange transfusion on cardiac function: an echocardiographic study. Pediatrics. 1985;76(6):909-13.
44. Ramamurthy RS, Brans YW. Neonatal polycythemia: I. Criteria for diagnosis and treatment. Pediatrics. 1981;68(2):168-74.
45. Shohat M, Merlob P, Reisner SH. Neonatal polycythemia. I. Early diagnosis and incidence relating to time of sampling. Pediatrics. 1984;73(1):7-10.
46. Pappas A, Delaney-Black V. Differential diagnosis and management of polycythemia. Pediatr Clin North Am. 2004;51(4):1063-86.
47. Sankar MJ, Agarwal R, Deorari A, Paul VK. Management of polycythemia in neonates. Indian J Pediatr. 2010;77(10):1117-21.
48. Tapia JL, Solivelles X, Grebe G, Legnes GE. Evaluation of different solutions for erythropheresis in the treatment of neonatal polycythemia. Pediatr Res. 1992;31:271A.
49. Goldberg K, Wirth FH, Hathaway WE, Guggenheim MA, Murphy JR, Braithwaite WR, et al. Neonatal hyperviscosity. II. Effect of partial plasma exchange transfusion. Pediatrics. 1982;69(4):419-25.
50. Black VD, Lubchenco LO, Koops BL, Poland RL, Powell DP. Neonatal hyperviscosity: randomized study of effect of partial plasma exchange transfusion on long-term outcome. Pediatrics. 1985;75(6):1048-53.
51. Maertzdorf WJ, Tangelder GJ, Slaaf DW, Blanco CE. Effects of partial plasma exchange transfusion on cerebral blood flow velocity in polycythaemic preterm, term and small for date newborn infants. Eur J Pediatr. 1989;148(8):774-8.
52. Villalta I, Pramanik AK, Krouskop R, Diaz Blanco J. Comparison of partial exchange transfusion with fresh frozen plasma versus saline in neonatal polycythemia. Pediatr Res. 1989;274A:1627.
53. Wong W, Fok TF, Lee CH, Ng PC, So KW, Ou Y, et al. Randomised controlled trial: comparison of colloid or crystalloid for partial exchange transfusion for treatment of neonatal polycythemia. Arch Dis Child Fetal Neonatal Ed. 1997;77(2):F115-8.
54. Supapannachart S, Siripoonya P, Boonwattanasoontorn W, Kanjanavanit S. Neonatal polycythemia: effects of partial exchange transfusion using fresh frozen plasma, Haemaccel and normal saline. J Med Assoc Thai. 1999;82 Suppl 1:S82-6.
55. Deorari AK, Paul VK, Shreshta L, Singh M. Symptomatic neonatal polycythemia: comparison of partial exchange transfusion with saline versus plasma. Indian Pediatr. 1995;32(11):1167-71.
56. Roithmaier A, Arlettaz R, Bauer K, Bucher HU, Krieger M, Duc G, et al. Randomized controlled trial of Ringer solution versus serum for partial exchange transfusion in neonatal polycythaemia. Eur J Pediatr. 1995;154(1):53-6.
57. Kumar A, Ramji S. Effect of partial exchange transfusion in asymptomatic polycythemic LBW babies. Indian Pediatr. 2004;41(4):366-72.
58. Dempsey EM, Barrington K. Short and long term outcomes following partial exchange transfusion in the polycythaemic newborn: a systematic review. Arch Dis Child Fetal Neonatal Ed. 2006;91(1):F2-6.
59. Schimmel MS, Bromiker R, Soll RF. Neonatal polycythemia: is partial exchange transfusion justified? Clin Perinatol. 2004;31(3):545-53, ix-x.

SECTION 3

Coagulation Disorders in Newborn

Section Editors

Mamta Vijay Manglani, Jagdish Chandra

CHAPTER

18

Congenital Coagulation Disorders in the Neonate

Mamta Vijay Manglani, Pooja Balasubramanian, Nimish Kulkarni, Snehavardhan Pandey

INTRODUCTION

Neonatal bleeding can be due to congenital or acquired disorders of various phases of hemostasis including vascular, platelet, coagulation as well as fibrinolytic pathway. This chapter will focus only on congenital coagulation disorders presenting in the neonatal period. While severe congenital hemostatic defects present with bleeding during the first few hours to days of life in an otherwise healthy newborn, acquired causes such as sepsis, disseminated intravascular coagulation (DIC), vitamin K deficiency, etc. are encountered in sick babies.[1,2] Milder defects may not be apparent until later in childhood. Among the various congenital causes of bleeding in a neonate, coagulation factor deficiencies are the most common, with factors VIII and IX being the most frequent defect encountered. Deficiency of prothrombin, factors V, VII, XI, XIII, fibrinogen and α2-antiplasmin deficiency are less common. Though von Willebrand disease (vWD) is one of the most common bleeding disorders in children, it rarely manifests in the neonatal period, except for severe forms. Bleeding in the neonatal period due to inherited coagulation factor deficiency is seen in 15–30% of children.[3]

Bleeding in a neonate due to any cause may lead to significant morbidity and mortality due to low blood volume. Hence, it is important to achieve early and correct diagnosis with a focus on immediate and appropriate treatment of the condition. Caution should be exercised while interpreting the laboratory values for tests of coagulation as, physiologically, a neonate has reduced levels of almost all coagulant proteins. While this would pose a higher risk of bleeding in a newborn, it is not so, due to the balance achieved by presence of lower anticoagulant proteins too! Reference ranges for neonates should be used for concluding the laboratory results.

INHERITANCE PATTERNS

Deficiencies of prothrombin, factors V, VII, X, XI, XIII, fibrinogen and α2-antiplasmin are all inherited as autosomal recessive disorders whereas hemophilia A and B (factors VIII and IX deficiencies) are both X-linked recessively inherited. Types 1 and 2 vWD are inherited as an autosomal dominant disorder, whereas, type 3 may be autosomal recessive. History of consanguinity assumes significance in all autosomal recessive disorders whereas family history of a similar disorder might be present in any of the congenital coagulation disorders. In vWD, parents as well as siblings could also be affected, whereas, in hemophilia, it would be present among maternal uncles and male maternal cousins as well as male siblings. All autosomal recessive conditions would have a history, if at all, of the same disorder among siblings. One-third of the cases are *de novo* mutations.

CLINICAL PRESENTATION

The common clinical manifestations of bleeding in a neonate include oozing from the umbilical cord, bleeding into the scalp (cephalhematoma) **(Fig. 18.1)**, bruising, intracranial bleeds, oozing from sites of venipuncture, delayed cord fall, excessive bleeding following circumcision in male babies. Bleeding following birth trauma may be exaggerated in presence of a bleeding disorder.

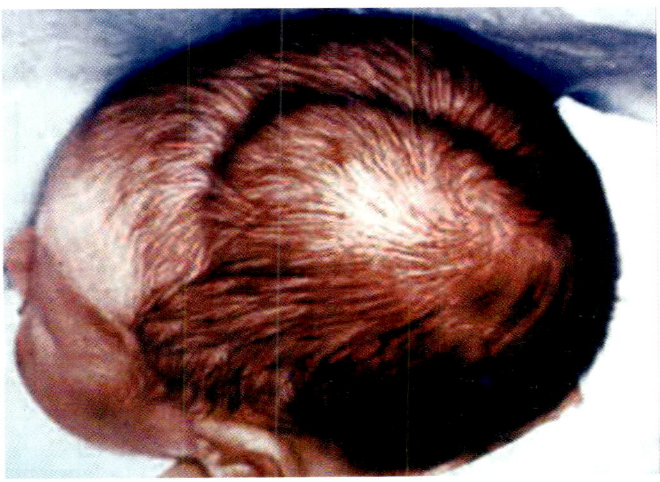

Figure 18.1 Cephalhematoma in a neonate with hemophilia A

The type of bleeding in neonatal period is different from that seen in older children with majority of bleeding occurring following a hemostatic challenge. Oozing and hematoma formation following venipuncture or intramuscular injection, circumcision site bleed, trauma during birthing process causing intracranial and extracranial bleeds are the common bleeding manifestations.[1,4,5]

Severe deficiencies of fibrinogen, factors VII, X and XIII more commonly present in the neonatal period. Persistent oozing from the umbilical stump, uncommon in hemophilia, is typically associated with fibrinogen defects and factor XIII deficiency.[4] Joint bleeds, seen often in older infants and children, are rare in newborns.[1] Intracranial hemorrhage (ICH) may be the first presentation in a few neonates with severe deficiencies of factors VII, X and XIII deficiency and less frequently factor VIII deficiency.[2,4] Most common location of ICH is subarachnoid, followed by subdural and parenchymal bleed and less commonly subgaleal hematoma.[1] Deficiencies of factor XII, prekallikrein and high molecular weight kininogens are of no clinical significance in newborns.[6] Hemorrhagic disease of the newborn (HDN) may be a most common manifestation of vitamin K deficiency in the neonate; however, congenital deficiency of vitamin K-dependent clotting factors deficiency (VKCFD) also may rarely present in the neonate with bleeding of varying intensity.

LABORATORY INVESTIGATIONS AND INTERPRETATION

Initial laboratory screening tests must include platelet count and morphology, prothrombin time (PT), activated partial thromboplastin time (aPTT), thrombin time (TT) and fibrinogen. Diagnosis may be challenging in neonates as PT, PTT and TT are prolonged compared to adult values. As mentioned earlier, this may be due to physiological "deficiencies" of the vitamin K-dependent factors (II, VII, IX and X) and contact factors (XI, XII, prekallikrein and high-molecular-weight kininogen) as well as the presence of fetal glycoforms of fibrinogen. Hence, knowledge of developmental hemostasis and age appropriate values is required to achieve a correct diagnosis of bleeding disorder in a newborn. Hence, referring to normal ranges for preterm and full-term neonates helps in identifying abnormal results. The absolute values of the tests are based on reagent and analyzer and, hence, all laboratories must have their own reference ranges for neonates of different gestational ages.

Algorithm for Interpreting the Laboratory Tests

If platelet counts are normal and platelets are seen in clumps on the peripheral blood smear, a coagulation defect is more likely the cause of bleeding. This could be congenital or acquired. If the baby is well, it is more likely to be a congenital disorder.

If PT is exclusively prolonged, it is likely to be factor VII deficiency. If the PTT is exclusively prolonged, then deficiency of factors VIII, von Willebrand factor (vWF), IX and XI need to be considered. But if both PT and PTT are prolonged, either combined deficiencies of intrinsic and common pathway or fibrinogen deficiency needs to be ruled out after acquired causes such as DIC, liver injury and HDN have been clinically ruled out. Fibrinogen deficiency would also depict a prolonged TT **(Fig. 18.2 and Flow chart 18.1)**.

Hypofibrinogenemia can then be confirmed by performing plasma fibrinogen assay. If levels are normal, in presence of prolonged TT, dysfibrinogenemia should be diagnosed. If all these tests are normal for age, then consider factor XIII deficiency.

Depending on the results of screening tests, factor assay may be done based on age-specific values. Levels of factor VIII, V and fibrinogen correlate well with normal adult values in term and preterm infants and hence a deficiency can be diagnosed in the neonatal period, irrespective of severity or gestational age.[4,6] Moderate and severe deficiencies of factors II, VII, IX and X can be identified while mild deficiency may be difficult to diagnose due to overlap with physiological values in newborns thus requiring repeat testing at 6 months of age to confirm diagnosis.[5,6]

Factor XIII deficiency should be excluded in the presence of typical bleeding pattern with normal tests for coagulation.[6] Screening test involves solubility of the fibrin clot produced by calcium or thrombin in either 5 mol/L urea or 1% monochloroacetic acid. Clots from patients with less than 1% factor XIII activity are soluble and hence mild deficiency may be missed.

Tests recommended for vWD include PTT, factor VIII assay, ristocetin cofactor assay to measure vWF activity, vWF antigen assay and ABO blood group typing. If these tests suggest vWD, vWF multimer analysis should be performed. Concentrations of vWF and the proportion of high-molecular-weight multimers of vWF are physiologically increased thus making diagnosis of types 1 and 2 vWD difficult in newborns and require repeat testing in infancy. Type 3 vWD can be diagnosed due to complete deficiency of the factor.[4]

Protein induced by vitamin K absence or antagonist-II (PIVKA-II) immunoassay, which specifically combines with undercarboxylated prothrombin reflects the vitamin K-deficient state seen in VKCFD or in acquired conditions like HDN.

Prenatal diagnosis by amniocentesis or chorionic villus biopsy may be done in families with known inherited coagulation disorders. This is commonly advised for severe hemophilia A and B, though deficiencies of factors V, VII, XIII and vWF can also be diagnosed prenatally. Early diagnosis allows for termination of pregnancy or timely intervention in affected fetuses.[4,6]

Molecular Diagnosis

Genetic defects identified in decreasing frequency are missense mutations (50–80%), insertion/deletion (20–30% of gene variations of the fibrinogen, *FV*, *MCFD2*, and *FXIII* genes; <15% of remaining coagulation factor mutations), splicing and nonsense mutations (5–15%), variants located in the 3' and 5' untranslated regions of the genes (<5% and found only

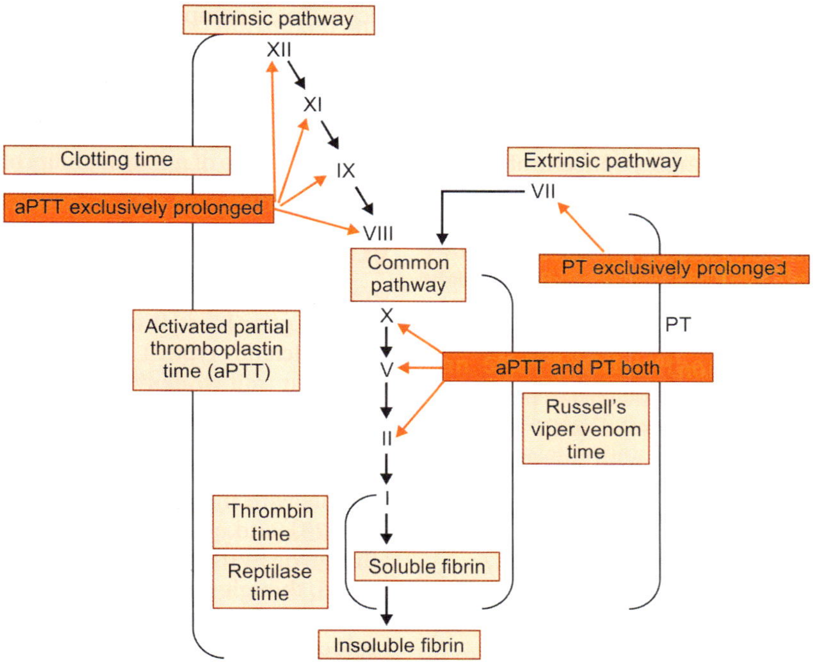

Figure 18.2 The interpretation of the laboratory tests for coagulation defects
Abbreviations: aPTT, activated partial thromboplastin time; PT, prothrombin time

Flow chart 18.1 The correction studies to interpret the prolonged activated partial thromboplastin time

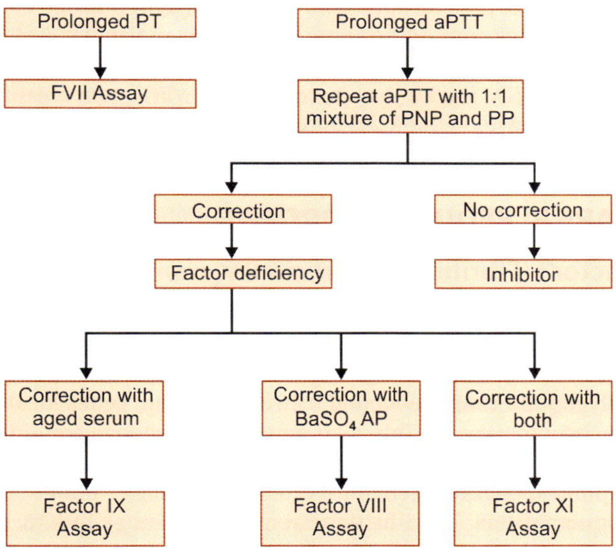

Abbreviations: aPTT, activated partial thromboplastin time; PNP, platelet neutralization procedure; PP, patient's plasma; $BaSO_4$ AP, barium sulphate adsorbed plasma

in fibrinogen, FVII, FXI and FXIII).[7] No identifiable genetic defect is found in 5–10% of patients with severe deficiencies.

These mutations are found in genes encoding corresponding coagulation factors.[8]

Exceptions are combined FV and FVIII deficiency and VKCFD with mutations in genes encoding proteins/enzymes involved in transport and metabolism.[8]

General Management

Antenatal care should be provided with a focus to the management of the suspected bleeding disorder (with a family history of bleeding disorder) in such cases. Delivery should be managed in a tertiary care hospital by an experienced team of obstetrician, neonatologist and pediatric hematologist. Bleeding manifestations may be enhanced with instrumentation, increasing the risk for ICH and therefore, should be avoided in known cases if possible.[3,9] Normal vaginal delivery may be generally safe for many babies with hemophilia,[9] however, the optimal mode of delivery for infants of hemophilia carrier mothers has yet to be determined.[3,9]

Prophylactic factor VIII replacement to prevent ICH as a routine practice is not recommended. It should be considered in known severe factors XIII, VII and X deficiency states where the risk of ICH is higher.[6] Hence, cranial ultrasound must be done within a few hours of birth in case of trauma during delivery or these factor deficiencies (XIII, VII and X).[2]

Acute episodes of bleeding in a suspected congenital coagulation factor deficiency may be treated with FFP at a dose of 10–15 mL/kg, while awaiting test results to confirm diagnosis.[6] The aim of treatment to raise the plasma concentration of the deficient factor to minimal hemostatic level, which depends on site/nature of bleeding and deficient protein.[5]

Factor XI Deficiency (Hemophilia C)

Factor XI deficiency is seen in 1 in 1 million population contributing to 26.5% of cases of rare bleeding disorders.[8,19] FXI is a homodimer composed of two identical chains bound together by disulfide bonds with the gene for FXI located on chromosome 4.[1]

Severe deficiency of factor XI is rare. The bleeding tendency is variable and may not correlate with plasma concentration of factor XI which differs from other bleeding disorders.[33] The bleeding risk is affected by site of injury with increased bleeding at sites of high fibrinolytic activity (urogenital tract, oral cavity).[34]

Two newborns have been reported with bleeding complications due to severe FXI deficiency. One newborn had bilateral subdural hemorrhage which was diagnosed prenatally while the other had bleeding from circumcision site 3 days after birth.[35,36]

Laboratory screening tests reveal prolonged PTT and normal PT and TT. Plasma derived factor XI concentrates (available in countries with high prevalence, e.g. Israel),[23] FFP at a dose of 10–20 mL/kg or cryoprecipitate can be used to treat bleeding episodes. The half-life of factor XI is over 48 hours.[20] Antifibrinolytic agents (ε-aminocaproic acid or tranexamic acid) may be used to control local bleeding. Cases with severe factor XI deficiency previously treated with FFP have been reported to develop inhibitors.[37]

Factor XIII (Fibrin-stabilizing Factor) Deficiency

Factor XIII deficiency is a rarer bleeding disorder accounting for 6.5% cases and is seen in 1 in 2 million of the world population.[8,19] Factor XIII is a tetramer consisting of two A subunits and two B subunits with the gene for the A subunit located on chromosome 6 and the gene for the B subunit located on chromosome 1.[1] The site of production of factor XIII-A subunit is bone marrow and factor XIII-B subunit is liver.[38] Deficiency of factor XIII inherited in autosomal recessive fashion is due to mutations in the A subunit.[5]

Bleeding due to FXIII deficiency is usually severe and delayed. Umbilical stump bleeding or/and ICH are the characteristic bleeding manifestations at birth.[39] Delayed wound healing, abnormal scar formation, and recurrent soft-tissue hemorrhage, with tendency to form hemorrhagic cysts are some of the clinical presentations of homozygous FXIII deficiency.[1] Approximately one-third of all affected patients may develop ICH even in the absence of a traumatic event.[40] Newborns with heterozygous defects are not clinically affected.

Laboratory screening tests reveal normal PT, PTT and TT. Screening tests such as clot solubility test with a low sensitivity may be done in resource limited settings. Quantitative estimation using specific amine incorporation assays are available in specialized research laboratories.[41]

Factor XIII deficient patients may be treated with FFP, cryoprecipitate, or FXIII concentrates (heat-treated, lyophilized, plasma-derived; Corifact).[42] Due to the high incidence of ICH, a prophylactic regimen of FXIII replacement should be given to newborns with known FXIII deficiency. Once-a-month therapy is sufficient due to the very long half-life of 5–7 days with hemostatic plasma concentrations of 2–3 U/dL.[20] Low doses of FFP (2–3 mL/kg) administered every 4–6 weeks, cryoprecipitate at a dose of 1 bag/10–20 kg every 3–4 weeks, or, preferably, FXIII concentrate at a dose of 10–20 U/kg every 4–6 weeks, may be used for prophylactic replacement therapy.[43]

HEREDITARY DEFICIENCIES OF MULTIPLE COAGULATION FACTORS

Only two infants with multiple factor deficiencies have been reported with bleeding in the neonatal period.[1] Congenital deficiencies of two or more coagulation factors have been described in various combinations.

Combined Factor V and Factor VIII Deficiency

This has been reported in over 50 families till date.[20] Mutations in the genes *LMAN1* and *MCFD2* encoding proteins involved in FV and FVIII intracellular transport have been identified.[8] Both coagulant factor V and VIII activity and antigen are decreased.[44] Clinical symptoms are mild with mostly mucocutaneous bleeds.[44] Regular prophylactic therapy is not required. DDAVP and FFP transfusion may be given during bleeds, along with factor VII concentrates in severe cases. The different half-lives of factors V and VIII must be considered during replacement therapy.

Vitamin K-dependent Clotting Factors Deficiency

Hereditary combined VKCFD is a rare congenital bleeding disorder with decreased levels of coagulation factors II, VII, IX and X as well as natural anticoagulants protein C, protein S and protein Z. It is an extremely rare autosomal recessive condition with less than 30 affected patients described in literature till date.[45] There are two subtypes of VKCFD depending on mutation of two enzymes of the vitamin K cycle: VKCFD type 1 is defined by defective gamma-glutamyl carboxylase (GGCX) activity[46] while VKCFD type 2 derives from functional deficiency of vitamin K 2, 3-epoxide reductase complex (VKORC).[47]

These enzymes are necessary for gamma-carboxylation, a post-translational modification required for normal activity of coagulation proteins and a few nonhemostatic proteins such as osteocalcin, PROX and matrix-Gla protein (MGP) expressed in the connective tissue.[48] Clinical bleeding may vary in severity from mild-to-severe, life-threatening episodes occurring either spontaneously or following a surgical intervention. Severe form of the disease usually presents in the neonatal period with fatal ICH reported, as seen in hemorrhagic disease of newborn due to acquired vitamin K deficiency.[49,50] Mucocutaneous bleeding is more common with occasional umbilical cord bleeding; hemarthrosis is rare.[49] Diagnosis may be delayed in milder cases.

Nonhemostatic manifestations include developmental and/or skeletal abnormalities resembling warfarin embryopathy and involve stippling of the long bones epiphyses and shortness of finger distal phalanges.[51] An increased rate of fetal loss has been observed due to bone impairment during embryogenesis.[51]

Laboratory screening tests reveal markedly prolonged PT and PTT with correction on mixing studies. Factor assay reveals variably reduced levels of factors II, VII, IX and X activity. PIVKA-II or/and undercarboxylated prothrombin are found to be increased, even after vitamin K or plasma administration due to its long half-life up to 70 hours.[52] It may not be able to differentiate VKCFD from other causes of vitamin K deficiency (e.g. liver disease); however it is more sensitive than measurement of activity levels of vitamin K-dependent factors. Molecular diagnosis is mandatory for confirmation of the condition. Although protein C, S and Z activities are also decreased in VKCFD, the risk of thrombosis is very low.[50]

Treatment includes oral or parenteral vitamin K1 supplementation. The response is variable with undercarboxylated forms of factors persisting despite massive vitamin K doses. Successful treatment with recombinant activated factor VII in an emergency surgical situation is possible.[53]

Major bleeding in neonates may be avoided by administration of vitamin K to women in the third trimester of pregnancy suspected to carry a child with VKCFD.[45] Hence, the benefit of prenatal diagnosis in a condition, which can be easily treated with vitamin K, needs to be established.

DEFECTS IN THE FIBRINOLYTIC PATHWAY

These rare defects include α2-antiplasmin deficiency and plasminogen activator inhibitor-1 (PAI-1) deficiency. They cause failure to control the fibrinolytic pathway and premature lysis of fibrin clot thereby presenting as bleeding disorders.[20]

Symptoms are mild and include umbilical stump bleeds, mucocutaneous bleeding and rarely joint hemorrhages. Laboratory screening tests reveal normal PT, PTT and TT. A measure of fibrinolytic activity, euglobulin clot lysis time, is shortened and specific assays for PAI-1 antigen and activity confirm the deficiency. Most bleeding episodes can be treated with use of antifibrinolytic agents, including ε-aminocaproic acid and tranexamic acid.[20]

CONCLUSION

Bleeding in the neonatal period is a common problem faced in neonatal intensive care unit (NICU) and nursery. It is important to evaluate the clinical condition of the bleeding neonate, i.e. whether the infant is a well baby or a sick baby. Generally, congenital coagulation deficiencies are seen in well babies with acute bleeding episodes. The gestational age is also of prime importance, as the laboratory tests for evaluating bleeding in these babies would be interpreted based on the normal reference ranges accordingly. Laboratory tests must be carried out in a stepwise manner with the knowledge of hemostatic features unique to neonates allowing a prompt diagnosis and appropriate management of these neonates.

REFERENCES

1. Albisetti M, Andrew M, Monagle P. Hemostatic abnormalities. In: de Alarcon PA, Werner E (Eds). Neonatal Hematology, 1st edition. United States of America: Cambridge University Press; 2005. pp. 310-48.
2. Girolami A, De Marc L, Dal Bo Zanon R, Patrassi G, Cappellato MG. Rarer quantitative and qualitative abnormalities of coagulation. Clin Hematol. 1985;14(2):385-411.
3. Kulkarni R, Ponder KP, James AH, Soucie JM, Koerper M, Hoots WK, et al. Unresolved issues in diagnosis and management of inherited bleeding disorders in the perinatal period: a White Paper of the Perinatal Task Force of the Medical and Scientific Advisory Council of the National Hemophilia Foundation, USA. Haemophilia. 2006;12(3):205-11.
4. Kenet G, Chan AK, Soucie JM, Kulkarni R. Bleeding disorders in neonates. Haemophilia. 2010;(16 Suppl 5):168-75.
5. Cantor AB. Hemostasis in the newborn and infants. In: Orkin SH, Nathan DG, Ginsburg D, Look AT, Fisher DE, Lux SE (Eds). Nathan and Oski's Hematology of Infancy and Childhood, 8th edition. Philadelphia, USA: Elsevier Saunders; 2015. pp. 128-50.
6. Williams MD, Chalmers EA, Gibson BE; Haemostasis and Thrombosis Task Force, British Committee for Standards in Haematology. The investigation and management of neonatal haemostasis and thrombosis. Br J Haematol. 2002;119(2):295-309.
7. Peyvandi F, Kunicki T, Lillicrap D. Genetic sequence analysis of inherited bleeding diseases. Blood. 2013;122(20):3423-31.
8. Peyvandi F, Palla R, Menegatti M, Mannucci PM. Introduction. Rare bleeding disorders: general aspects of clinical features, diagnosis, and management. Semin Thromb Hemost. 2009;35(4):349-55.
9. Chalmers E, Williams M, Brennand J, Liesner R, Collins P, Richards M, et al. Guideline on the management of haemophilia in the fetus and neonate. Br J Haematol. 2011;154(2):208-15.
10. United Kingdom Haemophilia Centre Directors Organisation Executive Committee. Guidelines on therapeutic products to treat haemophilia and other hereditary coagulation disorders. Haemophilia. 1997;3(1):63-77.
11. Kuhle S, Mitchell L, Massicotte P, Andrew M. Hemostatic disorders of the newborn. In: Taeusch HW, Ballard RA, Gleason CA (Eds). Avery's Diseases of the Newborn, 8th edition. Philadelphia, USA: Elsevier Saunders, 2005. pp. 1145-79.
12. Ljung RC. Prenatal diagnosis of haemophilia. Haemophilia. 1999;5(2):84-7.
13. Schulman I. Pediatric aspects of the mild hemophilias. Med Clin North Am. 1962;46:93-105.
14. Peyvandi F, Mannucci PM, Garagiola I, El-Beshlawy A, Elalfy M, Ramanan V, et al. A randomized trial of factor VIII and neutralizing antibodies in hemophilia A. N Engl J Med. 2016;374(21):2054-64.
15. Eikenboom JC, Reitsma PH, Peerlinck KM, Briët E. Recessive inheritance of von Willebrand's disease type I. Lancet. 1993;341(8851):982-6.
16. Katz JA, Moake JL, McPherson PD, Weinstein MJ, Moise KJ, Carpenter RJ, et al. Relationship between human development and disappearance of unusually large von Willebrand factor multimers from plasma. Blood. 1989;73(7):1851-8.
17. Gazengel C, Fischer AM, Schlegel N, Rothschild C, Torchet MF, Dautzenberg MD, et al. Treatment of type III von Willebrand's

disease with solvent/detergent-treated factor VIII concentrates. Nouv Rev Fr Hematol. 1988;30(4):225-7.
18. López-Fernández MF, López-Berges C, Corral M, García-Talavera JR, López Borrasca A, Batlle J. Assessment of multimeric structure and ristocetin-induced binding to platelets of von Willebrand factor present in cryoprecipitate and different factor VIII concentrates. Vox Sang. 1987;52(1-2):15-9.
19. Mannucci PM, Duga S, Peyvandi F. Recessively inherited coagulation disorders. Blood. 2004;104(5):1243-52.
20. Bauer KA, Sharda AV. Rare hereditary coagulation factor abnormalities. In: Orkin SH, Nathan DG, Ginsburg D, Look AT, Fisher DE, Lux SE (Eds). Nathan and Oski's Hematology of Infancy and Childhood, 8th edition. Philadelphia, USA: Elsevier Saunders; 2015. pp. 1055-61.
21. Acharya SS, Coughlin A, Dimichele DM; North American Rare Bleeding Disorder Study Group. Rare Bleeding Disorder Registry: deficiencies of factors II, V, VII, X, XIII, fibrinogen and dysfibrinogenemias. J Thromb Haemost. 2004;2(2):248-56.
22. Neerman-Arbez M, de Moerloose P. Hereditary fibrinogen abnormalities. In: Kaushansky K, Lichtman MA, Beutler E, Kipps T, Prchal J, Seligsohn U (Eds). William's Hematology, 8th Edition. New York, NY: McGraw-Hill; 2010. pp. 2051-68.
23. World Federation of Hemophilia (WFH).(2012). Registry of clotting factor concentrates, 9th edition. [online] Available from www1.wfh.org/publications/files/pdf-1227.pdf [Accessed July, 2016].
24. Lancellotti S, Basso M, De Cristofaro R. Congenital prothrombin deficiency: an update. Semin Thromb Hemost. 2013;39(6):596-606.
25. Kessler CM, Acs P, Mariani G. Acquired disorders of coagulation: the immune coagulopathies. In: Colman RW, Marder VJ, Clowes AW, George JN, Goldhaber SZ (Eds). Hemostasis and Thrombosis: Basic Principles and Clinical Practice, 5th edition. Philadelphia, USA: Lippincott Williams and Wilkins; 2006. pp. 1061-84.
26. Mariani G, Bernardi F. Factor VII deficiency. Semin Thromb Hemost. 2009;35(4):400-6.
27. Matthay KK, Koerper MA, Ablin AR. Intracranial hemorrhage in congenital factor VII deficiency. J Pediatr. 1979;94(3):413-5.
28. Levanon M, Rimon S, Shani M, Goldberg E, Ramot B. Active and inactive factor VII in Dubin-Johnson syndrome with factor-VII deficiency, hereditary factor-VII deficiency and on coumadin administration. Br J Haematol. 1972;23(6):669-77.
29. Seligsohn U, Shani M, Ramot B. Gilbert syndrome and factor-VII deficiency. Lancet. 1970;1(7661):1398.
30. Menegatti M, Peyvandi F. Factor X deficiency. Semin Thromb Hemost. 2009;35(4):407-15.
31. El Kalla S, Menon NS. Neonatal congenital Factor X deficiency. Pediatr Hematol Oncol. 1991;8(4):347-54.
32. Karimi M, Vafafar A, Haghpanah S, Payandeh M, Eshghi P, Hoofar H, et al. Efficacy of prophylaxis and genotype-phenotype correlation in patients with severe Factor X deficiency in Iran. Haemophilia. 2012;18(12):211-5.
33. Edson JR, White JG, Krivit W. The enigma of severe factor XI deficiency without hemorrhagic symptoms: distinction from Hageman factor and "Fletcher factor" deficiency; family study; and problems of diagnosis. Thromb Diath Haemorrh. 1967;18(3-4):342-8.
34. Kravtsov DV, Wu W, Meijers JC, Sun MF, Blinder MA, Dang TP, et al. Dominant factor XI deficiency caused by mutations in the factor XI catalytic domain. Blood. 2004;104(1):128-34.
35. Kitchens CS. Factor XI: a review of its biochemistry and deficiency. Semin Thromb Hemost. 1991;17(1):55-72.
36. Barozzino T, Sgro M, Toi A, Akouri H, Wilson S, Yeo E, et al. Fetal bilateral subdural haemorrhages. Prenatal diagnosis and spontaneous resolution by time of delivery. Prenat Diagn. 1998;18(5):496-503.
37. Salomon O, Zivelin A, Livnat T, Dardik R, Loewenthal R, Avishai O, et al. Prevalence, causes, and characterization of factor XI inhibitors in patients with inherited factor XI deficiency. Blood. 2003;101(12):4783-8.
38. Schroeder V, Kohler HP. Factor XIII deficiency: an update. Semin Thromb Hemost. 2013;39(6):632-41.
39. Merchant RH, Agarwal BR, Currimbhoy Z, Pherwani A, Avasthi B. Congenital factor XIII deficiency. Indian Pediatr. 1992;29(7):831-6.
40. Duckert F. Documentation of the plasma factor XIII deficiency in man. Ann N Y Acad Sci. 1972;202:190-9.
41. Lorand L, Urayama T, De Kiewiet JW, Nossel HL. Diagnostic and genetic studies on fibrin-stabilizing factor with a new assay based on amine incorporation. J Clin Invest. 1969;48(6):1054-64.
42. Inbal A, Oldenburg J, Carcao M, Rosholm A, Tehranchi R, Nugent D. Recombinant factor XIII: a safe and novel treatment for congenital factor XIII deficiency. Blood. 2012;119(22):5111-7.
43. Gootenberg JE. Factor concentrates for the treatment of factor XIII deficiency. Curr Opin Hematol. 1998;5(6):372-5.
44. Zheng C, Zhang B. Combined deficiency of coagulation factors V and VIII: an update. Semin Thromb Hemost. 2013;39(6):613-20.
45. Napolitano M, Mariani G, Lapecorella M. Hereditary combined deficiency of the vitamin K-dependent clotting factors. Orphanet J Rare Dis. 2010;5:21.
46. Soute BA, Ulrich MM, Watson AD, Maddison JE, Ebberink RH, Vermeer C. Congenital deficiency of all vitamin K-dependent blood coagulation factors due to a defective vitamin K-dependent carboxylase in Devon Rex cats. Thromb Haemost. 1992;68(5):521-5.
47. Oldenburg J, von Brederlow B, Fregin A, Rost S, Wolz W, Eberl W, et al. Congenital deficiency of vitamin K dependent coagulation factors in two families presents as a genetic defect of the vitamin K-epoxide-reductase-complex. Thromb Haemost. 2000;84(6):937-41.
48. Hauschka PV, Lian JB, Cole DE, Gundberg CM. Osteocalcin and matrix Gla protein: vitamin K-dependent proteins in bone. Physiol Rev. 1989;69(3):990-1047.
49. McMillan CW, Roberts HR: Congenital combined deficiency of coagulation factors II VII, IX, and X. Report of a case. N Engl J Med. 1966;274(23):1313-5.
50. Bhattacharyya J, Dutta P, Mishra P, Dixit A, Srinivas U, Kannan M, et al. Congenital vitamin K-dependent coagulation factor deficiency: a case report. Blood Coagul Fibrinolysis. 2005;16(7):525-7.
51. Pauli RM, Lian JB, Mosher DF, Suttie JW. Association of congenital deficiency of multiple vitamin K-dependent coagulation factors and the phenotype of the warfarin embryopathy: clues to the mechanism of teratogenicity of coumarin derivatives. Am J Hum Genet. 1987;41(4):566-83.
52. Shapiro AD, Jacobson LJ, Armon ME, Manco-Johnson MJ, Hulac P, Lane PA, et al. Vitamin K deficiency in the newborn infant:prevalence and perinatal risk factors. J Pediatr. 1986;109(4):675-80.
53. Lapecorella M, Napolitano M, Bernardi F, Pinotti M, Sbrighi PS, Marchetti G, et al. Effective hemostasis during minor surgery in a case of hereditary combined deficiency of vitamin K-dependent clotting factors. Clin Appl Thromb Hemost. 2010;16(2):221-3.

CHAPTER

19

Vitamin K Deficiency Bleeding

Jagdish Chandra, Piali Mandal

INTRODUCTION

Vitamin K deficiency bleeding (VKDB) in infancy is an acquired disorder of coagulation caused by reduction of VK1-dependent coagulation factors below the hemostatic levels. Intracranial hemorrhage is seen in 30–60% of the cases. Both oral and intramuscular routes have been tried but till date IM administration of VK at birth seems the most effective form of prophylaxis against all forms of VKDB.[1,2]

An unexpected association between IM VK and childhood cancer was reported in 1992,[3] which prompted a number of epidemiological studies which have yielded inconsistent results, though; most have been reassuring, the likelihood of a small risk remains.[4]

In later part of 19th century Charles Townsend had coined the term Hemorrhagic Disease of Newborn (HDN) describing bleeding in early neonatal period (under one week) where traumatic delivery, hemophilia, thrombocytopenia and birth asphyxia were excluded.[5] Though, later, it became apparent that the cause of this bleeding was VK deficiency resulting a fall in VK dependent coagulation factors, the term still continued to be used for neonatal period only. Subsequently, two more forms of disease were described—an early HDN—manifesting within 24 hours after birth and associated with certain maternal risk factors, and the second—late HDN—which was described to occur in late neonatal period and early infancy.[6,7] Since bleeding due to VK deficiency is not confined to neonatal period, as cases have been seen till late infancy, and neonatal bleeding is not always related to VK deficiency, the term VKDB-vitamin K deficiency bleeding was suggested to replace the term HDN.[1]

The tendency of the neonate to become VK deficient is in part due to the very small hepatic stores available at birth, stored almost exclusively in the form of vitamin K1. At birth, circulating vitamin K levels are low or undetectable often below the detection limit of 0.02 ng/mL. VK is poorly transferred across the placental barrier, though the reasons for this protection of the newborn from high levels of vitamin K are not well understood since no immediately clear biologic advantage has been implicated. Despite this, hemostasis is good and the vast majority of neonates do not have bleeding. Detectable levels of vitamin K are found after about 12 hours of birth and adult levels of 0.4 ng/mL are achieved by day 4, in breast-fed babies given no VK supplement.[8] Required amount of VK for neonate is around 1 μg/kg/day, whereas, breast milk often contains levels as low as 1–2 μg/L with even lower levels in colostrum. The situation is further worsened by intake of small volume of breast milk during the first few days of life and by the presence of a sterile gut initially. VK levels are approximately 10 times higher in those fed on formula milk than those found in exclusively breast-fed infants.[9] Thus formula-fed infants with some exceptions, like poor absorption or underlying liver diseases, are well protected against both classical and late VKDB. The trivial supply of VK in exclusively breastfed infants is reflected in lower VK levels and more frequent demonstration of PIVKA than in the formula-fed infants.[10] No difference in activity of the VK-dependent coagulation factors has been found.[8]

Vitamin K deficiency bleeding, though rarely seen, but holds importance in the set-up like India and other developing countries, where home deliveries (absence of vitamin K prophylaxis at birth), exclusive breastfeeding, frequent occurrence of diarrheal diseases, irrational use of antibiotics and very commonly unnoticed early signs of underlying liver disease, it becomes important to stress upon this entity. Late-onset VKDB has emerged as a major problem as most frequent presentation of this entity is central nervous system bleed which may be fatal. VKDB is, though not fully, but a preventable complication of inadequate vitamin K stores at birth.

EPIDEMIOLOGY

The historical perspective of use of VK has been very interesting, starting from its use for prophylaxis against HDN in selective neonates (complicated deliveries or preterms) to universal prophylaxis for all newborns, its later association with hemolytic anemia and childhood cancer. A paper in the *Lancet* in 1944 showed a fivefold reduction in death from bleeding in the first week of life when all the babies were given 1 mg of oral menadione at delivery in Göteborg, Sweden.[11] Following this, in 1948, Ethel Dunham proposed VK prophylaxis to all preterm neonates immediately after birth.[12]

Later, in 1953, the very first report of association between high dose of vitamin K and hemolytic anemia came into picture, and by 1956 it was proved beyond doubt that it can cause severe jaundice and death due to bilirubin encephalopathy.[13-15] *In 1961, AAP recommended routine prophylaxis for every baby (not just every preterm baby).*[16] Intramuscular route being universally adopted for routine prophylaxis, though reluctance to use it for all the babies persisted especially in United Kingdom, for the very reason of developing bilirubin encephalopathy due to VK administration. It was advocated to be used in "at-risk" babies: operative and preterm deliveries.

In 1983, Mc Ninch et al. from UK described resurgence of VKDB in babies older than one week who were exclusively breastfed and had not received VK prophylaxis.[17]

Followed by this, cases of L-VKDB started appearing in Indian literature and from other countries of south-east Asia. In 1987, Marwaha et al. reported the first Indian series followed by Merchant et al.[18-20] Though most cases of L-VKDB are seen up to 12 weeks of age, but the upper age limit was extended up to 6 months to include more such cases fulfilling the criteria for VKDB. In most of the Indian series, age of presentation for L-VKDB is under six month but disease has been seen to occur in infants as old as 12 months. A case series of L-VKDB from Delhi has reported occurrence in late infancy and beyond.[21] Further cases were reported from Italy in 1993 by Lulsegud et al. and in 1994 by Choo et al. from Malaysia.[22]

Classification and clinical manifestations of VKDB are based on the age of onset. Age criteria for VKDB has been kept revising. Pediatric and Perinatal Subcommittee of International Society on Thrombosis and Hemostasis (ISTH) has classified VKDB as early (onset within 24 hours), classical (onset in first week of life excluding first 24 hours), and late (onset after first week of life). The upper age limit of onset till 1993 as per ISTH was 12 weeks. Later in 1999 the cut-off was increased to six month.

As per Chochrane review in 2004, late disease was described with onset up to 12 weeks.[23]

The American Academy of Pediatrics (AAP) has classified the disease in two groups—early disease (onset from birth to 2 weeks) and late disease (onset at 2–12 weeks).[24]

Indian case series have described late VKDB with onset above 6 months also.

In a series from Delhi, out of 12 cases, 9 were aged 6 months and above with onset as old as 18 months.[21] Von-Kries et al. from Germany also have described cases with onset as old as 35 weeks.[25]

With various studies reporting L-VKDB in older infants and children as well, recommending an upper age limit for onset of L-VKDB does not hold any significance.

Incidence of classical VKDB is reported to vary between 0.01% and 1.5%, those not receiving vitamin K prophylaxis (0.25–1.5% in older reviews, 0.01–0.44% in recent reviews). Classic disease is more common in preterm and in breastfed babies.

Early VKDB occur in 6–12% babies of mothers on enzyme-inducing drugs such as anticonvulsants: phenytoin, phenobarbitone and barbiturates (not valproate) and antitubercular drugs: Rifampicin, isoniazid or VK antagonists like warfarin, procoumon.

Incidence of L-VKDB in infants without VK prophylaxis is estimated to be 4–10 per 100,000 births. These are the incidences in various countries with different forms of prophylaxis.[26]

In Germany, incidence was 1.8/100,000 with oral 1 mg × 3 oral prophylaxis, which further decreased to 0.72/100,000 with oral 2 mg × 3 oral prophylaxis.

In Switzerland, incidence in 1986–87 was 7.2/100,000. With oral two doses of mixed micellar preparation, the incidence dropped to 2.8/100,000 by 1995–98.

Australia had an incidence of 2.5/100,000 with oral 1 mg × 3 oral which became zero with IM 1 mg prophylaxis.

L-VKDB is believed to be more common in South East Asia, cause attributable to maternal malnutrition and increased incidence of diarrheal diseases in these geographical regions.[1,6,7] L-VKDB is more common in boys than in girls and in summer than winter months.[1,18,19]

ETIOLOGY

As discussed earlier, according to etiology, VKDB is divided into 2 groups: *idiopathic or secondary.*

In *idiopathic* VKDB, no cause other than breast-feeding can be established. Majority of breastfed infants have an adequate, though marginal, VK supply and do not bleed even if given no VK prophylaxis. It would seem that an added risk factor is required for further lowering of the VK-dependent factors and thus causing bleed.[27] But if no other cause is identified, the VKDB is termed idiopathic.

In *secondary* VKDB, additional factors impairing VK effect are present[2] such as poor intake of milk, malabsorption of VK (because of liver or bowel disease) or antagonism of VK by drugs.[28] In a study by Sutor AH et al. among 108 German cases of VKDB more than 60% had previously undiagnosed hepatobiliary disease, predominantly cholestasis.[27] Incidence of secondary disease is more common in western countries. These may reflect the extent of investigations done. These are the proportions of secondary cases in various studies:

- Merchant et al. 1989[20] secondary — Nil
- D'Souza et al. 2003[29] secondary — 2/14
- Chandra et al. 2003[21] secondary — Nil
- von Kries et al. 1999[30] secondary — 20/23
- Schubiger 1999[31] secondary — 8/11
- von Kries et al. 2003[25] secondary — 21/29

Risk factors for secondary VKDB are:

- Alpha-1 anti-trypsin deficiency
- Cystic fibrosis
- Hepatitis
- Biliary hypoplasia
- Intrahepatic cholestasis

- Byler disease
- Sclerosing cholangitis
- Bile duct atresia.

PATHOGENESIS

The blood procoagulant proteins namely factors II, VII, IX and X and the bone forming proteins osteocalcin and matrix Gla protein, needs post-transcriptional modification in the form of carboxylation of their glutamate side chain to gamma carboxyglutamate, to be functionally active **(Fig. 19.1)**. Vitamin K acts as a co-factor for the enzyme γ-glutamyl carboxylase. The resultant γ-carboxyglutamic acid is a calcium binding amino acid which is essential for the functioning of VK-dependent proteins. Function of coagulation proteins is the formation of a blood clot **(Fig. 19.2)** and the prevention of bleeding, whereas that of osteocalcin and matrix Gla protein is to ensure bone mineralization and thus prevention of pathological fractures. There are two proposed causes of VKDB in babies whose mothers are exposed to antiepileptic drugs during pregnancy, one is the fetal microsomal enzyme induction, which degrade VK and second is competitive inhibition of the calcium-binding gamma-carboxyglutamic acid residues synthesis to the precursors of the VK dependent procoagulant factors II, VII, IX, and X.

CLINICAL FEATURES

Each form of VKDB, different pathogenic mechanisms result in VK deficiency and therefore there are different implications for VK prophylaxis.

Early VKDB: Onset in less than 24 hours of age and is rare. It is almost exclusively due to transplacental transfer of maternal drugs which inhibit VK activity in the baby. The implicated drugs include anticonvulsants, antitubercular and vitamin K antagonists.[32,33] The incidence of early VKDB in newborns of mothers taking these drugs without VK supplementation varies from 6 to 12%.[34-36] Cephalhematoma, umbilicus, intracranial, intra-abdominal, intrathoracic, and gastrointestinal bleeds are seen with early VKDB. Life threatening bleeds (including intracranial) are more common compared to classic form. Early VKDB is not preventable by VK prophylaxis at birth. There is no adequate evidence that oral prenatal VK supplementation during last trimester in women with epilepsy diminished neonatal bleeding complications.

Hey E in 1999 reviewed 38 published cases of maternal anticonvulsant usage and VKDB in infants. Less than 1/3rd could be counted as established cases out of which 50% first presented at more than 48 hours age. Most had mild symptoms. Two had symptomatic bleeds despite VK administration at birth.[37]

Hey E (1999) studied 137 babies born to mothers taking anticonvulsants during pregnancy Only 14/105 with effective blood levels of antiepileptic drug had prolonged PT. None had overt bleeding. Abnormal PT was corrected quickly after VK administration. The author concluded that policy of giving VK to pregnant women being treated with anticonvulsants is not justified with the available evidences.[37]

Harden et al. evaluated the available literature published between 1985 and October 2007. They concluded that there is insufficient evidence to determine, if the newborns of women

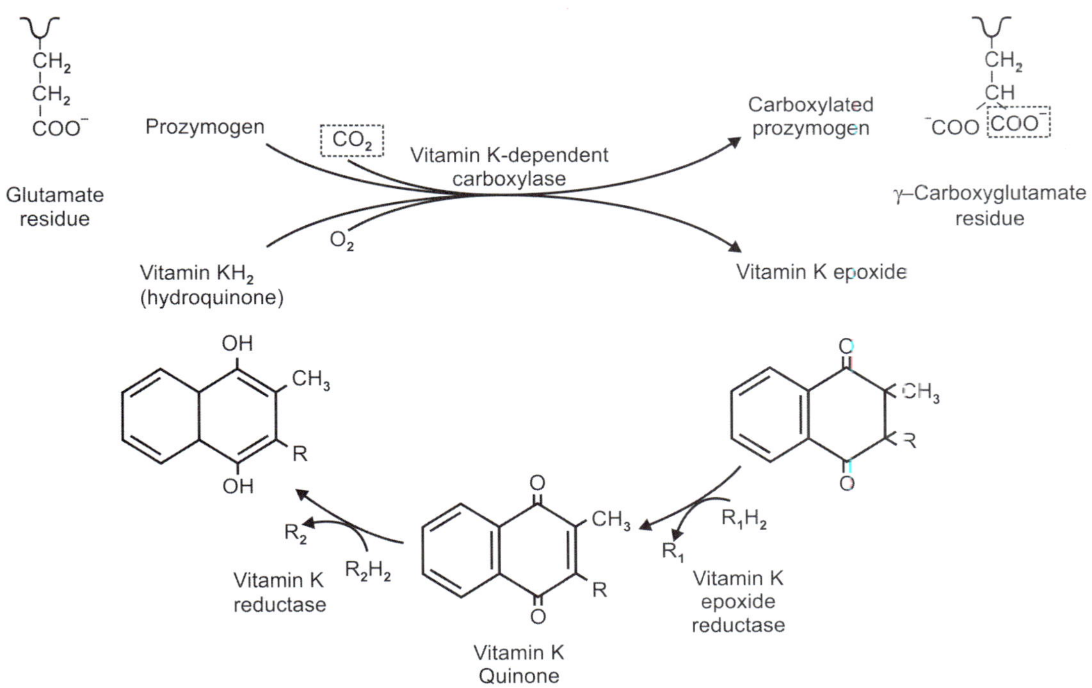

Figure 19.1 Role of vitamin K in carboxylation of vitamin K-dependent proteins

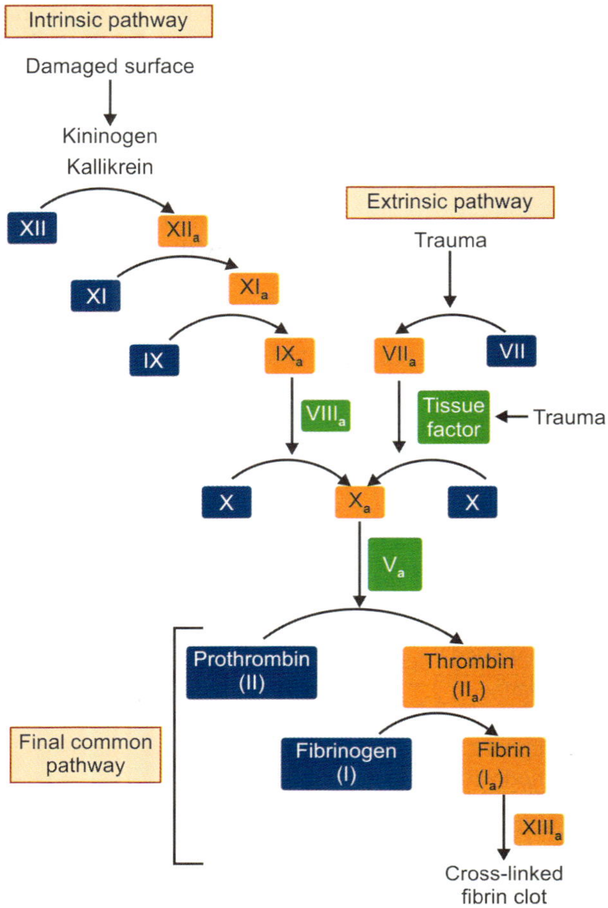

Figure 19.2 Coagulation cascade

with epilepsy taking AEDs have a considerably increased risk of hemorrhagic complications. There is no adequate evidence to support the role of oral prenatal VK supplementation in women with epilepsy in diminishing neonatal bleeding complications. This analysis further support the practice of routine VK prophylaxis at birth to newborns exposed to enzyme-inducing AEDs *in utero* as is being done for all newborns.[38]

Classical VKDB: Occurs in the first week of life, excluding the first 24 hours, usually between days 3 and 5 and usually in babies with delayed or inadequate feeding. More common in preterm than in term and in breastfed babies then top fed babies.

Incidence varies from 0.25 to 1.5% in older reviews (AAP 1961) and 0–0.44% in recent reviews.[39,40] Bleeding is usually from the umbilicus, the gastrointestinal tract, nose, skin punctures, hematuria and may cause significant blood loss. Surgical procedures such as circumcision unmask subclinical cases of VKDB.[41] Intracranial hemorrhage (ICH) is rare but can cause significant morbidity or death.

Late VKDB: VKDB of late onset has been described as late HDN or acquired prothrombin complex deficiency (APCD) from various parts of the world.[1,7] Late VKDB occurs almost exclusively or predominantly in breastfed infants, more often in boys than girls. It begins on or after day 8, most often between weeks 2 and 8, but cases have been reported to occur till late infancy and even beyond. Cases are seen mostly in those not receiving VK prophylaxis or given oral prophylaxis, as IM administration acts as a depot for slow and sustained release of vitamin K. Variable incidence can be explained by the racial variation including maternal diet, different VK prophylaxis regimens and compliance. According to etiology the disease can be divided in two groups based on the presence or absence of associated risk factors. L-VKDB is frequently associated with hepatobiliary disease. From western countries L-VKDB secondary to liver disease is reported in 73 and 87% cases.[39,40] In Indian series most cases are primary, except 15% reported to have secondary disease. One-third cases in Indian series[18,20] are associated with past or ongoing history of diarrheal illness.

Bleeding manifestations in these patients range from minor skin or mucus membrane bleeds, to epistaxis, bleeding from injection sites, umbilical ooze, gastrointestinal, intrathoracic, hematuria, retrobulbar hematoma and life-threatening central nervous system bleed. CNS bleeds can range from intracerebral hemorrhage, subdural, subarachnoid, intraventricular to cerebellar hemorrhage. Bleeding may occur following minor surgical intervention. Bleeding usually occurs in otherwise "well-looking child". Life-threatening intracranial bleed is relatively more frequent in L-VKDB than classical disease. Indian data reports intracranial bleeds in 20–90% cases, corresponding figure for which in western countries is 58–73%. Cases occurring after VK prophylaxis are likely to be older and are less likely to have intracranial bleed. Some babies might have minor "warning bleeds" such as mild bruises, nose bleeds or umbilical oozing, occurring few days before the intracranial or other life-threatening bleeds. Some might give history of diarrhea and receiving antibiotics.

Babies with secondary L-VKDB often have symptoms and signs of underlying liver disease (for example, prolonged jaundice, dark-colored urine and pale stools implying cholestasis, or failure to thrive suggesting malabsorption) long before bleeding begins. In fact, VKDB may be the first and the only manifestation of underlying disease. Earlier detection of signs and symptoms of underlying diseases predisposing to VKDB, and prompt investigation and treatment of "warning bleeds", help prevent the fatal consequences of VKDB.[40,42] Clinical profile and the frequency of bleeding at different sites, according to various Indian studies, are summarized in **Table 19.1**.

DIAGNOSIS

In any child with bleeding manifestation initial work-up would include complete blood count, including platelet count and estimation of PT and PTTK.

Coagulation defects: In VKDB, both late and classical type PT and APTT are prolonged. In early and milder forms prolonged PT may be the only abnormality. Platelet count is normal.

Table 19.1 Clinical profile of infants with L-VKDB			
	D'souza et al.[29]	*Pooni et al.*[43]	*Chandra et al.*[21]
Number of infants studied	14	42	12
Age group			
1–5 months	14 (100%)	32 (76%)	3 (25%)
> 6 months–1 year			8 (66.6%)
>1 year			1 (8.3%)
Sex			
Male	8	37	11
Female	6	5	1
Vitamin K prophylaxis	4 (28.4%)	None	None
Exclusive breast-fed	100%	100%	91.6%
Site of bleed			
Intracranial	92.8%	76.1%	16.6%
Skin bleed	NR	21.4%	100%
Umblical bleed	7%	NR	8.3%
Epistaxis	NR	NR	33.3%
GI bleed	NR	12%	25%
Prick-site bleed	NR	28.5%	NR
Gum bleed	NR	NR	8.3%
Retrobulbar Hematoma	NR	NR	8.3%

Abbreviation: NR, Not reported

There is decreased activity of the VK dependent coagulation factors (II, VII, IX, X) while levels of VK-independent factors are normal for age. Levels of fibrinogen are normal and fibrin degradation products and d-dimer assay will rule out disseminated intravascular coagulopathy. Circulating acarboxy proteins (PIVKA = Protein-induced in vitamin K absence) are present and since they have a long half-life, their presence is useful for diagnosis even after correction of coagulation defects.

For all practical purposes, any bleeding infant with an evidently prolonged prothrombin time (PT) [International Normalized Ratio (INR) >3.5] or low Quick-value (<20%) together with normal fibrinogen levels and normal platelet count is highly indicative of vitamin K deficiency.[27] Correction of these values (within 30–120 minutes) and/or cessation of bleeding after administration of VK is diagnostic.[44]

Diagnosis of VKDB is excluded, if the bleeding infant has a normal PT for age.

Since PT is prolonged, coagulopathies secondary to impaired production of procoagulant factors, due to hepatobiliary diseases must be excluded as L-VKDB may be the only initial manifestation in such cases. Children with hepatocellular dysfunction may have deficiencies of VK-independent factors also, for example of fibrinogen. Second important differential which needs exclusion is consumption coagulopathy. Along with prolonged PT, disseminated intravascular coagulopathy also features reduced fibrinogen, antithrombin (AT) and platelet count. The hereditary deficiencies of coagulation factors (hemophilia group) are excluded as they only have a prolonged APTT. Rare Deficiency of factors V, VII, or X may need to be excluded by analysis of individual factors (e.g. isolated factor VII deficiency has a normal PTT) but this investigation would be required, only if VK administration does not correct the PT. In contrast to all other above mentioned conditions which require exclusion, clinical improvement and cessation of bleeding with normalization or significant shortening of prothrombin time, after VK administration is seen only in VKDB.

Differential Diagnosis

This entity has to be differentiated from *disseminated intravascular coagulopathy*, resulting in consumption of coagulation factors and hence bleeding. Affected babies are often sick looking with clinical course characterized by infection, asphyxia, hypoxia, acidosis and shock. A normal platelet count and fibrinogen level would favor the diagnosis of VKDB, whereas presence of d-dimer and FDP would indicate DIC.

Clinical pattern similar to VKDB may also result from hereditary deficiency of clotting factors. Only 5–35% of cases with factor VIII and IX deficiency become clinically apparent in newborn period and only PTTK is prolonged in these deficiencies. In congenital deficiency of factor VII only PT is prolonged. Correction of congenital deficiencies of coagulation factors requires fresh frozen plasma or specific factor replacement.

THERAPY

Rapid and effective therapy is indispensable as VKDB carries a high risk of bleeding into central nervous system. VK should be administered either intravenously or subcutaneously (Dose 1–5 mg), to any bleeding infant suspected of having VKDB, even before laboratory confirmation of the diagnosis. Intramuscular injection should be avoided, since it may cause serious intramuscular bleeding. Intravenous VK should be given slowly because of the small theoretical risk of anaphylaxis.

Although the effect of parenteral VK is rapid, in very severe bleeding additional therapy needs to be given in the form of FFP and prothrombin complex concentrate.

As per British Committee for Standards in Hematology guidelines (BCSH) in cases of severe and life-threatening bleeding, FFP 10–20 mL/kg is indicated.

Prothrombin complex concentrate (PCC), should be considered for severe VKDB because of rapid reversibility of the abnormal coagulopathy, but currently there are not sufficient data-guiding dosage in this situation. At present, availability of these agents are only restricted to large pediatric centers and are thus not available to most pediatricians.[45]

Packed cell transfusion might be required following massive blood loss. Supportive care is given as for any other cause of bleeding.

Prevention

Intramuscular VK is administered for prophylaxis against vitamin K deficiency bleeding as far as prevention of VKDB in the first week is concerned[1,45] oral administration has also been found to be effective. Intramuscular VK administration as practiced in USA and Sweden had almost completely eliminated VKDB including the late onset type.[46,47] Since 1961, AAP recommends neonatal VK for prevention of VKDB.[16] National neonatology forum (NNF) of India recommends IM VK administration to every neonate at birth, in dose of 1 mg to term and 0.5 mg to preterm infants to prevent VKDB.

The mean plasma levels of vitamin K at 4 hours after IM VK (1 mg) is 20,000 times greater than age dependent normal levels.[8,48] After 2 weeks, VK levels are still 4 times, and by 4 weeks of life it is approximately 1.5 times the normal level in breastfed infants given no prophylaxis.[2] These sustained high levels of VK in the blood explain the longer protection conferred by IM VK as compared to that from single oral prophylaxis. High blood levels of VK following IM administration are reflected in the liver stores of VK. Neonates store VK in the form of VK1 up to second week of life, then starts accumulating VK2 in liver, whereas VK2 is the main storage form for adults. At birth, VK1 concentration in the liver is 1 ng/g which is about one fifth of adult levels and adult storage concentrations are reached after one month of life. Liver concentrations remain a thousand times higher for many days, following IM VK, than in infants not given VK prophylaxis.[49] The risk of exposing the blood and the liver to such high concentrations of VK is still unidentified.

Following a report in 1992, on possible and biologically plausible association of IM VK administration and risk of cancer in later childhood,[3] led many countries to change over to oral prophylaxis. A single oral prophylactic dose of 1 mg VK at birth leads to substantial rise in plasma levels of VK[50] and thus protects newborns against the classical form of VKDB.[28] Oral VK has short biological half-life, therefore in a normal breastfed infant given 1 mg oral VK, the levels of VK start declining very rapidly and by 2 weeks of life VK levels reaches to approximately 0.8 ng/mL, and then subsequently fall to unsupplemented levels.[51] Therefore, VKDB may occur in the most at risk babies following oral prophylaxis, if interval between oral VK doses is too long, which may enlighten the recurrence of late VKDB after VK prophylaxis was changed from intramuscular to three oral vitamin K (1 mg) doses.

There were different strategies for oral prophylaxis followed in various countries—1 mg dose × 3 (during neonatal period), 2 mg dose × 3, 1 mg in neonatal period followed by 25 μg daily oral dose to all breastfed babies till 13 weeks or 2 mg dose × 2 of mixed micellar preparation. Surveillance data on these forms of prophylaxis reveal that three oral doses of 1 mg dose is less effective than IM prophylaxis. Daily low dose oral administration following initial oral dose of 1mg is probably as effective as intramuscular prophylaxis. Using three 2 mg oral dose also did not offer complete protection against L-VKDB.[26,30,31] Due to failure of oral vitamin K in preventing L-VKDB, Australia subsequently reverted back to IM prophylaxis. In Sweden and Germany, fat-soluble oral VK was replaced by a new water-soluble mixed micellar analog of VK1. This preparation is better absorbed, even in presence of cholestasis.[26] This regimen is suitable for prophylaxis against VKDB, however, use of this preparation has also not completely eliminated L-VKDB, in infants with cholestatic disease.[30,31]

RISKS AND DISADVANTAGES OF DIFFERENT FORMS OF VK PROPHYLAXIS

The main disadvantages of oral VK prophylaxis are the erratic intake, poor absorption in unsuspected cholestasis and liver disease and short duration of action of each dose. Wide variation in plasma VK levels are seen after oral prophylaxis.[44] Thus one dose of oral VK does not appear to provide protection to all babies against late VKDB.[27,40,52]

The main disadvantages of IM VK prophylaxis are poor acceptance by parents, and relatively high cost and local trauma.[39] After IM-VK, rare complications such as injury to vessels and nerves, abscesses, osteomyelitis, and massive hemorrhage in infants with bleeding disorders have been reported.[2] There is a likelihood of potential unfavorable effect of extremely high blood levels of VK, on other VK dependent proteins and organs.[49]

Intramuscular Vitamin K and the Risk of Cancer in Childhood

Theoretical Background

VK-dependent Gla proteins act as ligands for receptor tyrosine kinases, establishing the role of VK in cell growth and transformation.[53] In animals, high concentrations of VK1 have been shown to increase sister chromatid exchange in lymphocyte suspensions and increase other forms of mutagenic activity. It has been postulated that the low levels of VK normally found in the fetus and neonate might be protective against potentially toxic and carcinogenic metabolites.[54]

From various epidemiological data, Golding et al. in 1992 suggested the possible association between IM VK and subsequent childhood cancer. The risk may be doubled by IM VK, but not with oral VK prophylaxis. This prompted many further studies to look for the possible link.

Cornelissen et al.[55] found that IM administration of 1 mg VK1 to six neonates did not lead to any increase in sister chromatid exchange or to chromosome aberrations.

At present, there is no convincing experimental evidence to suggest that VK is carcinogenic in humans. The attributable risk to the use of VK is not large but the possibility of some risk cannot be completely ruled out. "The risk, if any, attributable to the use of VK cannot be large... the possibility that there is some risk cannot be excluded".

CONCLUSION

Vitamin K deficiency bleeding (VKDB) is defined as bleeding due to insufficient activity of vitamin K (VK) dependent coagulation factors (II, VII, IX, X), which is correctable by VK replacement. Prolonged prothrombin time (PT) along with a normal fibrinogen level and platelet counts in a bleeding infant is almost diagnostic of VKDB; and rapid correction of the PT and/or cessation of bleeding after vitamin K administration further confirm the diagnosis. VKDB can be classified by age of onset into early (<24 hours), classic (days 1–7) and late (>1 week), and by etiology into idiopathic and secondary forms. Secondary VKDB has risk factors other than breastfeeding such as poor intake or poor absorption of VK and underlying hepatobiliary diseases. Common sites of bleeding for all the forms of VKDB are umbilical, gastrointestinal, nose, skin prick, circumcision and intracranial. Life-threatening and intracranial bleeding occur more commonly in early and late forms. Both oral and intramuscular (IM) VK (one dose of 1 mg) can effectively protects against classical VKDB, but intramuscular VK confers better protection against late onset VKDB, as it acts as depot for slow release of VK, for sustained levels of VK. The efficacy of oral prophylaxis can be augmented with use of triple rather than single dose, by using doses of 2 mg vitamin K rather than 1 mg and repeating the doses daily or weekly. In fact, repeated prophylaxis has efficacy equivalent to IM VK. Intramuscular VK has been implicated in leukemias, evidence for which are still inconclusive. Despite that, it is of utmost importance to provide prophylaxis as VKDB is a rare, but serious bleeding disorder with very high incidence of intracranial bleeding leading to fatal complications or long-term morbidity can be prevented by either one IM or multiple oral VK doses.

KEY MESSAGE

Vitamin K deficiency bleeding is a preventable entity, seen more commonly in exclusively breastfed infants, who have not received VK prophylaxis at birth. Bleeding in these cases can be serious and life-threatening. Early recognition of warning bleeds, instant diagnosis and treatment can help prevent serious bleeding and associated morbidity and mortality. VKDB can be the first symptom of underlying liver disease. This can be prevented or at least risk is minimized if prophylaxis recommendations are followed—single dose of intramuscular VK or oral VK regimens. In a bleeding infant, an evidently prolonged PT, normal fibrinogen levels and platelet count are highly suggestive of VKDB. Correction of these values (within 30–120 minutes) and/or cessation of bleeding after administration of VK is diagnostic.

REFERENCES

1. Sutor AH, Von Kries R, Marlies Conelissen EA, McNinch AW, Andrew M. Vitamin K deficiency bleeding (VKDB) in infancy. Thrombo Haemost. 1999;81:456-61.
2. Sutor AH. Vitamin K deficiency bleeding in infants and children. A status report. In: Sutor AH, Hathaway WE (Eds). Vitamin K in Infancy. Stuttgart, New York: Schattauer. 1995.pp.3-18.
3. Golding J, Greenwood R, Birmingham K, Mott M. Childhood cancer, intramuscular vitamin K, and pethidine given during labour. BMJ. 1992;305:341-6.
4. Passmore SJ, Draper G, Brownbill P, Kroll M. Case-control studies of relation between childhood cancer and neonatal vitamin K administration. Brit Med J. 1998;316:178-84.
5. Townsend CW. The haemorrhagic disease of newborn. Arch Paediatr. 1894. pp. 1747-52.
6. Narang A. Hemorrhagic disease of newborn. Indian Pediatr. 1989;26:523-4.
7. Von Kries R, Hanawa Y. Neonatal vitamin K prophylaxis. Thrombo Haemost. 1993 69:293-5.
8. Shearer M. Vitamin K metabolism and nutriture. Blood Reviews. 1992;6:92-104.
9. Cornelissen EAM, Kollée LAA, van Lith TGPJ, Motohara K, Monnens LAH. Evaluation of a daily dose of 25 mg Vitamin K 1 to prevent vitamin K deficiency in breast-fed infants. J Pediatr Gastroenterol Nutr. 1993;16:301-5.
10. Widdershoven J, Lambert W, Motohara K, et al. Plasma concentrations of vitamin K and PIVKA-II in bottle-fed and breast-fed infants with and without vitamin K prophylaxis at birth. Eur J Pediatr. 1988;19:354-7.
11. Lehmann J. Vitamin K as a prophylactic in 13,000 babies. Lancet. 1944;i:493-4 (see also i:506-8 and ii:737-8).
12. Dunham EC. Premature infants: a manual for physicians. Washington: Federal Security Agency. Children's Bureau Publication. 1948. p. 325.
13. Gasser C. Die hämolytische Frügeburtenamie mit spontaner Innerkörperbildung: Ein neues Syndrom, beobachten an 14 Fällen. Helvet Paediatr Acta. 1953;8:491-528.
14. Allison AC. Danger of vitamin K to newborn. [Letter] Lancet. 1955;i:669 (see also 819).
15. Mayer TC, Angus J. The effect of large doses of 'Synkavit' in the newborn. Arch Dis Child. 1956 31:212-5.
16. American Academy of Pediatrics. Committee on Nutrition. Vitamin K compounds and the water soluble analogues. Pediatrics. 1961;28:501-7.
17. McNinch AW, L'Orme R, Tripp JH. Haemorrhagic disease of the newborn returns. Lancet. 1983;i:1089-90.
18. Marwaha RK, Kumar A, Garewal G, Marwaha N, Walia BNS. Vitamin K deficiency related bleeding manifestations in older neonates and infants. Indian Pediatrics. 1987;24:307-11.
19. Merchant RH, Divekar RM. Late hemorrhagic disease with intracranial hemorrhage. Indian Pediatr. 1988;25:381-4.
20. Merchant RH, Divekar R, Shah MD. Late hemorrhagic disease of infancy. Indian Pediatr. 1989;26:553-8.
21. Chandra J, Naithani R. Chhetri A, Singh V, Sharma S. Serious and life threatening bleeding in late vitamin K deficiency. Annals of Tropical Peadiatrics. 2007;27:241-2.
22. Choo KE, Tan KK, Chuah SP, et al. Hemorrhagic disease in newborn and infants: a study of hospitalized children in Kelantan, Malayasia. Ann Trop Pediatr. 1994;15:231-7.
23. Puckett RM, Offringa M. Prophylactic vitamin K for vitamin K deficiency bleeding in neonates (Chochrane review). In: The Chochrane Library. Chichester, UK: John Wiley And Sons, Ltd. 2004;3.
24. American Academy of Pediatrics Committee on fetus and Newborn: Controversies concerning vitamin K and the newborn. J Pediatr. 2003;112:191-2.
25. von Kries R, Hachmeister A, Göbel U. Oral mixed micellar vitamin K for prevention of late vitamin K deficiency bleeding. Arch Dis Child Fetal Neonatal Ed. 2003;88:F109-F112.
26. Cornelissen M, Von Kries R, Loughnan P, Schubiger G. Prevention of vitamin K deficiency bleeding: Efficacy of

different multiple oral dose schedules of vitamin K. Eur J of Pediatr. 1997;156:126-30.

27. Sutor AH, Dagres N, Niederhoff H. Late form of vitamin K deficiency bleeding in Germany. Klin Pädiatr. 1995;207:89-97.
28. Von Kries R, Funda J, Shearer M, Göbel U. Late hemorrhagic disease of newborn: a case with increased vitamin K requirement. Acta Paediatr. 1992;81:728-30.
29. D'Souza IE, Subba Rao SD. Indian Pediatrics. 2003;40:226-9.
30. Von Kries R, Hachmeister A, Gobel U. Can 3 oral 2 mg doses of vitamin K effectively prevent late vitamin K deficiency in bleeding? Eur J Pediatr. 1999;158[Suppl 3(6)]:S183-6.
31. Schubiger G, Stocker C, Banziger O, Laubscher B, Zimmermann H. Oral vitamin K prophylaxis for newborns with a new mixed-micellar preparation of phylloquinone: 3 year experience in Switzerland. Eur J Pediatr. 1999;158:599-602.
32. Cornelissen EAM, Steegers-Theunissen R, Kollée LA, Eskes T, Vogels-Mentink G, Motohara K, De Abreu R, Monnens LA. Increased incidence of neonatal vitamin K deficiency resulting from maternal anticonvulsant therapy. Am J Obstet Gynecol. 1993;168:923-8.
33. Cornelissen EAM, Steegers-Theunissen R, Kollée LA, Eskes T, Motohara K, Monnens LA. Supplementation of vitamin K in pregnant women receiving anticonvulsant therapy prevents neonatal vitamin K deficiency. Am J Obstet Gynecol. 1993; 168:884-8.
34. Deblay MF, Vert P, Andre M, Marchal F. Transplacental vitamin K prevents haemorrhagic disease of infant of epileptic mother. Lancet. 1982;I:1242.
35. Mountain KR, Hirsh J, Gallus AS. Neonatal coagulation defect due to anticonvulsant drug treatment in pregnancy. Lancet. 1970;I:265-8.
36. Thorp JA, Parriot J, Ferrette-Smith D, Meyer BA, Cohen GR, Johnson J. Antepartum vitamin K and phenobarbital for preventing intraventricular hemorrhage in the premature newborn: a randomized, double blind, placebo-controlled study. Obstet Gynec. 1994;83:70-6.
37. Hey E. Effect of maternal anticonvulsant treatment on neonatal blood coagulation. Arch Dis Child (fetal and neonatal edition). 1999;81:F208-10.
38. Aleksey K, Renee CW, Mathew S, Gideon K. Antiepileptic drugs in pregnancy and hemorrhagic disease of the newborn 2010 Canadian Family Physician. Le Médecin de famille canadien. 2010;56:1291-2.
39. Von Kries R. Vitamin K prophylaxis—a useful public health measure? J Paediatric and Perinatal Epidemiology. 1992;6:7-13.
40. McNinch AW, Tripp JH. Haemorrhagic disease of the newborn in the British Isles: two year prospective study. Brit Med J. 1991;303:1105-9.
41. Sutherland JM, Glueck HI, Gleser G. Hemorrhagic disease of the newborn. Breast feeding as a necessary factor in the pathogenesis. Am J Dis Child. 1967;113:524-33.
42. Auerswald G, Sutor AH. Thirteen cases of Alpha-1-Antitrypsin deficiency presenting as a bleeding diathesis with intracranial hemorrhage in the newborn. In: Vitamin K in Infancy. Sutor AH, Hathaway WE (Eds). Stuttgart, New York: Schattauer. 1995. pp. 217-23.
43. Pooni PA, Singh D, Singh H, Jain BK. Intracranial Haemorrhage in Late Heamorrhagic Disease of newborn. Indian Pediatrics. 2003;40:243-8.
44. Sutor AH, Künzer W. Time interval between Vitamin K administration and effective hemostasis. In: Perinatal Thrombosis and Haemostasis. Suzuki S, Hathaway WmE, Bonnar J, Sutor AH (Eds). Berlin, Heidelberg, New York, London, Tokyo, Hong Kong: Springer. 1991. pp. 257-62.
45. British Committee for Standards in Haematology Transfusion guidelines for neonates and older children. B J Haematol. 2004(124);4:433-53.
46. Ekelund H. Vitamin K prophylaxis and vitamin K deficiency (VKD) bleeding in Sweden. In: Vitamin K in Infancy. Sutor AH, Hathaway WE (Eds). Stuttgart, New York: Schattauer. 1995. pp. 173-4.
47. Hathaway WE. Efficacy of vitamin K prophylaxis in the USA. In: Vitamin K in Infancy. Sutor AH, Hathaway WE (Eds). Stuttgart, New York: Schattauer. 1995. pp. 161-3.
48. McNinch AW, Upton C, Samuels M, Shearer MJ, McCarthy P, Tripp JH, Orme L'ER. Plasma concentrations after oral or intramuscular vitamin K1 in neonates. Arch Dis Child. 1985;60:814-8.
49. Shearer MJ. Chemistry, sources and metabolism of vitamin K with special reference to the newborn. In: Vitamin K in Infancy. Sutor AH, Hathaway WE (Eds). Stuttgart, New York: Schattauer. 1995. pp. 21-32.
50. McNinch AW, Upton C, Samuels M, Shearer MJ, McCarthy P, Tripp JH, Orme L'ER. Plasma concentrations after oral or intramuscular vitamin K1 in neonates. Arch Dis Child. 1985;60:814-8.
51. Cornelissen EAM, Kollée LA, de Abreu RA, Motohara K, Monnens LAH. Prevention of vitamin K deficiency in infancy by weekly administration of vitamin K. Acta Paediatr. 1993;82:656-9.
52. Von Kries R, Göbel U. Vitamin K prophylaxis and late hemorrhagic disease of the newborn. Acta Paediatr Scand. 1992;81:655-7.
53. Israels LG, Israels ED. Vitamin K deficiency in the fetus and newborn. Has nature made a mistake? In: Vitamin K in Infancy. Sutor AH, Hathaway WE (Eds). Stuttgart, New York: Schattauer. 1995. pp. 261-72.
54. Israels LG, Friesen E, Jansen AH, Israels ED. Vitamin K1 increases sister chromatid exchange in vitro in human leukocytes and in vivo in fetal sheep cells: a possible role for "vitamin K deficiency" in the fetus. Pediatric Research. 1987;22:405-8.
55. Cornelissen EAM, Smeets D, Merkx G, de Abreu RA, Kollee L, Monnens LAH. Analysis of chromosome aberrations and sister chromatid exchanges in peripheral blood lymphocytes of newborns after vitamin K prophylaxis at birth. Pediatr Res. 1991;30:550-3.

CHAPTER

20 Disseminated Intravascular Coagulation in the Neonatal Period

Anand Prakash, Shashidhar A

INTRODUCTION

Disseminated intravascular coagulation (DIC) can be defined as a systemic thrombohemorrhagic disorder seen in association with well-defined clinical situations and laboratory evidence of: (1) procoagulant activation, (2) fibrinolytic activation, (3) inhibitor consumption and (4) biochemical and clinical evidence of end-organ damage or failure.[1]

There is a lack of data in newborn population both nationally and internationally regarding the incidence, management and outcomes of neonatal DIC probably as a result of the complexity in establishing a concrete diagnosis without universally accepted clear criteria. However, older publications point toward a significant prevalence of DIC in neonates who die in the neonatal intensive care unit (NICU). Of all the DIC reported in children, half occurs during the neonatal period. Dairaku et al.[2] conducted 201 consecutive autopsies and documented the histopathological features of DIC as the presence of microthrombi in three or more organs in 24 of the neonates. However, only one of these cases was clinically suspected to suffer from DIC demonstrating its underestimation. Other studies suggest an even higher incidence of the condition: A report from Russia documented disseminated or local microthrombus formation in the majority of 120 deceased neonates in 1996.[3] Schmidt et al. found increased thrombin and plasmin generation in 57 of 100 neonates in the NICU.[4]

There is a paucity of Indian studies evaluating the incidence or the manifestations of this pertinent issue in this susceptible population.

ETIOLOGY

Neonates are innately predisposed to acquire DIC due to altered levels of coagulation and fibrinolytic proteins that differ markedly from those in adults.

The most common conditions that lead to DIC in the neonatal population are probably infection/sepsis and hypoxic-ischemia.

Sepsis

Sepsis is the most common cause of neonatal mortality; it is responsible for about 30–50% of the total neonatal deaths in developing countries.[5] It is estimated that up to 20% of neonates develop sepsis and approximately 1% die of sepsis-related causes. The incidence of neonatal sepsis according to the data from National Neonatal Perinatal Database (NNPD, 2002–2003) is 30 per 1,000 live births. Two different patterns of DIC syndrome in sepsis are described "decompensated" and "overcompensated".

Neonates with sepsis develop an acquired prothrombotic state due to increased consumption of already limited supplies of coagulation inhibitors. El Beshlawy et al. compared 30 term newborns suffering from sepsis with 30 age-matched controls and documented a significant decrease in antithrombin (AT), protein C, and protein S in all cases; one-third of the sepsis patients developed DIC and died.[6] The plasma activity of the fibrinolysis inhibitor plasminogen activator inhibitor-1 (PAI-1) is increased in sepsis, reducing the endogenous fibrinolytic potential.[7] Persistent consumption of coagulation factors and platelets resulting in microcirculatory thrombosis with impaired perfusion is a likely contributor to sepsis-induced multiorgan dysfunction.

Hypoxic Ischemia

As per NNPD (2002–2003) data, asphyxia was responsible for 28.8% of all neonatal deaths and reported perinatal asphyxia to be the most common cause of still-births, accounting for 45.1%.

The multiorgan dysfunction such as DIC is responsible for many of these fatalities and long-term morbidities associated with the condition. There is activation of the coagulation system at the time of delivery with increased fibrinolytic activity, which further is aggravated by marked hemostatic alterations that occur due to the endothelial injury, release of tissue thromboplastin and acidosis in hypoxic ischemia.

Levels of thrombin-antithrombin complex, D-dimer and fibrin degradation products (FDPs) are elevated in association to a marked decrease in the levels of AT, protein C and protein S, thrombocytopenia, prolonged prothrombin time and partial thromboplastin time (PTT) forms a fertile ground for DIC in these newborns.[8,9]

Other reported causes of DIC include:

- *Gastrointestinal*: Necrotizing enterocolitis
- *Vascular*: Giant hemangioma (Kasabach-Merritt syndrome), hemangiomatosis
- *Respiratory*: Respiratory distress syndrome, meconium or amniotic fluid aspiration
- *Obstetric complications*: Placental abruption, severe pre-eclampsia and dead twin
- *Liver dysfunction*: Hepatitis
- *Hematologic*: Homozygous protein C or protein S deficiency, erythroblastosis fetalis
- Hypothermia
- Shock of any etiology
- Birth trauma
- TORCH (Toxoplasmosis/*Toxoplasma gondii*, Other infections, Rubella, Cytomegalovirus, Herpes simplex virus-2 or neonatal herpes simplex) and viral infections
- *Metabolic*: Neonatal hemochromatosis, galactosemia and acidosis
- *Malignancy*: Congenital mesoblastic nephroma, sacrococcygeal teratoma, congenital neuroblastoma and hamartoma
- Surgical intervention.

PATHOGENESIS/PATHOPHYSIOLOGY

Although the common predisposing conditions for DIC are not the same in adults and children, the pathophysiology remains the same with an overwhelmed hemostatic system that is unable to cope with continuous thrombin activation and the consumption of coagulation factors and platelets. The underlying disease process often results in endothelial damage, which causes the release of cytokines such as interleukins-1, 6, and 8, platelet activating factor and tumor necrosis factor. Tissue factor activity is increased in response to certain cytokines. Through the normal mechanisms of the coagulation pathway, this increased activity favors the overproduction of thrombin and a decreased generation of natural anticoagulants including AT, protein C, and tissue factor pathway inhibitor, and consequently to extensive intravascular deposition of fibrin.

The simultaneous inhibition of the fibrinolytic pathway due to increased plasma concentration of PAI-1 prevents an adequate removal of fibrin from small vessels resulting in extensive thrombosis and organ failure. The process also leads to consumption of platelets and coagulation factors, which may cause severe hemorrhage. Increased sensitivity of newborns to all factors initiating DIC is associated with certain unique physiological characteristics of the hemostatic system in newborns. The mononuclear phagocytes of a neonate have a lower ability to clean the blood from clotting products, neonates have an immature liver and are unable to provide adequate compensatory synthesis of pro- and anticoagulants.

In neonates, AT levels are within the concentration range at which spontaneous thromboses could occur in adults. Protein C and protein S are reduced at birth to 30% of adult plasma concentrations and remain decreased during the 1st week of life. In addition, differences in plasma concentrations of fibrinolytic proteins may also contribute to predisposition for DIC.[10] At birth, newborn plasminogen levels are 58% of adult concentrations while plasma concentrations of PAI-1 and TPA are approximately twice adult concentrations and decrease to adult plasma concentration values by day 5 of life.[10] Impaired fibrin degradation due to high circulating levels of PAI-1 contributes to enhanced intravascular fibrin deposition. These microvascular thrombi in various organs can contribute to sequelae and diminished quality of life. For these reason, effective therapy for DIC would have tremendous impact.

CLINICAL PRESENTATION

Most of these infants are already sick, probably requiring ventilatory support and possibly cardiovascular support as well. These affected infants usually present with bleeding complications. An infant who continues to bleed after laboratory draws or venipuncture should raise suspicion. Hemorrhage can range from oozing of an umbilical line or wound to petechiae, purpura, ecchymoses, or hematomas to bleeding in the mouth, nose, or orogastric or endotracheal tube indicating a major gastrointestinal or pulmonary bleed, and in severe cases an intracranial bleed can be devastating.

Ischemic damage related to thrombosis could manifest as cyanosis, as well as specific organ failure, depending on the site of the clot **(Fig. 20.1)**.

DIAGNOSIS

Clinical criteria for diagnosis of DIC syndrome include the severity of the predisposing disease of the newborn at risk (i.e. situational assessment), accompanied by multiple organ dysfunction—the combination of disorders of the central nervous system, lungs, kidneys, liver, hemodynamic status and often thrombosis and hemorrhage.

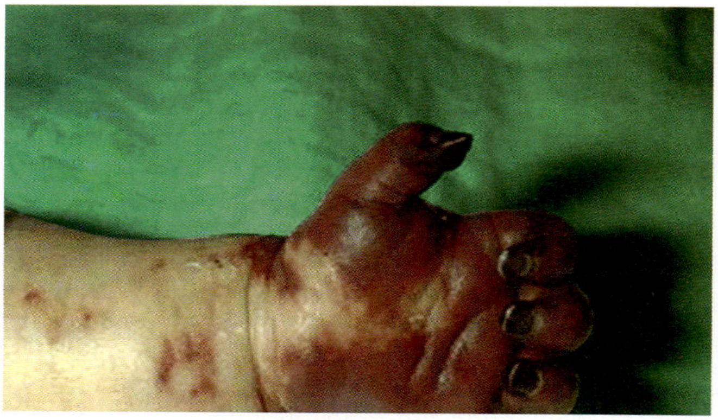

Figure 20.1 Hand with gangrene

Hemostasiological criteria of DIC syndrome include hypercoagulation and hypocoagulation shifts of activated partial thromboplastin time (aPTT), thromboplastin time (PT), consumption of procoagulants, antithrombin III, high-molecular-weight kininogen, plasminogen, FDP increasing and thrombocytopenia with failure of the aggregation platelet activity.[11]

The International Society on Thrombosis and Haemostasis (ISTH) DIC scoring system has not yet been validated in children or neonates born term and preterm. A DIC scoring system for very low-birth-weight preterms has been proposed.[12] Similar to the ISTH DIC score, this score includes platelet count, fibrinogen levels and fibrinogen degradation products. It presumes an underlying condition triggering DIC, bleeding symptoms, acidosis, hypotension, and tissue hypoxia, reflecting an impaired microcirculation. However, this score which was developed retrospectively and is currently not in widespread clinical use as its reliability and validity have not been proven. The correlation between abnormal laboratory parameters and the clinical picture remains indistinct and the relationship with mortality and morbidity uncertain. A study done in pediatric intensive care unit (PICU) patients showed that sequential measurement of parameters may be more beneficial and fibrinogen is relatively an excludable parameter.[13]

Platelets

Progressive thrombocytopenia is probably the most common sign a newborn with DIC presents with. A fall in platelet count below 1.5 lakh/mm^3 has a sensitivity of 39%, a specificity of 88% and positive and negative predictive values of 81% and 54%, respectively, indicating accelerated generation of thrombi as well as plasmin in term and preterm newborns, as revealed by increase in thrombin-antithrombin III (TAT) complexes and the plasmin-derived fibrinopeptide B beta 1–42.[4] However, this activation of the neonatal coagulation system does not necessarily mean a diagnosis of DIC.

Coagulation Tests

The PT and international normalized ratio (INR) in critically ill newborns are frequently abnormal due to the relative neonatal vitamin K deficiency. An INR more than 1.5 has a sensitivity of 11% and a specificity of 95% to detect increased thrombin and plasmin generation in sick infants.[14]

The APTT within the age-corrected normal (higher in newborns) range rules out impaired plasma coagulation with a high probability.

The APTT is prolonged if inhibitors are present that block the activity of certain coagulation factors (e.g. factor VIII) or if the patient is treated with new anticoagulants [hirudin, other FXa or thrombin inhibitors, activated protein C (APC)].

Fibrinogen

Together with thrombocytopenia, a low fibrinogen level can indicate DIC. However, plasma fibrinogen levels less than 1.5 g/L have a sensitivity of 12% and a specificity of 98% to detect increased thrombin and plasmin generation in sick newborn infants.[14] The fibrinogen level should always be interpreted in relation to levels of other acute-phase proteins (e.g. C-reactive protein), whose elevation indicate sepsis or an inflammatory process.

D-dimers

Elevated plasma levels of D-dimers are caused by the breakdown of fibrin by plasmin and are a sign of activation of the hemostatic and the fibrinolytic systems. However, the coagulation system is also activated in infections, malignancies and hypoxia; hence D-dimer values are elevated in these situations as well. Therefore, whereas elevation of D-dimers is nonspecific, this parameter is useful (and highly sensitive and specific) to rule out thromboembolic events: A negative D-dimer result fairly rules out DIC.

Protein C and Antithrombin

A decrease in plasma concentrations of the coagulation inhibitors protein C and AT have been shown to be moderately sensitive markers for DIC in adults. In neonates, sepsis and DIC are almost always associated with reduced protein C and AT levels.[7] In a study from India, low protein C plasma levels have been described as a marker of poor prognosis in preterm infants with sepsis.[15]

Other Investigations

The detection of thrombin generation by measuring prothrombin fragment 1 and 2, TAT, or the downstream products generated by thrombin formation (such as fibrinopeptide A and soluble fibrin) can reveal hidden DIC. But these are not available commercially yet and restricted blood and plasma volumes available for diagnostic investigations further limit the use of multiple assays in neonates, especially preterm.

Differential Diagnosis

The differential diagnosis for DIC should include hemorrhagic disease of the newborn severe liver disease and rarely Kasabach-Merritt syndrome. A careful history of the delivery can uncover the possibility of vitamin K deficiency related to not receiving the prophylactic dose at birth. The liver is the site of synthesis of all clotting factors except factor VIII; therefore in liver disease there will be prolonged values due to a lack of factor production. Transfusing the patient with fresh frozen plasma (FFP) and monitoring the PT and PTT can exclude liver disease. The values will normalize somewhat, then gradually become prolonged as the body uses the factors provided by the transfusion unlike in DIC. In a clinically well neonate or infant, where there is no evidence of sepsis or asphyxia, but hematological parameters suggest DIC, a careful search for vascular malformations is necessary. If there is no evident skin discoloration or edema on physical examination, a hidden malformation either in the cranium or the abdomen should be evaluated by imaging.

MANAGEMENT

The cornerstone of treatment of DIC in all patients remains the successful treatment of the underlying disease. Hence, early antibiotic therapy and identification and control of the source of disease in cases of necrotizing enterocolitis, sepsis, septic shock and improvement in oxygen delivery in the microcirculation are the mainstay. Treatment of the secondary hemostatic disorder may be helpful, but has to be considered as an adjuvant therapy and is of limited benefit.

These patients will need careful maintenance of their respiratory and cardiovascular systems, often requiring ventilator assistance and pressor support. Diligent monitoring of blood gases will dictate changes to correct hypoxia, hypercapnia and acidosis. Vital signs and physical assessment determine the need for vasopressor infusions and medications. Fluid and electrolyte balance and nutritional support as tolerated are important as always in this population.

Avoid any intramuscular injections or invasive procedures that may cause trauma or bleeding. Limit venipuncture and place a central line to avoid heelsticks for the frequent examination of laboratory values such as complete blood counts and coagulation studies.

However, in patients with overt DIC, coagulopathy can be self-sustaining, and hence persist even after the initial insult to the endothelium is eliminated and as such require specific therapy.

Specific treatment directed toward either the coagulation or fibrinolytic derangement has occasionally been attempted.

Clinically practical goals when treating newborns that are bleeding from DIC are to maintain the platelet count above 50×10^9/L, fibrinogen concentrations above 1.0 g/L, and PT and APTT values near normal values for age.

Fresh Frozen Plasma

Although there is no evidence for the benefit of FFP therapy to prevent bleeding in DIC, many guidelines and protocols of several working groups recommend the use of FFP in DIC to limit hemorrhage. As FFP may be beneficial in deficiencies of all clotting factors and inhibitors of coagulation in DIC, it is frequently administered as an empirical therapy. A small controlled study in 33 neonates with DIC[16] showed no difference in resolution of DIC or survival, regardless of whether DIC was treated with FFP, exchange transfusion, or without any specific coagulation management.

There is also no evidence for prophylactic use of FFP in DIC in the absence of bleeding or for impending invasive procedures. Furthermore, prophylactic use of FFP in preterm infants who are at high risk of hemorrhagic complications, especially intracranial hemorrhage, has not produced benefit. A meta-analysis of clinical studies in preterm infants, in whom FFP was administered routinely at birth, shows no advantage in survival or long-term outcome.[17]

Many critically ill neonates may not tolerate the volume of FFP required for ongoing replacement. In recent years, although recombinant and highly purified, viral-inactivated, plasma-derived proteins for more specific replacement therapy (factor XIII, factor XI, protein C and fibrinogen) are available, FFP remains the product of choice to replace factors V, XI, protein S and plasminogen. Most neonatologists would consider FFP in preterm neonates with extremely deranged coagulation tests even in the absence of acute hemorrhage, due to the high risk of bleeding in this population.

Heparin

In a case series on 10 newborns with DIC, after initial failure of isolated heparin therapy, fast improvement of DIC was observed after normalization of AT plasma levels, which can be depleted in advanced DIC by consumption.[18] In another old study of newborns, with DIC and respiratory distress syndrome, significantly shorter ventilation periods and a trend toward faster normalization of the coagulation parameters in the heparin-treated group was reported.[19] Larger randomized controlled studies on the use of heparin in DIC are unavailable even in adult and pediatric patients. Hence, due to an increased risk of bleeding complications in the newborn (especially preterm), the use of heparin in a neonate is currently restricted to those with clinically obvious thromboembolic events.

Antithrombin

Increased consumption or loss of AT results in reduced AT plasma levels, which by itself is a strong predictor of a severe course of disease. Providing the natural anticoagulant AT to interrupt the complex cycle of DIC and using the anti-inflammatory properties of AT that are independent from its anticoagulant characteristics has been tried.

Few adult studies have shown marginal benefit effect in terms of improvement of a DIC score, shortening of the duration of DIC, and improvement in organ function and it is recommended by some societies.

In neonates, AT replacement was used in a randomized trial of 122 infants with respiratory distress syndrome showing adverse effects of AT on ventilator parameters.[20] However, patients in this study were also exposed to a low dose of heparin (20 IU/kg/day) to keep arterial catheters patent. In a retrospective study on the use of AT in pediatric patients of different age groups with sepsis-associated DIC, administration of AT resulted in a normalization of age-related AT plasma activity levels and platelet counts as well as termination of DIC without severe adverse effects even in patients with very high AT plasma activity levels.[21] Combined therapy with AT and recombinant-tissue plasminogen activator (r-tPA) improved survival, degree of macroscopic and microscopic organ involvement and hematocrit in newborn piglet model of endotoxin-induced DIC compared with supportive care alone.[22]

Thus, the use of AT in neonates with DIC cannot be recommended in the absence of data from large randomized trials.

Human Protein C

Among the plasma proteins that have been evaluated in animal models and early clinical trials, protein C (PC) has emerged as the most promising inhibitor of coagulation as well as exaggerated inflammation and apoptosis triggered by a systemic inflammatory host response. Low plasma protein C activity levels act as an independent risk factor for death in low-birth-weight neonates[15] a finding that was described in adults.

Although large placebo-controlled trials on the use of human protein C (HPC) are lacking in adults and neonates, the positive effect of HPC on sepsis-induced coagulation disturbances in children is discussed in the surviving sepsis campaign guidelines.

For the want of further evidence, protein C substitution should be restricted to those patients with clinical symptoms of an acute protein C deficiency (e.g. purpura fulminans) **(Fig. 20.2)**.

Activated Protein C

Some case reports have described the use of activated protein C in neonates with sepsis and DIC.[23] However, there is a specific recommendation not to use recombinant human activated protein C in children and neonates because of an increased rate of intraventricular hemorrhage.

Double Volume Exchange Transfusion

In the most severe cases of DIC particularly associated with sepsis, a double volume exchange transfusion (DVET) may be useful.[8] Although this is a rare treatment, probably due to the associated complications and no definitive data, there are several benefits like replacement of clotting factors at adult content levels and removal of FDPs. The adult hemoglobin can improve oxygen delivery, and fluid overload from multiple transfusions can be avoided.

Thrombomodulin

Thrombomodulin (TM) is a glycoprotein expressed on vascular endothelial cells which binds to thrombin that has been produced as a result of intravascular hypercoagulation and stimulates the activation of protein C by thrombin. The resulting activated protein C uses protein S as a cofactor to inactivate factors Va and VIIIa. TM is also known to directly suppress inflammatory reactions by inhibiting the production of inflammatory cytokines such as interleukin-1β. Recombinant soluble human thrombomodulin-alpha (TM-α) is the first anticoagulant drug in the world shown to be superior to heparin in a randomized clinical trial of adult DIC patients with infection or hematological malignancy and in 60 Japanese newborns have shown high improvement rate and survival rate of DIC.[24] However, currently the drug is not available for commercial use in India.

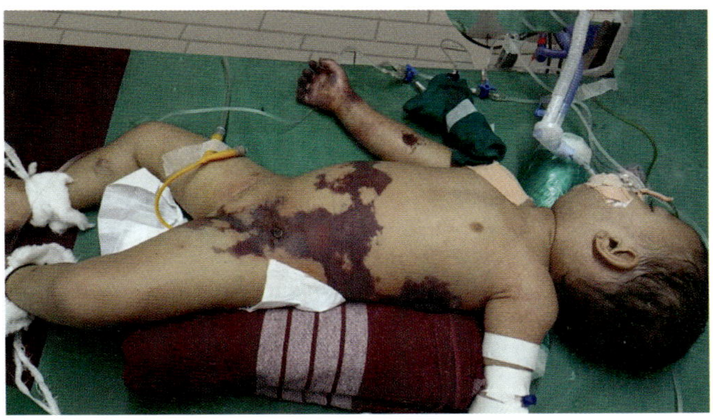

Figure 20.2 Suspected purpura fulminans

Recombinant Factor VIIa

In background of an injured endothelium that exposes tissue factor, enhanced fibrin deposition leads to widespread microvascular thrombosis and result in tissue necrosis. Currently, there is also evidence that recombinant factor VIIa (rFVIIa) binds to the endothelial protein C receptor, thus reducing binding and activity of protein C on the microcirculation. However, in the clinical scenario of life-threatening hemorrhage the use of rFVIIa has been described with varying success in achieving hemostasis.[25] Thus the use of rFVIIa is currently as a rescue in acutely life-threatening hemorrhage in which conventional measures have been unsuccessful.

Recombinant Tissue Plasminogen Activator

Recombinant tissue plasminogen activator has been used in children with DIC and purpura fulminans; however, a high rate of intracerebral hemorrhage limits its use in neonates to life-threatening local thromboembolic events.[26] A recommendation for the use of r-tPA in DIC does not exist presently.

OUTCOMES/PROGNOSTIC FACTORS

As with the treatment of DIC, the prognosis and outcomes are essentially dependent on the primary disease process. Historically, most infants with DIC have died. Avery and coworkers[27] report that the underlying disease and the ischemic damage caused by the cardiovascular collapse and DIC result in high mortality rates. In infants with DIC who experience severe bleeding, mortality rates are reported to 60–80%.[28] However, literature now states that the majority of infants with DIC survive due to the advances in neonatal medicine and its supportive care.[29,30]

CONCLUSION

Disseminated intravascular coagulation in the newborn though highly frequent, is an underdiagnosed entity that can significantly increase the mortality of the underlying pathology. Reversal of the underlying condition and supporting adequate blood flow and oxygen delivery remain the focus of therapy. Early recognition and intervention by the caregivers in the NICU can dramatically enhance the overall survival of these critically ill infants.

KEY POINTS

- Neonates are inherently susceptible to DIC.
- Screen for DIC in any sick newborn irrespective of underlying etiology.
- Supportive management and blood component therapy go hand in hand with the specific treatment of underlying disorder.

REFERENCES

1. Bick RL. Disseminated intravascular coagulation: a review of etiology, pathophysiology, diagnosis, and management: guidelines for care. Clin Appl Thromb Hemost. 2002;8(1):1-31.
2. Dairaku M, Sueishi K, Tanaka K. Disseminated intravascular coagulation in newborn infants. Prevalence in autopsies and significance as a cause of death. Pathol Res Pract. 1982;174(1-2):106-15.
3. Arkhangel' skiĭ AV, Masliakova GN. [Frequency and morphology of DIC-syndrome in children in early neonatal period]. Arkh Patol. 1996;58(5):61-3.
4. Schmidt B, Vegh P, Johnston M, Andrew M, Weitz J. Do coagulation screening tests detect increased generation of thrombin and plasmin in sick newborn infants? Thromb Haemost. 1993;69(5):418-21.
5. Bang AT, Bang RA, Baitule SB, Reddy MH, Deshmukh MD. Effect of home-based neonatal care and management of sepsis on neonatal mortality: field trial in rural India. Lancet. 1999;354(9194):1955-61.
6. El Beshlawy A, Alaraby I, Abou Hussein H, Abou-Elew HH, Mohamed Abdel Kader MS. Study of protein C, protein S, and antithrombin III in newborns with sepsis. Pediatr Crit Care Med. 2010;11(1):52-9.
7. Watanabe R, Wada H, Miura Y, Murata Y, Watanabe Y, Sakakura M, et al. Plasma levels of total plasminogen activator inhibitor-I (PAI-I) and tPA/PAI-1 complex in patients with disseminated intravascular coagulation and thrombotic thrombocytopenic purpura. Clin Appl Thromb Hemost. 2001;7(3):229-33.
8. Suzuki S, Morishita S. Hypercoagulability and DIC in high-risk infants. Semin Thromb Hemost. 1998;24(5):463-6.
9. El Beshlawy A, Hussein HA, Abou-Elew HH, Abdel Kader MS. Study of protein C, protein S, and antithrombin III in hypoxic newborns. Pediatr Crit Care Med. 2004;5(2):163-6.
10. Edstrom C, Christensen RD, Andrew M. Developmental aspects of blood hemostasis and disorders of coagulation and fibrinolysis in the neonatal period. In: Christensen RD (Ed). Hematologic Problems of the Neonate. Philadelphia, PA: WB Saunders Company; 2000. pp. 239-71.
11. Ivanov D, Shabalov N, Petrenko Y, Shabalova N, Treskina NA. The specific characteristics of DIC syndrome vary with different clinical settings in the newborn. J Matern Fetal Neonatal Med. 2014;27(11):1088-92.
12. Shirahata A, Shirakawa Y, Murakami C. Diagnosis of DIC in very low birth weight infants. Semin Thromb Hemost. 1998;24(5):467-71.
13. Soundar EP, Jariwala P, Nguyen TC, Eldin KW, Teruya J. Evaluation of the International Society on Thrombosis and Haemostasis and institutional diagnostic criteria of disseminated intravascular coagulation in pediatric patients. Am J Clin Pathol. 2013;139(6):812-6.
14. Schmidt B, Vegh P, Johnston M, Andrew M, Weitz J. Do coagulation screening tests detect increased generation of thrombin and plasmin in sick newborn infants? Thromb Haemost. 1993;69(5):418-21.
15. Venkataseshan S, Dutta S, Ahluwalia J, Narang A. Low plasma protein C values predict mortality in low birth weight neonates with septicemia. Pediatr Infect Dis J. 2007;26(8):684-8.
16. Gross SJ, Filston HC, Anderson JC. Controlled study of treatment for disseminated intravascular coagulation in the neonate. J Pediatr. 1982;100(3):445-8.
17. Osborn DA, Evans N, Kluckow M. Clinical detection of low upper body blood flow in very premature infants using blood pressure, capillary refill time, and central-peripheral temperature difference. Arch Dis Child Fetal Neonatal Ed. 2004;89(2):F168-73.
18. von Kries R, Stannigel H, Göbel U. Anticoagulant therapy by continuous heparin-antithrombin III infusion in newborns with disseminated intravascular coagulation. Eur J Pediatr. 1985;144(2):191-4.
19. Göbel U, von Voss H, Jürgens H, Petrich C, Pothmann R, Sprock I, et al. Efficiency of heparin in the treatment of newborn infants with respiratory distress syndrome and disseminated intravascular coagulation. Eur J Pediatr. 1980;133(1):47-9.
20. Schmidt B, Gillie P, Mitchell L, Andrew M, Caco C, Roberts R. A placebo-controlled randomized trial of antithrombin therapy in neonatal respiratory distress syndrome. Am J Respir Crit Care Med. 1998;158(2):470-6.
21. Nowak-Göttl U, Groll A, Kreuz WD, Brand M, Breddin HK, von Loewenich V, et al. [Treatment of disseminated intravascular coagulation with antithrombin III concentrate in children with verified infection]. Klin Padiatr. 1992;204(3):134-40.
22. Davis-Jackson, Correa H, Horswell R, Sadowska-Krowicka H, McDonough K, Debata C, et al. Antithrombin III (AT) and recombinant tissue plasminogen activator (R-TPA) used singly and in combination versus supportive care for treatment of endotoxin-induced disseminated intravascular coagulation (DIC) in the neonatal pig. Thromb J. 2006;4:7.
23. Frommhold D, Birle A, Linderkamp O, Zilow E, Pöschl J. Drotrecogin alpha (activated) in neonatal septic shock. Scand J Infect Dis. 2005;37(4):306-8.
24. Shirahata A, Mimuro J, Takahashi H, Kitajima I, Tsuji H, Eguchi Y, et al. Recombinant soluble human thrombomodulin (thrombomodulin alfa) in the treatment of neonatal disseminated intravascular coagulation. Eur J Pediatr. 2014;173(3):303-11.
25. Fischer D, Schloesser R, Buxmann H, Veldman A. Recombinant activated factor VII as a hemostatic agent in very low birth weight preterms with gastrointestinal hemorrhage and disseminated intravascular coagulation. J Pediatr Hematol Oncol. 2008;30(5):337-42.
26. Zenz W, Zoehrer B, Levin M, Fanconi S, Hatzis TD, Knight G, et al. Use of recombinant tissue plasminogen activator in children with meningococcal purpura fulminans: a retrospective study. Crit Care Med. 2004;32(8):1777-80.
27. Veldman A, Fischer D, Nold MF, Wong FY. Disseminated intravascular coagulation in term and preterm neonates. Semin Thromb Hemost. 2010;36(4):419-28.
28. Avery GB, Fletcher MA, MacDonald MG. Neonatology: Pathophysiology and Management of the Newborn, 5th edition. Philadelphia, PA: Lippincott Williams &Wilkins; 1999.
29. Christensen RD. Hematologic Problems of the Neonate, 1st edition. Philadelphia, PA: WB Saunders Company; 2000. p. 453.
30. Trotter L. Disseminated intravascular coagulation in the neonatal period. Newborn Infant Nurs Rev. 2004;4(4):176-80.

CHAPTER

21

Thrombophilia in Newborns

Satyendra Katewa

INTRODUCTION

Thrombophilia is used to define a group of conditions where there is an increased tendency, often recurrent and often over an extended period of time, for excessive clotting. The process of making a blood clot is called thrombosis. The vascular system includes both the venous system and the arterial system. Thrombotic episodes may occur in either system. The symptoms depend on the part of the vascular system thrombosed, the extent of the clot and whether the clot breaks off and travels to another part of the body (e.g. the lungs-pulmonary embolus, the brain-embolic stroke, etc.). Although we are now able to determine the underlying cause in some patients and families for this tendency to an increased risk of excessive blood clotting, we are still not able to make this determination in all cases. This means that there is still more to understand about why some persons and families have increased clotting tendency.

Thromboembolism (TE) thought relatively common in newborns but is still regarded as a rare event in childhood and therefore knowledge of diagnostics, therapy and prophylaxis is limited among general pediatricians. During the past two decades, besides the greater awareness, an objective increase in childhood thrombosis is due to the medical progress in the treatment of critically ill patients. This is primarily secondary to the use of central catheters and invasive interventional procedures in the treatment of premature infants, neonates and older children who are critically ill, suffering from complex cardiac defects, and from malignant disease, respectively. The increasing knowledge of exogenous and endogenous thrombophilic risk factors has initiated a number of studies to assess the impact of such factors with respect to their contribution to the thrombophilic state, both individually but also in concert with other factors. In addition to their impact on a first thrombotic event, much of the interest is now focused on their importance for thrombotic relapses.

EPIDEMIOLOGY

The reported annual incidence of TE in childhood in general is considerably lower than in adults. The reasons for the lower incidences of TE in children compared to adults are not completely understood; an intact vascular endothelium, the lower capacity of thrombin generation and elevated levels of β_2-macroglobulin (an inhibitor of thrombin) are possible age-dependent modifying factors in children. Arterial TE in children is less common than venous thrombosis[1] with the exception of stroke. The estimated yearly incidence of stroke in childhood is between 3 and 8 per 100,000.[2,3] The highest incidence of 25–35 per 100,000 livebirths has been reported for neonates.[4] There are two age-related peaks in the frequency of thromboembolic disorders in children and adolescents: the first peak corresponds to the perinatal/neonatal period, with the highest relative incidence, and the second is observed postpuberty in adolescents, with a higher frequency in females.[1,5]

ETIOLOGY

Heritable Thrombophilia

Many of the causes of a long-term increased risk of venous thrombosis have been associated with a heritable abnormality of one of the many plasma proteins. **Table 21.1** summarizes the common inherited causes of thrombophilia and the risk associated with these causes.

Hereditary Prothrombotic Factors

The most important factors involved in the genetic predisposition to thrombophilia are the factors of the coagulation cascade and in particular their natural inhibitors. Certain metabolic defects also cause thrombophilia. **Figure 21.1** shows the normal coagulation cascade and its feedback control through anticoagulation system.

Table 21.1 Common causes of heritable thrombophilia and associated risks of thrombus formation

	Increased risk of thrombosis	*Prevalence in patients with venous thromboembolism (VTE) (%)*	*Prevalence in normal population (%)*
• Factor V Leiden heterozygous (activated protein C resistance)	3–8 ×	25–50	5.0
• Prothrombin G20210A	3 ×	6	2.0
• Antithrombin deficiency	25–50 ×	1	0.02
• Protein C deficiency	10–15 ×	3	0.3
• Protein S deficiency	10 ×	3	2.0
• Dysfibrinogenemia	Variable	Low	Rare

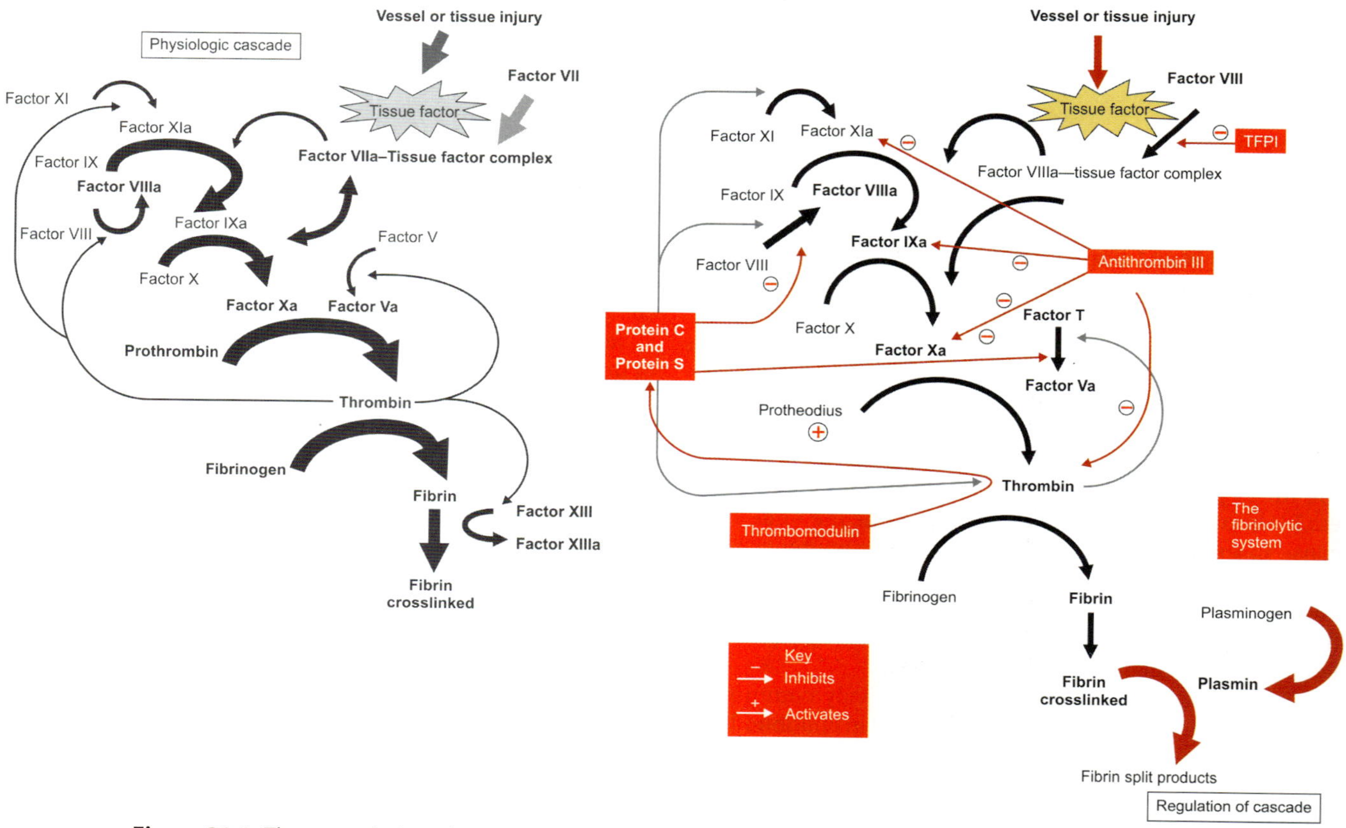

Figure 21.1 The normal physiological coagulation cascade and its control through anticoagulation systems

- *Coagulation factors*
  - *Fibrinogen (FI)*: In addition to being the final substrate for thrombin, FI is also an acute-phase protein that may lead to acquired thrombophilia and may also contribute to the risk of arterial TE.[6]
  - *Prothrombin (FII)*: Heterozygosity for the 20210A allele of the common FII polymorphism 20210G/A in the prothrombin (FII) gene 14 is found at a prevalence of 2.7% in the normal Caucasian population. This mutant correlates with slightly elevated FII levels, suggesting a quantitative contribution to thrombophilia.
  - *Factor V*: The factor V (FV) mutation Arg506 to Gln506 (R506Q or FV Leiden) causes relative resistance against cleavage by the activated protein C (PC) complex.[7,8] It has been identified as the most common significant genetic risk factor for thrombosis. In newborns and children with venous thrombosis, FV Leiden was identified in up to 30%.[9]
  - *Factor VIII*: Elevated factor VIII (FVIII) seems to contribute to the risk of TE in newborns and children. Furthermore, persistence of elevated FVIII after TE may also predict an unfavorable prognosis.[10]
  - *von Willebrand factor (vWF)*: Due to its key position in platelet adhesion and aggregation under conditions of high shear forces, vWF plays a most important hemostatic role in arterial vessels and in the microcirculation[11] and thereby to arterial TE and to microangiopathies such as thrombotic

thrombocytopenic purpura (TTP). In neonates, supra large vWF multimers (which are most active in primary hemostasis) are quantitatively more than later in life and correlate with a very effective platelet-dependent function of vWF.[12] It can be speculated if these large multimers contribute to the higher rate of stroke in the perinatal period, but respective data have not been reported yet.

- *Inhibitors of coagulation:* The hemostatic process is tightly regulated by specific inhibitors that act on coagulation factors and on the factors of primary hemostasis. Functionally, most important are tissue factor pathway inhibitor, the protein C system, antithrombin (AT) and the vWF cleaving protease ADAMTS13. Clinically, only the later three are important.
  1. *Protein C system (PC system)*: The protein C system comprises protein C, protein S (PS) and FV as cofactors. Protein C is activated to activated protein C (APC) by thrombin, which changes its substrate specificity from FI to protein C by being bound to thrombomodulin at the endothelial cell surface. Activated protein C cleaves and inactivates activated FV and activated FVIII, thereby regulating the formation of thrombin. Severe protein C deficiency as well as severe protein S deficiency correlates with purpura fulminans in newborns, a life-threatening thromboembolic disorder.
  2. *Antithrombin*: Antithrombin when bound to heparan sulfate on endothelial cells inhibits not only thrombin but also aFXI, aFIX and aFX. Its action on thrombin is enhanced 1,000 fold by heparin through an allosteric conformational change. In contrast, low-molecular-weight heparin (LMWH) makes AT more aFX specific. These effects are the basis for prophylactic or therapeutic anticoagulation by heparin. Even mild hereditary deficiency of AT function may correlate with thrombophilia with a penetrance higher than in protein C and protein S deficiency.
  3. *ADAMTS13*: *ADAMTS13* regulates the size of vWF multimers and thereby its functional activity in primary hemostasis. Its deficiency has clearly been established as the main etiology in TTP.[13] An acquired form caused by autoantibodies against ADAMTS13 and an inherited form called Upshaw-Schulman syndrome (USS) due to mutations in the gene exist. Lack of the protease correlates with persistence of supra large vWF multimers and, on an adequate trigger (infection, stress and hypoxia), these large multimers will induce platelet adhesion and aggregation in the microcirculation with subsequent microangiopathy, finally resulting in organ failure and death in 80% of cases when untreated.
- *Metabolic factors*
  - *Methylene tetrahydrofolate reductase (MTHFR) polymorphism 677C/T*: The rare condition of classical homocystinuria is most often caused by a deficiency of either cystathionine-synthetase or 5-methyltetrahydrofolate-homocysteine-methyltransferase and correlates with frequent TE due to severe homocysteinemia causing endothelial cell damage.
  - *Lipoprotein*: Lipoprotein (a) [LP(a)] is considered a significant venous and arterial risk factor for TE in newborn children.[14,15] However, other reports could not confirm these findings.[16]
- *Acquired prothrombotic risk factors*
  - *Central venous catheters (CVCs)*: CVCs have become an important tool to deliver effective medical and supportive management to newborns. These catheters bear many serious complications namely thrombotic occlusion, CVC-associated deep vein thrombosis (DVT) and systemic infections. CVCs seem to be the most important risk factor for DVT. The reported CVC-related DVT ranges from 1% to nearly 70%, reflecting the problem of different definitions, diagnostic methods and alertness.[17,18] However, the estimated contribution of CVCs to all thromboembolic events in newborns is as high as 90% and even over 50% in older children.[19]
  - *Childhood cancer*: Thromboembolism is a well-known complication in adult patients with cancer. TE in cancer is the result of complex interactions of a variety of factors such as the malignancy itself, chemotherapy and its side effects including infections or dehydration, CVCs, the unbalanced hemostatic system with predominant hypercoagulability as well as possible inherited acute lymphoblastic leukemia (ALL). The knowledge about TE in childhood cancer is very limited but the overall estimated risk comes around 16%.[20]
  - *Thrombosis and antiphospholipid syndrome*: Antiphospholipid syndrome (APS) is an antibody-mediated thrombophilic state characterized by clinical manifestations of venous, arterial or small vessel TE at any site as well as the presence of antiphospholipid antibodies (APA) in the blood. In newborns, it can present with acute ischemic stroke or transient ischemic attacks. APS is often associated with a number of autoimmune disorders.[21] APS is classified as primary and secondary; the clinical picture, however, is the same. Patients with no underlying disease are diagnosed as primary APS. Secondary APS refers to patients with underlying autoimmune (mainly rheumatologic) disorders as well as viral and bacterial infections or cancer. All proposed pathophysiological mechanisms share the binding of the APA to anionic protein-phospholipid complexes, leading to activation of endothelial cells, platelets and prothrombin, interference with natural inhibitory pathways and fibrinolysis, and disruption of the binding of annexin V to phospholipids coating the vascular system.[22,23] APA along with decreased activity of various coagulation factors, mainly FXII, are found in about 50% of otherwise healthy children with multiple viral infections, screened

Table 21.2 Prothrombotic predisposing factors in neonates and children

Commoner in newborns	*Usually in older children*
• Indwelling vascular catheters • Trauma • Infections • Surgery • Vascular anomalies • Polycythemia • Primary antiphospholipid antibody syndrome • Congenital heart disease • Prosthetic cardiac valves	• Causes in the newborns • Rheumatoid arthritis • Crohn's disease • Ulcerative colitis • Malignancy • Sickle cell anemia and other hemoglobinopathies • Chemotherapy with L-asparaginase • Renal disease • Diabetes mellitus • Appendicitis • Systemic lupus erythematosus • Systemic inflammatory response syndrome

for prolonged activated partial thromboplastin time (aPTT) preceding tonsillectomy or adenotomy.[24,25]

- *Heparin-induced thrombocytopenia type 2*: The overall incidence of heparin-induced thrombocytopenia (HIT) type 2 is estimated around 1% of patients hospitalized in the neonatal and pediatric intensive care units.[26,27]
- *Other acquired prothrombotic conditions*: Perinatal asphyxia, systemic infections/sepsis/disseminated intravascular coagulation (DIC), congenital heart disease (CHD) and hypovolemia are the main risk factors in neonates, the latter particularly prone to arterial events in association with CHD and/or arterial catheters frequently used in an intensive care setting.[28] There are additional factors in older children: trauma, major surgery, immobilization, estrogen-containing contraceptives in adolescent girls, corticosteroid therapy, nephrotic syndrome, hemolytic-uremic syndrome, inflammatory bowel disease, and rheumatic and other chronic disorders. **Table 21.2** shows the commoner prothrombotic risk factors in newborn and children.

PATHOPHYSIOLOGY

The basic events in thrombosis are as follows:

Vessel injury → abnormal platelet adhesiveness (aggregation) → activated coagulation mechanism → defective or deficient anticoagulation system → dysfunctional fibrinolytic mechanism → thrombus persists and propagates → and reduced blood flow leads to organ perfused and → complication mainly TE.

CLINICAL FEATURES

The clinical presentation primarily depends on the site of the thrombus and the organ involved. Inferior vena cava (IVC) thrombosis manifests with prominent cutaneous veins and possibly liver or renal dysfunction depending on the site and extension of the thrombus. Superior vena cava thrombosis leads to cyanosis and swelling of the head and upper thorax with prominent collateral veins and may finally result in acute cardiac failure. Portal vein thrombosis (PVT) in most cases due to central catheters may present with liver dysfunction including a failure, and renal vein thrombosis (RVT) presents with hematuria and possibly even renal failure.

An international registry of symptomatic venous TE in neonates reported an incidence of 25–35 per 100,000 admissions to neonatal intensive care units, almost all of which are secondary to CVCs. The mechanisms by which CVC causes TE include damage to vessel walls, poor blood flow, infusion of substances such as total parenteral nutrition that damage endothelial cells and thrombogenic catheter materials.[4] The true incidence of venous TE in neonates is difficult to find because of the less accurate diagnostic strategies. There are no well-designed comparative studies to compare commonly used noninvasive techniques (ultrasound) to invasive techniques like venogram or magnetic resonance venography (MRV). Ultrasound's sensitivity is only around 20% for upper system CVC in comparison to venography. The low pulse pressure and presence of CVC make compressibility difficult to assess, which ultimately reduce the sensitivity of ultrasound in newborns and that is why venogram is considered the gold standard for diagnostic imaging of venous TE in newborns but still not exercised widely because of difficult intravenous access, poor neonatal glomerular filtration rate (GFR) and limited availability of MRV. Post-thrombotic syndrome (PTS) is one of the bad long-term complications of venous TE, which has been recently recognized in a number of children with a history of neonatal thrombosis.[29] Neonates are particularly at increased risk of this complication due to impaired fibrinolytic degradation of clot, as the fibrinolytic pathways are physiologically suppressed in this age group. Clinically, PTS presents as chronic edema, skin discoloration, poor wound healing/impaired tissue viability, pain and limitation of limb function.

Renal vein thrombosis is the most common noncatheter-related TE in newborns. It accounts for 10% of venous TE. Increased risk of RVT in neonates is secondary to hyperviscous, hyperosmolar, and hypercoagulable states in association with reduced renal blood flow. The other neonatal problems like sepsis, dehydration, acidosis, hypotension, congenital cardiac disease, hyperinsulinism, asphyxia, polycythemia and asphyxia make RVT the most common spontaneous TE in newborns. Clinically, it presents as palpable flank mass, hematuria, proteinuria, consumptive thrombocytopenia and renal impairment. Bilateral RVT occurs in approximately 24% of cases, and if unilateral RVT then the right and left renal veins are equally affected.[29] Ultrasound is the current modality of choice to diagnose RVT. Clinical findings of edematous lower limbs with temperature variation and cyanosis suggest thrombus extension into IVC. In a retrospective study, extension into the IVC has been reported to be around 50% of the cases. In a small retrospective case series, 17% of the patients were found to be hypertensive later in the life. The incidence of long-term renal dysfunction was significantly lower in the treated group (30%) versus 100% in the nontreated group. Survival in the acute phase of RVT has improved significantly in the last decade with medical treatment including observation, anticoagulation and thrombolysis, as opposed to previous surgical therapy such as nephrectomy/embolectomy.[29] The true incidence of one other neonatal thrombotic problem, PVT is unknown, because thrombus in this location is usually clinically silent. Risk of PVT due to the use of umbilical venous catheter (UVC) remains controversial and ranges from 1% to 40%. Its incidence is increased, if UVC is complicated with umbilical sepsis or omphalitis. Diagnosis of PVT is usually made by ultrasound. Computed tomography and magnetic resonance imaging (MRI) are not better than ultrasound. Spontaneous resolution of asymptomatic PVT is also known but the most important clinical consequence of UVC-associated PVT is portal hypertension which may present even years after the actual insult.[29]

Swelling, discoloration and pain (older children) of extremities are acute symptoms of DVT. Acute dyspnea and pain (older children) could suggest pulmonary embolism. Signs of central nervous insults such as irritability, cerebral convulsions, signs of venous congestion and headache and or visual impairment (older children) may indicate sinus venous thrombosis. Childhood arterial ischemic stroke (AIS) manifests in neonates preferentially with seizures and abnormalities of muscle tone, whereas in elder children hemiparesis is the most frequent neurologic sign.[30] Acquired or inherited severe deficiencies of protein S and protein C are disorders involving both the microcirculation and arterial vessels, and may manifest with characteristic symptoms such as deep skin necrosis (purpura fulminans), blindness due to retinal vessel occlusion and arterial embolism followed by necrosis of distal extremities or whole limbs. TTP, a severe microangiopathic disorder, is characterized by nonimmunologic hemolytic anemia and thrombocytopenia, neurologic symptoms, and renal, pulmonary and cardiac involvement. Signs and symptoms of CVC-associated DVT are loss of CVC patency, the need for local thrombolytic therapy or CVC replacement, CVC-related sepsis, or prominent collateral circulation over chest, neck and head.

DIAGNOSIS

Lab Diagnosis

Every thrombotic event initiates a particular response to reestablish the balance of the hemostatic system, e.g. by fibrinolysis. Subsequently, markers of fibrinolysis such as D-dimers can be detected in the circulation. The specificity of these markers is low; however, the negative predictive value of the D-dimer test to correctly exclude DVT is as high as 89%. In a study on the outcome of TE in newborns and children, elevated D-dimer and/or FVIII:C were found in around 67% of the patients; however, elevations of these markers at diagnosis and during follow-up are significantly correlated with persistence or recurrence of TE and/or a PTS. Recommendation for the phasic evaluation of thrombophilia is given here.

Imaging

Color Doppler ultrasound, conventional and MRI angiography, lineograms and echocardiography are the diagnostic means of imaging the occlusion of vessels. Pulmonary embolism of proximal pulmonary arteries can be visualized by echocardiography and by CT scan; however, the specificity and sensitivity are low in detecting more distal clots. In such cases, ventilation and perfusion scintigraphies are the recommended techniques for children. Transcranial Doppler ultrasound is used to assess the risk of stroke in patients with sickle cell disease. All techniques can be regarded as equally specific, sensitive and precise; their application, however, differs with respect to the region of interest, age and therapeutic options. **Table 21.3** summarizes the indications

Table 21.3 Indications and imaging techniques used for thromboembolism (TE) in neonate and children[31]

Circumstances in young infants that require a laboratory work-up for thrombophilia		
• Unprovoked and/or recurrent thrombosis at any age		
• Thrombosis at unusual sites such as cerebral, mesenteric, portal, or hepatic veins		
• Positive family history for thrombosis		
• Thrombosis during pregnancy, oral contraceptives, or hormone replacement therapy (HRT)		
• Unexplained abnormal laboratory test such as prolonged PTT		
Common diagnostic methods and their limitations		
Method	*Indication*	*Limitation*
Lineograms	CVC-related thrombosis	Only clots at the tip of the CVC and the distal adjacent vessel wa l
Color Doppler ultrasound	DVT, SVT*	Exception—subclavian vein, use venography
Lateral venography	DVT, SVT	Exception—juglar vein use color Doppler USG or MRI
Echocardiography	CVC-related thrombosis, intracardiac thrombus, pulmonary embolism (PE)	Distal clots in PE
Scintigraphy	Pulmonary embolism	

*In young infants through the patent fontanelle.

Abbreviations: CVC, central venous catheter; DVT, deep vein thrombosis; PPT, partial thromboplastin time; SVT, sinus venous thrombosis

Table 21.4 Recommendations for laboratory testing in children with thrombosis*

Level I	*Level II*	*Level III*
Basic evaluation for all newborns and children	Extended evaluation for children with normal level I values and recurrent thrombosis, a positive family history for thrombosis or severe thrombosis	Currently under investigation
• Complete blood count with hematocrit, white blood count and platelet count • Antithrombin III • Protein C activity • Free and total protein S antigen • Factor V G1691A and/or functional activated protein C resistance assay • Prothrombin G20210A • MTHFR T677T and/or fasting homocysteine level • Lipoprotein (a) • Lupus anticoagulant • Anticardiolipin antibodies • *Sickle cell:* Screen or hemoglobin electrophoresis	• Euglobulin clot lysis time (ELT) • Plasminogen • *Dysfibrinogenemia evaluation:* Fibrinogen activity, antigen, thrombin time, reptilase time, fibrin degradation products, consider crossed immunoelectrophoresis • Plasminogen activator inhibitor (PAI) • Heparin cofactor II • Paroxysmal nocturnal hemoglobinuria (PNH) (sucrose hemolysis) • If not previously performed • Functional activated protein C resistance (modified assay) • Fasting homocysteine level • Hemoglobin electrophoresis • Erythrocyte sedimentation rate (ESR) • C-reactive protein (CRP)	• Factor VIII • Factor XII • Factor XI • von Willebrand factor (vWF) level and multimers • Spontaneous platelet aggregation • Platelet receptor polymorphisms • Tissue plasminogen activator (TPA) • Tissue factor pathway inhibitor (TFPI)

*Guidelines issued by Subcommittee for Perinatal and Pediatric Haemostasis of the Scientific Standardization Committee of the International Society for Thrombosis and Haemostasis.

and different techniques used with their limitations, and **Table 21.4** details the stepwise evaluation of thrombotic episode in newborns and children.

MANAGEMENT

Irrespective of an underlying disease, most of the thromboembolic events in the newborns should be evaluated for a possible treatment, aiming at the complete recanalization of the occluded vessel and stopping the thrombotic process. In the vast majority of cases, thrombosis will resolve with heparin given for 5–14 days. Other therapy options with a higher risk such as thrombolytic therapy or surgical embolectomy should be limited for patients with extensive thrombosis and/or threatened organ function. As LMWH shows considerable advantages over unfractionated heparin (UFH) for therapeutic as well as prophylactic purposes, the following recommendations are in favor of LMWH. Yet evidence shows no difference in the antithrombotic efficacy.

Commonly Used Anticoagulants

Heparin

Mechanism of action: Heparin enhances the rate by which antithrombin-III neutralizes the activities of several activated clotting proteins especially—factor Xa and thrombin (common pathway coagulation factors). Half-life of heparin is dose-dependent, increases with increasing dose. The short half-life of UFH ranges from 25 minutes in neonates to 1 hour in adolescents. Heparin is of two types:

1. *Unfractionated heparin*: Intravenous UFH should only be given in the initial phase of antithrombotic therapy and then switched to LMWH. The following disadvantages should be considered when using UFH.
   - Need for venous access for therapy and monitoring
   - Age-dependent unpredictable pharmacokinetics
   - Normal AT levels required
   - Monitoring by aPTT is prone to preanalytic errors
   - Risk for bleeding
   - Risk for HIT.
2. *Low-molecular-weight heparin*: Low-molecular-weight heparin is prepared by enzymatic or chemical cleavage of UFH, and the advantages with the use are as follows:
   - Easy subcutaneous administration once daily without need of venous access
   - Predictable pharmacokinetics
   - Minimal monitoring
   - Minimized bleeding complications
   - Reduced risk of HIT.

Low-molecular-weight heparin must be withheld for 24 hours prior to invasive procedure, especially lumbar puncture. It is cleaved by kidneys, so dose should be reduced in renal failure. Important side effects are reversible increase in serum glutamic oxaloacetic transaminase (SGOT) and serum glutamic pyruvic transaminase (SGPT). Infants less than 5 kg required about 50% higher doses than older children to reach equivalent anti-FXa levels. As a general guideline

Table 21.5 Recommended dosing of unfractionated heparin (UFH) and low-molecular-weight heparin (LMWH) in neonates and children[31]

	Neonates < 5 kg	*Children > 5 kg*	*Target at 48 hours*
Unfractionated heparin (UFH) via intravenous (IV) route			
Loading dose Maintenance dose	75 units/kg over 10 minutes 25–30 units/kg	75 units/kg over 10 minutes 20 units/kg	aPTT: 60–85 sec†
Low-molecular-weight heparin (LMWH; enoxaparin*) via subcutaneous (SC) route			
Initial treatment dose	1–2 mg/kg/day	1–1.5 mg/kg/day	Anti-Xa: 0.4–0.8 units/mL
Initial prophylaxis dose	1–1.5 mg/kg/day	1.0 mg/kg/day	Anti-Xa: <0.4 units/mL

*1 mg enoxaparin = 110 anti-FXa units

- *For UFH:* aPTT 4 hours after loading dose and 4 hours after each dosage adjustment, at least once daily; keep antithrombin (AT) levels within normal range; daily blood count (platelets)
- *For LMWH:* Anti-Xa activity 4 hours after injection

†Dose adjustments based on aPTT

- aPTT < 60 sec—increase heparin dose by 10%
- aPTT < 50 sec—repeat bolus by 50 U/kg and increase the dose by 10%
- aPTT > 90 sec—stop infusion for 30 minutes and then restart with 10% reduced dose.

Table 21.6 Indications, contraindications of thrombolysis and recommendation during systemic thrombolysis in neonates and children[31]

Indication			
Extensive and/or life/organ-threatening thrombosis			
Contraindications			
Strong	≤10 days after hemorrhage or major surgery ≤7 days after severe asphyxia ≤3 days after invasive procedure		
Soft	≤48 hours after cerebral convulsion Prematurity < 32 weeks of gestation Sepsis Active minor hemorrhage Refractory thrombocytopenia and hypofibrinogenemia		
Recommendations during thrombolysis			
• Keep fibrinogen > 0.5 g/L and platelets > 50 g/L • Increasing D-dimers indicate effective fibrinolysis • Dose reduction or cessation of rt-PA, if major bleeding occurs • Minor bleeding treated with local pressure • Optimal duration of rt-PA therapy uncertain, mostly up to 7 days, short/longer courses			
Systemic thrombolysis in newborns and young infants			
Therapy	Loading dose	Maintenance	Monitoring
rt-PA	0.1–0.2 mg/kg/10 min	0.8–2.4 mg/kg/24 hour	FI, platelets, D-dimers
UFH	None	5–10 U/kg/hour	aPTT

use LMWH with therapeutic anti-Xa levels for 4-6 weeks, followed by prophylactic dosage up to less than or equal to 6 months. The recommended dosing of UFH and LMWH are given in **Table 21.5**.

Thrombolytic Agents

The agent of choice is recombinant plasminogen activator (rt-PA). Streptokinase should not be used because of its allergic reactions. rt-PA may be indicated, if thrombosis is extensive or organ/life-threatening. **Table 21.6** summarizes the indications, contraindications and recommendations of thrombolysis in newborns and young infants.

Vitamin K Antagonists

Warfarin and phenprocoumon are usually administered for oral anticoagulation and inhibit gamma carboxylation

Table 21.7 Recommended dosing of oral anticoagulants (OAC) in neonates and children[31]

Oral anticoagulant	Day 1	Day 2	Day 3 onward	Target International normalized ratio (INR)*
• Warfarin	0.2 mg/kg	0.2 mg/kg	0.1–0.3 mg/kg	2.0–3.0
• Phenprocoumon	6 mg/m^2	3 mg/m^2	1–2 mg/m^2	2.0–3.0
Reversal of oral anticoagulation therapy				
• No bleeding, slow reversal		Vitamin K 0.5–2.0 mg orally, SC, IV		
• No bleeding, rapid reversal		Vitamin K 0.5–2.0 mg SC, IV		
• Significant bleeding (not life-threatening)		Vitamin K 0.5–2.0 mg SC, IV Injection fresh frozen plasma (FFP 20 mL/kg)		
• Significant bleeding (life-threatening)		Vitamin K 5.0 mg IV over 20 min (risk of anaphylactic shock) + Prothrombin concentrate 50 u/kg IV		
Coumarin therapy should always begin with concomitant heparin therapy (UFH or LMWH). To stop heparin, INR should be within therapeutic range for at least 2 days. We should keep a close watch for multiple drug interactions.				

*Suggested dose adjustments to achieve target INR
- INR 1.1–1.4—increase the dose by 20%
- INR 1.5–1.9—increase the dose by 10%
- INR 3.2–3.5—decrease the dose by 20%
- INR >3.5—withhold until INR < 3.5, then restart at 20% less than previous dose.

of vitamin K-dependent proteins (factors II, VII, IX and X). It also reduces protein C and S. Vitamin K antagonists should be administered in cases of prophylaxis exceeding 6 months. **Table 21.7** summarizes the recommendation regarding the dosing of oral anticoagulants in young infants.

Infusion of Deficient Inhibitors of Hemostasis

In cases of thrombosis with hereditary or acquired deficiencies of coagulation inhibitors, replacement therapy may be an option. Concentrates of AT and protein C are commercially available and are lifesaving in conditions of purpura fulminans due to inhibitor deficiency. Protein C concentrate also proved to be effective in heterozygous or acquired protein C deficiency.[31]

New Anticoagulants

The limitations of the traditional anticoagulants are particularly obvious in pediatrics; hence, the promotion of the new drugs, which are already approved in adults, is necessary. Yet there is but individual experience in children with the following substances: the pentasaccharides fondaparinux and idraparinux, and the direct thrombin inhibitors hirudin, bivalirudin, argatroban; ximelagatran has been withdrawn from the market because of hepatic toxicity.[32,33]

Special Conditions

Prophylaxis of Central Venous Catheter Occlusion

Unfractionated heparin: Prophylactic UFH seems to significantly decrease CVC-related DVT as well as bacterial colonization of the catheter.[34] Heparin-bonded catheters do not reduce clot formation and bacterial colonization beyond 24 hours after CVC insertion.

Thrombolytic agents (urokinase, rt-PA): Thrombolytic therapy is widely and safely used for the management of occluded catheters. Some studies show a substantial benefit of thrombolytic agents over UFH or no prophylaxis[34] whereas others get contradictory results.[35,36]

Low-molecular-weight heparin: Prophylactic use of LMWH has been efficient and safe in the treatment and prevention of DVT in children with cancer.[20,37,38] However, LMWH to maintain CVC-latency and prevent CVC-related DVT has to remain an individual decision.

Oral Anticoagulation with Vitamin K Antagonists

There are no data for children on using low-dose oral anticoagulation to prevent CVC-associated DVT and to maintain catheter patency. **Table 21.7** summarizes the recommendation regarding the dosing of oral anticoagulants in young infants.

Management of Thrombosis in Children with Cancer

The main challenge is to keep the balance of benefit and risk of an antithrombotic treatment, as most children are being treated with chemotherapy with intermittent thrombocytopenia and an unbalanced hemostatic system, both of which lead to potential bleeding complications. It is therefore strongly recommended not to use antithrombotic agents with potentially serious side effects such as thrombolytic agents, UFH or vitamin K antagonists.

Prophylaxis of Thromboembolism in Children with Cancer

Though, there is a lack of clear evidence-based indications but the following conditions for primary prophylaxis may be considered:

- Children with hereditary thrombophilia under intensive chemotherapy
- Adolescents with additional risk factors such as major surgery or immobilization
- Patients with prior TE in their history and
- Children with tumors compressing large vessels.

Because ALL carries the highest risk for TE an efficient prophylaxis would be of major importance. To date there are no controlled trials that allow the extrapolation of prophylactic strategies.

Antithrombotic Therapy for Antiphospholipid Syndrome

Long-term prognosis depends on the risk of recurrent TE which seems to be the highest within 6 months of discontinuation of anticoagulation.[39] Duration and intensity of therapy are still controversial at least for subgroups. After the first DVT, secondary prophylaxis for 12 months is indicated. Lifelong anticoagulation is to be considered after a very serious first event and recurrent TE with persistence of APA. After arterial TE the optimal secondary prophylaxis remains controversial.[39,40]

CONCLUSION

Thromboembolism in young children is a serious occurrence that may adversely affect the child's further development. Almost 90% of neonatal thrombosis are secondary to vascular access devices and a very high index of clinical suspicion is required to detect thrombosis in neonates with central venous access device (CVAD) *in situ*. Among the laboratory investigations, angiography remains the best diagnostic test for thrombosis in neonates. When it comes to treatment, thrombophilia work-up usually does not change the acute management of vascular access-related thrombosis. Bilateral RVT or even unilateral thrombosis with extension into the IVC is likely to benefit from antithrombotic therapy. The pharmacokinetics of antithrombotic agents is vastly different in neonates compared to adults, and age-specific dosing protocols need to be used. Since these thrombotic events have an impact on the ultimate outcome of children's development, we need better predictors of prognosis in relation to risk factors and therapy and we also need to emphasize the importance of prophylaxis in this vulnerable age group. The large number of established and less established, known and also hitherto unknown risk factors for TE do not allow us to predict outcome or prognosis at an individual level. The latest data on the prognostic value of FVIII and D-dimers are promising but we need more exhaustive and well-planned studies before we conclude. Research will also help to define the optimal duration of anticoagulation at an individual patient level based on the better defined risk profiles.

However, one should always remember the overall low risk of TE in children compared to the adults. This means that in a developing country like ours, it is of paramount importance to think about the concerning costs and possible overinterpretation of laboratory tests before we order them. The investigations of the risk factors in the individual patient should be limited according to their usefulness in that particular setting.

REFERENCES

1. Kuhle S, Massicotte P, Chan A, Adams M, Abdolell M, de Veber G, et al. Systemic thromboembolism in children. Data from the 1-800-NO-CLOTS Consultation Service. Thromb Haemost. 2004;92(4):722-8.
2. Giroud M, Lemesle M, Gouyon JB, Nivelon JL, Milan C, Dumas R. Cerebrovascular disease in children under 16 years of age in the city of Dijon, France: a study of incidence and clinical features from 1985 to 1993. J Clin Epidemiol. 1995;48(11):1343-8.
3. Lynch JK, Hirtz DG, deVeber G, Nelson KB. Report of the National Institute of Neurological Disorders and Stroke workshop on perinatal and childhood stroke. Pediatrics. 2002;109(1):116-23.
4. Chalmers EA. Perinatal stroke: risk factors and management. Br J Haematol. 2005;130(3):333-43.
5. Stein PD, Kayali F, Olson RE. Incidence of venous thromboembolism in infants and children: data from the National Hospital Discharge Survey. J Pediatr. 2004;145(4):563-5.
6. Rothwell PM, Howard SC, Power DA, Gutnikov SA, Algra A, van Gijn J, et al. Fibrinogen concentration and risk of ischemic stroke and acute coronary events in 5113 patients with transient ischemic attack and minor ischemic stroke. Stroke. 2004;35(10):2300-5.
7. Dahlbäck B, Carlsson M, Svensson PJ. Familial thrombophilia due to a previously unrecognized mechanism characterized by poor anticoagulant response to activated protein C: prediction of a cofactor to activated protein C. Proc Natl Acad Sci USA. 1993;90(3):1004-8.
8. Bertina RM, Koeleman BP, Koster T, Rosendaal FR, Dirven RJ, de Ronde H, et al. Mutation in blood coagulation factor V associated with resistance to activated protein C. Nature. 1994;369(6475):64-7.
9. Aschka I, Aumann V, Bergmann F, Budde U, Eberl W, Eckhof-Donovan S, et al. Prevalence of factor V Leiden in children with thrombo-embolism. Eur J Pediatr. 1996;155(12):1009-14.
10. Goldenberg NA, Knapp-Clevenger R, Manco-Johnson MJ. Mountain States Regional Thrombophilia Group. Elevated plasma factor VIII and D-dimer levels as predictors of poor outcomes of thrombosis in children. N Engl J Med. 2004;351(11):1081-8.
11. Ruggeri ZM, Ruggeri ZM. Platelet and von Willebrand factor interactions at the vessel wall. Hamostaseologie. 2004;24(1):1-11.
12. Rehak T, Cvirn G, Gallistl S, Leschnik B, Köstenberger M, Katzer H, et al. Increased shear stress- and ristocetin-induced binding of von Willebrand factor to platelets in cord compared with adult plasma. Thromb Haemost. 2004;92(4):682-7.

13. Lämmle B, Kremer Hovinga JA, Alberio L. Thrombotic thrombocytopenic purpura. J Thromb Haemost. 2005;3(8): 1663-75.
14. Nowak-Göttl U, Strater R, Heinecke A, Junker R, Koch HG, Schuierer G, et al. Lipoprotein (a) and genetic polymorphisms of clotting factor V, prothrombin, and methylenetetrahydrofolate reductase are risk factors of spontaneous ischemic stroke in childhood. Blood. 1999;94(11):3678-82.
15. Nowak-Göttl U, Junker R, Hartmeier M, Koch HG, Münchow N, Assmann G, et al. Increased lipoprotein (a) is an important risk factor for venous thromboembolism in childhood. Circulation. 1999;100(7):743-8.
16. Revel-Vilk S, Chan A, Bauman M, Massicotte P. Prothrombotic conditions in an unselected cohort of children with venous thromboembolic disease. J Thromb Haemost. 2003;1(5):915-21.
17. Mitchell LG, Andrew M, Hanna K, Abshire T, Halton J, Anderson R, et al. A prospective cohort study determining the prevalence of thrombotic events in children with acute lymphoblastic leukemia and a central venous line who are treated with L-asparaginase: results of the Prophylactic Antithrombin Replacement in Kids with Acute Lymphoblastic Leukemia Treated with Asparaginase (PARKAA) Study. Cancer. 2003;97(2):508-16.
18. Male C, Chait P, Andrew M, Hanna K, Julian J, Mitchell L, et al. Central venous line-related thrombosis in children: association with central venous line location and insertion technique. Blood. 2003;101(11):4273-8.
19. Parasuraman S, Goldhaber SZ. Venous thromboembolism in children. Circulation. 2006;113(2): e12-6.
20. Wiernikowski JT, Athale UH. Thromboembolic complications in children with cancer. Thromb Res. 2006;118(1):137-52.
21. Miyakis S, Lockshin MD, Atsumi T, Branch DW, Brey RL, Cervera R, et al. International consensus statement on an update of the classification criteria for definite antiphospholipid syndrome (APS). J Thromb Haemost. 2006;4(2):295-306.
22. Levine JS, Branch DW, Rauch J. The antiphospholipid syndrome. N Engl J Med. 2002;346(10):752-63.
23. Rand JH. The antiphospholipid syndrome. Annu Rev Med. 2003;54:409-24.
24. Kenet G. Perinatal/Pediatric Haemostasis Subcommittee of the SSC of the ISTH, Minutes and Annual Reports 2006, 52nd Annual SSC meeting of the ISTH, Oslo 2006.
25. Mizumoto H, Maihara T, Hiejima E, Shiota M, Hata A, Seto S, et al. Transient antiphospholipid antibodies associated with acute infections in children: a report of three cases and a review of the literature. Eur J Pediatr. 2006;165(7):484-8.
26. Klenner A, Lubenow N, Raschke R, Greinacher A. Heparin-induced thrombocytopenia in children: 12 new cases and review of the literature. Thromb Haemost. 2004;91(4):719-24.
27. Newall F, Barnes C, Ignjatovic V, Monagle P. Heparin-induced thrombocytopenia in children. J Paediatr Child Health. 2003;39(4):289-92.
28. Albisetti M, Schmugge M, Haas R, Eckhardt BP, Bauersfeld U, Baenziger O, et al. Arterial thromboembolic complications in critically ill children. J Crit Care. 2005;20(3):296-300.
29. Greenway A, Massicotte MP, Monagle P. Neonatal thrombosis and its treatment. Blood Rev. 2004;18(2):75-84.
30. Steinlin M, Pfister I, Pavlovic J, Everts R, Boltshauser E, Capone Mori A, et al. The first three years of the Swiss Neuropaediatric Stroke Registry (SNPSR): a population-based study of incidence, symptoms and risk factors. Neuropediatrics. 2005;36(2):90-7.
31. Schneppenheim R, Greiner J. Thrombosis in infants and children. Hematology Am Soc Hematol Educ Program. 2006. pp. 86-96.
32. Balsa VV. New anticoagulants: a pediatric perspective. Pediatr Blood Cancer. 2005;45(6):741-52.
33. Kuhle S, Lau A, Bajzar L, Vegh P, Halton J, Cherrick I, et al. Comparison of the anticoagulant effect of a direct thrombin inhibitor and a low molecular weight heparin in an acquired antithrombin deficiency in children with acute lymphoblastic leukaemia treated with L-asparaginase: an in vitro study. Br J Haematol. 2006;134(5):526-31.
34. Hentschel R, Sutor AH. Catheter-related thrombosis and its prevention in infancy. Hamostaseologie. 2002;22(4):167-73.
35. Aquino VM, Sandler ES, Mustafa MM, Steele JW, Buchanan GR. A prospective double-blind randomized trial of urokinase flushes to prevent bacteremia resulting from luminal colonization of subcutaneous central venous catheters. J Pediatr Hematol Oncol. 2002;24(9):710-13.
36. Solomon B, Moore J, Arthur C, Prince HM. Lack of efficacy of twice-weekly urokinase in the prevention of complications associated with Hickman catheters: a multicentre randomised comparison of urokinase versus heparin. Eur J Cancer. 2001;37(18):2379-84.
37. Elhasid R, Lanir N, Sharon R, Weyl Ben Arush M, Levin C, Postovsky S, et al. Prophylactic therapy with enoxaparin during L-asparaginase treatment in children with acute lymphoblastic leukemia. Blood Coagul Fibrinolysis. 2001;12(5):367-70.
38. Massicotte P, Julian JA, Gent M, Shields K, Marzinotto V, Szechtman B, et al. An open-label randomized controlled trial of low molecular weight heparin for the prevention of central venous line-related thrombotic complications in children: the PROTEKT trial. Thromb Res. 2003;109(2-3):101-8.
39. Lim W, Crowther MA, Eikelboom JW. Management of antiphospholipid antibody syndrome: a systematic review. JAMA. 2006;295(9):1050-7.
40. Ortel TL. Thrombosis and the antiphospholipid syndrome. Hematology Am Soc Hematol Educ Program. 2005. pp. 462-8.

SECTION 4

Platelets, Platelet Disorders and Approach to Bleeding in Newborn

Section Editors

Nitin K Shah, Amita Mahajan

CHAPTER

22 Approach to Neonatal Thrombocytopenia

Nitin K Shah

NEONATAL MEGAKARYOPOIESIS AND THROMBOPOIESIS

INTRODUCTION

After birth, the platelets are produced by megakaryocytes in the bone marrow and have a life of 9–10 days. In the fetus, they are produced predominantly in the liver. Platelets appear in the circulation in a fetus by 5–6 weeks of gestational age and platelet count steadily rises to 159 ± 34 × 10^9/L by 10–17 weeks of gestation and 240 ± 60 × 10^9/L by 18 weeks of gestation, remaining constant at that level, thereafter, until birth and beyond. Hence, the lower limit of the platelet count in a newborn, irrespective of the gestational age, remains at the adult level, i.e. more than 150 × 10^9/L. Thrombocytopenia in a newborn is defined as platelet count lower than 150 × 10^9/L, though clinical bleeding is usually seen with platelet count less than 50 × 10^9/L or even lower. Spontaneous and severe bleeding is usually seen when the platelet count drops to less than 20 × 10^9/L. Presence of significant bleeding at higher platelet counts should arouse suspicion of associated platelet dysfunction as is seen in cases with inherited thrombocytopenia, e.g. Bernard-Soulier syndrome.

A minimum platelet count of 7 × 10^9/L is required for maintenance of the vascular integrity, and in that sense a normal platelet count of more than 150 × 10^9/L provides a lot of reserve functional capacity. Similarly, 30% of the circulating platelets are stored in the spleen which can be brought into the circulation during the need or stress. Normal bone marrow contains 6 × 10^6 megakaryocytes/kg body weight. The normal daily platelet production is approximately 35,000 ± 4,300 platelets per microliter of blood to maintain steady levels of about 250,000 ± 100,000 platelets/mL. Normal bone marrow can respond by increasing the platelet production by 7–8 folds during periods of thrombocytopenia.

Platelets are required at each stage of hemostasis. With the help of von Willebrand factor, they adhere to the exposed endothelial cells at the site of injury and help form the primary platelet plug. They secrete granules that contain the factors to help aggregate further platelets and coagulation factors that help form a clot locally. They secrete vasoactive amines that lead to vasospasm to prevent further blood loss. Platelet membrane provides the surface required for the coagulation to proceed.

There are several growth factors that are required for the formation of platelets from megakaryocytes in the bone marrow. These include interleukin (IL)-3, IL-6, IL-11, stem cell factor, leukemia inhibitory factor, erythropoietin (EPO) and the most important thrombopoietin (Tpo). Tpo, discovered in 1994, is a polypeptide glycoprotein that binds to its receptor c-mpl (named after its cell of discovery, i.e. acute myeloproliferative leukemic cell) expressed on the megakaryocytes, megakaryocytic precursors, hematopoietic precursor cells and platelets. Tpo acts to commit early precursor cells to lineage-specific differentiation and enhances production and release of platelets in the circulation. It acts via further signal conduction pathway and prevents apoptosis in the target cells. It also appears to play a role as pan-hematopoietic growth factor which explains why defects in its metabolism ultimately leads to total bone marrow failure, as seen in rare cases of congenital amegakaryocytic thrombocytopenia. Tpo levels are inversely proportional to the total megakaryocytic mass. High levels of Tpo indicate aregenerative type of thrombocytopenia.

The bone marrow in neonates is very sensitive to insults like hypoxia which leads to suppression of the megakaryocytes more than other precursor cells. This explains why thrombocytopenia is more common than other cytopenias in neonate, especially following hypoxic stress.

INCIDENCE

There are very few prospective studies which have specifically looked at the incidence of thrombocytopenia in newborns. Recent prospective studies have shown that 0.5–4.1% of the neonates have thrombocytopenia. Around 30% of the babies admitted to the neonatal intensive care unit (NICU) have platelet counts less than 150×10^9/L and around 10% of the babies will have counts less than 100×10^9/L. Fortunately, most of the episodes of thrombocytopenia in NICU are mild to moderate but 20% of them (6% of the neonatal admissions) will have severe thrombocytopenia with counts less than 50×10^9/L who are at a risk of severe bleeding including intracranial bleeds. Around 80% of these babies with severe bleeds are sick, preterms who have sepsis or necrotizing enterocolitis (NEC).

CAUSES OF NEONATAL THROMBOCYTOPENIA

While traditionally one can classify the causes of neonatal thrombocytopenia into those caused by reduced production, increased destruction or consumption, sequestration, dilutional or a combination of these, it does not help while approaching a case of neonatal thrombocytopenia as most of the causes listed are rare. It is easy to group the cases as per their onset, the nadir of counts, the type of recovery, their mechanism of disease, their associated findings, presence of physical anomalies, presence of immunodeficiency and syndromes which helps to narrow down the differential diagnosis. The causes of neonatal thrombocytopenia are shown in **Box 22.1**.

Patterns of Neonatal Thrombocytopenia

While there are many etiological causes of neonatal thrombocytopenia, most of the patients fall into two types of patterns. This helps us narrow down the etiology. Around 75% of the neonatal thrombocytopenia cases fall into the early onset type and the remaining into the late onset type.

Early Onset Type

This accounts for 75% of the total cases. Most babies have low platelet at birth or soon after birth in the first 72 hours of life. The causes include thrombocytopenia due to chronic or acute hypoxia like in preterm, intrauterine growth restriction (IUGR) baby risk factors like perinatal asphyxia, maternal diabetes, placental insufficiency, maternal hypertension or pre-eclampsia. The platelet counts in low normal in the first 2–3 days, falls to a nadir at 4–5 days and recovers by 7–8 days. The counts rarely drop below 50×10^9/L. If the pattern of recovery does not follow this path, one has to think of other causes of early onset thrombocytopenia like chromosomal anomalies, congenital or perinatal infections, inherited causes or immune causes.

Late Onset Type

This accounts for the remaining 25% of the cases and is usually associated with late onset sepsis with or without NEC. The counts drop to a low level and there may be significant bleeding in these babies.

Box 22.1 Causes of neonatal thrombocytopenia

- *Perinatal hypoxia*:
  - Maternal diabetes
  - Maternal hypertension, pre-eclampsia
  - IUGR
- *Immune causes*:
  - Alloimmune
  - Autoimmune
- *Infections*:
  - *Perinatal infections*: Bacterial, TORCH, HIV
  - Late onset sepsis or NEC
- *DIC*:
  - Asphyxia
  - Infections
  - Mismatched transfusions
  - Congenital TTP
- *Aneuploidy*:
  Trisomy 18, trisomy 13, trisomy 21, Turner's syndrome
- *Inherited*:
  - *Giant platelets*: Bernard-Soulier syndrome, May-Hegglin's anomaly, Sebastian syndrome, Fechtner syndrome, Epstein syndrome, Alport's syndrome, Montreal platelet syndrome, Quebec syndrome, Gray platelet syndrome
  - *Immunodeficiency*: Wiskott-Aldrich syndrome
  - X-linked thrombocytopenia
  - Hemophagocytic lymphohistiocytosis
  - *Bone marrow failure*: Fanconi's anemia, TAR syndrome, congenital amegakaryocytic thrombocytopenia
  - *Pre-malignant*: Monosomy 7
- *Others*:
  - *Consumption*: Kasabach-Merritt syndrome, vascular thrombosis, hepatic hemangioendothelioma
  - *Metabolic*: Propionic academia, methylmalonic acidemia
  - *Miscellaneous*: Congenital leukemia, exchange transfusions, Rh disease of newborn, subcutaneous fat necrosis of the neonate

Abbreviations: DIC, disseminated intravascular coagulation; IUGR, intrauterine growth restriction; NEC, necrotizing enterocolitis; Rh, Rhesus; TTP, thrombotic thrombocytopenic purpura

Neonatal Alloimmune Thrombocytopenia

This is the platelet equivalent of the Rhesus (Rh) disease where alloantibodies are produced by the mother against the paternal platelets antigens inherited by the newborn from the father which are missing in the mother. These antibodies pass across the placenta and destroy the baby's platelets resulting in often moderate to severe thrombocytopenia. Unlike in Rh disease, in more than 50% of cases the first-born babies are also affected. In 80% of cases, the missing platelet antigen in the mother is human platelet antigen (HPA)-1a (also known as PlA1), in 10–15% it is HPA-5b and in the rest, it is HPA-3a, HPA-1b or some other unknown and rare antigen. In Asian communities, it is usually the HPA-4 antigen. Development of the alloantibodies in HLA-1A negative women is strongly associated with HLA DRB3 0101 (odds ratio of 140).

1:350 pregnancies are associated with maternal antiplatelet antibodies, but only 1:1000 livebirths are associated with neonatal alloimmune thrombocytopenia proving that a good number of them are silent or unnoticed. The affected neonates, who otherwise look well, present with purpura, bruising, mucosal bleeds and thrombocytopenia at birth or immediately after birth. The platelet count is usually less than 30×10^9/L. Around 20% of the affected neonates develop severe bleeding including intracranial bleeds. Around 20–50% of the intracranial bleeds start in the intrauterine life and 20% of the survivors develop long-term neurodevelopmental sequelae. The diagnosis is done by laboratory testing for the antiplatelet antibodies.

Treatment of the mildly affected babies without mucosal bleeds or with platelet count above 30×10^9/L is conservative. Those with significant mucosal bleeds, evidence of intracranial bleeds or platelet count less than 30×10^9/L need specific treatment including platelet transfusions, intravenous immunoglobulin (IVIg) and steroids. HPA compatible platelets need to be transfused. While one can use washed mother's platelets (which obviously will be negative for the missing platelets), HPA-1a negative platelets are usually stored and easily available in major centers in the West. If severe thrombocytopenia persists in spite of the platelet transfusions, one need to give IVIg in the dose of 2 g/kg body weight over 2–5 days and/or IV methyl prednisolone in the dose of 1 mg/kg 8 hourly. The treatment is required for 1–6 weeks till the platelet counts is in the safe range.

The severity depends on the maternal antibody titers. The second born neonate is usually severely affected if the first baby was symptomatic or had intracranial bleeds especially with intrauterine onset. In such cases, fetal monitoring of the platelet counts is advocated and the mother is given IVIg in the dose of 1–2 g/kg/week with prednisolone in the dose of 0.5–1 mg/kg/day. The fetus can also be given in-utero HPA compatible platelet transfusions if the maternal treatment alone dose not help. Elective lower segment cesarean section (LSCS) is also advocated to prevent trauma to head.

Neonatal Autoimmune Thrombocytopenia

This occurs due to transplacental transfer of the antiplatelet autoantibodies. It is suspected because of the prior history of thrombocytopenia in the mother due to idiopathic thrombocytopenic purpura (ITP), systemic lupus erythematosus (SLE) or some such autoimmune disease. The platelet count in the mother may be normal even when the antibodies persist, especially following splenectomy. The antibodies are formed against the common platelet antigens like gp1b/IX or gpIIb/IIIa. The disease is generally milder than the alloantibody-mediated neonatal thrombocytopenia. The newborn is usually normal at birth with even normal platelet count which drops after few days. Less than 10–15% of the babies have platelet counts less than 50×10^9/L and the bleeding is usually milder. Intracranial bleeds occur in less than 1–2% of babies. In most, the platelet counts recover in the next 2–3 weeks though rarely they may take a longer time. There is no role of antenatal treatment or LSCS. After birth, treatment is required in presence of significant bleeding or platelet counts less than 30×10^9/L. The treatment consists of IVIg and or steroids as in the case of alloimmune thrombocytopenia. Like in ITP, there is no role of platelet transfusions as the autoantibodies will react with all the platelets as the target antigens are common to all the donors. The prognosis is usually excellent.

Thrombocytopenia Following Hypoxia

This is the most common cause of early onset pattern of thrombocytopenia. The newborn is usually a preterm or an IUGR baby who has risk factors like maternal diabetes, maternal hypertension or pre-eclampsia or perinatal asphyxia. The counts are 100×10^9/L in first few days, fall to a nadir of 50×10^9/L at 4–5 days and recover by 7–8 days. The counts often recover above the normal levels. They may also have neutropenia and polycythemia besides thrombocytopenia. Though platelet destruction is an important cause, especially in acute hypoxia where disseminated intravascular coagulation (DIC) with thrombocytopenia is seen in 50% of such babies, in most with chronic hypoxia there is decreased production too as the major contributing factor. Less than 10% of such babies have evidence of DIC and the Tpo levels are high suggestive of aregenerative type of thrombocytopenia. There is evidence of increased erythropoiesis with increased levels of EPO and circulating normoblasts. This with increased Tpo levels suggests preferential differentiation toward erythropoiesis with depressed megakaryopoiesis. This is because the megakaryocytes are sensitive to hypoxia and are suppressed with hypoxia temporarily. The bleeding is usually mild. Most do not need any specific treatment. Those who are symptomatic need platelet transfusions.

Thrombocytopenia due to Neonatal Infections

Perinatal Sepsis

Perinatal bacterial sepsis can occur in 1–2/1,000 livebirths. The common organisms include group B sepsis or *E. coli* in the West and gram-negative organisms like Klebsiella or *E. coli* in our country. Around 50% of the sepsis cases develop thrombocytopenia and DIC are important cause of low platelet counts. The platelet counts are low early in life and recover with the treatment of the primary cause.

Congenital Infections

TORCH group of infection can lead to thrombocytopenia. Most, but not all, will have other signs like jaundice, anemia, congenital defects, hepatosplenomegaly, etc. Cytomegalovirus (CMV) is a common cause of such thrombocytopenia. About

0.5–1% of all newborns develop congenital CMV infection and though only 10–15% of them are otherwise symptomatic, 75% of them have low platelet counts. There may be associated neutropenia and the thrombocytopenia may persist for several months. Similarly, 40% of those infected with toxoplasma can develop low platelet counts. Another common cause in our country is perinatal HIV infection and rubella infection as MMR (Measles, mumps and rubella) vaccine is still not a part of our national schedule.

Late Onset Sepsis

A common cause of late onset of thrombocytopenia is late onset of sepsis with or without NEC. Thrombocytopenia may be the first sign of infection, though usually other signs of infection are also present. The platelet counts fall after the first 72 hours and may take around 7–8 days to recover after the treatment for sepsis is started and is effective. Less than 10% of these patients have DIC. The Tpo levels are high suggesting aregenerative type of thrombocytopenia. This is also evident by the fact that thrombocytopenia persist even after the infection is under control. This suggests that the cause of low platelet is less production due to suppression of the megakaryocytes. The counts are usually less than 30×10^9/L and 15–20% of the patients have significant bleeding. Platelet transfusions are required for the symptomatic patients.

Consumption of Platelets

Disseminated intravascular coagulation: Consumption and destruction of platelets occur in DIC which usually occurs following perinatal asphyxia or neonatal infection. The newborn will have the signs of the primary disease and will have severe thrombocytopenia with significant bleeding. The patient may have the signs of thrombosis like gangrene. The prothrombin time and activated partial thromboplastin time will be prolonged and D-dimers or the fibrinogen split products (FDP) will be raised. The peripheral smear will show evidence of microangiopathic hemolytic anemia along with low platelet counts. Treatment will include use of platelets along with fresh frozen plasma besides treatment of the primary cause.

Kasabach-Merritt syndrome: Large hemangioma can occur over extremities, trunk, neck or in internal organs. Platelets can get trapped in the slow circulation within the hemangioma and can lead to local consumption or localized DIC with consumption of other coagulation factors too. There may be multiple afferent and feeders to the hemangioma. The mass may not be restricted to the defined anatomical layers and usually infiltrates deep into the tissues making it difficult to excise the hemangioma. The diagnosis is obvious when the hemangioma is seen externally, whereas it can be difficult if the hemangioma is in some organ. Very low platelet counts, evidence of microangiopathy, raised D-dimers or FDP levels and high retic count will suggest the diagnosis. Imaging and vascular studies will help define the extent of the lesion which may be actually much widespread than appearing visibly. Medical treatment includes use of FFP followed by antifibrinolytic agents hoping to induce thrombosis of the important feeding vessels. Interferon therapy and vincristine can help shrink the lesion permanently; however, they have their own side effects. Surgery often is mutilating and may land up into amputation.

Congenital and Inherited Thrombocytopenia

This includes causes like chromosomal anomalies and rare inherited causes of low platelet count. The counts are low at or soon after the birth. In most, but not all, there are other features of the basic disease. The platelet count can be very low in some of them needing platelet transfusions and other treatment. The counts take a long to recover and may be low for months. Those with associated thrombasthenia bleed a lot at relative higher platelet counts. Some of them will have typical platelet morphology on smear examination.

Chromosomal Anomalies

The incidence of thrombocytopenia in various aneuploidy cases varies from 86% in trisomy 18–31% in trisomy 13, 6% in trisomy 21 and 31% in Turner's syndrome. Usually the thrombocytopenia is not severe and many a times it is associated with neutropenia and polycythemia as seen in placental insufficiency. The mechanism of thrombocytopenia may also be similar to that seen in placental insufficiency.

Inherited Thrombocytopenia

Inherited thrombocytopenias are a rare but interesting group of disorders which provided some insight into the molecular mechanisms for megakaryopoiesis. For some of these disorders, the molecular defects have been identified, like mutation of the c-mpl in congenital amegakaryocytic thrombocytopenia, defect in transduction pathway after binding of Tpo to c-mpl in TAR (thrombocytopenia with absent radius) syndrome, mutations in CBFA2 (core-binding factor subunit alpha-2) transcription factor gene *RUNX1* (*AML1*) in familial platelet syndrome with predisposition to acute myeloid leukemia (AML), mutation in GATA-1 transcription factor (xp 11) in X-linked thrombocytopenia with microcytosis, mutation in myosin heavy chain A gene (*MYH9*) in giant platelet syndromes including May-Hegglin anomaly and mutations in the WASP gene in Wiskott-Aldrich syndrome and X-linked thrombocytopenia. Most, but not all, have associated congenital anomalies to point to the possible diagnosis. Many of them have abnormal platelet morphology like giant platelet on peripheral smear examination. Some have associated platelet dysfunction leading to more bleeding than expected for the platelet count.

Inherited Thrombocytopenia with Giant Platelets

This group includes the disorders like Bernard-Soulier syndrome; May-Hegglin syndrome and its variants like Sebastian syndrome, Fechtner syndrome, Epstein syndrome and Alport syndrome; Montreal platelet syndrome; Quebec syndrome and Gray platelet syndrome.

Bernard-Soulier Syndrome: It is an autosomal recessive disorder. The platelet count is moderately low but the bleeding is quite significant. The platelets can be as large as 20 microns in diameter with cytoplasmic vacuoles. The defect is in the demarcation membrane system. This results in defect in gpIb-V-IX complex leading to poor adhesion. Diagnosis is made by absent response to ristocetin in platelet function study. A close differential with similar results is von Willebrand disease which can be differentiated by normal von Willebrand factor levels and pattern. Treatment includes platelet transfusions for significant bleeding. Stem cell transplant will be curative in this condition.

May-Hegglin Anomaly: This is an autosomal dominant condition characterized by thrombocytopenia, giant platelets, large inclusions in granulocytes and monocytes known as Dohle bodies and presence of physical defects like hearing loss, renal failure and cataract. The platelet count is moderately low in the range of 80–100,000/mm^3 but with significant bleeding due to associated platelet dysfunction. The defect is in the *MYH9* gene that codes for Myosin II-A, which is the only protein expressed in platelets and neutrophils, which explains the characteristic defects seen in platelets and neutrophils. Desmopressin (DDAVP), antifibrinolytic agents, helps to control bleeding. Platelet transfusions are rarely required.

Gray platelet syndrome: It is an autosomal recessive disorder with mild thrombocytopenia and significant bleeding. The platelets are unable to store alpha granule proteins. This leads to poor aggregation especially with thrombin, adenosine diphosphate and collagen. The platelets appear large, gray and bland with vacuolations. The treatment is platelet transfusion for significant bleeding.

Inherited Thrombocytopenia with Immunodeficiency

This includes Wiskott-Aldrich syndrome and hemophagocytic lymphohistiocytosis.

Wiskott-Aldrich syndrome: This is an X-linked disorder characterized by thrombocytopenia, eczema and immunodeficiency. It is caused by mutations in the WASP gene located at Xp11-12 band. The Wiskott-Aldrich syndrome protein is known to be involved in the signal transduction and it regulates actin filament assembly in platelets as well as lymphocytes affecting their cytoskeleton. This explains the association of thrombocytopenia and immunodeficiency. Patients present with thrombocytopenia early in life with more bleeding than expected based on the platelet counts. The platelets are small in volume and the mean platelet volume is characteristically low (as is also seen in patients with TORCH group of infection). Patient usually has lower GI bleeding. Eczema and immunodeficiency develop as the child grows. Some patients have milder phenotype with minimal immunodeficiency as the defect is restricted only to the platelets even when they have the same WASP gene mutations (though restricted only to the exon 2 of the gene), these patients are grouped as X-linked thrombocytopenia. Often these patients are mistaken as ITP later in the life.

The treatment of Wiskott-Aldrich syndrome includes control of bleeding with platelet transfusions and treatment of infections. In those with difficulty, splenectomy will also help as also IVIg at times. Bone marrow transplantation is the only curative treatment possible at present. Around 10% of the patients can progress to develop lymphoma later in their life.

Hemophagocytic lymphohistiocytosis: This is a rare but interesting disease caused by mutations in the genes for perforin or granzymes involved in the killing of phagocytosed material by the phagosomes of the macrophage-monocyte series and natural killer cells. Absence of effective killing by the phagosomes leads to unnecessary stimulation of the macrophages and monocytes leading to production of cytokines by these cells leading to what is described as cytokine storm which leads to all the symptoms like hemophagocytosis, cytopenias, liver dysfunction, central nervous system (CNS) changes, fever, DIC, increased triglycerides levels, etc. It is an autosomal recessive disorder which can present even at or soon after the birth with fever, thrombocytopenia, convulsions, hyperbilirubenemia and cytopenias. The diagnosis is made by high index of suspicion and demonstrating hemophagocytes in the bone marrow or organs like liver, spleen or lymph nodes. Sometimes hemophagocytes are also seen on the peripheral blood smears. The treatment includes use of steroids and VP-16 to induce remission. Bone marrow transplant will cure those who do not respond to conservative management.

Inherited Thrombocytopenia with Bone Marrow Failure

This includes three disorders, i.e. congenital amegakaryocytic thrombocytopenia, TAR syndrome and Fanconi's anemia.

Congenital amegakaryocytic thrombocytopenia: This is a rare autosomal recessive disorder presenting as neonatal thrombocytopenia which progresses over the time to total bone marrow failure. It presents with bleeding and thrombocytopenia in the first few days to weeks of life where it may be confused with many other common etiologies especially alloimmune thrombocytopenia. Around 20% of the patients can develop intracranial hemorrhage. 10–30% of them can have associated orthopedic or CNS anomalies. It is only when the patient dose not recover that a bone marrow is ordered which will pick up absent or grossly reduced megakaryocytes with normal granulopoietic and erythropoietic elements. It is caused by mutations in the c-mpl genes which results in marked maturation of the megakaryocytes and its precursors. As the action of Tpo via c-mpl is vital for maturation of other hemopoietic cells, even the other series will get affected with time including the stem cells due to lack of preservation of apoptosis induced by Tpo. This explains why there is total bone marrow failure with time. While platelet transfusions help controlling

from immunodeficiency, autoimmunity and malignancy carrying a score of 1. The most severe disease manifesting with all of the above symptom carry a score of 5 while the least severe ones are those presenting with only neutropenia or myelodysplasia carry a score of 0.

Investigations reveal small platelets on smear (<7 fL), lymphopenia, poor T-cell response to mitogens, reduced levels of immunoglobulin (IgG), IgA, IgM and raised levels of IgE. Flow cytometry-based WASp expression is used as a screening tool for the diagnosis, which can be confirmed by *WAS* gene sequencing.

Management principles include prevention of infection and major bleeding till the patient is taken up for an allogeneic hematopoietic stem cell transplant. This includes regular administration of intravenous immunoglobulin (IVIg), avoidance of live attenuated vaccines, aggressive treatment of any infection, septran prophylaxis and antivirals prophylaxis; in case, someone has a history of documented viral infection and limiting use of platelet transfusions for situations like perioperative needs or treatment of severe mucosal hemorrhages to prevent alloimmunization. The definite cure lies in a matched related or unrelated stem cell transplant. Human leukocyte antigen (HLA) typing should be done for the entire family as soon as the diagnosis is established. If no matched family donor is identified, a search for an unrelated donor is initiated. Other forms of transplants like haploidentical transplant is still in experimental stage for patients with WAS. The unique post-transplant complications include development of autoimmunity, severe viral infection and higher chances of development of malignancies.

Thrombocytopenia with Absent Radius Syndrome[2,3]

Thrombocytopenia-absent radius syndrome is characterized by bilateral radial aplasia with thrombocytopenia. The feature that distinguishes this disorder with Fanconi's anemia is presence of thumb in both hands. Severe forms of disease can have absence of humerus or more severe limb anomalies like phocomelia and lower limb involvement as well.

Patient may also have short stature, facial dysmorphology and renal or cardiac abnormality. Young children with this disorder are often found to have cow's milk allergy and this worsens the thrombocytopenia. Discontinuation of cow's milk often resolves the symptoms of diarrhea. Thrombocytopenia improves with age and some adults have normal platelet counts.

Congenital Amegakaryocytic Thrombocytopenia[3]

This is a serious condition characterized by bleeding manifestations within 1st week of life. Platelet size and morphology is normal. The degree of thrombocytopenia is usually severe and worsens with age. By 2nd decade of life these children develop aplastic anemia. There is a poor response to usage of IVIg. Bone marrow examination reveals absence of megakaryocytes. The only cure for this condition is bone marrow transplant preferable from a matched family donor.

May-Hegglin Anomaly[4]

This is a type of *MYH9*-related disorder (*MYH9*-RD) characterized by macrothrombocytopenia from birth with autosomal inheritance. May-Hegglin anomaly, Epstein syndrome, Fechtner syndrome or Sebastian syndrome once considered different identities are now known to be heterozygous pathogenic variants in *MYH9* and regarded as one disorder known as *MYH9*-RD. Blood counts reveal thrombocytopenia and peripheral smear examination shows large-sized platelets. Neutrophils may show Döhle like bodies, which are light blue inclusion like material. *MYH9* protein aggregates in cytoplasm of neutrophils can be demonstrated by immunofluorescence of the peripheral smear.

The nonhematological manifestations worsen with age and include a spectrum of sensorineural hearing loss, glomerulopathy, presenile cataract and hepatitis. Most patients have stably low platelet counts throughout the life but some patients present with intermittent mucocutaneous bleeding. Occasional individuals can have severe bleeding manifestations. Treatment of bleeding comprises of local measures and usage of tranexamic acid or desmopressin. Platelet transfusions are reserved only for severe cases to avoid alloimmunization.

Bernard-Soulier Syndrome[5]

This is characterized by an absent or dysfunctional (Bolzano variant) glycoprotein (Gp) Ib-IX-V receptor on platelets that lead to their poor adhesion to subendothelial von Willebrand factor (vWF). The usual presentation is that of a bleeding child with thrombocytopenia, giant platelets and markedly prolonged bleeding time. Bleeding can range from bruises to mucosal bleeds, severe menorrhagia or even intracranial bleeds. The diagnosis is based on an absent ristocetin-induced platelet aggregation assay. Treatment mainly consists of platelet transfusions at the time of severe bleeding or perioperatively. As with other inherited platelet disorders, if possible HLA-matched platelets should be administered to avoid alloimmunization.

Velocardiofacial Syndrome[5]

Abnormal pharyngeal arch development due to a microdeletion at chromosome 22q11.2 leads to this syndrome. Platelet receptor gene GpIb also located on same chromosome is also deficient in these individuals leading to macrothrombocytopenia. Patients commonly present with palatal abnormalities, facial defects, congenital heart disease, immunodeficiency and thymic defects.

Storage Pool Disorders[6]

The two main types associated with thrombocytopenia are the (1) alpha-granule and (2) the dense-granule disorders.

Alpha-granule Disorders

Gray platelet syndrome gets its name from their appearance on staining with Wright-Giemsa stain. The underlying problem is deficiency of alpha-granules that makes the platelets look large and gray. Patients have mild-to-moderate thrombocytopenia with bleeding tendency.

Other form of alpha-granule disease is Paris-Trousseau syndrome due to deletion of long arm of chromosome 11. It has autosomal inheritance and presents with low platelets, bleeding tendencies, developmental lag, cardiac and craniofacial anomalies along with short stature.

Quebec platelet disorder is a rare but unique bleeding disorder characterized by delayed onset bleeding after trauma. There is increased fibrinolysis due to overexpression of urokinase-type plasminogen activator in platelets that degrades alpha-granule proteins and causes clot lysis.

Arthrogryposis, renal dysfunction, and cholestasis (ARC) syndrome presents with persistent joint contractures secondary to degeneration of anterior motor neurons. Mild-to-moderate bleeding tendency is because of platelet alpha-granule deficiency leading to poor aggregation. Most patients die in infancy secondary to the neuronal disease and renal tubular dysfunction.

Dense-granule Disorders

Hermansky-Pudlak syndromes and Chédiak-Higashi syndromes are dense-granule disorders but have normal platelet counts and hence not discussed in this section. Griscelli syndrome is characterized by silver gray hair with albinism, immunodeficiency, mild neutropenia and thrombocytopenia, hepatosplenomegaly and neurological abnormalities.

Fanconi Anemia[7,8]

Fanconi anemia is the most common inherited bone marrow failure syndrome. It presents with a wide variety of hematological disorders. Most patients have normal blood counts in newborn period. Macrocytosis is usually the first abnormality in the blood counts followed by thrombocytopenia and then pancytopenia due to bone marrow failure that develops at a median age of 7 years. Bleeding in newborn period is rare. Patients with Fanconi anemia often present with skeletal abnormalities like radial ray, scoliosis, vertebral anomalies, skin pigmentation, café-au-lait spots, short stature, hearing and visual defects, microphthalmia, mental retardation, genitourinary and gastrointestinal defects, etc. Chromosomal breakage analysis using diepoxybutane or mitomycin C picks up the chromosomal fragility characteristic of this disorder. Genetic and prenatal diagnosis is now available for diagnosis of Fanconi anemia. These children usually die in early age due to untreated marrow failure syndrome or hematological malignancies or later in adulthood secondary to squamous cell neoplasms of head and neck area. Bone marrow transplant from a matched donor offers the only chance of cure of hematological issues in these children.

Trisomy 21 (Down's Syndrome)[9]

This is the most common malformation syndrome seen in children. It is characterized by typical facies, hypotonia, epicanthic eye folds, mental retardation, typical dermatoglyphics, congenital heart disease and many other malformations of varying severity. These children have predisposition for hematological abnormalities in form of neutrophilia, thrombocytopenia, thrombocytosis, anemia, transient myeloproliferative syndrome and cancers. Thrombocytopenia is usually mild, however 6% of children can have platelets less than 50,000/mm^3 in their 1st week of life. This is usually self-resolving. Thrombocytopenia associated with transient abnormal myelopoiesis is also self-limiting in most cases; however, the severe forms especially those associated with significant organ infiltration may need low-dose chemotherapy. These children are more likely to develop leukemia's at a later age.

Trisomy 18 (Edward Syndrome)[10]

This is the second most common malformation syndrome characterized by mental retardation, clenched hand, tendency of overlapping index finger over the third, fifth finger over the fourth, prominent occiput, short sternum, narrow pelvis, absent supraorbital ridges, hypertonia, cardiac defects and characteristic dermatoglyphics.

Trisomy 13 (Patau Syndrome)[10]

This is characterized by holoprosencephaly, cleft lip or cleft palate, sloping forehead, defects of eyes and nose, polydactyly, narrow hyperconvex nails and posterior scalp defects.

Most children die within the 1st month of life and are not investigated in detail. However, a study done on hematological parameters in children with above two syndromes during the 1st week of life showed thrombocytopenia to be the most common abnormality with incidence of 83% in trisomy 18 and 75% in children with trisomy 13.

Kasabach-Merritt Syndrome[11]

This is an association between giant hemangiomas and thrombocytopenia secondary to entrapment and destruction of platelets in the hemangioma The usual presentation is that of a young infant with significant thrombocytopenia and an obvious hemangiomas. However, sometimes a hemangiomas is detected on investigations being done for an undiagnosed symptomatic thrombocytopenia. Treatment comprises of management of hemangiomas either by surgery, radiotherapy, steroids, interferon or vincristine. Surgery is often not possible and radiotherapy carries serious long-term side effects.

CONCLUSION

Thrombocytopenia is a fairly common hematological disorder in newborns. However, syndromic thrombocytopenia is a rare condition leading to low platelets in a newborn with an underlying genetic disorder. A good clinical examination and basic tests like karyotyping helps to identify the underlying disorder in most newborns.

KEY POINTS

- Syndromic thrombocytopenia is diagnosed when a newborn with an underlying syndrome has low platelets and other causes of thrombocytopenia such as sepsis have been ruled out.
- A good clinical examination and basic genetic tests are enough to diagnose these rare conditions.
- A genetic consult helps appropriately manage and counsel these families.

REFERENCES

1. Buchbinder D, Nugent DJ, Fillipovich AH. Wiskott-Aldrich syndrome: diagnosis, current management, and emerging treatments. Appl Clin Genet. 2014;7:55-66.
2. Greenhalgh KL, Howell RT, Bottani A, Ancliff PJ, Brunner HG, Verschuuren-Bemelmans CC, et al. Thrombocytopenia-absent radius syndrome: a clinical genetic study. J Med Genet. 2002;39(12):876-81.
3. Ballmaier M, Germeshausen M. Congenital amegakaryocytic thrombocytopenia: clinical presentation, diagnosis, and treatment. Semin Thromb Hemost. 2011;37(6):673-81.
4. Fatima S. May-Hegglin anomaly: rare entity with review of literature. Indian J Hematol Blood Transfus. 2012;28(1):58-60.
5. Diz-Küçükkaya R. Inherited platelet disorders including Glanzmann thrombasthenia and Bernard-Soulier syndrome. Hematology Am Soc Hematol Educ Program. 2013;2013:268-75.
6. Salles II, Feys HB, Iserbyt BF, De Meyer SF, Vanhoorelbeke K, Deckmyn H. Inherited traits affecting platelet function. Blood Rev. 2008;22(3):155-72.
7. Soulier J. Fanconi anemia. Hematology Am Soc Hematol Educ Program. 2011;2011:492-7.
8. Tischkowitz MD, Hodgson SV. Fanconi anaemia. J Med Genet. 2003;40(1):1-10.
9. Henry E, Walker D, Wiedmeier SE, Christensen RD. Hematological abnormalities during the first week of life among neonates with Down syndrome: data from a multihospital healthcare system. Am J Med Genet A. 2007;143A(1):42-50.
10. Wiedmeier SE, Henry E, Christensen RD. Hematological abnormalities during the first week of life among neonates with trisomy 18 and trisomy 13: data from a multi-hospital healthcare system. Am J Med Genet A. 2008;146A(3):312-20.
11. Croteau SE, Liang MG, Kozakewich HP, Alomari AI, Fishman SJ, Mulliken JB, et al. Kaposiform hemangioendothelioma: atypical features and risks of Kasabach-Merritt phenomenon in 107 referrals. J Pediatr. 2013;162(1):142-7.

CHAPTER

24

Qualitative Platelet Disorders

Purvi Kadakia Kutty

INTRODUCTION

Platelets play a crucial role in hemostasis. Platelet dysfunction due to congenital and acquired etiologies is one of the common causes of bleeding encountered in clinical practice. Mucocutaneous bleeding of variable severity in a newborn with a normal platelet count suggests a disorder of platelet function. In this chapter, etiology, pathophysiology of the main inherited and acquired platelet qualitative defects are reviewed with highlights on newer investigations and approach to treatment. An attempt has been made to summarize the spectrum of clinical manifestations of these disorders and their management.

PATHOPHYSIOLOGY

Platelets are instrumental in the process of forming primary hemostatic plug by interacting with the subendothelium-bound von Willebrand factor (vWF) via the membrane glycoprotein (GP) complex GP Ib. This leads to further recruitment of platelets mediating platelet aggregation via GP IIb/IIIa complex. This is followed by platelet activation and release of proaggregatory substances, which act to consolidate the initial hemostatic plug and lead to restoration of normal vessel architecture.

Disruption in any of the events and biochemical processes may lead to platelet dysfunction, which may be either inherited or acquired.

ETIOLOGY

Platelet dysfunction disorders broadly fall in two categories:

1. Hereditary:
   - Glanzmann's thrombasthenia (GT)
   - Bernard-Soulier syndrome (BSS)
   - *Platelet release disorders:* (a) Membrane defect, (b) Defect of metabolic pathway of release reaction, (c) Storage pool defect (SPD) and (d) Associated with von Willebrand disease (vWD)
   - Alport syndrome
   - May-Hegglin syndrome
   - Gray platelet syndrome
   - Ehlers-Danlos syndrome
   - Osteogenesis imperfecta (OI)
   - Marfan syndrome
   - Pseudoxanthoma elasticum
   - Miscellaneous.
2. Acquired.

CLINICAL FEATURES OF PLATELET FUNCTIONAL DEFECTS

The initial diagnosis of a platelet function disorder relies on careful evaluation of clinical findings and a detailed medical history, including family history. Most of the inherited platelet function disorders present in childhood. Following are some of the typical features, which help to make a clinical diagnosis of qualitative platelet disorders:

- *Age at presentation*: The inherited platelet disorders of the severe type usually present in early childhood.
- *Type of bleeding*: Milder variants may be asymptomatic, bleeding may range from mild bruising, epistaxis, gingival bleeding, trauma or surgery provoked bleeding to severe life-threatening mucocutaneous hemorrhage.
- *Site of bleeding*: Mucocutaneous, rarely GT, visceral and intracranial hemorrhage have been reported.
- Family history.
- *Drug history*: To rule out acquired causes of platelet dysfunction.
- *Syndromic association*: Oculocutaneous albinism in CHS, hyperextensible joints in Ehlers-Danlos syndrome, cataracts in MH19 disorders.

HEREDITARY PLATELET DYSFUNCTION DISORDERS

Glanzmann's Thrombasthenia

Glanzmann thrombasthenia is a genetic platelet disorder in which the platelets have qualitative or quantitative deficiencies of the fibrinogen receptor $\alpha_{IIb}\beta_3$. It is a rare autosomal recessive platelet function disorder, named after the Swiss pediatrician Dr Eduard Glanzmann, who first described it in 1918. The genes of the $\alpha_{IIb}\beta_3$ or the GP-IIb/IIIa complex are located on the chromosome 17. The $\alpha_{IIb}\beta_3$ GP is a calcium-dependent heterodimer receptor complex, which binds platelets to fibrinogen. About 80,000 GP IIb/IIIa receptors are present on the platelet surface and 50% activity of the protein is enough to support platelet aggregation. More than 70 mutations are described that affect platelet aggregation and thus prolong bleeding time (BT). The clinical picture is characterized by mucosal bleeding typically presenting early in infancy and is known to have a slightly higher female preponderance.

Prognosis

Bleeding problems can be variable in severity in patients with GT, but the prognosis remains good with appropriate supportive care. The bleeding is primarily mucocutaneous in nature. Generally, bleeding incidence decreases with age.

The work-up for GT may include complete blood cell count, prothrombin time and activated partial thromboplastin time. Flow cytometry and monoclonal antibodies confirm the diagnosis. Treatment of GT includes preventive measures such as avoidance of antiplatelet agents [e.g. aspirin and nonsteroidal anti-inflammatory drugs (NSAIDs)], iron or folate supplementation for anemia, and vaccination for hepatitis B due to the infectious risks associated with multiple transfusions.

Treatment

Patients with GT who are bleeding require platelet transfusions. Because patients are likely to require multiple transfusions during their lifetime, they should receive leukocyte-depleted blood products in order to avoid alloimmunization.

Patients with Glanzmann thrombasthenia who require surgical intervention should receive platelet transfusions preoperatively to prevent excessive bleeding during surgery. Further platelet transfusions are considered, based on maintaining hemostasis.

Alternatively, recombinant activated factor VII (rFVIIa) may be useful for preventing or controlling perioperative bleeding.

Recombinant activated factor VII has been used in patients with antibodies to platelet GP-IIb/IIIa and/or human leukocyte antigen (HLA) that render transfusions ineffective. In July 2014, The Food and Drug Administration (FDA) approved rFVIIa for treatment of bleeding episodes and perioperative management in adults and children with GT that is refractory to platelet transfusions with or without antibodies to platelets.

Bernard-Soulier Syndrome

Bernard-Soulier syndrome (BSS) is a rare autosomal recessive bleeding disorder characterized by deficiency of GP Ib/IX/V complex, the receptor for vWF, which mediates the initial interaction of platelets with the subendothelial components. Thrombocytopenia, prolonged BT and abnormally large platelets characterize it.

This defect results in deficient binding of vWF to the platelet membrane resulting in defective platelet adhesion. Platelets with decreased sialylated GP Ib are associated with reduced survival and this leads to thrombocytopenia. BSS platelets do not aggregate ristocetin. This is not corrected by the addition of normal plasma as seen in vWD. As with other inherited platelet function defects, BSS presents with early childhood onset of mucocutaneous bleeds, easy bruising, epistaxis and abnormally prolonged bleeding from small injury disproportionate to the degree of thrombocytopenia.

Life-threatening bleeds are associated with major trauma or surgery. Dental extraction may be troublesome. Women often suffer with menorrhagia and severe bleeding may occur after childbirth. Diagnostic evaluation must include a complete blood count and a peripheral smear examination, which shows giant platelets. BT is nearly always prolonged with delayed closure time on the platelet function analyzer-100 (PFA-100).

A definitive diagnosis is conducted by flow cytometry measurement using CD61 antibodies. The bleeding tendency is variable and needs to be assessed individually. In addition to the investigations mentioned above patients should have liver function tests, blood group and iron status measured as children, adolescents, and women are often anemic and iron-deficient requiring supplementation. Many of these children are misdiagnosed as immune thrombocytopenia or alloimmune thrombocytopenia in infancy, leading to inappropriate steroid therapy, hence BSS should be distinguished from other causes of thrombocytopenia and giant platelet syndromes. Infants with thrombocytopenia may present a diagnostic challenge. Consanguinity of the parents may be an important indicator of a possible autosomal recessive condition. In the affected infant with BSS, normally no treatment is needed unless there is bleeding or in rare cases where the platelet count is low, and there is danger of spontaneous hemorrhage.

Disorders of Platelet Release Reaction

This group includes membrane defects, abnormalities of platelet granules, SPDs and defects of secretion and thromboxane (TX) synthesis.

Platelet Granule Disorders

Platelet dysfunction can result from deficiencies of the storage organelles, granule content and a biochemical or structural defect in the secretory pathway. These disorders are associated with systemic manifestations and may occasionally present with a mild bleeding diathesis. These include:

- Hermansky-Pudlak syndrome (HPS)
- Chédiak-Higashi syndrome (CHS)
- Idiopathic dense-granule deficiency.

Dense granules are a lysosome-related organelle that are part of a family of highly specialized, cell-type-specific organelles that include melanosomes and lytic granules of cytotoxic T lymphocytes and natural killer cells. In general, the platelet defect in dense-granule disorders causes a mild-to-moderate bleeding defect with easy bruising, epistaxis and menorrhagia, but the possibility of significant surgical- or trauma-induced bleeding.

Hermansky-Pudlak Syndrome

Hermansky-Pudlak syndrome is a recessively inherited autosomal disease, which is a genetically, clinically and biologically diverse disorder. It was first described by two Czechoslovakian pathologists, Hermansky and Pudlak in 1959, and is characterized by tyrosinase-positive oculocutaneous albinism, bleeding diathesis due to platelet dysfunction and systemic complications associated to lysosomal dysfunction, including pulmonary fibrosis, granulomatous colitis, neutropenia and mild immunodeficiency.

Patients with HPS are known to have mutations of either HPS1 or HPS4, which are located on chromosome 10(10q2). All the proteins encoded by the HPS genes are involved in intracellular vesicular trafficking, controlling processes such as protein sorting, vesicle docking and fusion. The course of the disease is usually poor.

Chédiak-Higashi Syndrome

Chédiak-Higashi syndrome is an autosomal recessive dense granule that arises from a mutation of a lysosomal trafficking regulator protein, which is associated with oculocutaneous albinism, recurrent pyogenic infections and a lymphoproliferative accelerated phase in the majority of patients with death usually occurring in the 1st decade. The accelerated phase is associated with fever, bleeding episodes, sepsis and multiorgan failure. The pathognomonic feature in this condition is very large peroxidase-positive cytoplasmic granules or "giant inclusion bodies" in hematopoietic (neutrophils) and nonhematopoietic cells. There is no specific treatment option for CHS. Bone marrow transplant may be the only curative modality of treatment.

Idiopathic Dense-granule Disorder

Idiopathic dense-granule disorder is a group of qualitative platelet defect, with an unclear genotypic variant and a mild phenotypic variant. The bleeding manifestations are due to deficiency in the dense granules.

Diagnostic features of dense-granule disorders: In SPDs, there is a reduction or absence of dense bodies leading to a reduction in the total amount of adenosine triphosphate (ATP) and adenosine diphosphate (ADP) and a marked increase in the ratio of ATP to total platelet ADP.

A defect in platelet dense granule content or release is common to HPS, CHS and the idiopathic dense-granule disorders.

Hermansky-Pudlak syndrome and CHS have in common oculocutaneous albinism, but can be distinguished by the large peroxidase-positive cytoplasmic granules in neutrophils in CHS. In addition, CHS is usually lethal within the 1st decade.

Characteristic features of dense-granule deficiency on light transmission aggregometry (LTA) are: (1) high concentrations of ADP elicit full and irreversible aggregation, (2) the absence of second wave aggregation to adrenaline, (3) a delayed and impaired response to collagen and (4) impaired aggregation to arachidonic acid and ristocetin.

A marked reduction in both the content of ADP and ratio of ADP to ATP or an absence of release of ATP is diagnostic of a platelet dense-granule disorder. Decreased numbers or absence of dense granules can be confirmed by electron microscopy (EM).

Treatment: The treatment principles for dense-granule disorders are generally supportive and include preventive and local measures as outlined for mild platelet function defects. Some disorders, like CHS, HPS, the only curative option is bone marrow transplantation.

Alpha-granule Disorders

Genetic deficiencies of alpha-granules cause congenital bleeding disorders, which are termed as storage pool deficiencies. The most common SPD described is Gray platelet syndrome (GPS). Few others described include Paris-Trousseau or Jacobsen syndrome. Quebec platelet syndrome and arthrogryposis-renal dysfunction-cholestasis (ARC).

Gray Platelet Syndrome

This is an extremely rare bleeding disorder caused by absence of alpha granules in platelets with less than 100 cases reported worldwide. GPS is characterized by thrombocytopenia and abnormally large agranular platelets in peripheral smear.

Both autosomal recessive and autosomal dominance patterns of inheritance have been described. The defect in GPS is due to the failure of megakaryocytes to package secretory proteins into the alpha granules. Mild-to-moderate bone marrow myelofibrosis has been described. The appearance of "gray", misshapen and slightly large platelets on a blood film is characteristic. Patients are affected by mild-to-moderate bleeding tendencies. EM of platelets demonstrates reduced or absence of alpha granules.

Paris-Trousseau or Jacobsen Syndrome

Paris-Trousseau or Jacobsen syndrome is an autosomal dominant inherited disorder characterized by relatively mild bleeding diathesis. FL1 gene deletion on chromosome 11q, a transcription factor essential for megakaryocytopoiesis is responsible for the defect. In addition to the mild bleeding tendency these patients have dysmegakaryopoiesis and abnormal platelets with giant granules detected by EM. These children are also known to have craniofacial malformations and cardiac defects.

Quebec Platelet Syndrome (or Factor V Quebec)

Quebec platelet syndrome is an autosomal dominant, extremely rare disorder, which was originally described in a family from the province of Quebec in Canada. The genetic cause of this disorder has been recently identified as a mutation involving an extra copy of *uPA* (urokinase plasminogen activator) gene that accelerates blood clot breakdown. This is the reason why bleeding responds to fibrinolytic inhibitors. Individuals are at risk of a number of bleeding events including joint bleeds and hematuria. There is no characteristic morphological or platelet aggregometry features, so many cases may be undiagnosed.

Arthrogryposis-Renal Dysfunction-Cholestasis

Arthrogryposis-renal dysfunction-cholestasis is an autosomal recessive multisystem disorder associated with platelet dysfunction caused by a deficiency in platelet alpha granules. This is a very rare disorder characterized by joint contractures, kidney dysfunction and cholestasis and is associated with a poor prognosis.

Disorders of Platelet Receptors and Signal Transduction Pathways

The disorders of platelet receptors and pathways of signaling are still incompletely understood. Platelet adhesion receptors are the key initiators of platelet activation at the site of vascular injury. A common platelet response to all agonists is secretion of granule contents and secretion-dependent signal amplification. Defects in the above mentioned signaling pathways contribute to platelet dysfunction.

The affected individuals present with mild bleeding defects due to compensatory effect of other membrane receptors and pathways.

Diagnostic Criteria

These disorders are associated with normal platelet count and morphology. Platelets usually show a decrease in primary aggregation to one or more agonists, along with absence of secondary aggregation in response to standard laboratory agonists. This group of disorders may be distinguished from SPDs by the demonstration of normal platelet nucleotide content and nucleotide release.

Defects in Thromboxane A2 Formation or Thromboxane A2 Receptor Function

Thromboxane A2 (TXA2) is a type of TX that is produced by activated platelets, which stimulates platelet aggregation. Hence a defective TXA2 receptor function is associated with impaired platelet aggregation to arachidonic acid and a variable response to other agonists, sometimes comprising a reduced primary wave and absent secondary wave. The clinical picture may be variable.

Adenosine Diphosphate Receptor Defects

Adenine nucleotides act on platelets through two G protein-coupled receptors for ADP, P2Y1 and P2Y12. The P2Y1 initiates platelet aggregation. The P2Y12 receptor is the molecular target for clopidogrel and is responsible for completion of aggregation to ADP. Both the receptors play a role in signal transduction pathways in response to ATP or ADP.

Collagen Receptor Defects

The exact principal by which collagen receptor defects affect platelet activation is unclear. It may be due to a secondary factor, such as, e.g. immune thrombocytopenia or the presence of a myeloproliferative disorder. Very few cases have been described so far.

Adrenoceptor Defects

Aggregation response to adrenaline may be impaired in a subset of individuals of the normal population who remain asymptomatic. This feature has to be differentiated from selective absence of an aggregation response to adrenaline, which has been described as a heritable trait in association with easy bruising and reduced expression of platelet α2-adrenoceptors.

Scott Syndrome and Related Disorders

Scott syndrome is a rare congenital bleeding disorder. It was originally described in 1979. Later it was demonstrated that the defect is inherited in an autosomal recessive pattern. In Scott syndrome, the mechanism for translocating phosphatidylserine (PS) to the platelet membrane is defective leading to a significantly reduced ability to promote both tenase and prothrombinase activity on the platelet surface. This leads to impaired thrombin formation. Recently, a novel missense mutation has been found in the gene that encodes the lipid transporter ABCA1, which resulted in altered protein trafficking and reduced PS translocation in a patient with Scott syndrome. Clinically patients present postinjury or procedure bleeds, which may be severe. The prothrombin consumption index is a useful screening test for Scott syndrome; mainstay of treatment is platelet transfusions.

A similar clinical condition, termed as Stormorken syndrome, has also been described in one family that presented with platelets with so-called "inverse Scott syndrome". The molecular basis for Stormorken syndrome is not yet known. This disorder is characterized by mild bleeding tendency, thrombocytopenia, asplenia, miosis and muscular dystrophy. Scott syndrome and Stormorken syndrome can be easily diagnosed using flow cytometry.

ACQUIRED PLATELET FUNCTION DEFECTS

This group of disorder is more frequently encountered in clinical practice. Platelet disorder is due to secondary disease or condition and affects platelet function with variable bleeding manifestations **(Box 24.1)**.

Box 24.1 Causes of acquired platelet dysfunction
• Drugs • Herbal supplements and foods • Liver disease • Renal failure • Cardiopulmonary bypass and extracorporeal membrane oxygenation • Myeloproliferative disorders • Myelodysplastic syndromes • Dysproteinemia • Diabetes mellitus • Trauma • Platelet antibody-induced platelet dysfunction

Antiplatelet drugs are the most common cause of acquired platelet defects leading to bleeding. Aspirin, clopidogrel and integrin receptor antagonists are well known prototypes of antiplatelet drugs. Widely used NSAIDs, antibiotics, certain foods, spices, and vitamins have been reported to impair platelet function. In contrast to inherited platelet disorders, acquired platelet function defects are much more frequent in clinical practice. Platelet dysfunction has also been reported in patients with uremia, liver dysfunction, cardiac bypass procedures, sepsis or infections, leukemia and conditions including disseminated intravascular coagulation (DIC). Their pathogenesis is widespread and heterogeneous. Clinically acquired platelet dysfunction can present at any age and range in severity from mild to life-threatening bleeding manifestations. However, laboratory findings may not be correlated with clinical risk. Knowledge of which factors affect bleeding risk is important in optimizing patient care. Treatment approaches and prognosis vary according to the underlying cause of platelet dysfunction and the associated disease.

INVESTIGATIONS

The approach to a patient with suspected platelet function defect requires a detailed clinical assessment of bleeding history including any significant family history and drug intake, followed by physical examination and an appropriate battery of investigations. The diagnostic evaluation of platelet disorders is complex, poorly standardized and time consuming. This coupled with the wide spectrum of a known range of disorders some of which are very rare, presents a significant challenge to even the best diagnostic laboratory.

Laboratory investigations of platelet number and function are therefore recommended in any patient where bleeding symptoms cannot be fully explained by standard clinical tests.

RECOMMENDATIONS FOR SPECIMEN COLLECTION AND PROCESSING

Similar for other tests of hemostasis, the investigation of platelet function defects is vulnerable to preanalytical variables. It is recommended that samples are collected either in syringes or evacuated tubes. The sample should be collected in 3.2% sodium citrate tubes. A blood or citrate ratio of 9:1 is recommended; higher concentration of citrate over chelates Ca^{++} and subsequently interferes with later platelet function. It must be received within 2 hours of collection. All samples must be gently inverted, and maintained at room temperature (20–25°C) during transport and storage. The samples with low hematocrits less than 35% or low platelet counts less than 100,000 may exhibit false positive results. Clotted samples and an elevated erythrocyte sedimentation rate (ESR) may also interfere with results. Pneumatic tube system should not be used to transport the sample.

Laboratory panel for platelet function defects includes:

- Platelet number, size and morphology
- Global screening tests of platelet hemostatic function
- Specific assays of platelet function.

Platelet Number, Size and Morphology

A complete blood count with review of peripheral blood smear should be the first step in the evaluation of a platelet function disorder.

The measurement of platelet number and size using automated cell counters and blood film analysis is highly sensitive and specific for numerical platelet disorders and is therefore valuable to eliminate thrombocytopenia. Giant platelets on peripheral smear may be supportive of BSS. Absent clumping is supportive of GT. Large inclusion granules in white cells are visible on smears in CHS.

Global Screening Tests of Platelet Hemostatic Function

The most widely performed tests for screening platelet function disorders are currently the template BT and the PFA-100 closure time. If normal results they rule out diagnosis of platelet function disorders so that further specialized testing can be avoided.

Other commercial platelet function assay systems are also available, including those designed to measure the effect of antiplatelet drugs. Thromboelastography (TEG) and rotational thromboelastometry (ROTEM) provide global tests of hemostasis and platelet function and are mainly used within the surgical setting.

Bleeding Time

The BT described by Duke in 1912 is the oldest test of platelet function. It measures:

- Vessel integrity
- Platelet integrity
- Protein/platelet interaction.

Methods

- Duke (1912): Earlobe
- Ivy (1941): Volar surface of forearm with blood pressure (BP) cuff inflated to 40 mm Hg
- Meckel (1969): Standardized template device
- Simplate or Surgicutt method (modification of Ivy).

The greatest source of variation in the interpretation of the BT is due to standardization, patient variables and operator dependency. Hence, it is useful only as a screening test for platelet plug formation and capillary integrity. It is not a gold standard diagnostic tool for platelet function defects. It is not recommended due to poor sensitivity and specificity.

Closure Time by the Platelet Function Analyzer

PFA-100 system was designed to measure primary hemostasis in vitro by uniquely simulating the in vivo hemodynamic condition of platelet adhesion, activation and aggregation.

Assay Principle

The PFA-100 device is a test system in which citrated whole blood is aspirated at high shear rates (5,000–6,000s^{-1}) through disposable cartridges containing an aperture coated with either collagen and epinephrine (CEPI) or collagen and ADP (CADP). These agonists trigger platelet adhesion, activation and aggregation leading to rapid occlusion of the aperture and cessation of blood flow. The end-points for each test are time to occlusion of blood flow closure time (CT) or nonclosure if the CT exceeds 300 seconds. The PFA-100 assay system requires small quantities of citrated venous blood (0.8 mL per cartridge) and is therefore useful for studying pediatric samples. Accordingly, the PFA-100 device is widely used as a screening tool to measure global platelet hemostatic function.

Factors that influence PFA-100 closure time: The choice of anticoagulant, specimen collection and transportation techniques and time between sampling and analysis all have critical effects on CT results.

Knowledge of the full blood count is critical for interpreting CT results from the PFA-100. Thrombocytopenia (<100 × 10^9/L) and anemia (<20% hematocrit) often result in prolongation of the CT. CT also correlates inversely with plasma vWF activity in normal subjects and may therefore be longer in patients with blood group O. Cyclooxygenase-1 (COX-1) inhibitors such as aspirin, usually prolong the CEPI CT, but not the CADP CT.

PFA-100 closure time and vWD: Abnormal CT on both cartridges are typical for types 2A, 2B, 2M and 3vWD with a sensitivity of more than 98%.

PFA-100 CT and inherited platelet function disorders: In severe platelet function defects, such as GT, Bernard-Soulier syndrome and platelet type or pseudo-vWD, nonclosure is typical. In many less severe platelet function defects, the CT may be either normal or prolonged; abnormal results are more frequently reported with the CEPI than the CADP cartridge. Thus, the sensitivity of the PFA-100 for mild inherited platelet function defects is difficult to estimate. If the clinical suspicion of a platelet function defect is high, then a PFA result should be confirmed with specific assays of platelet function **(Table 24.1)**.

Specific Assays for Platelet Hemostatic Function

Light Transmission Aggregometry

Light transmission aggregometry (LTA) was invented in the early 1960s and is still regarded as the gold standard for platelet function testing. Platelet aggregation testing measures the ability of various agonists to induce in vitro activation. ADP, epinephrine, collagen, arachidonic acid and ristocetin are the traditional baseline panel of agonists for LTA. A recommended baseline example panel comprises: 2.5 mM ADP, 1.25 mg/mL collagen, 5 mM epinephrine, 1.2 mg/mL ristocetin and 1.0 mM arachidonic acid. LTA patterns seen in platelet function defects are described below, although in clinical practice many of these are rare. Due to natural variations in adrenoreceptors, even a small proportion of normal samples may not have a full aggregation response. Clinical and drug history must also be taken in detail before interpretation of the LTA result. If the initial aggregation results with ADP, collagen or epinephrine are abnormal then retesting should be done with higher to supranormal concentrations of the agonist(s) to confirm a specific defect. If the aggregation to ristocetin is normal then retesting should additionally be performed with low dose (0.5–0.7 mg/mL) ristocetin to check for hyperfunction or gain of function (associated with type 2B and platelet type vWD). If results with 1.2 mg/mL ristocetin are absent then retesting can be performed with addition of an external source of vWF (e.g. cryoprecipitate or a vWF concentrate) to confirm either a vWF or GP-Ib defect. Interpretation of LTA trace may be difficult in various disorders. All abnormal results should be repeated and confirmed with flow cytometry, nucleotide assay or genetic testing if available **(Fig. 24.1)**.

Flow cytometry: Analysis of platelet surface GPs by flow cytometry is a rapid and sensitive technique for the definitive diagnosis of disorders, like GT, Bernard-Soulier syndrome and Scott syndrome, and may also be used to investigate abnormalities in the collagen (GP VI and GP Ia/IIa) and thrombin receptors (PAR-1). The test requires a small sample volume and so is readily applicable to the neonate. Multiple platelet receptors can be analyzed simultaneously.

Platelet nucleotide assays: Lumi-aggregometry is a modification of LTA which measures ATP release from dense granules and provides an important diagnostic tool for determining whether there is any specific deficiency in dense granule numbers or their content (e.g. SPD) or specific defect in degranulation (e.g. release defects).

Table 24.1 Platelet function analyzer (PFA)-100

PFA-100				
	Normal	*Aspirin*	*vWD*	*GT*
CEPI	<140 S (N)	AB	AB	AB
CADP	<100 S (N)	N	AB	AB

Abbreviations: CEPI, collagen and epinephrine; CADP, collagen-adenosine diphosphate; vWD, von Willebrand disease

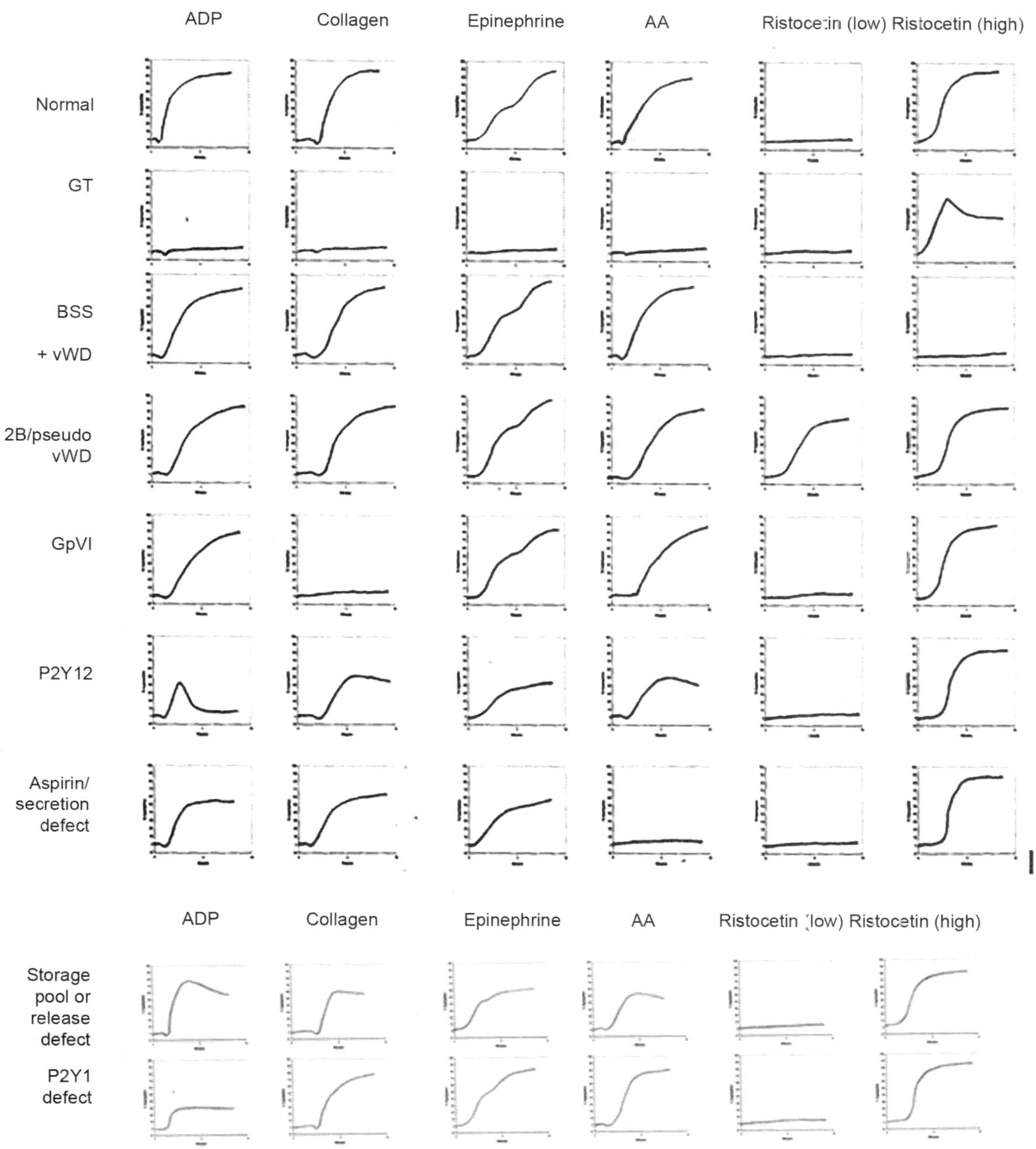

Fig. 24.1 Light transmission aggregometry (LTA) patterns in platelet function defects
Abbreviations: GT, Glanzmann's thrombasthenia; BSS, Bernard-Soulier syndrome; vWD, von Willebrand disease; GP, glycoprotein; ADP, adenosine diphosphate; AA, arachidonic acid

Electron microscopy: The electron microscope is a useful tool in the diagnostic process of syndromes originating from platelet organelle, cytoskeleton and membrane leading to platelet dysfunction. This is available in only few specialized laboratories. It has a role in assessing patients with MHY-9 defects, Paris-Trousseau syndrome, storage pool diseases and Wiskott-Aldrich syndrome (WAS). Whole mount EM is particularly useful for quantifying dense-granule numbers. In HPS, the dense granules are completely absent **(Table 24.2)**.

Table 24.2 Minimal diagnostic criteria for various platelet defects. The pattern of expected platelet function test results are listed for the most common platelet disorders. The result for a potential P2Y1 defect are hypothetical as none described yet

Disorder	*Platelet count/Morphology*	*PFA*	*LTA pattern*	*Nucleotides*	*Flow cytometry*	*Other*
Type 1, 2A and 3 vWD	Normal	CADP/CEPI both equally prolonged. Very prolonged in 2A and 3.	Defective response to high dose ristocetin (correctable by VWF source).	Normal	Normal	vWF panel will confirm subtype
Platelet type or type 2B vWD	Mild thrombocytopenia	Both abnormal	Platelets aggregate on addition of plasma or cryoprecipitate. Gain of function with low-dose ristocetin	Normal	Increased VWF binding to platelets	Abnormal vWF panel in type 2B vWD/Loss of high molecular weight vWF in platelet type vWD
GT	Normal	CADP/CEPI both very prolonged	Profound impairment to all agonists except high-dose ristocetin	Normal	Significantly reduced copy number of $\alpha_{IIb}\beta_3$ (variants, heterozygotes or defective functioning can be investigated)	
BSS	Mild-to-moderate macrothrombocytopenia	CADP/CEPI both very prolonged	Defective aggregation to high-dose ristocetin (not correctable by addition of VWF source)	Normal-to-high levels	Significantly reduced copy number of GpIb (heterozygotes can also be measured)	
Dense granule defects	Low-to-normal count Reduced electron dense granules by whole mount EM	CADP normal CEPI sometimes prolonged	Decreased secondary aggregation to ADP and epinephrine	*Increased ATP:* ADP ratio with reduced ADP level. Reduced ATP release by luminoaggregometry	Reduced Mepacrine uptake and release	Reduced serotonin release Hermansky–Pudlak and Chediak-Higashi syndromes are autosomal recessive and associated with oculocutaneous albinism
Secretion defect	Normal	CADP normal CEPI sometimes prolonged	Decreased secondary aggregation to ADP and epinephrine	Normal but with defective release. Reduced ATP release by luminoaggregometry	Normal mepacrine uptake but defective release	

Contd...

Contd...

Disorder	*Platelet count/Morphology*	*PFA*	*LTA pattern*	*Nucleotides*	*Flow cytometry*	*Other*
Aspirin-like defect	Normal	CADP normal CEPI normally prolonged (NB can by bypassed by high VWF levels)	Absent arachidonic acid response but normal to U46619. Decreased secondary aggregation to ADP and epinephrine	Normal		Retest or defer for 10 days if patient taking aspirin or NSAIDs
Thromboxane receptor defect	Normal	CADP normal CEPI sometimes prolonged	Absent arachidonic acid and U46619 response	Normal		
Giant platelet syndrome	Macrothrombocytopenia	Sometimes normal	Normal response to ristocetin	Normal to high	Normal-High receptor copy numbers per platelet	
Collagen receptor defects	Normal	Both abnormal	Decreased collagen aggregation. Decreased CRP response if GpVI defect	Normal	Low GpIa/IIa or GpVI levels by flow cytometry	
P2Y12 defect	Normal	Normal	Decreased ADP aggregation. Reversible response at high doses. Reduced secondary responses	Normal	Low P2Y12 copy number using radioligand-binding assay	Retest or defer, if patient taking clopidogrel or other anti-P2Y12 drugs
P2Y1 defect	Unknown	Unknown	Decreased response to ADP—no shape change and curves not reversible	Normal		
Scott syndrome	Normal	Normal	Normal	Normal	Reduced expression of phosphatidyl serine on activated platelets by flow cytometry using Annexin-V	Reduced PCI and ETP

Abbreviations: ATP, adenosine triphosphate; BSS, Bernard-Soulier syndrome; CADP, collagen adenosine diphosphate; CEPI, collagen and epinephrine; CRP, C-reactive protein; ETP, endogenous thrombin potential; GT, Glanzmann's thrombasthenia; LTA, light transmission aggregometry; PCI, prothrombin consumption index; PFA, platelet function disorder; vWD, von Willebrand disease; vWF, von Willebrand factor

CHALLENGES IN DIAGNOSING PLATELET FUNCTION DISORDERS IN INFANTS

Severe platelet disorders such as GT and BSS usually present in infancy or early childhood but the diagnosis of these disorders in the very young is more challenging than in older children or adults for a number of reasons, mainly preanalytical. Pediatricians commonly take blood using heelpricks, fingerpricks or a standard venipuncture needle inserted into a vein, collecting the drops from the end of the needle. None of these methods is appropriate for assessment of platelet function, which should be done on a free-flowing venipuncture sample. The minimum volume of blood required for full platelet LTA and nucleotide testing is usually 20 mL; this may be 8–10% of the blood volume in neonates and could cause hypovolemic symptoms.

The available literature suggests that in infancy the platelets are generally hyporeactive (except to ristocetin and variably collagen) but beyond infancy reactiveness of platelets, both aggregation and nucleotide release reactions, is very similar to that in adults.

Therefore, the usual and pragmatic approach is to assess platelet function in children more than 1 year of age using adult controls and normal ranges. Family testing may also be useful not only to confirm a given defect but also to discern the potential inheritance pattern.

TREATMENT OF QUALITATIVE PLATELET DEFECTS

Treatment of platelet function defects comprises both preventive measures and treatment of bleeding events.

Preventive measures include avoidance of antiplatelet agents commonly used over the counter NSAIDs, aspirin and to maintain good dental hygiene as it lessens the risk of gingival bleeds.

Hepatitis B vaccination and specific presurgical care to be ensured as a comprehensive preventive strategy.

Local Care

Many local hemostatic agents such as gelfoam, fibrin sealants, topical thrombin and antifibrinolytic agents are used for management of local oral or nasal bleeds. Nasal packs and postprocedure antifibrinolytic mouthwashes are effective in controlling oral bleeds.

Treatment Modalities in Platelet Dysfunction

Antifibrinolytic Agents

These agents include epsilon aminocaproic acid (EACA) and tranexamic acid, which are used as adjuvant therapy in platelet function defects. They are used in menorrhagia and control of local oral mucosal bleeds spontaneous or postsurgical, e.g. from tonsillectomy site or dental extractions. These agents inhibit the activation of plasminogen to plasmin, prevent the break-up of fibrin and maintain clot stability.

Tranexamic acid (15–25 mg/kg orally every 6–8 hours or 10 mg/kg intravenously every 8 hours) has an important role in primary and secondary prevention of hemorrhage.

Tranexamic acid and EACA may be used as a mouthwash for control of local oral bleeding such as from tonsillectomy site or from dental extractions.

Desmopressin

Desmopressin (1-deamino-8-D-argine vasopressin, DDAVP) has been proven to have a role in the treatment of bleeding episodes in patients with platelet function defects. It exerts hemostatic effect by release of vWF from its storage sites in the endothelial cells. This provides a more efficient platelet adhesion through platelet-vWF interaction.

Dosing and Administration: Desmopressin is given at a dose of 0.3 µg/kg administered intravenously in 30–50 mL of normal saline over 30 minutes. Peak action of DDAVP is usually seen after 30 minutes of infusion. Same dose can be given subcutaneously once daily.

Intranasal preparation is available in a concentrated form (150 µg per dose) to be administered at one puff/150 µg for a child (20–50 kg) once daily. DDAVP is the preferred modality in mild platelet function defects where local measures alone are ineffective. Side effects of DDAVP include flushing, hypotension, fluid retention and caution to be exercised while its use in infants due to risk of hyponatremic seizures.

The therapeutic efficacy of DDAVP decreases significantly after the first dose (tachyphylaxis). The initial response can be reproduced after 1 week. Clinical response assessment is used to monitor the effect of DDAVP as laboratory parameters may be unreliable.

Platelet Transfusions

Platelet transfusions are the most efficient mode of therapy for bleeding episodes and prophylaxis in severe platelet function disorders. However, they carry risks of transfusion-transmitted infections and allergic reactions. A major concern regarding use of platelet transfusions in qualitative disorders is potential development of alloimmune antibodies against HLA antigens and/or the missing platelet GPs. It is hence recommended to transfuse HLA and ABO-matched platelets to prevent sensitization. Alternatively, use of single donor platelet transfusions diminishes the risk of refractoriness. In children the conventional dose of platelets is 10–15 mL/kg.

Recombinant Factor VIIa (rFVIIa)

The use of rFVIIa has been approved for GT patients refractory to platelet transfusion or those who have developed antiplatelet antibodies. The mechanism by which rFVIIa arrests bleeding is due to increase in thrombin generation by a tissue factor independent process, enhanced platelet adhesion and restoration of platelet aggregation. The dose recommended should be at least 90–120 µg/kg administered intravenously. Its use carries a theoretical risk of ischemic stroke and venous thromboembolism.

Splenectomy

Splenectomy has shown significant hemostatic benefit by improving platelet count in patients with WAS. However, there is no role of splenectomy in any other inherited or acquired platelet function disorders.

Hematopoietic Stem Cell Transplantation

Bone marrow transplant may have a role in severe disorders such as GT, WAS, Chédiak-Higashi in reversing hematologic and immune dysfunction. Each individual must be assessed for risk-benefit ratio prior to this modality of treatment.

CONCLUSION

Platelets play a key role in primary hemostasis. Platelet function defects are heterogeneous group of disorders, which vary in genotypic and phenotypic expression. Bleeding manifestations may be diverse ranging from mild mucocutaneous bleeds to life-threatening hemorrhage. Hence a good clinical acumen is essential for diagnosis. Despite recent advances in the biology of platelet structure and signaling pathways treatment options are limited to platelet transfusions and fibrinolytic drugs. Stem cell therapy is curative in some conditions.

BIBLIOGRAPHY

1. Bolton-Maggs PH, Chalmers EA, Collins PW, Harrison P, Kitchen S, Liesner RJ, et al. A review of inherited platelet disorders with guidelines for their management on behalf of the UKHCDO. Br J Haematol. 2006;135(5):603-33.
2. Brewer DB. Max Schultze (1865), G. Bizzozero (1882) and the discovery of the platelet. Br J Haematol. 2006;133(3):251-8.
3. George JN. Platelets. Lancet. 2000;355(9214):1531-9.
4. Harrison P, Mackie I, Mumford A, Briggs C, Liesner R, Winter M, et al. Guidelines for the laboratory investigation of heritable disorders of platelet function. Br J Haematol. 2011;155(1):30-44.
5. Konkle BA. Acquired disorders of platelet function. Hematology Am Soc Hematol Educ Program. 2011;2011:391-6.
6. Michelson AD. Platelets, 2nd edition. Philadelphia, PA, USA: Academic Press; 2006.

CHAPTER

25

Approach to a Bleeding Neonate

Gaurav Tripathi, Amita Mahajan

INTRODUCTION

Bleeding in a neonate is a common scenario in clinical practice that causes considerable anxiety to the parents and can sometimes pose difficulties for the practicing pediatrician in making a definite diagnosis due to unavailability of sophisticated laboratory tests especially in developing world. Approach to the diagnostic workup of a bleeding neonate requires understanding of the concept of developmental hemostasis and the differences in the coagulation and fibrinolysis pathways of neonates. Developmental hemostasis balances procoagulant and anticoagulant forces to protect uncontrolled bleeding as well as prevents excessive clotting after a vessel wall injury. Coagulation factors are synthesized and begin to appear at 10 weeks of gestational age.[1] Hemostasis system is incompletely developed in a neonate and gradually matures until adulthood causing differences in coagulation factor levels compared to older children and adults. Also, concentrations of coagulation proteins are further lower in premature infants compared to full term and gradually increase with time.[2]

In the neonate, vitamin K-dependent coagulation factors (II, VII, IX, X) and contact factors (XI, XII, Prekallikrein, high molecular weight Kininogen) are about half of the adult values.[2] Above all, the capacity of neonates to generate thrombin is also reduced.[3] Platelet count in a healthy neonate is same as that of adult values but platelet function evaluation is difficult and requires special tests.[4] Decreased receptors, impaired signal transduction and low thromboxane synthesis make neonatal platelets hyporeactive which was confirmed in some studies.[5] Bleeding times in neonates are shorter than older children because of higher hematocrit and high von Willebrand factor (VWF) levels.

The onset of bleeding in a healthy term or late preterm newborn may be due to thrombocytopenia or inherited bleeding disorder. The causes in a sick neonate may be due to sepsis, asphyxia, nonaccidental injuries or disseminated intravascular coagulation (DIC).

Occasionally, neonates are referred due to prolonged prothrombin time (PT) and activated partial thromboplastin time (APTT) without any evidence of bleeding. These tests may have been done as part of preoperative workup for surgery as for hernia. It is important to remember that the normal values for these tests especially APTT are vastly different from that in older children and adults and the reports must be interpreted keeping the age and gestation of the newborn in mind. Equally, not every child with bleeding has a bleeding or coagulation disorder. Other causes such as hypoxia, trauma, pulmonary causes or enterocolitis may in fact be the cause of bleeding.

EPIDEMIOLOGY

Vitamin K deficiency bleeding (VKDB) accounts for the major burden of bleeding in neonatal period. The main exogenous source of vitamin K in neonates, which is almost exclusively milk, cannot adequately compensate for deficient endogenous production, since human breast milk contains between 1 μg/L and 4 μg/L of vitamin K1 (and a much lower concentration of vitamin K2). The incidence of early VKDB in neonates in western world without vitamin K supplementation is about 6–12%[6] and classic VKDB accounts for 0.44%[7] in recent reviews. In exclusively breastfed infants who did not receive vitamin K at birth, the incidence of late VKDB is reported to be about 1/15,000. Neonates with cholestasis and malabsorption are at higher risk and incidence of intracranial hemorrhage and neurological sequelae is also higher ranging from 20 to 50%. Neonatal thrombocytopenia is seen in about 5–10% of newborns which can be as high as 20–25% in neonates admitted in neonatal intensive care due to DIC, sepsis, etc.[8]

There is a paucity of published data on bleeding in newborns from India and other Asian countries. In some studies, it was found that the incidence of late VKDB is higher than Western world and ranges from 25 to 80 per

100,000 births out of which intracranial hemorrhages are seen in about two-thirds of neonates and infants.[9]

PATHOPHYSIOLOGY

It is very important to understand the hemostasis mechanism to be able to correctly diagnose and manage a bleeding newborn effectively. There are three phases of hemostasis which occur simultaneously and confined to the area of injury.

1. *Vascular phase:* This phase is mediated by the release of vasoactive substances locally causing vasoconstriction leading to reduction in blood flow. Procoagulant proteins such as tissue factor, collagen, and von Willebrand factors (VWF) play a major role in this phase.
2. *Platelet phase:* Platelets bind to vWF forming a layer over the subendothelium referred as platelet adhesion. The platelets get activated, alter their shape and release Thromboxane A2, serotonin and adenosine diphosphate (ADP) leading to further vasoconstriction and platelet plug formation.
3. *Plasma phase:* In this phase, tissue factor (TF) binds to and activates factor VII (FVII) to form TF-FVIIa complex which further activates factor X. Factor Xa converts prothrombin to thrombin which in turn leads to thrombin burst which is essential for normal clot formation. Thrombin then cleaves fibrinogen to fibrin strands which are stabilized by factor XIII to form a stable clot.

The hemostatic system has two major inhibitors: (1) Antithrombin, and (2) Protein C-Protein S complex which prevents thrombosis.

Disorders leading to bleeding in a neonate can be due to deficiency or malfunction of any of these components of hemostasis secondary to congenital or acquired conditions. Circulating levels of most of the coagulation proteins except fibrinogen are lower in the neonatal period but levels of factor VIII and vWF are higher in circulation in neonates. Platelet counts are same to that of adult levels but platelet function is found to be deficient in aggregation studies of newborns. A relatively small change in these factors can lead to large effect on this balance making a neonate more vulnerable for bleeding.

ETIOLOGY

The causes of bleeding in a neonate can be broadly divided into two categories depending upon the clinical status of the baby. The etiology in a well, otherwise healthy neonate is likely to be different from that in a sick newborn.

Healthy Neonate

Vitamin K Deficiency Bleeding

It can be early VKDB (within first 24 hours of birth), classic VKDB (4 hours to 7 days of life) or late VKDB (beyond 2 weeks of life)

Disorders of Primary Hemostasis (Platelet-Vessel Interaction)

A number of disorders with quantitative and qualitative defects have been reported in children. They are listed briefly below but enumerated in separate sections.

Quantitative defects in platelet number:
- Thrombocytopenia absent radii (TAR) syndrome
- Autosomal dominant thrombocytopenia: May-Hegglin anomaly, macrothrombocytopenia
- Amegakaryocytic thrombocytopenia
- Wiskott-Aldrich syndrome
- Fanconi anemia

Qualitative defect in platelet function:
- Bernard-Soulier syndrome
- Glanzmann thrombasthenia
- Collagen receptor deficiency
- Gamma (dense) granule deficiency
- Alpha-gamma storage pool deficiency

Inherited defect in platelet-vessel interaction:
- von Willebrand disease (VWD)
- *Connective tissue disorders*: Ehler-Danlos syndrome (EDS), Marfan syndrome, osteogenesis imperfecta

Acquired decrease in platelet number:
- Decreased production of platelets as in aplastic or hypoplastic anemia, congenital leukemia, myelodysplastic syndrome, or severe folate, vitamin B_{12} deficiency
- Peripheral destruction of platelets
  - Maternal immune thrombocytopenic purpura (ITP)
  - Neonatal alloimmune thrombocytopenia (NAIT)
  - Maternal systemic lupus erythematosus (SLE)
  - Heparin induced thrombocytopenia (HIT)

Disorders of Secondary Hemostasis

The disorders of secondary hemostasis (fibrin clot formation) are as follows:

Hereditary disorders:
- X-linked factor VIII (hemophilia A) and factor IX (hemophilia B) deficiency
- Autosomal
  - Factor XI deficiency (hemophilia C)
  - Combined factor V or factor VIII deficiency
  - Factor X deficiency
  - Dysprothrombinemia (factor II deficiency)
  - Factor XIII deficiency
  - Afibrinogenemia or dysfibrinogenemia

Acquired disorders:
- Vitamin K deficiency
- Maternal autoantibodies to procoagulant factors

Disorders of increased fibrinolysis
- Plasminogen activator inhibitor type 1 (PAI-1) deficiency
- Alpha2-antiplasmin deficiency.

Bleeding with thrombocytopenia:
- Sepsis or infections
- Severe rhesus (Rh) disease
- Disseminated intravascular coagulation (DIC)
- Kasabach-Merritt syndrome
- Drugs and toxins
- Viral infections.

Bleeding without thrombocytopenia:
- Liver diseases
- Hypoxia-perinatal asphyxia
- Birth trauma
- Pulmonary hemorrhage (PDA, mechanical ventilators) or gastrointestinal hemorrhage without underlying bleeding diathesis.

CLINICAL PRESENTATION

The neonate may manifest with any of the following symptoms:
- Bleeding into the skin (petechiae, purpura, ecchymosis)
- Bleeding related to birth injury
- Persistent oozing from umbilical stump (defective fibrinogen production or factor XIII deficiency)
- Cephalohematomas
- Intracranial hemorrhage (ICH)
- Bleeding from IV cannula sites
- Large hematoma formation at intramuscular injection sites
- Gastrointestinal bleeding from mouth or in stools.

Bleeding isolated to a single organ or system is usually due to some iatrogenic cause. Hemoptysis, hematemesis and hematuria are rarely seen in a healthy newborn as a result of bleeding disorder. These may, however, be seen in sick neonates with DIC, liver disease or vitamin K deficiency. In a small number of infants with severe coagulation factor deficiencies, ICH may be the first manifestation.[10]

Asphyxiated neonates can develop thrombocytopenia, reduced platelet function, survival and even DIC.[11] The cause of bleeding in these neonates is, therefore, multifactorial. In sepsis, coagulopathy secondary to liver failure and thrombocytopenia can cause DIC and severe bleeding.[12] Preterm and very low-birth weight babies are at high-risk of intraventricular hemorrhage (IVH) due to immaturity of cerebral vascular system, especially in the first week of life.[13]

Neonates with thrombocytopenia or platelet function defects usually present with mucocutaneous bleeds in the form of bruising at birth injury sites, petechiae, purpura or ecchymosis. Around 20–25% of neonates with NAIT may manifest with ICH at presentation.

In coagulation factor deficiencies, the clinical presentation is highly variable and usually associated with positive family history and can be suspected in advance. In severe deficiencies, they can have intra- or extra-cranial bleeding, prolonged bleeding from venipuncture or heel puncture sites, after circumcision, hematomas at sites of intramuscular injection.

DIAGNOSIS OF BLEEDING IN A NEONATE

The approach to a bleeding neonate includes thorough history taking, detailed clinical examination of the neonate, baseline investigations and a logical step-wise approach to reach a definite diagnosis.

History

- Detailed family history of bleeding diathesis
- History of maternal medications like phenytoin, phenobarbitone, carbamazepine, aspirin, cephalosporins, rifampicin, isoniazid
- Any previous sibling with bleeding diathesis and sex of that sibling
- History of any complications in pregnancy, i.e. hypertension, diabetes mellitus, antepartum hemorrhage, placenta previa, maternal hemorrhage, intrauterine growth restriction (IUGR), maternal rash
- History of collagen vascular disorder in mother
- History of medications and any procedure done to the neonate
- Detailed information regarding the location, frequency, pattern and duration of bleeding in the neonate
- History of vitamin K supplementation at birth after delivery to the neonate.

Examination

It is very important to assess whether the newborn is clinically "well" or "sick". In an otherwise well-looking neonate, the possible causes of bleeding are vitamin K deficiency bleeding, birth trauma or congenital deficiencies of coagulation factors. In case of gastrointestinal bleeding in a well-neonate, Apt test can be done to rule out ingested maternal blood before doing the other screening tests. Presence of jaundice or splenomegaly may indicate liver disease in a well-looking baby.

In a sick child the common causes of bleeding are perinatal asphyxia, sepsis, or DIC due to other factors.

Laboratory Screening

In a bleeding neonate, some baseline laboratory screening tests are required to reach at the likely cause of bleeding. Based on the results of these screening tests, further approach to a definite diagnosis is formulated. The common screening tools in a bleeding neonate includes:
- Complete hemogram
- Peripheral smear
- Platelet count
- Prothrombin time (PT)
- Activated partial thromboplastin time (APTT)
- Fibrinogen
- D-dimer
- Bleeding time (BT).

Based on the results of the above mentioned tests, following conclusions can be drawn in a bleeding newborn (**Table 25.1**).

Table 25.1 Interpretations of laboratory screening in a bleeding neonate

Laboratory findings	*Well neonate*	*Sick neonate*
• Normal platelets • Normal PT • Normal APTT	• Local trauma • Mild GI hemorrhage • Factor XIII deficiency • Alpha2-antiplasmin deficiency • Platelet function disorders	• Hypoxia-acidosis • Birth weight < 1,000 g • Pulmonary hemorrhage, hyperosmolarity
• Low platelets • Normal PT • Normal APTT	• Autoimmune thrombocytopenia (ITP) • Neonatal alloimmune thrombocytopenia (NAIT) • Cryptic thrombus • TAR syndrome • Wiskott-Aldrich syndrome • Bernard-Soulier syndrome • Bone marrow hypoplasia (rare)	• Infections (bacterial or viral) • Sepsis • Severe Rh disease, TORCH infections • NEC • Renal vein thrombosis
• Normal platelets, prolonged PT • Prolonged APTT	Vitamin K deficiency (HDN)	Severe liver disease
• Low platelets • Prolonged PT • Prolonged APTT	Hypofibrinogenemia	• DIC • Kasabach-Merritt syndrome, liver failure
• Normal platelets • Normal PT • Prolonged APTT	• Congenital deficiency of Factor VIII, IX, XI, XII • Heparinization • von Willebrand disease	

Abbreviations: APTT, activated partial thromboplastin time; DIC, disseminated intravascular coagulation; GI gastrointestinal; HDN, hemolytic disease of the newborn; ITP, immune thrombocytopenic purpura; NAIT, neonatal alloimmune thrombocytopenia; NEC, necrotizing enterocolitis; PT, prothrombin time; Rh, rhesus; TAR, thrombocytopenia with absent radius; TORCH, toxoplasmosis, other (syphilis, varicella-zoster, parvovirus B19), rubella, cytomegalovirus (CMV), and herpes

The stepwise approach to a bleeding neonate can be illustrated in the following algorithm **(Flow chart 25.1)**.

RECENT DEVELOPMENT IN THE DIAGNOSTICS

Most of the congenital severe factor deficiencies can be diagnosed prenatally by the examination of fetal DNA obtained through chorionic villous biopsy or amniocentesis. In families with hemophilia, it helps in prevention either by early intervention and therapy or by termination of pregnancy.

In special cases, pregenetic determination (PGD) together with in vitro fertilization (IVF) can be used for selection of healthy embryos prior to actual pregnancy.

Recently, the Perinatal and Pediatric Hemostasis Subcommittee (SCC) of International Society of Thrombosis and Hemostasis (ISTH) has given a consensus recommendation for laboratory reporting of pediatric samples. All laboratories processing pediatric samples should have age, analyzer and reagent appropriate reference ranges to make interpretations more meaningful.[14]

MANAGEMENT

In a newborn or infant with bleeding, the management depends on the underlying medical conditions. Therapeutic options and treatments of some common clinical conditions causing bleeding are as follows:

Vitamin K Deficiency Bleeding

Vitamin K deficiency bleeding is one of the most common causes of bleeding in a neonate. The basic principles of management of VKDB are:

- Any patient suspected to have vitamin K deficiency should be treated with vitamin K while awaiting laboratory results. The preferred route of administration is subcutaneously as intramuscular injections have risk of hematoma formation. Intravenous vitamin K can be associated with anaphylactoid reactions due to presence of polyethoxylated castor oil.[15]
- A dose of 1 mg is given, however, doses up to 2–5 mg can be given.
- In significant bleeding, fresh frozen plasma (FFP) 10–15 mL/kg can be infused which promptly increases the vitamin K dependent factors level to 10–20 IU/dL.
- Patients with life-threatening bleeds may also require prothrombin complex concentrate of 50 U/kg accordingly.[16]
- Packed red cell transfusion may be needed in case of significant blood loss.

Thrombocytopenia

Neonatal alloimmune thrombocytopenia has a high risk of ICH as high as 20%, so the target platelet count has to be maintained above 50,000/cumm in first 2 weeks of life.

Flow chart 25.1 Stepwise approach to a bleeding neonate

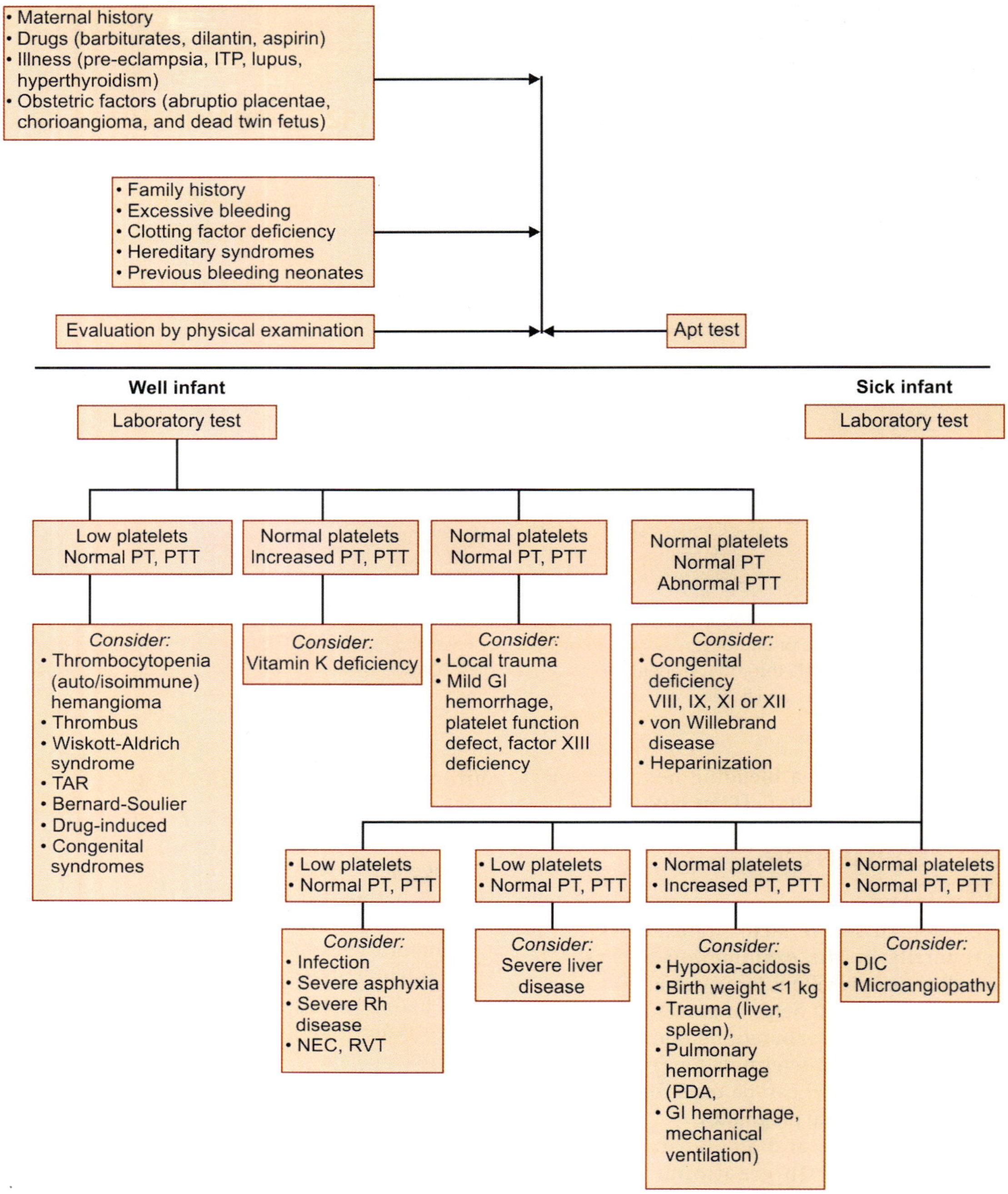

Abbreviations: DIC, disseminated intravascular coagulation; GI, gastrointestinal; ITP, immune thrombocytopenic purpura; NEC, necrotizing enterocolitis; PT, prothrombin time; Rh, rhesus; TAR, thrombocytopenia with absent radius

- Management starts from antenatal period with percutaneous umbilical blood sampling of fetus and high-dose intravenous immunoglobulin (IVIG) to the mother to prevent ICH in neonates.
- All neonates with NAIT should undergo cranial ultrasonography (USG) to detect ICH. Washed maternal platelets or random donor platelets can be used for transfusions to the newborn to reduce further antibody-mediated platelet destruction.
- In milder cases, higher dose of IVIG may be helpful alone or with transfusions to maintain platelet count in safer range in the first 48 hours of life.
- In neonates with platelet count above 50,000/cumm and no bleeding a watchful approach may be opted.

Neonatal autoimmune thrombocytopenia is seen in cases of maternal ITP or SLE due to transplacental transfer of IgG against neonatal platelets. Unlike NAIT, the platelet counts may be normal at birth and bleeding may be mild. Serial platelet counts may be required to detect thrombocytopenia.

- This condition is self-limiting and platelet counts normalize in 2–3 months.
- IVIG in the dose of 2 g/kg for 2–5 days is effective in cases of platelet counts less than 50,000/cumm in majority of patients.
- Platelet transfusion is only required in cases of life-threatening bleeds.

Nonimmune causes of thrombocytopenia are usually seen in sick neonates and are usually associated with low-birth weight, asphyxia, sepsis, necrotizing enterocolitis (NEC), respiratory distress syndrome (RDS) and acidosis.

- In most of these conditions, thrombocytopenia occurs as a part of generalized coagulopathy due to DIC or sometimes as isolated thrombocytopenia.
- Reduced production, increased destruction, and increased splenic sequestration play a role simultaneously in thrombocytopenia.
- The management of the underlying disease is the mainstay of treatment.
- Platelet transfusion is indicated in cases of clinical bleeding with thrombocytopenia or very low platelet counts (<30,000/cumm) **(Table 25.2)**.

Platelet Function Disorders

- Desmopressin (DDAVP) is used to improve platelet functions in many congenital disorders. It increases the circulating levels of factor VIII and vWF in plasma.
- Recombinant factor VIIa is also recommended for use in patients with Glanzmann's thrombasthenia.
- Antifibrinolytic agents are also used as an adjunctive therapy.
- Platelet transfusion is only indicated in cases of life-threatening bleeds to prevent the risk of alloimmunization.

Clotting Factor Deficiencies

- Various specific factor concentrates are used for the treatment of specific factor deficiencies.
- Recombinant or plasma-derived factor VIII or factor IX is used in the management of hemophilia A and B respectively.
- Prothrombin complex concentrates.
- FXIII concentrate is used for factor XIII deficiency.
- Recombinant activated factor VII (in hemophilia patients with inhibitors, factor VII deficiency, Glanzmann's thrombasthenia).
- Cryoprecipitate can be used in hemophilia A, vWD, fibrinogen disorders and factor XIII deficiency when specific concentrates are not available.

PROGNOSTIC FACTORS

Prognosis in a bleeding neonate depends largely upon the severity, site of bleed as well as associated medical conditions.

- Neonates with isolated thrombocytopenia have excellent outcomes provided severe life-threatening bleeds like ICH were not the presentations. Conditions like NAIT, ITP are self-limiting and completely resolve with time. ICH may lead to poor neurological sequelae in future.
- Prognosis of nonimmune thrombocytopenia largely depends upon the outcome of associated medical conditions like asphyxia, sepsis, RDS, NEC, etc.
- In clotting factor deficiencies, timely administration of specific factor concentrates may cause good future

Table 25.2 Guidelines for platelet transfusion in neonates[17]

Platelet count (per cumm)	*Nonbleeding neonate (1st week)*	*Nonbleeding neonate (2nd week)*	*Bleeding neonate*	*Autoimmune thrombocytopenia*	*NAIT (suspected)*	*NAIT (known)*
<30,000	Transfuse all	Transfuse all	Transfuse all	Transfuse if bleeding present or IVIG unavailable	Transfuse using HPA1a/5b negative platelets	Transfuse using compatible platelets
30–49,000	Transfuse if: • Weight <1000 g • Clinically unstable • Previous major bleeding tendency • Surgery or exchange transfusion • Concurrent coagulopathy	Do not transfuse	Transfuse	Do not transfuse, if stable and not bleeding	Transfuse using HPA1a/5b negative platelets	Transfuse using compatible platelets
50–99,000	Do not transfuse	Do not transfuse	Transfuse	Do not transfuse	Transfuse using HPA1a/5b negative platelets	Transfuse using compatible platelets

Abbreviations: HPA, human platelet antigen; IVIG, intravenous immunoglobulin; NAIT, neonatal alloimmune thrombocytopenia outcome. Development of inhibitors in hemophilia can worsen the prognosis and lead to developmental arthropathy in children.

- Administration of vitamin K can prevent as well as treat the VKDB in the neonates. It also prevents against the late VKDB which is often associated with ICH and thus, poor prognosis in children.

PREVENTION

Most of the cases of neonatal bleeding can be prevented by the regular antenatal examinations, institutional monitoring and deliveries as well as vitamin K prophylaxis.

VKDB, which accounts for a major burden of bleeding in neonatal and infantile period, can be prevented by administration of 1 mg of intramuscular vitamin K1 to the newborn babies immediately after birth. Intramuscular (IM) vitamin K soon after birth can prevent early, classic and late VKDB and also more effective than oral vitamin K prophylaxis. It is easily available, cost effective and safe in neonates. Children receiving antibiotics for more than one week should also receive vitamin K prophylactically. In high-risk conditions like cholestasis, malnutrition, chronic liver disease and chronic diarrhea, vitamin K is recommended monthly till the condition resolves.

In patients with known family history of coagulation disorders, the early diagnosis and institution of disease-specific therapy can prevent bleeding episodes in neonates and infants and also can prevent the long-term sequelae of bleeding episodes.

History of NAIT in previous sibling and presence of ICH warrant antenatal monitoring of fetus and institution of IVIG to the mother from 18 weeks of gestation to prevent ICH in the subsequent delivery. Delivery of baby at 32–34 weeks of gestation and lower segment cesarean section (LSCS) delivery are other methods to prevent bleeding in the neonates. All newborns should undergo cranial USG to detect any ICH.

CONCLUSION

Majority of bleeding disorders in neonates in developing countries can be prevented by administration of vitamin K1 at birth. Thorough history and clinical assessment of the bleeding neonate plays a vital role in diagnosing the cause of bleeding. The possible etiology depends on whether the neonate is well or sick. Baseline screening tests like platelet count, PT, APTT, fibrin degradation products (FDP) can guide the treating physician to the diagnosis of bleeding in most of the cases. The management has to be individualized depending upon the underlying cause.

KEY POINTS

- Majority of bleeding disorders in neonates in developing countries can be prevented by administration of vitamin K1 at birth.
- Thorough history and clinical assessment of the bleeding neonate plays a vital role in diagnosing the cause of bleeding.
- The possible etiology depends on whether the neonate is well or sick.
- Baseline screening tests like platelet count, PT, APTT, fibrin degradation products (FDP) can guide the treating physician to the diagnosis of bleeding in most of the cases.
- The management has to be individualized depending upon the underlying cause.
- Prognosis depends upon the cause, site, and severity of bleeds at the time of presentation.

REFERENCES

1. Reverdiau-Moalic P, Delahousse B, Bardos P, Body G, Leroy J, Gruel Y. Evolution of blood coagulation activators and inhibitors in the healthy human fetus. Blood. 1996;88(3):900-6.
2. Andrew M, Vegh P, Johnston M, Bowker J, Ofosu F, Mitchell L. Maturation of the hemostatic system during childhood. Blood. 1992;80(8):1998-2005.
3. Cvirn G, Gallistl S, Muntean W. Effects of antithrombin and protein C on thrombin generation in newborn and adult plasma. Thromb Res. 1999;93(4):183-90.
4. Saxonhouse MA, Sola MC. Platelet function in term and preterm neonates. Clin Perinatol. 2004;31(1):15-8.
5. Rajasekhar D, Barnard MR, Bednarek FJ, Michelson AD. Platelet hyporeactivity in very low birth weight neonates. Thromb Haemost. 1997;77(5):1002-7.
6. Deblay MF, Vert P, Andre M, Marchal F. Transplacental vitamin K prevents hemorrhagic disease of infants of epileptic mother. Lancet. 1982;1(8283):1247.
7. Von Kries R. Vitamin K prophylaxis: a useful public health measure? Pediatr Perinat Epidemiol. 1992;6(1):7-13.
8. Roberts I, Stanworth S, Murray NA. Thrombocytopenia in the neonate. Blood Rev. 2008;22(4):173-86.
9. Pooni PA, Singh D, Singh H, Jain BK. Intracranial hemorrhage in late hemorrhagic disease of newborn. Indian Pediatr. 2003;40(3):243-8.
10. Kenet G, Chan AK, Soucie JM, Kulkarni R. Bleeding disorders in neonates. Haemophilia. 2010;16(Suppl 5):168-75.
11. Baumen ME, Cheung PY, Messicotte MP. Hemostasis and platelet dysfunction in asphyxiated neonates. J Pediatr. 2011;158(2):e35-9.
12. Sola-Visner M, Sallmon H, Brown R. New insights into the mechanisms of nonimmune thrombocytopenia in neonates. Semin perinatal. 2009;33(1):43-51.
13. Owens R. Intraventricular hemorrhage in the premature neonate. Neonatal Netw. 2005;24(3):55-71.
14. Ignjatovic V, Kenet G, Monagle P. Perinatal and Paediatric Haemostasis Subcommittee of the Scientific and Standardization Committee of the International Society on Thrombosis and Haemostasis. Developmental hemostasis: recommendations for laboratories reporting pediatric samples. J Thromb Haemost. 2012;10(2):298-300.
15. Hey E. Vitamin K: what, why, and when. Arch Dis Child Fetal Neonatal Ed. 2003;88(2):F80-3.
16. Williams MD, Chalmers EA, Gibson BE. The investigation and management of neonatal hemostasis and thrombosis. Br J Haematol. 2002;119(2):295-309.
17. Roberts I, Stanworth S, Murray NA. Thrombocytopenia in the neonate. Blood Rev. 2008;22(4):173-86.

SECTION 5

Neutrophil Disorders

Section Editors

Bharat Agarwal, Tulika Seth

- Neutrophilia
  Bhavna Dhingra, Bharat Choudhary
- Important Causes of Neutropenia Including Inherited Conditions: Diagnosis and Work-up
  Nitin Gupta, Rahul Arora
- Neutrophil Function Defects
  Praveen Narsaria, Sushil K Kabra, Rakesh Lodha
- Management of Neutropenia and Infections
  Sangeeta Mudaliar, Bharat Agarwal

CHAPTER

26

Neutrophilia

Bhavna Dhingra, Bharat Choudhary

INTRODUCTION

Neutrophilia is defined as an increase in the absolute neutrophil count (ANC). Neutrophilia is a nonspecific response of innate immune system in neonates, especially in preterm babies. Unlike in older children and adults, there is no specific magic number, which can draw a line between normal ANC and neutrophilia. In neonates, neutrophilia is defined as ANC count more than 95th percentile for that gestational age.

NEUTROPHIL COUNTS IN NEWBORN

Complete blood count is one of the most frequent investigation ordered in neonatal intensive care unit (NICU), generally done in view of suspected sepsis. Clinician wants to look for changes in neutrophil and platelet counts to pickup sepsis at the earliest. Unlike in adults, neutrophil count in newborn varies with age so it is very difficult to interpret ANC values. Care should be taken to make any decision solely based on the neutrophil count.

Neutrophil reference range is still a debate because various studies quote different reference ranges. Manroe et al. mentioned neutrophil count for normal term babies **(Figs 26.1 to 26.3)**.[1]

Neutrophils increase after birth reaching peak between 12–14 hours ranging from 7800–14500 cell/mm^3 and thereafter numbers slowly decline and reaches to a stable count after 60 hours and remains stable up to 28 days.

In very low-birth-weight babies, the reference range is much wider (though the upper limit remains same) and the rise in neutrophil count happens gradually around 18–20 hours **(Figs 26.3 to 26.5)**.[2] Babies born at high altitudes have more wider reference range (2,700–13,500 mm^3) for unknown reasons.[3] Hence, a single value may be normal for a neonate and abnormal for other.

MECHANISM OF NEUTROPHILIA IN NEWBORNS

Neutrophil production takes place in the bone marrow. The main storage pools of neutrophils are: bone marrow, circulating blood and peripheral tissues. During neutrophilia, increase in the count occurs due to shift from one pool to another. There are four main mechanism underlying neutrophilia:

1. *Demargination*: Demargination is shift of peripheral neutrophils to circulation. It takes few minutes for this process. This happens due to any stressful situation leading to release of epinephrine. Epinephrine leads to β2-receptors activation on neutrophils, production of cyclic adenosine monophosphate (cAMP) and result into decreased chemotaxis and decreased adhesion.
2. *Mobilization*: Mobilization is shift of preformed neutrophils from the marrow. This also occurs in response to acute stress, secondary to release of catecholamines. This process takes few hours.
3. *Proliferation*: As the name suggests, it occurs secondary to increased production of neutrophils and release into the circulating pool. This leads to release of premature form of neutrophils along with mature ones. Infection, inflammation and chromosomal disorder like Down syndrome lead to neutrophilia with this mechanism.

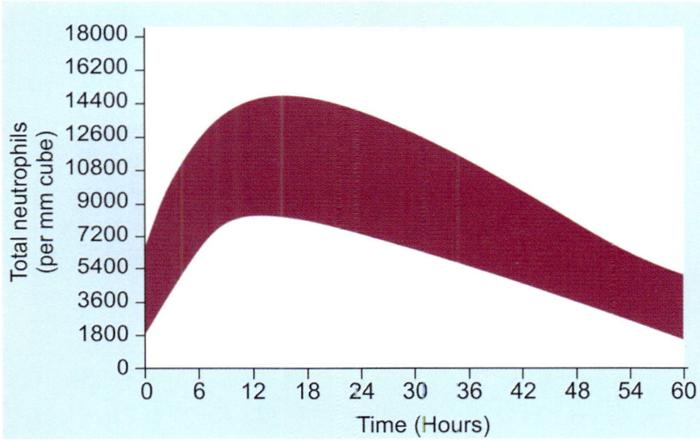

Figure 26.1 Reference range of neutrophils in first 60 hours
Modified from Source: Manroe BL, Weinberg AG, Rosenfeld CR, Browne R. The neonatal blood count in health and disease I. Reference values for neutrophilic cells. J Pediatr. 1979;95(1):89-98.

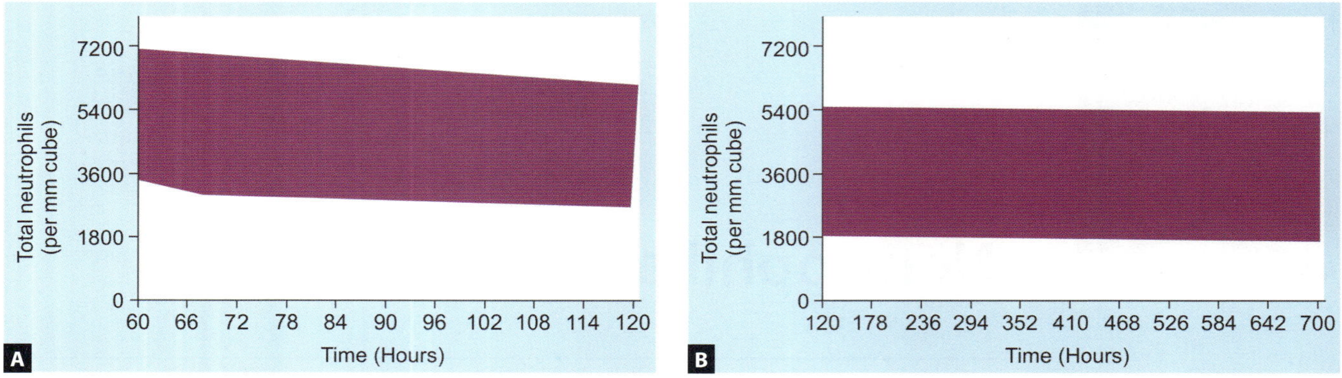

Figures 26.2A and B Neutrophil reference range in neonate from 60 hours to 28 days of life

Modified from Source: Manroe BL, Weinberg AG, Rosenfeld CR, Browne R. The neonatal blood count in health and disease I. Reference values for neutrophilic cells. J Pediatr. 1979;95(1):89-98.

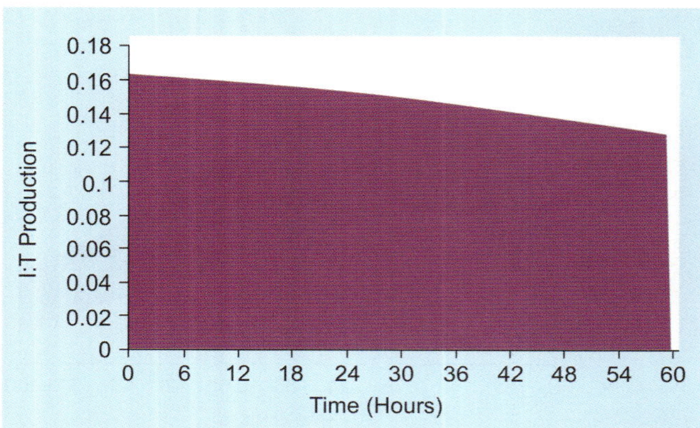

Figure 26.3 Reference range for immature to total ANC (I:T ratio) in term neonates up to 60 hours

Modified from Source: Manroe BL, Weinberg AG, Rosenfeld CR, Browne R. The neonatal blood count in health and disease I. Reference values for neutrophilic cells. J Pediatr. 1979;95(1):89-98.

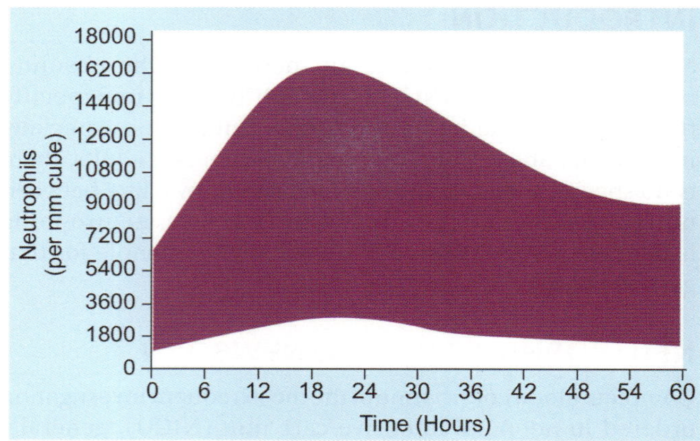

Figure 26.4 Reference range for neutrophil count up to 60 hours in very low birth weight babies

Modified from Source: Mouzinho A, Rosenfeld CR, Sánchez PJ, Risser R. Revised reference ranges for circulating neutrophils in very-low-birth-weight neonates. Pediatrics. 1994;94(1):76-82.

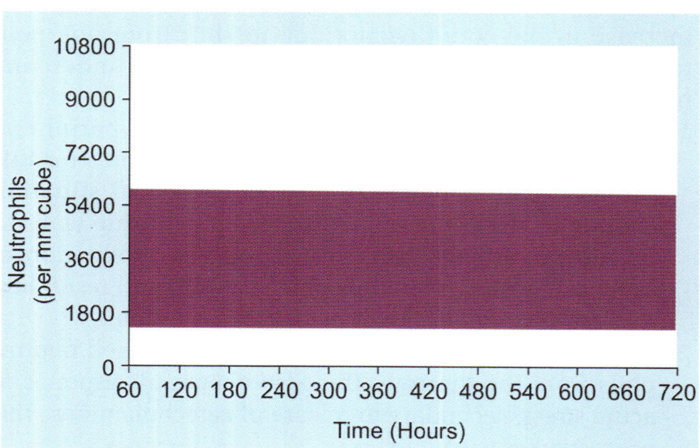

Figure 26.5 Reference range for very low birth weight babies from 60 hours to 28 days

Modified from Source: Mouzinho A, Rosenfeld CR, Sánchez PJ, Risser R. Revised reference ranges for circulating neutrophils in very-low-birth-weight neonates. Pediatrics. 1994;94(1):76-82.

4. *Decreased demargination*: Due to underlying deficiency of adhesion molecules, most of the neutrophils remain in the circulatory pool.

Though these mechanism are not specific to a single disorder, various mechanisms add together leading to neutrophilia. The various cause of neutrophilia are mentioned in **Box 26.1**.[4]

FACTORS AFFECTING NEUTROPHIL COUNTS

There are various physiological conditions, which can affect neutrophil counts. Some of these factors are:[3,5,6]

- Site of sampling
- Amount of sample
- Hours of life at which sample drawn
- Birth weight
- Sex of the child
- Excessive crying
- Mode of delivery.

Box 26.1 Causes of neutrophilia in neonates

- *Accelerated neutrophil production:*
  - Sepsis
  - TORCH infection
  - Down's syndrome, Trisomy 21 mosaicism
  - Treatment with r-GCF, r-GMCF
  - Hereditary neutrophilia (autosomal dominant, hepatosplenomegaly, increased ALP, Gaucher-type histiocytes)
  - Associated amegakaryocytic thrombocytopenia with congenital deformities such as TOF, absent radii
- *Accelerated release of neutrophils from the bone marrow into the blood:*
  - Corticosteroid administration
  - Epinephrine administration
  - Sepsis
  - Stress of delivery/labor, neutrophilic response last 3 days
  - Postsurgical
- *Neutrophil demargination:*
  - Epinephrine
  - Crying
  - Sepsis
  - Stress of delivery/labor, neutrophilic response last 3 days
  - Postictal phase
  - Erythrocyte transfusion
- *Diminished egress of neutrophils from the blood into the tissues:*
  - Adhesion molecule deficiency (LAD)
  - Corticosteroid therapy
- *Spurious neutrophilia* (platelets clumps read as neutrophil by automatic counters)

Abbreviations: ALP, alkaline phosphate; GCF, granulocyte-colony stimulating factor; GMCF, granulocyte-monocyte colony-stimulating factor; TOF, tetralogy of Fallot

Modified from Source: Nittala S, Subbarao GC, Maheshwari A. Evaluation of neutropenia and neutrophilia in preterm infants. J Matern Fetal Neonatal Med. 2012;25(Suppl 5):100-3.

There are considerable differences in the neutrophil count between capillary, venous and arterial sample. Samples obtained from the skin puncture, i.e. capillary blood has more number of neutrophils compared to venous and arterial one. Schmutz et al. had found a significant difference of 2,000 ANC count/mm^3 between female and male children with female children having higher counts. They also observed that neonates born by normal delivery had higher neutrophil counts compared to babies born by cesarean section and also those mothers who underwent labor before cesarean had babies with higher ANC counts as compared to mothers who directly underwent cesarean section.[3]

DISORDERS WITH NEUTROPHILIA

Sepsis

Neutrophilia is nonspecific response to stress. In case of suspected sepsis it is believed to be an early marker in older children and adults, but the same does not hold true for neonates and especially for very low-birth-weight or preterm neonates. In neonates, neutropenia is a more specific marker for sepsis rather than neutrophilia.

In view of any stress, there occurs release of preformed neutrophils. Along with it, the bone marrow gets stimulated and starts producing neutrophils from its precursors. As a result, immature neutrophils, i.e. band forms, myelocytes and promyelocytes come into the circulation. In newborns, neutrophil progenitor and precursor storage pools are less in number resulting in early neutrophil depletion and neutropenia.

The absolute number of immature cell in the circulation is also not of much help for early prediction of sepsis. It is the immature cell to total neutrophil count ratio (I:T ratio, ranges from 0.12 to 0.16 up to 60 hours), which is more specific than ANC especially in setting of neutropenia.[7] The incidence of neutrophilia in the presence of sepsis and without sepsis is same. It has been seen that neutrophilia and platelet count are not of much value in diagnosis of sepsis whereas neutropenia and increased I:T ratio have more specificity and high likelihood ratio for sepsis.[8]

Mikhael et al. developed neutrophil value score (NVS) for predicting risk of early onset sepsis (EOS) based on serial total leukocyte counts (TLCs) counts at 0–6, 10–16 and 22–28 hours.[9] Score produced on the values of absolute total neutrophil (ATN), absolute total immature (ATI) and I:T ratio based on reference range. The maximum NVS score is of 9. The NVS score had AUC (area under curve of receiver operating curve) of 0.9 and 0.81 for proven and proven plus suspected sepsis respectively to predict no EOS. The specificity for NVS score of 6, 7 and 8 is 100% for no EOS and for proven plus suspected sepsis is 78%, 92% and 97%, respectively.

Down Syndrome

Down syndrome is known for various congenital anomalies as well as hematological abnormalities. The most common of hematological abnormality is neutrophilia. It has been observed that 80% of children with trisomy 21 have neutrophil count in the range above 95th percentile for gestation age as mentioned in Manroe's charts.[10] This abnormality is transient and usually recovers after 1st week of life.

Leukocyte Adhesion Deficiency

Leukocyte adhesion deficiency (LAD) is a rare group of neutrophil function disorder characterized by mutation in the adhesion molecules resulting in decreased migration ability leading to neutrophilia and immunodeficiency. There are three main type of LAD:

1. Leukocyte adhesion deficiency type I is caused by mutation of ITGb2 (integrin β2), which leads to absent or decreased production of β2 integrin.[11] This leads to defective adhesion to vessel wall and migration. It is characterized by delayed separation of umbilical cord and leukocytosis.
2. Leukocyte adhesion deficiency type II is caused due to defective fucosylation of various cell surface glycoproteins,

which function as ligands for selectin. These patients also lack H and Lewis blood group antigen leading to Bombay blood group.
3. LAD type III is caused due to inside out activation defect of β2 integrin.

Hereditary Neutrophilia

It is an autosomal dominant condition leading to neutrophilia and presents as leukocyte counts chronically in the 20,000 to more than 100,000/μL range. Splenomegaly, often massive, elevated leukocyte alkaline phosphatase scores and widened diploë of the skull. The neutrophil function and CD18/CD11b surface expression are normal. Some patients may have a platelet dysfunction.[12]

Pelger-Huët Anomaly

This is a benign dominantly inherited defect of terminal neutrophil differentiation with a frequency at birth of 1:6,000, due to mutations in the lamin β-receptor gene. It can give rise to an apparent increase in neutrophil band forms, which is often confused with a left shift. Most neutrophils in heterozygotes have nuclei with only two lobes joined by a thin bridge that is much thinner than that seen in a normal band form, and excessively coarse clumping of nuclear chromatin. In the homozygous state, the neutrophils contain a single round eccentric nucleus with clumped chromatin.[13,14]

Congenital Anomalies and Leukemoid Reaction

Leukemoid reactions have been associated with amegakaryocytic thrombocytopenia and with congenital deformities such as tetralogy of Fallot, dextrocardia and absent radii and rudimentary little toes.[15,16] Asplenia is associated with moderate neutrophilia.

Rac2 Deficiency or Neutrophil Immunodeficiency Syndrome

This is a syndrome of global neutrophil dysfunction that presents as delayed separation of the umbilical cord, poor pus formation, leukocytosis, neutrophilia, and nonhealing perirectal and periumbilical abscesses. Rac2 (Ras-related C3 botulinum toxin substrate 2) is a Rho-GTPase that is essential for several important neutrophil functions like rolling via L-selectin, F-actin assembly, chemotaxis, and superoxide generation in response to some agonists. Neutrophils in Rac2 deficiency have defects in rolling on endothelium, chemotaxis and phagocytosis.[17-22]

CONCLUSION

- Neutrophil counts vary widely in the newborn period.
- Sepsis is the most common cause of neutrophilia.
- LAD and Down syndrome should be suspected in cases of persistent neutrophilia.

KEY MESSAGE

Age appropriate curves should be used in neonatal period to define neutrophilia.

REFERENCES

1. Manroe BL, Weinberg AG, Rosenfeld CR, Browne R. The neonatal blood count in health and disease. I. Reference values for neutrophilic cells. J Pediatr. 1979;95(1):89-98.
2. Mouzinho A, Rosenfeld CR, Sánchez PJ, Risser R. Revised reference ranges for circulating neutrophils in very-low-birth-weight neonates. Pediatrics. 1994;94(1):76-82.
3. Schmutz N, Henry E, Jopling J, Christensen RD. Expected ranges for blood neutrophil concentrations of neonates: the Manroe and Mouzinho charts revisited. J Perinatol. 2008;28(4):275-81.
4. Nittala S, Subbarao GC, Maheshwari A. Evaluation of neutropenia and neutrophilia in preterm infants. J Matern Fetal Neonatal Med. 2012;25(Suppl 5):100-3.
5. Kayiran SM, Ozbek N, Turan M, Gürakan B. Significant differences between capillary and venous complete blood counts in the neonatal period. Clin Lab Haematol. 2003;25(1):9-16.
6. Christensen RD, Rothstein G. Pitfalls in the interpretation of leukocyte counts of newborn infants. Am J Clin Pathol. 1979;72(4):608-11.
7. Newman TB, Puopolo KM, Wi S, Draper D, Escobar GJ. Interpreting complete blood counts soon after birth in newborns at risk for sepsis. Pediatrics. 2010;126(5):903-9.
8. Hornik CP, Benjamin DK, Becker KC, Benjamin DK Jr, Li J, Clark RH, et al. Use of the complete blood cell count in early-onset neonatal sepsis. Pediatr Infect Dis J. 2012;31(8):799-802.
9. Mikhael M, Brown LS, Rosenfeld CR. Serial neutrophil values facilitate predicting the absence of neonatal early-onset sepsis. J Pediatr. 2014;164(3):522-8.
10. Henry E, Walker D, Wiedmeier SE, Christensen RD. Hematological abnormalities during the first week of life among neonates with Down syndrome: data from a multihospital healthcare system. Am J Med Genet A. 2007;143A(1):42-50.
11. Van de Vijver E, Maddalena A, Sanal Ö, Holland SM, Uzel G, Madkaikar M, et al. Hematologically important mutations: leukocyte adhesion deficiency (first update). Blood Cells Mol Dis. 2012;48(1):53-61.
12. Herring WB, Smith LG, Walker RI, Herion JC. Hereditary neutrophilia. Am J Med. 1974;56(5):729-34.
13. Hoffmann K, Dreger CK, Olins AL, Olins DE, Shultz LD, Lucke B, et al. Mutations in the gene encoding the lamin B receptor produce an altered nuclear morphology in granulocytes (Pelger-Huët anomaly). Nat Genet. 2002;31(4):410-4.
14. Best S, Salvati F, Kallo J, Garner C, Height S, Thein SL, et al. Lamin B-receptor mutations in Pelger-Huët anomaly. Br J Haematol. 2003;123(3):542-4.
15. Emery JL, Gordon RR, Rendleshort J, Varadi S, Warrack AJ. Congenital amegakaryocytic thrombocytopenia with congenital deformities and a leukemoid blood picture in the newborn. Blood. 1957;12(6):567-76.
16. Dignan PS, Mauer AM, Frantz C. Phocomelia with congenital hypoplastic thrombocytopenia and myeloid leukemoid reactions. J Pediatr. 1967;70(4):561-73.
17. Dharmawardhane S, Bokoch GM. Rho GTPases and leukocyte cytoskeletal regulation. Curr Opin Hematol. 1997;4(1):12-8.

18. Knaus UG, Heyworth PG, Evans T, Curnutte JT, Bokoch GM. Regulation of phagocyte oxygen radical production by the GTP-binding protein Rac 2. Science. 1991;254(5037):1512-5.
19. Roberts AW, Kim C, Zhen L, Lowe JB, Kapur R, Petryniak B, et al. Deficiency of the hematopoietic cell-specific Rho family GTPase Rac2 is characterized by abnormalities in neutrophil function and host defense. Immunity. 1999;10(2):183-96.
20. Ambruso DR, Knall C, Abell AN, Panepinto J, Kurkchubasche A, Thurman G, et al. Human neutrophil immunodeficiency syndrome is associated with an inhibitory Rac2 mutation. Proc Natl Acad Sci USA. 2000;97(9):4654-9.
21. Williams DA, Tao W, Yang F, Kim C, Gu Y, Mansfield P, et al. Dominant negative mutation of the hematopoietic-specific Rho GTPase, Rac2 is associated with a human phagocyte immunodeficiency. Blood. 2000;96(5):1646-54.
22. Kurkchubasche AG, Panepinto JA, Tracy TF Jr, Thurman GW, Ambruso DR. Clinical features of a human Rac2 mutation: a complex neutrophil dysfunction disease. J Pediatr. 2001;139(1):141-7.

CHAPTER 27

Important Causes of Neutropenia Including Inherited Conditions: Diagnosis and Work-up

Nitin Gupta, Rahul Arora

INTRODUCTION

Neutropenia is a frequent finding in the neonatal period, particularly in very low birth weight (VLBW) neonates during the 1st week of life. Neutrophil function of neonates, particularly preterm neonates, is less robust than that of adults and might also contribute to the increase in propensity to infection. In premature infants, early-onset neutropenia is caused by sepsis, maternal hypertension, intrauterine growth restriction, severe asphyxia and periventricular hemorrhage. Some varieties of neutropenia in the neonates are very common and others are extremely rare. The most common causes of neutropenia have an underlying cause that is often evident, and require little diagnostic evaluation. Persistent neutropenia, although uncommon, should prompt evaluation even if it is of moderate severity. The laboratory tests to consider should include hemogram with peripheral smear examination and a complete blood count of the mother. Maternal neutrophil antigen typing and an antineutrophil antibody screen should be done, if maternal neutrophil count is normal. A bone marrow biopsy should be done in patients with prolonged, unusual or refractory neutropenia. The clinical significance of neutropenia depends on the level of depression of the absolute neutrophil count (ANC). Mild neutropenia-neutrophil counts of 1,000–1,500 cells/µL and moderate neutropenia-neutrophil counts of 500–1,000 cells/µL are not generally clinically significant but may warrant evaluation to determine the underlying cause. Severe neutropenia refers to ANCs below 500 cells/µL with the term "agranulocytosis" usually reserved for counts below 200 cells/µL predisposes to increased risk of infection and sepsis. Both recombinant granulocyte stimulating factor and recombinant granulocyte macrophage-colony-stimulating factor (rGM-CSF) have been used in neonatal neutropenia with variable success.

DEFINITION AND CLASSIFICATION

Neutropenia is defined as an absolute decrease in the number of circulating neutrophils in blood. Normal neutrophil levels should be stratified for age, race and other factors. For whites, the lower limit of normal neutrophil counts (neutrophils and bands) is 1,000 cells/µL in infants between 2 weeks and 1 year of age; after infancy it rises to 1,500 cells/µL.[1] In general, neutropenic syndromes are broadly classified as intrinsic, or caused by defects in myelopoiesis, or as acquired and caused by extrinsic factors such as drugs, infections, or autoantibodies **(Table 27.1)**.

SYMPTOMS OF NEUTROPENIA

The hallmark of neutropenia is increased susceptibility to bacterial and fungal infection; neutropenia by itself does not diminish host defense against viral or parasitic infections.

Common Pediatric Presentation

The most frequent types of pyogenic infections in patients with significant neutropenia are cellulites, furunculosis, superficial or deep cutaneous abscesses, pneumonia and septicemia.[2] Endogenous bacteria are the most frequent cause of infections, but colonization or infection may occur with a variety of nosocomial and opportunistic organisms. The most commonly isolated organisms from neutropenic patients are *Staphylococcus aureus* and gram-negative bacteria, but almost any organisms can be isolated, particularly in hospitalized patients or those receiving frequent or prolonged courses of antibiotics. The usual symptoms and signs of local infection such as exudates, fluctuation, ulceration, and regional adenopathy may be less evident in neutropenic patients than in normal individuals.[3]

Neutropenia in the Neonatal Intensive Care Unit

Neutropenia is a relatively frequent finding in the neonatal intensive care unit (NICU) with an overall incidence reported at about 8% of all patients at some time during their NICU stay.[4,5] Neutropenia is more common in VLBW neonates (VLBW<1,500 g) affecting up to 50% in the 1st week of life, which might place these neonates at higher risk for sepsis

Table 27.1 Common causes of neonatal neutropenia

Neutropenia caused by decreased neutrophil production	• Infants of hypertensive women • Donors of twin-twin transfusions • Neonates with Rh hemolytic disease • Bone marrow failure syndromes (Kostmann syndrome, Reticular dysgenesis, Barth syndrome, Shwachman-Diamond syndrome, cartilage-hair hypoplasia, cyclic neutropenia) • Inherited errors of metabolism (organic acidemias, glycogen storage disease type 1b) • Viral infections (Rubella, Cytomegalovirus) • Copper deficiency • Alloimmune neutropenia • Cyclic neutropenia • Familial benign neutropenia • Albinism or neutropenia syndromes (including Chédiak-Higashi syndrome)
Neutropenia caused by increased utilization	• Sepsis • Necrotizing enterocolitis • Alloimmune neonatal neutropenia • Neonatal autoimmune neutropenia • Autoimmune neutropenia (AIN) of infancy • Drug-induced neutropenia • Chronic idiopathic neutropenia

and mortality.[6] Blood neutrophil counts of normal neonates change considerably over the 1st day following birth. Reference ranges for ANCs in neonates were described by Manroe et al.[7] and later modified for VLBW neonates by Mouzinho et al.[8] Neutrophil count increase during the first 12 hours of life and then gradually decline toward a steady 2,000–6,000/µL range between 2 days and 3 days. Higher neutrophil count is seen in neonate born at higher altitude, in females, and after birth following labor versus section delivery.[9,10] The significance of minimally reduced neutrophil counts (such as below 1,500/µL) is not clear.

Most neutropenic episodes in neonates occur in the first postnatal week and are transient. Only 10–20% persists longer than 5–7 days.[11] Neutropenia can result from a combination of decreased neutrophil production, increased utilization or destruction, or excessive margination of neutrophils in the microvascular endothelium. In general, a large left shift (elevated proportion of bands and metamyelocytes) suggests the mechanism of accelerated neutrophil destruction or usage and lack of a left shift suggests reduced production. A rare but very important variety of neonatal neutropenia is termed "severe chronic neutropenia" (SCN). This is a cluster of diagnoses that bear the common feature of very low circulating neutrophil concentrations from birth.[12] These are particularly important because these neonates tend to do well if recognized and treated with recombinant granulocyte-colony stimulating factor (G-CSF).

Neutropenia in Premature Infants

In premature infants, early-onset neutropenia is correlated with sepsis, maternal hypertension, intrauterine growth restriction, severe asphyxia, and periventricular hemorrhage and might be associated with an increase in the incidence of early-onset sepsis nosocomial infection and *Candida* colonization.[13]

"Idiopathic neutropenia of prematurity" is a condition, which occurs late in the hospital course of anemia, infants born prior to 30 weeks gestation when they are 4–10 weeks old and experience an increase in erythropoiesis. These infants are otherwise well and this condition is thought to be due to stem-cell competition between erythropoiesis and granulocytopoiesis. This resolves spontaneously.[14]

Neutropenia is relatively common among neonates with severe necrotizing enterocolitis (NEC) particularly among preterm neonates.[15] Neutropenia associated with pregnancy-induced hypertension (PIH) is mediated by a circulating inhibitor of granulocytopoiesis of placental origin.[11,16] It can occur in up to 50% of exposed infants, and generally resolves completely by 1 week of life. The ANC can be very low, sometimes less than 500/µL, but generally rises spontaneously within the 1st day and is almost always greater than 1,000/µL by day 3. Due to the transient nature of this phenomenon, it probably does not predispose to infections.[17,18] Neutropenia associated with severe intrauterine growth restriction seems to be mechanistically identical to that associated with PIH. No difference was found in onset, duration, or severity of neutropenia in small for gestational age (SGA) neonates versus neonates born after PIH have been reported.[19]

NEUTROPENIA BY ETIOLOGY

Neutropenia Caused by Decreased Neutrophil Production

Reticular Dysgenesis

The selective failure of stem cells committed to myeloid and lymphoid development leads to reticular dysgenesis, one of the rarest and most severe forms of combined immunodeficiency.[20] It is characterized by severe leukopenia, including both agranulocytosis and lymphopenia; defective cellular and humoral immunity; and absence of lymph nodes, tonsils, Peyer's patches and splenic follicles. Erythroid and megakaryocyte development is normal. All reported infants have died of bacterial or viral infections within the 1st week of life, except a few treated by hematopoietic stem cell transplantation (HSCT).[21]

Cyclic Neutropenia

Cyclic neutropenia is a sporadic or autosomal dominant disorder characterized by regular periodic oscillations approximately every 21 days in the number of peripheral blood neutrophils with a nadir of less than 200 cells/μL.[22] The incidence has been estimated at 0.5–1 case per million population. During the neutropenic nadir of each cycle, patients may suffer malaise, fever, oral ulcers, gingivitis and pharyngitis associated with lymph node enlargement. Symptoms typically begin during the 1st year of life but may not commence until adulthood. More serious complications are uncommon. Many patients experience improvement in symptoms as they grow older. In these individuals, the cycles tend to become less noticeable as the neutrophil nadir rises to a more functionally adequate level. Mortality of up to 10% has been reported with the most frequent causes of death being pneumonia and peritonitis complicated by clostridial sepsis. Neutrophil counts often fall to 0 at some time during the nadir and remain below 200 cells/μL for at least 3–5 days. In most patients, monocytosis occurs when neutrophil counts are at their lowest. The myeloid series may show hypoplasia with "maturation arrest" at the myelocyte stage during the declining phase of neutrophil oscillation, but normal or hyperplastic myelopoiesis during neutrophil recovery. Patients with both sporadic and autosomal dominant forms of cyclic neutropenia have been shown to have mutations in the *ELA2* gene encoding neutrophil elastase, similar to severe congenital neutropenia.[23] Management of patients with cyclic neutropenia includes careful attention to identification and treatment of infections acquired when these patients are neutropenic. G-CSF is effective in improving peripheral blood neutrophil counts in this disorder. Most patients still experience cycles but with shortened cycle periods and increased neutrophil counts at the nadir.[24] Cases of myelodysplastic syndrome (MDS) or acute myelogenous leukemia (AML) have not been reported in cyclic neutropenia patients, including those treated with G-CSF.

Severe Congenital Neutropenia

Severe congenital neutropenia was first described by Kostmann in 1956 as an autosomal recessive disorder associated with severe neutropenia. Since then other forms of SCN have been identified with sporadic occurrence with autosomal recessive or autosomal dominant inheritance. The incidence of SCN is approximately two cases per million population. Most patients are diagnosed in the first 3 months of life with severe neutropenia and often present with extremely low ANCs of less than 200 cells/μL.[25] Frequent episodes of fever, skin infections (including omphalitis), stomatitis, pneumonia and perirectal abscesses typically appear during the 1st month of life. Infections often disseminate to the blood, meninges and peritoneum, and are usually caused by *S. aureus*, *Escherichia coli* and *Pseudomonas* species. Before the current era of G-CSF therapy, most patients died in the first 1–2 years of life, and survivors were known to be at risk for the development of MDS and AML.[26] In addition to severe neutropenia, moderate to marked monocytosis, eosinophilia and secondary changes such as anemia and thrombocytosis are seen. G-CSF production in SCN patients appears to be normal. Bone marrow examination characteristically shows a myeloid "maturation arrest" at the myelocyte stage of development with normal to increased numbers of promyelocytes but few if any more mature forms.[2] Megakaryocytes are normal in number and morphology. The genetic basis of 60–80% of SCN cases derives from mutations in the *ELA2* gene,[27] which encodes neutrophil elastase and is also responsible for the related but distinct disorder cyclic neutropenia (discussed earlier). Neutrophil elastase is a serine protease synthesized in promyelocyte stage of neutrophil development and stored in primary granules. It is hypothesized that ELANE mutation leads to cytoplasmic accumulation of defective protein, which triggers apoptosis. *ELA2*-related SCN may be sporadic or inherited in an autosomal dominant Mendelian pattern. Bone marrow of SCN patients shows evidence of accelerated apoptosis of neutrophil precursors.[28] Mutations in most autosomal recessive SCN patients including ones originally studied by Kostmann have been identified in the *HAX1* gene,[29] which encodes a mitochondrial protein. More than 95% of SCN patients respond to G-CSF treatment with an increase in the ANC to greater than 1,000/μL, along with a documented reduction in infections. There is often a delay of 7–10 days before the rise of peripheral blood neutrophil counts at the start of treatment. G-CSF has revolutionized the treatment of this disorder although doses of G-CSF needed are higher than those needed for cyclic or idiopathic neutropenia.[30]

Conversion to MDS or AML and bacterial sepsis remains the most serious complications of SCN. Now, longer survivors appear to be at increased risk for the development of MDS, which almost invariably progresses to AML, whereas death from sepsis has become rarer. During long-term G-CSF therapy, some SCN patients acquire mutations in the G-CSF receptor gene (G-CSFR), then myelodysplasia characterized by monosomy 7, and finally myeloid leukemia. Cytogenetic abnormalities may precede and predict leukemic conversion. For this reason, the Severe Chronic Neutropenia International Registry (SCNIR) recommends yearly bone marrow surveillance including karyotyping and chromosome 7 fluorescence in situ hybridization (FISH) for all SCN patients. In the SCNIR analysis of 374 SCN patients, many monitored for 10 or more years, the cumulative incidence of death from sepsis was 8% after 10 years of G-CSF therapy. In contrast, the cumulative incidence of MDS or AML was 21% after

10 years of G-CSF therapy and 36% after 12 years. There is an increasing risk for MDS or AML as patients receive G-CSF for longer periods.[31]

Myelokathexis and WHIM Syndrome

The acronym WHIM refers to warts, hypogammaglobulinemia, infections and myelokathexis. Myelokathexis is an uncommon form of moderate to SCN in which mature neutrophils are retained in bone marrow leading to peripheral blood neutropenia. Bone marrow shows granulocyte hyperplasia with degenerating neutrophils with cytoplasmic vacuoles, prominent granules, and nuclear hypersegmentation with very thin filaments connecting pyknotic-appearing nuclear lobes.[32] Recurrent warts and hypogammaglobulinemia [low immunoglobulin G (IgG) and occasionally low IgM and IgA] have often been reported in patients in whom myelokathexis has been diagnosed. Patients develops recurrent sinopulmonary infections and other bacterial infections, however, early deaths related to infection have not been reported, and affected patients are capable of mobilizing increased numbers of neutrophils into peripheral blood during infectious episodes.[33]

The genetic basis of WHIM syndrome is a truncating mutation in the gene encoding chemokine receptor 4 (CXCR4) leading to hyperactivity of CXCR4 leading to retention of neutrophils in bone marrow.[34] The neutropenia and excessive granulocyte apoptosis associated with WHIM syndrome are partially corrected by G-CSF. Immunoglobulin levels also return to normal in patients treated with G-CSF.

Shwachman-Diamond Syndrome

Shwachman-Diamond syndrome, a rare multiorgan disease inherited as an autosomal recessive trait, includes clinical findings of neutropenia, pancreatic exocrine insufficiency, short stature and metaphyseal chondrodysplasia. The pancreatic acini are largely replaced by fatty tissue with relative sparing of the pancreatic ducts and islets. Patients are at risk for the development of progressive bone marrow failure and eventual conversion to MDS or AML.[35] Patients may be seen in infancy due to recurrent infections. Pancreatic insufficiency is typically manifest in early infancy as steatorrhea, weight loss and failure to thrive. Later in childhood, pancreatic function may improve, thus rendering the clinical diagnosis difficult. Common skeletal abnormalities include metaphyseal dysostosis in about 50% of affected children, most often involving the femoral head but generally asymptomatic. Neutropenia is the most common hematologic manifestation of the syndrome, although anemia or thrombocytopenia can also occur.[36] Neutrophil counts fall below 1,000 cells/μL in approximately two-thirds of patients with no reciprocal monocytosis, but the neutropenia may be intermittent. Around 90% of cases are due to mutations in the Shwachman-Bodian-Diamond syndrome gene (SBDS), which functions in ribosomal RNA maturation. Treatment includes pancreatic enzyme replacement. Steatorrhea tends to diminish with time, although the pancreatic insufficiency persists. The bacterial infections generally respond to appropriate antibiotics. G-CSF may be used in patients with persistently severe neutropenia and recurrent or life-threatening infections. However, aplastic anemia or MDS develops in up to a fourth to a third of patients.

Albinism-Neutropenia Syndromes

This group of rare primary immunodeficiency syndromes derives from autosomal recessive defects in the biogenesis or trafficking of lysosomes and related late endosomal organelles.[37] As a result, they share varying degrees of overlap in phenotype including defects in the formation of melanosomes (hence partial albinism), abnormal platelet function and immunologic defects involving not only neutrophil but also B-lymphocytes and cytotoxic T lymphocytes.

Chédiak-Higashi syndrome (CHS) is a rare genetic disorder characterized by partial oculocutaneous albinism, giant lysosomes in many cell types, including granulocytes and neuropathy. Most patients have moderate neutropenia, apparently caused by ineffective granulopoiesis, and are at high risk for the development of hemophagocytic lymphohistiocytosis (HLH). Available data suggest that the pathophysiology of CHS involves defective trafficking of proteins to organelles. Neutropenia is also seen in similar disorders like Hermansky-Pudlak syndrome type 2, Griscelli's syndrome.[38]

Familial Benign Neutropenia

Chronic benign neutropenia is a heterogeneous group of disorders sharing the common features of chronic neutropenia with little if any increased risk of infection in an otherwise healthy patient. Both familial and nonfamilial forms of this disorder are described. Familial benign neutropenia has been described in Yemenite Jews, American and African blacks, and Germans, French, Americans and South Africans. Affected family members demonstrate moderate-to-severe neutropenia without associated leukopenia, relative monocytosis and lymphocytosis with variable eosinophilia. Bone marrow studies reveal normal cellularity with reduced mature granulocytes. The presumed defect is faulty release of mature neutrophils from the bone marrow.[39]

Neutropenia associated with immune dysfunction: Primary disorders of immunoglobulin production have been associated with neutropenic syndromes. A third of males with X-linked agammaglobulinemia, hyper-IgM immunodeficiency syndrome, common variable immunodeficiency and isolated IgA deficiency have neutropenia at sometime during the course of their disease. Immunoglobulin replacement therapy abolished the neutropenia in some, but not all of these patients.[40]

Autoimmune lymphoproliferative syndrome (ALPS), which reflects a family of defects in lymphocyte apoptosis, is characterized by lymphadenopathy, splenomegaly, and a variety of autoimmune disorders, including immune thrombocytopenia, anemia and neutropenia. The neutropenia associated with ALPS tends to be chronic and because of the unique pathophysiology of the underlying disorder represents one of the few forms of neutropenia treated by immunosuppression with corticosteroids or mycophenolate mofetil.[41]

Cartilage-hair hypoplasia, an autosomal recessive disorder found frequently in the Amish population, is characterized by short-limbed dwarfism, fine hair, moderate neutropenia (100–2,000 cells/μL) and impaired cell-mediated immunity.[42] Autoimmune disorders such as systemic lupus can be associated with antibody- or immune complex-mediated destruction of neutrophils or their precursors. G-CSF therapy is effective but may precipitate flares of the underlying disease.[43] In patients with human immunodeficiency virus (HIV) infection, neutropenia is common and has multiple causes, including antiretroviral drugs, cellular immune dysfunction, ineffective hematopoiesis, antineutrophil antibodies, an hypersplenism.[44]

NEUTROPENIA ASSOCIATED WITH METABOLIC DISEASES

Significant neutropenia, often with a relative monocytosis, occurs in Barth's syndrome, a distinctive X-linked disorder also associated with dilated cardiomyopathy, growth retardation and 3-methylglutaconic aciduria.[45] Symptoms develop in infancy or childhood in affected boys, and neutropenia can precede the development of cardiac abnormalities. Children suffering from hyperglycinemia, isovaleric acidemia, propionic acidemia, methylmalonic acidemia and tyrosinemia may also have significant neutropenia.[46] Neutrophils in patients with glycogen storage disease type IB are not only diminished in number with neutrophil counts commonly less than 500 cells/μL but also are functionally defective.[47] Macrocytic anemia, often accompanied by neutropenia or thrombocytopenia, is a hematologic hallmark of Pearson's syndrome, a rare and fatal congenital disorder involving not only the hematopoietic system but also the exocrine pancreas, liver and kidneys. The bone marrow shows normal cellularity, but striking abnormalities include vacuolization of erythroid and myeloid precursors, hemosiderosis and ringed sideroblasts.[48]

NUTRITIONAL DEFICIENCIES

Ineffective granulopoiesis is part of the megaloblastic marrow pathology observed in patients with nutritional deficiencies of vitamin B12 or folic acid. Neutropenia also occurs with starvation in such conditions as anorexia nervosa and marasmus in infants, as well as occasionally in patients maintained by parenteral feeding. In addition, neutropenia and marrow megaloblastosis have been observed in patients thought to have copper deficiency because these patients responded promptly to copper replacement.[49] Notably, these nutritional deficiencies do not cause isolated neutropenia; anemia is virtually universal and thrombocytopenia is an occasional additional finding.

NEUTROPENIA CAUSED BY EXTRINSIC FACTORS

Infection

The most common cause of transient neutropenia in childhood is viral infection. Viruses commonly causing neutropenia include cytomegalovirus, Epstein-Barr virus, hepatitis A and B, HIV, influenza A and B, measles, respiratory syncytial virus, parvovirus B19, rubella and varicella. Neutropenia develops during the first 24–48 hours of the illness and may persist for 3–6 days. Significant neutropenia may occur during typhoid, paratyphoid, tuberculosis, brucellosis, tularemia and rickettsial infections.[2,50] Sepsis is one of the more serious causes of neutropenia. The neutropenia in patients with bacteremia and endotoxemia may result from excessive destruction of neutrophils and depletion of the bone marrow reserve pool. Significant neutropenia occurs most commonly in neonatal bacterial sepsis. Newborns can exhaust their neutrophil reserves during overwhelming bacterial infection because their neutrophil storage pool is small and neutrophil production is already near a maximum.[50]

Drug-induced Neutropenia

Drug-induced neutropenia is a disorder characterized by a severe and selective reduction in levels of circulating blood neutrophils (usually to levels of less than 200 cells/μL) and is due to an idiosyncratic reaction to the offending drug. Although the majority of patients will recover, drug-induced neutropenia is a serious disorder with high morbidity but most deaths occur in patients who are elderly or have metabolic complications such as shock or renal failure.[51]

The most common drug classes include antimicrobial agents, particularly sulfonamides and penicillins; antithyroid drugs; antipsychotics such as phenothiazines and clozapine; antipyretics, particularly aminopyrine; antirheumatics, including gold, levamisole and penicillamine; and sedatives, including barbiturates and benzodiazepines. Although the underlying mechanisms for most drug-induced neutropenia are unknown, most studies suggest that they can be classified as leading to toxic suppression of neutrophil formation or immune destruction of mature cells. Neutropenia secondary to drug-induced myelosuppression is usually insidious in onset and may be asymptomatic. Oral mucositis may be the first clinical sign before infectious complications occur. Drug-induced immune neutropenia is characterized by an abrupt onset (often with fever, chills and prostration) 7–14 days after the first exposure to the drug or immediately after reexposure. The duration of drug-induced neutropenia is highly variable. Acute idiosyncratic drug reactions may last only a few days. By contrast, immune-mediated neutropenia usually lasts for 6–8 days. Once neutropenia occurs, the most important therapeutic action is, of course, to withdraw all suspected drugs. During recovery from drug-induced neutropenia, rebound leukocytosis accompanied by a left-shifted marrow and circulating immature leukocytes can occur. G-CSF therapy may hasten neutrophil recovery.[52]

IMMUNE NEUTROPENIA

Autoimmune Neutropenia

Many cases of chronic idiopathic neutropenia in children and adults are now recognized as being secondary to autoimmunity directed against neutrophils. In primary autoimmune neutropenia (AIN), low circulating neutrophil counts are the only hematologic finding, and associated diseases or other factors that cause neutropenia are absent. The peak incidence of AIN occurs in infants and young children,[53] where it is generally a benign disorder that remits spontaneously as discussed in the following section. Patients with AIN may have variable neutrophil count ranging from mild neutropenia (ANC < 1,000 cells/μL) to agranulocytosis (ANC < 200 cells/μL). Mild splenomegaly is occasionally present. It may predispose to cutaneous and respiratory infections but serious infections are generally uncommon. Spontaneous remission occurs in most infants but occurs less commonly in older children. Neutrophil-specific cell surface antigens identified as targets of autoantibodies include NA1 and NA2, NB1, ND1 and NE1. To detect antineutrophil antibodies, a combination of an indirect granulocyte immunofluorescence test (GIFT) and granulocyte agglutination test (GAT) appears to result in optimal sensitivity and specificity. In the GIFT assay, a panel of heterologous donor granulocytes is incubated with serum or plasma from patients and controls, and bound immunoglobulins are detected by a fluorescent dye-labeled antihuman immunoglobulin antibody and quantitated by fluorescence microscopy or flow cytometry. The GIFT assay is analogous to the indirect antiglobulin (Coombs) test for erythrocyte antibodies.[54] Importantly, the standard laboratory test for antineutrophil cytoplasmic antibody (ANCA) does not detect the antibodies responsible for AIN. The neutropenia of AIN is presumed to primarily be due to peripheral destruction of antibody-coated neutrophils, which may also be augmented by the deposition of C3. Infections tend to be less frequent in patients with immune neutropenia than in those with the corresponding degree of neutropenia from other causes, probably because granulopoiesis is intact in most cases. G-CSF, starting at low doses of 1–2 μg/kg/day, has been successful in increasing the neutrophil count to the normal range or even higher in patients with primary AIN, including secondary immune neutropenia and Felty's syndrome.[53] The initial response may be apparent within days of starting therapy, but up to 2 weeks may be required. G-CSF therapy should be reserved for those with serious or recurrent infections or multiple hospitalizations for febrile neutropenia.

Chronic Benign Neutropenia and Autoimmune Neutropenia of Childhood

Autoimmune neutropenia of childhood occurs predominantly in children younger than 3 years. The median age at diagnosis is 8–11 months with a range of 2–54 months.[54] There is a slight female preponderance. Although AIN of childhood is the most common cause of chronic neutropenia in the pediatric age group with an incidence of approximately 1 in 100,000 children per year. The initial ANC is often in the severe range (<200 cells/μL) and may approach zero, usually with a relative monocytosis or eosinophilia, or both. Transient increases in circulating neutrophil counts can occur in response to infection.

Antineutrophil antibodies can be detected in almost all patients when combinations of immunofluorescence and agglutination assays are used. However, absence of detectable antibody does not exclude the diagnosis and a positive result does not exclude SCN. As the neutropenia resolves, antibodies gradually become undetectable. Some, but not all patients will manifest an increase in the peripheral neutrophil count in response to hydrocortisone or prednisone.

Bacterial infections in AIN of childhood are often increased in frequency but are mild (e.g. skin infections, upper respiratory infections, otitis media, gingivitis) and responsive to standard antibiotics. Spontaneous remission occurs in almost all patients with neutropenia persisting for a median duration of 20 months.[55] The diagnosis of AIN of childhood is generally straightforward if the signs and symptoms occur within the first 2 years of life; there is no history of serious infections over a period of several months of observation, and neutrophil morphology and other peripheral counts are otherwise normal. Evaluation of immunoglobulin levels should be performed to exclude hypogammaglobulinemia. Bone marrow examination should always be performed if hematologic abnormalities other than neutropenia are present, if the child's age falls outside the usual range for AIN of infancy, or if the patient has an unusual or deep-seated infection. Administration of G-CSF results in an increased peripheral neutrophil count in childhood AIN and is the treatment of choice for the rare child with AIN who manifests very severe or recurrent major infections.

Neonatal Immune Neutropenia

Immune-mediated neutropenia in the newborn may be alloimmune and be due to maternal immune response to fetal alloantigens or may be isoimmune and be due to passive transfer of maternal autoantibody. Neonatal alloimmune neutropenia, an immunologic disorder analogous to Rh hemolytic disease, results from maternal sensitization to fetal neutrophils bearing antigens that differ from the mother's. Maternal IgG antibodies cross the placenta and result in an immune-mediated neutropenia that can be severe and last from several weeks to as long as 6 months.[56]

Neutrophil antibodies are found in the serum of the mother and the infant and are frequently directed to the neutrophil-specific NA antigen system. The NA1 and NA2 antigens are two isotypes of the neutrophil FcγRIII receptor. Affected infants may be asymptomatic or can exhibit omphalitis, cutaneous infections, pneumonia, sepsis and meningitis. Because neonatal sepsis can itself be associated with profound neutropenia, the underlying immune-mediated neutrophil destruction may not be appreciated immediately in affected newborns with sepsis. The initial management of neonatal alloimmune neutropenia should include parenteral antibiotics, even if signs of infection are absent, because of the association of neutropenia with neonatal sepsis. Intravenous gamma globulin may sometimes be effective in increasing neutrophil counts.[56] Treatment with G-CSF should be considered for very profound neutropenia or when serious infections develop in infants with alloimmune neutropenia.

Neonatal immune neutropenia can also occur in infants of mothers with AIN. Transplacental passage of an IgG antineutrophil antibody can react with the infant's neutrophils bearing the inciting antigen and result in a profound neutropenia lasting 2–4 weeks.[57] Treatment is similar to that for isoimmune neutropenia. Leukoagglutinating antibodies directed against HLA antigens are frequently found in multiparous women and their newborn children's sera; these antibodies are not associated with neutropenia and thus need to be distinguished from neutrophil-specific antibodies in laboratory assays.[58]

Reticuloendothelial Sequestration

Splenic enlargement as a result of portal hypertension, intrinsic splenic disease, or splenic hyperplasia can lead to neutropenia. The usual picture is one of moderate neutropenia, usually accompanied by similar degrees of thrombocytopenia and anemia. The neutropenia is usually mild and may be ameliorated by successful treatment of the underlying disease. Bed rest alone may lead to restoration of the neutrophil counts because of a reduction in portal pressure. In certain selected situations, splenectomy may be necessary to restore the neutrophil count to normal. Histiocytic disorders may also cause reticuloendothelial hyperplasia leading to neutropenia and anemia secondary to the ingestion of neutrophils and red cells.[59]

Hemophagocytic Lymphohistiocytosis

Hemophagocytic lymphohistiocytosis is characterized by fever, neurologic findings, hepatosplenomegaly, pancytopenia, liver and coagulation abnormalities and elevated triglyceride and ferritin levels. Mutation in several genes have been found among patients with familial HLH. The cause of cytopenia is multifactorial hemophagocytosis of cells, cytokine storm, etc. The neonate will mostly present with primary HLH. Specific therapy is required and most patients will also require allogeneic hematopoietic stem cell transplant.

Bone Marrow Infiltration

Malignancies, including leukemia, lymphoma, and solid tumors that infiltrate the bone marrow result in a myelophthisic picture characterized by leukoerythroblastic peripheral blood smears with neutropenia, usually accompanied by other cytopenias. Neutropenia can also result from bone marrow involvement in granulomatous infections, lysosomal storage disease, or osteopetrosis.[60-62]

Chronic Idiopathic Neutropenia

Chronic idiopathic neutropenia represents a group of disorders that by definition are poorly understood and cannot be placed in any of the aforementioned categories. Overall, the clinical features, bone marrow findings, and natural history of chronic idiopathic neutropenia are variable but generally milder than those of congenital neutropenia;[63] it is likely that many of the patients described in older studies had antibody-mediated neutrophil destruction and normal bone marrow reserve. Treatment, when necessary, should be based on the severity of symptoms; G-CSF has proved effective at lower doses than needed for SCN and without any reported increase in risk for MDS or AML.

Approach to a Neonates and Infants with Neutropenia

Some varieties of neutropenia in the neonates are very common and others are extremely rare. The most common causes of neutropenia in the neonates have an underlying cause that is often evident like sepsis, SGA and PIH. Additional evaluation should be considered if neutropenia persists more than 2–3 days in a neonate with sepsis, or for more than 5 days in neonatal neutropenia accompanying SGA or PIH.[6] In fact, the risk of infection increases with duration and severity. The presence of neutropenia or autoimmune disease in the mother can suggest the presence of transplacental transfer of antineutrophil autoantibodies. Neutropenia associated with maternal hypertension usually is observed at birth. Congenital bone marrow failure syndromes also can present early. Idiopathic neutropenia of prematurity and neutropenia associated with inborn errors of metabolism can occur late in the hospital course.

The basic approach to an infant with neutropenia includes a history and physical examination with emphasis on (1) related phenotypic abnormalities; (2) determination of whether bacterial infection is present (including evaluation of the gingiva and perineum); (3) evaluation of lymphadenopathy, hepatosplenomegaly, and any other signs of an underlying associated chronic illness and (4) a history of recent infection and drug exposure. The frequency and duration of symptoms are important and a history of periodontitis, dental abscesses, or tooth loss is particularly suspicious for significant chronic or recurrent neutropenia. The family history may reveal other individuals with recurrent infection. Unexplained deaths in children younger than 1 year and the race and ethnic background of each patient should be noted. In the laboratory evaluation of neonatal neutropenia the first tests that must be ordered are a peripheral blood film, a complete blood count on the mother, and, if her blood neutrophil concentration is normal, maternal neutrophil antigen typing and an antineutrophil antibody screen.[6] Direct and indirect antiglobulin (Coombs) tests should be performed to evaluate the presence of red cell autoantibodies and serum immunoglobulins (IgG, IgA, and IgM, but not IgE) should be measured to detect associated immunoglobulin abnormalities. HIV testing is also indicated in chronic cases. Bone marrow aspiration and biopsy with cytogenetics should be part of the initial evaluation if leukoerythroblastosis, anemia, macrocytosis, or thrombocytopenia is present and should be performed eventually if the diagnosis remains obscure despite initial testing.[64] If SCN is suspected, bone marrow analysis with cytogenetic screening for monosomy 7 should be performed both to establish the diagnosis and to provide a baseline before G-CSF therapy. Other laboratory tests that should be considered depending on the clinical situation include evaluation for collagen vascular disease, exocrine pancreatic insufficiency and metabolic disorders (e.g. organic acidurias) as well as measurement of vitamin B_{12}, folate and copper levels. Radiographic studies of the femoral heads, rib cage, and spine may be useful in the diagnosis of Shwachman-Diamond syndrome.

THERAPY FOR NEONATAL NEUTROPENIA

Both recombinant granulocyte-colony-stimulating factor (rG-CSF) and rGM-CSF have been used with variable success. rG-CSF increases the number of circulating neutrophils by stimulating the release of neutrophils from bone marrow and inducing myeloid proliferation.[65] rG-CSF treatment is recommended when SCN is diagnosed, but in other varieties of neonatal neutropenia the benefit of rG-CSF is doubtful. In a large (n = 200), multicenter, randomized, placebo-controlled trial in France, rG-CSF recipients had only a transient (2-week) period of fewer infections, but did not have an overall improvement in infection-free survival.[66]

Early studies suggested that rG-CSF was helpful in the neutropenia of PIH but, since neutropenia due to maternal hypertension is transient with few clinical consequences, this treatment should probably be reserved for the few cases where the ANC is less than 500 cells/μL for several days.[64] We suggest the same practice for neonates with neutropenia associated with severe intrauterine growth retardation, twin-twin transfusion syndrome and Rh hemolytic disease.[67] Two infection-related strategies have been proposed for rG-CSF and rGM-CSF usage among neonates: treatment of active infections and prophylaxis against developing infections. In a Cochrane review, Carr and colleagues examined both potential uses, concluding that evidence is insufficient to support either practice.[68] No studies have focused specifically on rG-CSF usage for neutropenic neonates with fungal infections or with NEC.

Chronic idiopathic neutropenia of prematurity is benign condition and requires no treatment. Calhoun and colleagues proposed a guideline for diagnosing and treating neutropenia in neonates.[65] All patients identified with SCN should be treated with rG-CSF using a dose of 10 mg/kg subcutaneously, once per day for 3 consecutive days. Thereafter, doses are given as needed to titrate the ANC to around 1,000 cells/μL.

In most situations, the response is evident within 24–48 hours. rG-CSF should not be used routinely in neutropenia related to sepsis because it usually is a transient phenomenon, and endogenous levels frequently are high in these patients. Neonates who have immune-mediated neutropenia warrant rG-CSF treatment only if they have severe and persistent neutropenia. They generally respond well and need treatment for only 2–4 weeks.

In short-term rG-CSF treatment may lead to low-grade irritability after the first few doses. Long-term rG-CSF therapy is not advisable in view of reports of leukemic transformation (described in Kostmann syndrome), anti-G-CSF antibodies and osteopenia.[69,70] rGM-CSF has been evaluated in neonates and the results are similar to those obtained with rG-CSF. Carr and associates reported that early postnatal prophylactic rGM-CSF corrects neutropenia but does not reduce sepsis or improve survival.[69]

Intravenous immunoglobulin (IVIG) has been tested as a means of preventing or treating neonatal sepsis among neonates with neutropenia. In theory, IVIG should improve the preterm neonate's capacity to defend against infections. A systematic review suggests that IVIG therapy in infants with sepsis may improve outcome,[71] however, its prophylactic use has produced inadequate clinical benefits.

Corticosteroids have also been tried in the management of immune-mediated neonatal neutropenia and in the congenital bone marrow failure syndromes. The inconsistent response does not encourage a larger use in neutropenic neonates. Current evidence does not show a clear beneficial role for granulocyte transfusions in septic neutropenic neonates.[72] A recent meta-analysis concluded that evidence from randomized controlled trials is insufficient to confirm or refute the use of granulocyte transfusions in neutropenic, septic neonates.[73]

Gamma interferon (IFN-γ) has been claimed to have potential for correcting abnormalities of cell movement and bacterial killing *in vitro*,[74] raising the possibility that increasing IFN-γ levels might be beneficial, but no studies have focused on using IFN-γ among neutropenic neonates.

CONCLUSIONS AND KEY POINTS

Neutropenia is common problem in neonatal intensive care units, specially in very low birth weight babies. Common causes of neutropenia are sepsis, pregnancy induced hypertension and intrauterine growth restriction. Moreover in most cases neutropenia is transient and do not predispose to sepsis. Prolonged severe neutropenia (more than 5–7 days) requires diagnostic work up to exclude underlying hematologic disorder as it has been seen to be associated with sepsis and increased mortality. Diagnosis is made by clinical features, peripheral smear and bone marrow examination. Specific genetic mutations identification is helpful in making and confirming the diagnosis.

REFERENCES

1. Hsieh MM, Everhart JE, Byrd-Holt DD, Tisdale JF, Rodgers GP. Prevalence of neutropenia in the U.S. population: age, sex, smoking status, and ethnic differences. Ann Intern Med. 2007;146(7):486-92.
2. Boxer L, Dale DC. Neutropenia: causes and consequences. Semin Hematol. 2002;39(2):75-81.
3. Sickles EA, Greene WH, Wiernik PH. Clinical presentation of infection in granulocytopenic patients. Arch Intern Med. 1975;135(5):715-9.
4. Christensen RD. Expected hematologic values for term and preterm neonates. In: Christensen RD (Ed). Hematologic Problems of the Neonate. Philadelphia, PA, (USA): WB Saunders Co; 2000. pp. 117-36.
5. Funke A, Berner R, Traichel B, Schmeisser D, Leititis JU, Niemeyer CM. Frequency, natural course, and outcome of neonatal neutropenia. Pediatrics. 2000;106(1 Pt 1):45-51.
6. Christensen RD, Calhoun DA, Rimsza LM. A practical approach to evaluating and treating neutropenia in the neonatal intensive care unit. Clin Perinatol. 2000;27(3):577-601.
7. Manroe BL, Weinberg AG, Rosenfeld CR, Browne R. The neonatal blood count in health and disease. I. Reference values for neutrophilic cells. J Pediatr. 1979;95(1):89-98.
8. Mouzinho A, Rosenfeld CR, Sánchez PJ, Risser R. Revised reference ranges for circulating neutrophils in very-low-birth-weight neonates. Pediatrics. 1994;94(1):76-82.
9. Schmutz N, Henry E, Jopling J, Christensen RD. Expected ranges for blood neutrophil concentrations of neonates: the Manroe and Mouzinho charts revisited. J Perinatol. 2008;28(4):275-81.
10. Lambert RM, Baer VL, Wiedmeier SE, Henry E, Burnett J, Christensen RD. Isolated elevated blood neutrophil concentration at altitude does not require NICU admission if appropriate reference ranges are used. J Perinatol. 2009;29(12):822-5.
11. Koenig JM, Christensen RD. Incidence, neutrophil kinetics, and natural history of neonatal neutropenia associated with maternal hypertension. N Engl J Med. 1989;321(9):557-62.
12. Christensen RD, Calhoun DA. Congenital neutropenia. Clin Perinatol. 2004;31(1):29-38.
13. Del Vecchio A, Christensen RD. Neonatal neutropenia: what diagnostic evaluation is needed and when is treatment recommended? Early Hum Dev. 2012;88(Suppl 2):S19-24.
14. Juul SE, Calhoun DA, Christensen RD. "Idiopathic neutropenia" in very low birth weight infants. Acta Paediatr. 1998;87(9):963-8.
15. Juul SE, Haynes JW, McPherson RJ. Evaluation of neutropenia and neutrophilia in hospitalized preterm infants. J Perinatol. 2004;24(3):150-7.
16. Fraser SH, Tudehope DI. Neonatal neutropenia and thrombocytopenia following maternal hypertension. J Paediatr Child Health. 1996;32(1):31-4.
17. Procianoy RS, Silveira RC, Mussi-Pinhata MM, Souza Rugolo LM, Leone CR, de Andrade Lopes JM, et al. Sepsis and neutropenia in very low birth weight infants delivered of mothers with preeclampsia. J Pediatr. 2010;157(3):434-8.
18. Cetinkaya M, Ozkan H, Köksal N, Karali Z, Ozgür T. Neonatal outcomes of premature infants born to preeclamptic mothers. J Matern Fetal Neonatal Med. 2010;23(5):425-30.
19. Christensen RD, Henry E, Wiedmeier SE, Stoddard RA, Lambert DK. Low blood neutrophil concentrations among extremely low birth weight neonates: data from a multihospital health-care system. J Perinatol. 2006;26(11):682-7.
20. De Vaal O, Seynhaeve V. Reticular dysgenesia. Lancet. 1959;2(7112):1123-5.
21. Levinsky RJ, Tiedeman K. Successful bone-marrow transplantation for reticular dysgenesis. Lancet. 1983;1(8326 Pt 1):671-2.
22. Wright DG, Dale DC, Fauci AS, Wolff SM. Human cyclic neutropenia: clinical review and long-term follow up of patients. Medicine (Baltimore). 1981;60(1):1-13.
23. Horwitz M, Benson KF, Person RE, Aprikyan AG, Dale DC. Mutations in ELA2, encoding neutrophil elastase, define a 21-day biological clock in cyclic haematopoiesis. Nat Genet. 1999;23(4):433-6.
24. Hammond WP 4th, Price TH, Souza LM, Dale DC. Treatment of cyclic neutropenia with granulocyte colony-stimulating factor. N Engl J Med. 1989;320(20):1306-11.
25. Kostmann R. Infantile genetic agranulocytosis. A review with presentation of ten new cases. Acta Paediatr Scand. 1975;64(2):362-8.
26. Gilman PA, Jackson DP, Guild HG. Congenital agranulocytosis: prolonged survival and terminal acute leukemia. Blood. 1970;36(5):576-85.
27. Bellanné-Chantelot C, Clauin S, Leblanc T, Cassinat B, Rodrigues-Lima F, Beaufils S, et al. Mutations in the ELA2 gene correlate with more severe expression of neutropenia: a study of 81 patients from the French Neutropenia Register. Blood. 2004;103(11):4119-25.
28. Dinauer MC, Lekstrom-Himes JA, Dale DC. Inherited Neutrophil Disorders: Molecular Basis and New Therapies. Hematology Am Soc Hematol Educ Program; 2000. pp. 303-18.
29. Klein C, Grudzien M, Appaswamy G, Germeshausen M, Sandrock I, Schäffer AA, et al. HAX1 deficiency causes autosomal recessive severe congenital neutropenia (Kostmann disease). Nat Genet. 2007;39(1):86-92.
30. Dale DC, Cottle TE, Fier CJ, Bolyard AA, Bonilla MA, Boxer LA, et al. Severe chronic neutropenia: treatment and follow-up of patients in the Severe Chronic Neutropenia International Registry. Am J Hematol. 2003;72(2):82-93.
31. Rosenberg PS, Alter BP, Bolyard AA, Bonilla MA, Boxer LA, Cham B, et al. The incidence of leukemia and mortality from sepsis in patients with severe congenital neutropenia receiving long-term G-CSF therapy. Blood. 2006;107(12):4628-35.
32. Latger-Cannard V, Bensoussan D, Bordigoni P. The WHIM syndrome shows a peculiar dysgranulopoiesis: myelokathexis. Br J Haematol. 2006;132(6):669.
33. Gorlin RJ, Gelb B, Diaz GA, Lofsness KG, Pittelkow MR, Fenyk JR Jr. WHIM syndrome, an autosomal dominant disorder: clinical, hematological, and molecular studies. Am J Med Genet. 2000;91(5):368-76.
34. Christopher MJ, Link DC. Regulation of neutrophil homeostasis. Curr Opin Hematol. 2007;14(1):3-8.
35. Dror Y, Durie P, Ginzberg H, Herman R, Banerjee A, Champagne M, et al. Clonal evolution in marrows of patients with Shwachman-Diamond syndrome: a prospective 5-year follow-up study. Exp Hematol. 2002;30(7):659-69.
36. Shimamura A. Shwachman-Diamond syndrome. Semin Hematol. 2006;43(3):178-88.
37. Dell'Angelica EC. Bad signals jam organelle traffic. Nat Med. 2007;13(1):31-2.
38. Huizing M, Anikster Y, Gahl WA. Hermansky-Pudlak syndrome and Chediak-Higashi syndrome: disorders of vesicle formation and trafficking. Thromb Haemost. 2001;86(1):233-45.

39. Shoenfeld Y, Alkan ML, Asaly A, Carmeli Y, Katz M. Benign familial leukopenia and neutropenia in different ethnic groups. Eur J Haematol. 1988;41(3):273-7.
40. Winkelstein JA, Marino MC, Ochs H, Fuleihan R, Scholl PR, Geha R, et al. The X-linked hyper-IgM syndrome: clinical and immunologic features of 79 patients. Medicine (Baltimore). 2003;82(6):373-84.
41. Rao VK, Straus SE. Causes and consequences of the autoimmune lymphoproliferative syndrome. Hematology. 2006;11(1):15-23.
42. Lux SE, Johnston RB Jr, August CS, Say B, Penchaszadeh VB, Rosen FS, et al. Chronic neutropenia and abnormal cellular immunity in cartilage-hair hypoplasia. N Engl J Med. 1970;282(5):231-6.
43. Vasiliu IM, Petri MA, Baer AN. Therapy with granulocyte colony-stimulating factor in systemic lupus erythematosus may be associated with severe flares. J Rheumatol. 2006;33(9):1878-80.
44. Israel DS, Plaisance KI. Neutropenia in patients infected with human immunodeficiency virus. Clin Pharm. 1991;10(4):268-79.
45. Barth PG, Valianpour F, Bowen VM, Lam J, Duran M, Vaz FM, et al. X-linked cardioskeletal myopathy and neutropenia (Barth syndrome): an update. Am J Med Genet A. 2004; 126A(4):349-54.
46. Sweetman L. Branched chain organic acidurias. In: Scriver CR, Beaudet AL, Sly WS, Valle D (Eds). The Metabolic Basis of Inherited Disease. New York, USA: McGraw-Hill Medical Publisher; 1989. pp. 791-819.
47. Beaudet AL, Anderson DC, Michels VV, Arion WJ, Lange AJ. Neutropenia and impaired neutrophil migration in type 1B glycogen storage disease. J Pediatr. 1980;97(6):906-10.
48. Pearson HA, Lobel JS, Kocoshis SA, Naiman JL, Windmiller J, Lammi AT, et al. A new syndrome of refractory sideroblastic anemia with vacuolization of marrow precursors and exocrine pancreatic dysfunction. J Pediatr. 1979;95(6):976-84.
49. Huff JD, Keung YK, Thakuri M, Beaty MW, Hurd DD, Owen J, et al. Copper deficiency causes reversible myelodysplasia. Am J Hematol. 2007;82(7):625-30.
50. Strauss RG. Granulopoiesis and neutrophil function in the neonate. In: Stockman JA, Pochedley C (Eds). Developmental and Neonatal Hematology. New York, USA: Raven Press; 1988.
51. Andersohn F, Konzen C, Garbe E. Systematic review: agranulocytosis induced by nonchemotherapy drugs. Ann Intern Med. 2007;146(9):657-65.
52. Dinauer MC. The phagocyte system and disorders of granulopoiesis and granulocyte function. In: Orkin SH, Fisher DE, Look TA, Lux SE, Ginsburg D, Nathan DG (Eds). Nathan and Oski's Hematology of Infancy and Childhood, 7th edition. Philadelphia, PA, USA: WB Saunders-Elsevier. pp. 1137-57.
53. Bruin M, Dassen A, Pajkrt D, Buddelmeyer L, Kuijpers T, de Haas M. Primary autoimmune neutropenia in children: a study of neutrophil antibodies and clinical course. Vox Sang. 2005;88(1):52-9.
54. Stroncek D. Neutrophil alloantigens. Transfus Med Rev. 2002;16(1):67-75.
55. Lalezari P, Khorshidi M, Petrosova M. Autoimmune neutropenia in infancy. J Pediatr. 1986;109(5):764-9.
56. Cartron J, Tchernia G, Cleton JL, Damay M, Cheron G, Farrokhi P, et al. Alloimmune neonatal neutropenia. Am J Pediatr Hematol Oncol. 1991;13(1):21-5.
57. Van Leeuwen EF, Roord JJ, DeGast GC, Vander Plas-Van Dalen C. Neonatal neutropenia due to maternal autoantibodies against neutrophils. Br Med J (Clin Res Ed). 1983;287(6385):94.
58. McFarland JG. Platelet and neutrophil alloantigen genotyping in clinical practice. Transfus Clin Biol. 1998;5(1):13-21.
59. Risks of agranulocytosis and aplastic anemia. A first report of their relation to drug use and special reference to analgesics. The International Agranulocytosis and Aplastic Anemia Study. JAMA. 1986;256(13):1749-57.
60. Goldblatt J. Type I Gaucher disease. J Med Genet. 1988; 25(6):415-8.
61. Loría-Cortés R, Quesada-Calvo E, Cordero-Chaverri C. Osteopetrosis in children: a report of 26 cases. J Pediatr. 1977;91(1):43-7.
62. Wessels G, Schaaf HS, Beyers N, Gie RP, Nel E, Donald PR, et al. Haematological abnormalities in children with tuberculosis. J Trop Pediatr. 1999;45(5):307-10.
63. Papadaki HA, Eliopoulos AG, Kosteas T, Gemetzi C, Damianaki A, Koutala H, et al. Impaired granulocytopoiesis in patients with chronic idiopathic neutropenia is associated with increased apoptosis of bone marrow myeloid progenitor cells. Blood. 2003;101(7):2591-600.
64. Maheshwari A, Christensen RD. Neutropenia in the neonatal intensive care unit. Neo Reviews. 2004;10:e431-42.
65. Calhoun DA, Christensen RD, Edstrom CS, Juul SE, Ohls RK, Schibler KR, et al. Consistent approaches to procedures and practices in neonatal hematology. Clin Perinatol. 2000;27(3):733-53.
66. Kuhn P, Messer J, Paupe A, Espagne S, Kacet N, Mouchnino G, et al. A multicenter, randomized, placebo-controlled trial of prophylactic recombinant granulocyte-colony stimulating factor in preterm neonates with neutropenia. J Pediatr. 2009;155(3):324-30.
67. Koenig JM, Christensen RD. Neutropenia and thrombocytopenia in infants with Rh hemolytic disease. J Pediatr. 1989; 114 (4 Pt 1):625-31.
68. Carr R, Brocklehurst P, Doré CJ, Modi N. Granulocyte-macrophage colony stimulating factor administered as prophylaxis for reduction of sepsis in extremely preterm, small for gestational age neonates (the PROGRAMS trial): a single-blind, multicentre, randomised controlled trial. Lancet. 2009;373(9659):226-33.
69. Taniguchi S, Shibuya T, Harada M, Niho Y. Decreased levels of myeloid progenitor cells associated with long-term administration of recombinant human granulocyte colony-stimulating factor in patients with autoimmune neutropenia. Br J Haematol. 1993;83(3):384-7.
70. Yakisan E, Schirg E, Zeidler C, Bishop NJ, Reiter A, Hirt A, et al. High incidence of significant bone loss in patients with severe congenital neutropenia (Kostmann's syndrome). J Pediatr. 1997;131(4):592-7.
71. Jenson HB, Pollock BH. Meta-analyses of the effectiveness of intravenous immune globulin for prevention and treatment of neonatal sepsis. Pediatrics. 1997;99(2):E2.
72. Mohan P, Brocklehurst P. Granulocyte transfusions for neonates with confirmed or suspected sepsis and neutropaenia. Cochrane Database Syst Rev. 2003;(4):CD003956.
73. Pammi M, Brocklehurst P. Granulocyte transfusions for neonates with confirmed or suspected sepsis and neutropenia. Cochrane Database Syst Rev. 2011;5(10):CD003956.
74. Hill HR, Augustine NH, Jaffe HS. Human recombinant interferon gamma enhances neonatal polymorphonuclear leukocyte activation and movement, and increases free intracellular calcium. J Exp Med. 1991;173(3):767-70.

CHAPTER

28

Neutrophil Function Defects

Praveen Narsaria, Sushil K Kabra, Rakesh Lodha

INTRODUCTION

Neutrophils are phagocytic granulocytes, which are most abundant white blood cells (WBCs) in circulation and play important role in defense against bacteria and fungus. Children with primary neutrophil function defects usually present with low-grade chronic bacterial or fungal infections. Skin and mucosal infections, lymphadenitis, and abscesses are among the infections commonly seen. In this chapter, we will discuss disorders of neutrophil dysfunction related to adhesion, chemotaxis, ingestion and degranulation and microbicidal metabolism. The exact incidence of primary immunodeficiency is not known in India.[1]

DISORDER OF ADHESION

The adhesion of neutrophils to endothelium is essential for their migration from bloodstream to site of infection. The interaction between the endothelium and WBC glycoprotein is very important for this adhesion.

Leukocyte Adhesion Defect

The migration of neutrophils from bloodstream through endothelium to the site of inflammation or infection is mediated through a number of adhesion molecules and their ligands. Integrins are heterodimer protein containing an alpha and beta chain present on surface of all neutrophils. Three alpha-subunits (CD11a, CD11b and CD11c) combine with a beta-subunit (CD 18) to form an integrin dimer. Integrins are essential for adhesion of neutrophils to endothelium. Any molecular defect in these subunits leads to lack of function integrin on neutrophil surface. This leads to ineffective adhesion and transmigration of neutrophils across endothelium and thus development of leukocyte adhesion defect (LAD). Thus, neutrophils do not accumulate in extravascular space despite inflammation and hence, lack of pus formation is a constant feature of all types of LAD. Also, all of the patients with LAD have leukocytosis during infection-free periods, which is an important laboratory pointer toward this disease. Three types of LAD are known, inheritance of LAD I and II are autosomal recessive and of LAD III is not clear **(Table 28.1)**. The incidence of LAD I is about 1 in 10 million.[2]

Genetics

Mutation in gene encoding beta 2 subunit of integrin molecule located on chromosome 21 leads to LAD I.[3] LAD II is characterized by mutation on chromosome 11 involving specific Golgi GDP-fucose transporter.[4] LAD III involves defect in integrin activation.[5]

Management of Leukocyte Adhesion Defect

Most important component of management is control of infection. The organisms are similar to those found in neutropenia. Cotrimoxazole prophylaxis and broad-spectrum empiric antibiotic at times of infection should be used. Early allogeneic hematopoietic stem cell transplantation in severe LAD I and LAD III are curative.[6] High-dose oral fucose supplementation has shown benefit in patients in LAD II.[7,8] Children with LAD III may require platelet and packed red blood cell (PRBC) transfusion for control of bleeding and blood loss related anemia respectively.

Prenatal Diagnosis

Cordocentesis can be done to see the expression of CD18 by 20 weeks of gestation[9] for diagnosis of LAD I. Also Bombay phenotype can be detected at 20 weeks of gestation for LAD II in families with history of LAD. If the exact molecular or genetic defect is known in previous family members then diagnosis can be made earlier by 10–11 weeks of gestation. No prenatal diagnosis is possible yet for LAD III.

Prognosis

Prognosis largely depends on infections and their complications. Also children with severe forms of LAD I die in infancy or if they survive have life-threatening infections.

Table 28.1 Characteristics of different leukocyte adhesion defects

Disorder	*Genetic defect or function defect*	*Clinical features*	*Diagnosis*
LAD I *Severe:* <0.3% of normal amount of beta-2 microglobulin *Moderate:* Express 2–7% of normal amount)	AR, absence of CD11/18 (beta-2 integrin) on WBC membrane; decreased adhesion and transmigration of neutrophils	Persistent neutrophilia, recurrent bacterial infection with lack of pus formation; delayed fall of umbilical cord (>3 weeks)	Flow cytometry for CD11b/CD18
LAD II	AR, defect in GDP-fucose transporter protein; decreased adhesion and transmigration of neutrophils	Similar to LAD I but less severe, developmental delay, short stature	Flow cytometry for CD15s (SLeX) and Bombay phenotype (hh) in RBC typing
LAD III	AR, integrin activation defect; decreased adhesion of neutrophils and platelets	Similar to LAD I with bleeding tendency, delayed separation of umbilical cord	Functional assays for platelet and neutrophil adhesion (diagnosis of LAD III should be considered in patients with clinical features of LAD I with normal beta-2 integrin expression)

Abbreviations: LAD, leukocyte adhesion defect; AR, autosomal recessive

DISORDERS OF CHEMOTAXIS

Disorder of neutrophil chemotaxis is seen in multiple conditions, and it is not necessary that this decreased chemotaxis always has clinical impact on immunity. In general patients, these conditions have normal adhesive properties.

Enhanced Motile Response (Familial Mediterranean Fever)

Patients present with recurrent episodes of fever, polyserositis (arthritis, peritonitis, pleuritis) and amyloidosis. Mutation causing this condition is seen in Mediterranean fever (MEFV) gene, which produces pyrin. This protein is mainly expressed in neutrophils and there is a heightened response to endotoxin due to mutated pyrin protein. This leads to increased accumulation of neutrophils at site of inflammation with increased production of interleukins.

Depressed Motile Response

Immunoglobulin G (IgG) deficiency and deficiency of production of complement C3 and properdin factors due to genetic reasons may lead to decreased generation of chemotactic factors and hence, depressed neutrophil motility in response to inflammation.

Hyper IgE syndrome (Job syndrome) is a rare primary immunodeficiency disorder of elevated serum IgE level with recurrent episodes of cold *Staphylococcus* abscess and chronic dermatitis beginning early in childhood. The chemotactic response to mitogens amongst neutrophils is impaired.

DISORDERS OF DEGRANULATION

Chédiak-Higashi Syndrome

This is a rare disorder characterized by oculocutaneous albinism, immunodeficiency with recurrent infection, hematologic disorder and neurologic manifestations. The genetic defect leads to abnormal membrane targeting in secretary lysosomes and hence uncontrolled granule fusion. This leads to formation of large lysosome granules within WBCs and other cells. These abnormal granules cannot fuse with phagosomes and thus the phagocytosed bacteria are not killed. These large granules are seen in peripheral blood granulocytes and in their precursor cells in bone marrow.

These patients also have neutropenia due to death of myeloid precursors in bone marrow and impaired chemotaxis (due to intrinsic neutrophil defects). Natural killer (NK) cell dysfunction is related to abnormal granules and can be responsible for development of malignancy later on. Pigmentary abnormality is due to abnormal migration of giant melanosomes.[10] Neurologic defects are due to failure of decussation of optic and auditory nerve.

Genetics

This is an autosomal recessive syndrome caused by mutation in *LYST* (lysosomal trafficking regulator; CHS1) gene, present on the long arm of chromosome 1 (1q42.1-q42.2).

Clinical Features

This syndrome is characterized by oculocutaneous albinism, immunodeficiency, bleeding tendency and neurologic manifestation. The most life-threatening complication of Chédiak-Higashi syndrome (CHS) development of accelerated phase, a lymphoproliferative infiltration of bone marrow and reticuloendothelial system.

- *Partial oculocutaneous albinism*: Pigmentary changes involve skin, hair and eyes. In classic form, patients have silvery hair, light skin and photosensitivity with rotary nystagmus (due to reduced iris pigmentation). Visual acuity varies from moderate to normal vision.[11,12]
- *Immunodeficiency*: Infections are frequent and involve the mucous membranes, skin and respiratory tract. Children are susceptible to bacterial infection, especially *Staphylococcus* and *Streptococcus* species.[11] Viral and fungal infections are also seen.
- *Bleeding tendency*: Patients have prolonged bleeding time with normal platelet count due to platelet aggregation defect from deficiency of dense granules (containing serotonin and adenosine phosphate). Patients have mucosal or gum bleeding and easy bruising. These bleeding manifestations are mild and sometimes might not require treatment.
- *Neurologic manifestations*: Neuropathy is motor and sensory type with ataxia. It is generally seen in early adulthood and is not amenable to allogeneic hematopoietic stem cell transplantation (HSCT) as are hematologic and immunologic manifestations.[13]
- *Exacerbation phase*: This occurs in 85% of patients and can occur at any age. It is characterized by fever, jaundice, lymphadenopathy, hepatosplenomegaly and pancytopenia. The accelerated phase is now believed to be a genetic form of hemophagocytic lymphohistiocytosis (HLH). Most of the patients after entering this phase die within several months.[14]

Diagnosis

The mean age of diagnosis is 6 years and almost quarter of patients are diagnosed after 10 years of age.[11]

- The presence of large peroxidase positive inclusion granules in nucleated blood cells. Neutrophilic giant granules are pathognomonic, but these might not be seen in peripheral blood smear, but are easily identified on bone marrow examination **(Fig. 28.1)**. These patients might also develop anemia, thrombocytopenia and neutropenia.
- *Genetic assessment*: Identification of *LYST/CHS1* gene mutation located on chromosome 1.
- *Antenatal diagnosis*: Identification of gene mutation can be offered in at-risk families at time of pregnancy.

Management

Primary Disease

Stable phase: High-dose ascorbic acid (200 mg/day for infants and 2,000 mg/day for adults) can be used, but safety of high doses is a concern. Antibiotics and blood components are used as and when needed. Allogeneic HSCT is curative but does not take care of neurologic manifestations. The most favorable outcomes of transplantation are achieved if done before development of accelerated phase. G-CSF can be used in phase for neutropenia and can decrease infection rate.[15]

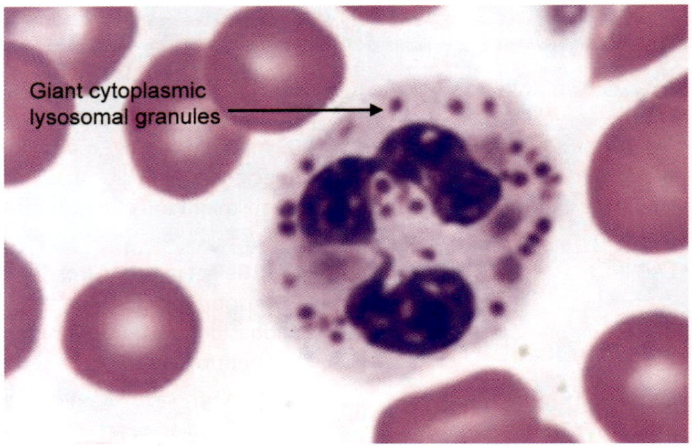

Figure 28.1 Giant cytoplasmic granules in Chédiak-Higashi syndrome (CHS) seen on blood film

Accelerated phase: Treatment protocols for accelerated phase are same as that of familial HLH, involving combination therapy of etoposide, cyclosporine, dexamethasone and intrathecal methotrexate and prednisolone. Remission is achieved in majority but relapses are common and response to therapy after each relapse decreases. So, it is recommended to do HSCT in remission phase.

Associated Complications

- *Ocular abnormalities:* Correction of refractive errors and protection of eyes from ultraviolet (UV) light.
- *Skin hypopigmentation*: Use of sunscreen lotion to prevent skin damage and skin cancer.
- *Bleeding*: Intravenous vasopressin or intranasal desmopressin can be given prior any invasive procedure and platelets can be transfused in case of extensive bleeding due to trauma. Use of drugs, which interfere with platelet function, should be avoided.

Prognosis: Prognosis depends on early diagnosis, as late diagnosis reduces success rate of HSCT. Overall this is a disease of poor prognosis and with universal fatality without treatment.

Specific Granule Deficiency

This congenital disorder is characterized by increased skin and deep tissue recurrent bacterial and fungal infection without increased incidence of viral infections.[16] Specific (secondary) granule contain leukocyte adhesion molecule, various enzymes involved in inflammatory cascade and oxidase system.[17] Neutrophils deficient in specific granules lack these secondary granules and are also deficit in defensins and lactoferrins leading deranged regulation of synthesis of lysosomal proteins. This results in abnormal chemotaxis and

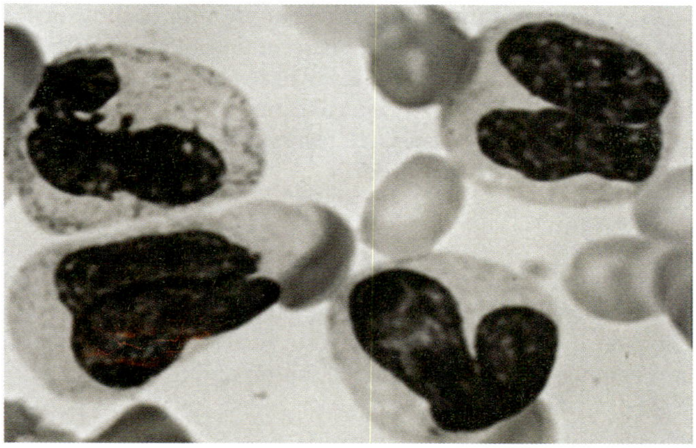

Figure 28.2 Bilobed nuclei in neutrophils seen in specific granule deficiency

impaired oxygen-free radical synthesis leading to deficient bactericidal activity.[16]

Genetics

This is an autosomal recessive disorder resulting from functional loss of myeloid transcriptional factor due to a mutation or reduced expression of *Gfi-1* or *C/EBPε*, which regulates specific granule formation.[2]

Clinical Manifestations

Specific granule deficiency neutrophils have severely impaired chemotaxis (due to lack of leukocyte adhesion molecules) and also deficiency of microbicidal molecules (lactoferrin, defensins and components of oxidase system) leads to recurrent and frequent bacterial and fungal infections (deep seated abscesses) starting from early infancy.[2,16] The common sites of infections are skin and lung.

Diagnosis

The neutrophils in peripheral smear are bilobed **(Fig. 28.2)** and lack secondary granule on Wright stain. Diagnosis is confirmed by demonstrating lack of B12 binding proteins, defensins or lactoferrins. Also, impaired neutrophil chemotaxis and respiratory burst can be demonstrated.

Treatment

Treatment includes good infection surveillance and use of prophylactic antibiotics. Also prompt recognition and aggressive control of infection is very important in determination of survival.

DISORDERS OF MICROBICIDAL METABOLISM

Chronic Granulomatous Disease

Chronic granulomatous disease (CGD) is characterized by the inability of phagocytic cells (neutrophils and monocytes) to kill catalase-producing microorganisms due to defect in generation of respiratory burst in the phagocytic cells.[18,19] This leads to frequent bacterial and fungal infection with granulomatous inflammatory lesions in histological specimens as a hallmark of disease. The incidence of CGD is estimated to be 4–5 cases per million individuals.[2]

Genetics or Pathogenesis

Under normal conditions the phagocytosis of opsonized microorganism leads to activation of metabolic activation of hexose monophosphate shunt with increased consumption of oxygen and glucose known as the "respiratory burst". This respiratory burst is mainly mediated by an enzyme system known as nicotinamide adenine dinucleotide phosphate (NADPH) oxidase. This enzyme system forms superoxide ion (O_2^-), which is then converted to reactive oxygen products (hydrogen peroxide and hypochlorous acid) within the phagosome by superoxide dismutase and lysosomal myeloperoxidase (MPO) respectively. These reactive oxygen products are involved in killing of microorganisms.

The NADPH enzyme system is made of four structural proteins, two membrane bound (gp91^{phox} and p22^{phox}) and two cytosolic (p47^{phox} and p67^{phox}).[20] Mutations in gene for any of these structural protein leads to four genetic subgroups of CGD. In addition to the structural components, the NADPH oxidase system also has critical regulatory proteins p40^{phox} and Rac. Mutation in *p40^{phox}* and *Rac* gene is yet to be associated with any CGD phenotype.[21,22] X-linked CGD is the most common type and is due to mutation in *gp91^{phox}*.[21,22] This is the clinically most severe form of CGD. Most cases are of autosomal recessive inheritance and arise due to mutation in other three protein genes. Amongst the autosomal recessive forms, mutation in gene for p47^{phox} is most common.

Clinical Features

Majority of patients are diagnosed before the age of 2 years, but a few can also be diagnosed in adulthood, which can be seen in autosomal recessive forms of disease. Patients have recurrent episodes of infections, which are difficult to treat and with unusual catalase positive organisms involving mostly skin, lung, bones and lymph nodes (other sites are also involved), leading to failure to thrive and granulomatous inflammation. Typically the infections are purulent bacterial infections (such as pneumonias, liver abscess, multiple site osteomyelitis, etc.) or necrotizing fungal infection of deep tissues. Patients may also present with severe or life-threatening infection and bacterial or fungal infections. Patients commonly have a family history of males being affected in early life with recurrent or life-threatening infections. The most common pathogen is *Staphylococcus aureus*, although other catalase positive organisms are also common (e.g. *Salmonella, Burkholderia cepacia, Candida, Aspergillus*, etc.). Granulomatous inflammation of gastrointestinal and genitourinary tract is common in CGD. In CGD, granulomatous inflammation of gastrointestinal tract may mimic Crohn's disease[20] and may develop functional gastric outlet obstruction, bladder outlet obstruction or ureter obstruction due to granulomas. In patients with falling counts and splenomegaly, possibility of macrophage activation syndrome should be kept.

Diagnosis

The possibility of CGD should be suspected in patients with severe or recurrent pulmonary or hepatic infections including abscess formation, isolation of unusual organisms, e.g. *Aspergillus, Serratia*. Granulomatous inflammation involving gastrointestinal and genitourinary tract should also prompt to investigate for CGD. On laboratory evaluation, patients have anemia, polyclonal hypergammaglobulinemia and elevated acute phase reactant proteins. The diagnosis of CGD is made by measurement of oxidative burst in neutrophils in response to stimulation. Dihydrorhodamine (DHR) test is a quantitative flow cytometric analysis of DHR 123. In this test DHR is used as a fluorescent marker of oxidase activity. This test has replaced the traditional NBT (nitro blue tetrazolium) test as it is easy to perform, can distinguish between X-linked and autosomal recessive forms and is more sensitive.[23] False positive DHR test can be seen in MPO deficiency,[20] SAPHO syndrome[24] and severe glucose 6-phosphate dehydrogenase (G6PD) deficiency.[25] In patients with severe G6PD deficiency also have features of chronic hemolysis; in MPO deficiency, the NBT and ferricytochrome C test results are normal. Molecular testing for specific genetic mutations (CYBB gene on X-chromosome for gp91^{phox}, NCF1 gene on chromosome 7 for p47phox, NCF2 on chromosome 1 for p67phox and CYBA on chromosome 16 for p22phox) is helpful in prenatal diagnosis and genotype or phenotype correlation for prognosis.

Treatment

Management of CGD involves reduction in frequency of infection and their prompt recognition and management. Oral and perianal hygiene should be maintained. Antibacterial mouth wash helps prevention of oral infections. Infections should be managed aggressively with broad-spectrum antibiotics along with antifungals. In case of severe infection, granulocyte transfusion may also be used. Parenteral antibiotics should be continued for at least 1 week after normalization of erythrocyte sedimentation rate (ESR) to prevent recurrence of infection after stoppage of antibiotics.

Prophylaxis against infection is achieved with cotrimoxazole prophylaxis (5 mg/kg/day of trimethoprim),[20] itraconazole (5 mg/kg/day), or voriconazole[26] and subcutaneous interferon gamma injections 50 µg/m^2 three times per week[26,27] are recommended.

Definitive treatment: Allogeneic HSCT is strongly recommended for all patients with CGD if suitable donor is found.

Prenatal Diagnosis

Prenatal diagnosis is offered in families in which the gene mutation is known for the family. In case of clinical suspicion with genetic mutation not known screening of mother for X-linked CGD for career state can be done using DHR test. In the carrier state, the DHR test will reveal a mosaic pattern of oxidase positive and negative neutrophils. In case of autosomal recessive case, DHR test may be normal and direct mutation analysis is required.

Prognosis

Prognosis has improved with better infection control and availability of HSCT. Highest mortality is amongst young children and the key to improved survival is on good infection surveillance and its prompt recognition and treatment.

Myeloperoxidase Deficiency

Myeloperoxidase is a minor phagocytic enzyme involved in intracellular killing of microorganisms and hypochlorous acid is major product of MPO. Hypochlorous acid is a reactive oxygen species and is involved in intracellular microbicidal activity. MPO deficiency theoretically should lead to inadequate microbicidal activity and increased propensity to infection. MPO deficiency is most common amongst the inherited disorders of phagocytes. This disease occurs at a frequency of 1 per 2,000 individuals.[2]

Genetics

It is an autosomal recessive disorder and there are two forms of disease with total and partial deficiency of MPO. Multiple restriction fragment length polymorphism has been suggested as a reason for partial and complete absence of MPO.[28] The gene for MPO is located on chromosome 17 at q22-q23 and MPO deficiency results from deranged post-translational processing of abnormal precursors.[28]

Clinical Features

Paradoxically, MPO deficiency is clinically silent.[2,29] In MPO-deficient individuals other reactive oxygen species (e.g. superoxide, hydrogen peroxide, hydroperoxyl radical, peroxynitrite) are present in microbicidal concentration and hence can account for its minor clinical effects.[30] Some patients may rarely develop disseminated candidiasis in association with other diseases like diabetes mellitus[31] or other compromises in immune function.

Diagnosis

The diagnosis is made by histochemical staining of neutrophils and monocytes for MPO. In severe deficiency of MPO a false-positive DHR test may be seen, but eosinophils will test normal for DHR test.

Treatment

As patients are asymptomatic, no antibiotic prophylaxis is indicated and aggressive treatment with antifungals to cover *Candida* is provided at times of infection. Also adequate management of associated diseases, which increase chances of candidiasis is indicated. Prognosis and survival is good.

Severe Glucose 6-Phosphate Dehydrogenase Deficiency

Glucose 6-phosphate dehydrogenase deficiency is an X-linked disease and its effect on RBCs is well known. Very little is known about the effects of its deficiency in neutrophils on their function and clinical impact. When NADPH enzyme system is activated on exposure to microorganisms, there is production of oxygen-free radicals from respiratory burst which has microbicidal activity. NADPH is the primary substrate of NADPH oxidase enzyme for generation of oxygen-free radicals. This NADPH is generated from first two steps of hexose monophosphate shunt pathway, catalyzed by G6PD and 6-phosphogluconate dehydrogenase (6PGD). In severe G6PD deficiency (neutrophil G6PD level < 5% of normal), supply of NADPH oxidase substrate is hindered and thus a CGD like state of impaired microbicidal killing develops.[32]

Clinical Features

The clinical status is like that of hemolytic anemia in most cases. Clinical signs and symptoms appear in first 2 years of life. Lymphadenopathy is seen in almost all cases and hepatic and perihepatic abscess may the first manifestation.[33]

Diagnosis

The diagnosis is made by demonstration of severe deficiency or absence of G6PD in RBCs and neutrophils with clinical features of hemolysis and CGD.

Treatment

Management mostly relies on prevention of hemolysis. In severe deficiency, management is similar to CGD with supportive care for hemolytic anemia. Granulocyte transfusion may be used in severe infections.

Rac2 Deficiency

There are three forms of Rac proteins in mammals, Rac1, 2 and 3. Rac1 and 3 proteins are abundantly expressed in different tissues, whereas Rac2 is expressed only in hematopoietic cells. In neutrophils Rac GTPase proteins have important role in activation of NADPH oxidase system for generation of oxygen-free radicals.[34] Rac2 is also known to play role in leukocyte migration and ingestion.[35] Thus an autosomal

Flow chart 28.1 Diagnostic approach to neutrophil function defects

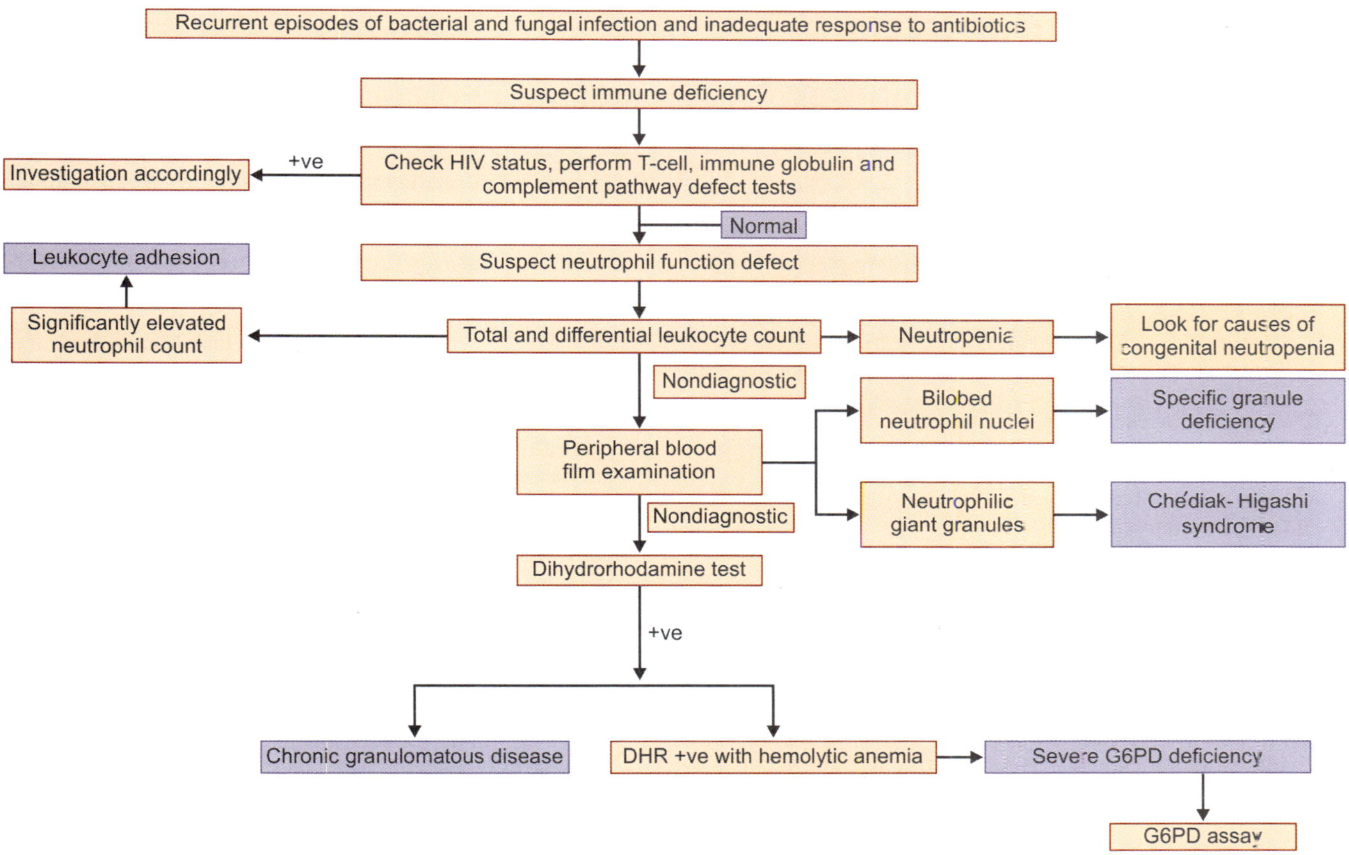

Abbreviations: DHR, dihydrorhodamine; HIV, human immunodeficiency virus

Table 28.2 Characteristics of neutrophil function defect disorders

Common diseases	*Clinical features*	*Screening test*	*Confirmatory test*
Leukocyte adhesion defect (LAD)	Recurrent infection, no pus formation and history of delayed fall of umbilical cord	Persistent PMN leukocytosis in interinfection periods also	Flow cytometry for CD11b/CD18/CD15
Chédiak-Higashi syndrome	Recurrent infection with oculocutaneous albinism, silvery hair and bleeding tendency	Neutrophilic giant granules in peripheral blood smear or bone marrow aspirate	Neutrophilic giant granules Identification of LYST/CHS 1 gene mutation located on chromosome 1
Specific granule deficiency	Recurrent infections deep-seated abscesses	Bilobed neutrophil on peripheral smear	Absence of specific granules on Wright's stain Lack of B_{12} binding proteins, defensins or lactoferrins
Chronic granulomatous disease	Recurrent episodes of abscess formation or pulmonary or hepatic infections especially affecting male members of family	DHR test	DHR test Identification of genetic mutation
Severe G6PD deficiency	Recurrent infections with clinical suspicion of hemolytic anemia	Absence or severe deficiency of G6PD	Demonstration of severe deficiency or absence of G6PD in RBCs and neutrophils with clinical features of hemolysis and CGD

Abbreviations: DHR, dihydrorhodamine; PMN, polymorphonuclear; CGD, chronic granulomatous disease

dominant mutation in Rac2 leads to a complex clinical picture showing features of LAD and CGD.

APPROACH TO THE DIAGNOSIS OF NEUTROPHIL FUNCTION DEFECTS

Flow chart 28.1 provides the diagnostic approach to neutrophil function defects. **Table 28.2** provides the features of different neutrophil function defects.

REFERENCES

1. Verma S, Sharma PK, Sivanandan S, Rana N, Saini S, Lodha R, et al. Spectrum of primary immune deficiency at a tertiary care hospital. Indian J Pediatr. 2008;75(2):143-8.
2. Coates TD. Disorders of phagocyte function. In: Kliegman RM, Stanton BM, Geme JS, Schor NF (Eds). Nelson Textbook of Pediatrics, 20th edition. Philadelphia, PA, USA: Elsevier; 2016. pp. 1040-6.
3. Vihinen M, Arredondo-Vega FX, Casanova JL, Etzioni A, Giliani S, Hammarström L, et al. Primary immunodeficiency mutation databases. Adv Genet. 2001;43:103-88.
4. Lühn K, Wild MK, Eckhardt M, Gerardy-Schahn R, Vestweber D. The gene defective in leukocyte adhesion deficiency II encodes a putative GDP-fucose transporter. Nat Genet. 2001;28(1):69-72.
5. Kinashi T, Aker M, Sokolovsky-Eisenberg M, Grabovsky V, Tanaka C, Shamri R, et al. LAD-III, a leukocyte adhesion deficiency syndrome associated with defective Rap1 activation and impaired stabilization of integrin bonds. Blood. 2004;103(3):1033-6.
6. van de Vijver E, van den Berg TK, Kuijpers TW. Leukocyte adhesion deficiencies. Hematol Oncol Clin North Am. 2013;27(1):101-16.
7. Marquardt T, Lühn K, Srikrishna G, Freeze HH, Harms E, Vestweber D. Correction of leukocyte adhesion deficiency type II with oral fucose. Blood. 1999;94(12):3976-85.
8. Yakubenia S, Wild MK. Leukocyte adhesion deficiency II. Advances and open questions. FEBS J. 2006;273(19):4390-8.
9. Weening RS, Bredius RG, Wolf H, van der Schoot CE. Prenatal diagnostic procedure for leukocyte adhesion deficiency. Prenat Diagn. 1991;11(3):193-7.
10. James WD, Berger TG, Elston DM. Disturbances of pigmentation. Andrew's Diseases of the Skin, 10th edition. Philadelphia, PA, USA: WB Saunders; 2006. pp. 853-68.
11. Barak Y, Nir E. Chediak-Higashi syndrome. Am J Pediatr Hematol Oncol. 1987;9(1):42-55.
12. BenEzra D, Mengistu F, Cividalli G, Weizman Z, Merin S, Auerbach E. Chediak-Higashi syndrome: ocular findings. J Pediatr Ophthalmol Strabismus. 1980;17(2):68-74.
13. Introne WJ, Westbroek W, Golas GA, Adams D. Chediak-Higashi syndrome In: Pagon RA, Adam MP, Ardinger HH, Wallace SE, Amemiya A, Bean LJ, et al. (Eds). GeneReviews®. Seattle, WA, USA: University of Washington, Seattle; 2015.
14. Pullarkat ST. Accelerated phase of Chédiak-Higashi syndrome. Blood. 2012;119(1):5.
15. Baldus M, Zunftmeister V, Geibel-Werle G, Claus B, Mewes D, Uppenkamp M, et al. Chédiak-Higashi-Steinbrinck syndrome (CHS) in a 27-year-old woman: effects of G-CSF treatment. Ann Hematol. 1999;78(7):321-7.
16. Gallin JI. Neutrophil specific granule deficiency. Annu Rev Med. 1985;36:263-74.
17. Boxer LA, Smolen JE. Neutrophil granule constituents and their release in health and disease. Hematol Oncol Clin North Am. 1988;2(1):101-34.
18. Borregaard N. Activation of phagocytes. Eur J Clin Invest. 1985;15(5):240-1.
19. Phagocytic defects II: Abnormalities of the respiratory burst. Hematol Oncol Clin North Am. 1988;2(2):185-336.
20. Seger RA. Modern management of chronic granulomatous disease. Br J Haematol. 2008;140(3):255-66.
21. Roos D. The genetic basis of chronic granulomatous disease. Immunol Rev. 1994;138:121-57.
22. Kinnon C, Levinsky R. The molecular basis of X-linked immunodeficiency disease. J Inherit Metab Dis. 1992;15(4): 674-82.

cytoplasmic granules. The disorder is caused by mutations in the *RAB27A* gene. Uncontrolled T-lymphocyte and macrophage activation syndrome occurs because of their immune abnormalities.[26]

Hemophagocytic Lymphohistiocytosis

Hemophagocytic lymphohistiocytosis (HLH) is characterized by fever, neurologic findings, hepatosplenomegaly, pancytopenia, liver and coagulation abnormalities and elevated triglyceride and ferritin levels. Mutation in several genes have been found among patients with familial HLH.

Autoimmune Lymphoproliferative Syndrome

In this disorder, neutropenia is a frequent finding and is often associated with other autoimmune disorders. In some patients defects in genes associated with lymphocyte apoptosis have been identified.

WHIM Syndrome

Neutropenia in this autosomal dominant syndrome characterized by Warts, Hypogammaglobulinemia, Infections, and Myelokathexis (WHIM)) may result from a defective release of marrow cells into the peripheral blood.

Stress, fever and possibly G-CSF administration may temporarily overcome the confinement of neutrophils to the marrow.[27]

Reticular Dysgenesis

It is one of the rarest and most extreme forms of neutropenia. This disorder is associated with severe combined immunodeficiency (SCID) and is characterized by congenital agranulocytosis, lymphopenia and lymphoid and thymic hypoplasia. G-CSF administration usually does not help in improving neutrophil counts and the patients often die within the first weeks of life. Hematopoietic stem cell transplantation may be help.

CLINICAL EVALUATION OF NEUTROPENIA IN NEONATES

Common causes of neonatal neutropenia are sepsis, maternal hypertension, twin-twin transfusion, hemolytic disease and allo-immunization. A careful history of maternal hypertension with evidence of growth restriction of fetus, disparity between twins in case of multiple gestation or infectious illness during pregnancy should be carefully elicited as it may be diagnostic. The infants born to mothers with pregnancy induced hypertension have incidence of neutropenia as high as 49%. The severity of growth restriction has been correlated to severity of neutropenia. Maternal history of chorioamnionitis or prolonged rupture of membranes, with neutropenia in a neonate can indicate increased risk of early onset sepsis. Transient neutropenia occurs with sepsis, and resolves with recovery from sepsis. But in critically ill neonates, neutropenia is a sign of severe sepsis and bone marrow depression.

A maternal drug history and a maternal neutrophil count should be obtained to exclude maternal illness (e.g. systemic lupus erythematosus) as a cause of neutropenia. A careful family history specifically about family members with documented neutropenia or a history of unusual or severe infections or early neonatal deaths should be elicited. Early neonatal deaths may be secondary to severe neutropenia and may be an important clue to the possibility of an inherited neutropenic syndrome (e.g. Kostmann syndrome). A careful physical examination will help to suggest or exclude hypersplenism and congenital viral infections as the likely cause of neutropenia. Neonatal alloimmune neutropenia should be considered in well appearing infants with-out apparent cause for the neutropenic state.

LABORATORY EVALUATION OF NEUTROPENIA IN NEONATES

Many of the underlying causes for neutropenia are clear- prematurity, sepsis, syndromes, etc. and do not need detailed diagnostic evaluation. Any persistent neutropenia needs evaluation, even if of moderate severity. Laboratory tests necessary are CBC and a blood film, mothers' CBC to check her neutrophil count. If the mother's neutrophil counts are normal, check maternal neutrophil antigen typing and an antineutrophil antibody screen.

The peripheral blood smear should be carefully examined for morphology of the neutrophils, vacuolization, Döhle bodies, or toxic granulations. The band to segmented neutrophil ratio should be determined. Is this a bone marrow failure with pancytopenia (inherited bone marrow failure syndrome), or bicytopenia (WAS) or only isolated neutropenia.

The immature to total neutrophil (I:T) ratio:

$$\frac{(\text{Bands} + \text{Metamyelocytes} + \text{Myelocytes})}{(\text{Segmented neutrophils} + \text{Bands} + \text{Metamyelocytes} + \text{Myelocytes})}$$

In the term neonate the mean value is 0.16 (SD 0.10), (with a 10–90th percentile range from 0.05 to 0.27). An elevated I:T ratio (≥ 0.3), with neutropenia, indicates a depletion of the neutrophil storage pool in the bone marrow, due to either increased peripheral destruction or pooling of neutrophils at the site of infection.

Decreased neutrophil production is indicated by a normal/low I:T ratio in a neutropenic infant. In preterm infants, the I:T ratio has a discriminatory value and can be employed along with tests for sepsis such as C-reactive protein concentration.[27,28]

In presence of prolonged neutropenia, more than two weeks or if neutropenia is severe a bone marrow biopsy should be considered. The bone marrow evaluation gives valuable information on the number and maturation stage or arrest of granulocytic cells in the bone marrow. Decreased marrow production is suggested by reduction in granulocytic cell precursors, while increased numbers of proliferative precursors, but with a depleted storage pool is indicative of increased peripheral destruction of neutrophils (alloimmune, hypersplenism, etc.). If alloimmune neutropenia is suspected then evaluation of neutrophil antibodies in a sample of mother and/or infant's serum and neutrophil-specific antigen typing of parents is possible.

CLINICAL MANAGEMENT OF A NEONATE WITH NEUTROPENIA

In unwell neonates with neutropenia, sepsis should be considered as foremost differential and a presumptive course of antibiotics should be started pending the cultures reports.[30] A history of prolonged rupture of membranes or chorioamnionitis in a newborn infant with neutropenia can indicate increased risk of early-onset sepsis. Sepsis-induced neutropenia is usually transient and resolves with recovery from sepsis, but in a critically-ill infant with multisystem dysfunction, neutropenia could be a sign of overwhelming sepsis and bone marrow depression.

When neonatal sepsis is suspected, treatment should be initiated immediately because of the neonate's relative immunosuppression. Begin antibiotics as soon as diagnostic tests are performed. A neonate with sepsis may also require treatment aimed at the overwhelming systemic effects of sepsis that is cardiopulmonary support, intravenous fluids, ionotropic support, DIC management and intravenous nutrition. Adequate monitoring of blood pressure, vital signs, hematocrit, platelets, and coagulation studies is vital, for proper management. Search for pathogen is very important to direct the treatment. Blood product transfusion, is necessary to manage the sick newborn hence packed red blood cells (PRBCs), platelets, and fresh-frozen plasma (FFP), are given as necessary. Follow the region specific guidelines for treatment of early-onset neonatal sepsis—IV aminoglycoside and expanded-spectrum penicillin antibiotic therapy for Gram-positive organisms, especially group B *Streptococcus* (GBS), and Gram-negative bacteria, such as *Escherichia coli*. It is important to know the hospital sensitivity and resistance patterns to guide therapy till blood culture reports are obtained. In nosocomial infections it is even more important to know the sensitivity and resistance patterns of common hospital-acquired infections, including *Staphylococcus aureus, Staphylococcus epidermidis*, and *Pseudomonas* species, and initiate early intervention, while awaiting reports.

Culture reports may not yield valuable information if the mother received antibiotics outside or cultures were taken after starting antibiotic treatment. This may result in false negative culture results in infants bacteremia or sepsis: follow all reports to give a clue to etiology of sepsis:

- Clinical status
- Complete blood cell (CBC) count and differential
- Culture results
- Maternal and intrapartum risk factors
- CSF results
- C-reactive protein (CRP) trend
- Radiographs or other imaging
- Clinical progress.

TREATMENT

Treatment may be indicated if strong case of suspicion, even if culture reports are negative. If there is no clinical or laboratory evidence of infection, other causes of neutropenia must be considered **(Table 29.1)**. However, until another cause is identified broad-spectrum antibiotic coverage may be continued.

To treat neonatal neutropenia, Recombinant G-CSF is frequently used, earlier Granulocyte-Macrophage-Colony stimulating factor (GM-CSF) was used, but now less frequently. GM-CSF generates both granulocyte and macrophage colonies from precursor cells[29] while G-CSF stimulates only neutrophil production and release from the bone marrow, and reduces neutrophil apoptosis. GM-CSF can be induced in inflamed tissues to promote neutrophil and macrophage maturation but may not play a major role in steady state conditions unlike G-CSF, which is the main systemic regulator of neutrophils.[30] In the clinical setting, both G-CSF and GM-CSF increase neutrophil counts, although G-CSF may be more efficacious in raising neutrophil counts than GM-CSF.[31] Use of growth factors as a routine standard of care for very low-birth-weight or extremely low-birth-weight is not recommended, even though many studies exist, but evidence based guidelines do not support the routine use of G-CSF to prevent or treat neutropenia in the setting of sepsis.

In immune-mediated neutropenias, the use of G-CSF is also very effective. Apart from its effect on delaying apoptosis and neutrophil production, G-CSF also renders neutrophils less vulnerable to circulating antibodies by downregulating antigen expression, and corrects some of the functional impairments in neutrophils induced by anti-neutrophil antibodies.

In many patients with congenital neutropenias, G-CSF is effective. It is highly effective in most patients with Kostmann syndrome. Treatment with G-CSF increases neutrophil counts and prevents infection in 90% of cases with Kostmann syndrome. Patients not responding to G-CSF alone may benefit with addition of low dose prednisone to the G-CSF regimen, or allogeneic hematopoietic stem cell transplantation.[32] G–CSF helps in to reduce the number of days of neutropenia in patients with cyclic neutropenia, which is a rare hematological disorder characterized by drop in absolute neutrophil counts (ANCs) at intervals of 3 weeks to levels as low as 250/μL. Bone marrow shows maturational arrest during or just before the onset of neutropenia but is normal during periods of normal ANCs.

Neutropenia related to maternal hypertension is usually self-limiting, the risk of infections in such patients is unclear, if needed, G-CSF can be used to correct neutropenia in these patients.

Idiopathic neutropenia of prematurity, can be severe and prolonged, the infants may be neutropenic at or shortly after

Table 29.1 Causes of neutropenia in newborn infants and their treatment

Decreased neutrophil production	
Infants of hypertensive mothers (unknown; possible causes include presence of a placenta-derived inhibitor of neutrophil production)	Supportive care
Donors of twin-twin transfusions	
Neonates with Rh hemolytic disease (precursors diverted towards erythroid differentiation to increase RBC production)	Supportive care
Viral infections (infection of neutrophil progenitors, hypersplenism)	
Cytomegalovirus	Ganciclovir
Rubella	Supportive care
Congenital neutropenias (Bone marrow failure syndromes)	
Kostmann syndrome	G-CSF Hematopoietic stem cell transplant (HSCT)
Wiskott-Aldrich syndrome (WAS) gene	Supportive care, prevention of infections, HSCT
Other gene mutations may involve anti-apoptotic genes *HAX1*, G6PC3	HSCT
Reticular dysgenesis	HSCT
Shwachman-Diamond syndrome	Supportive care, prevention of infections, management of pancreatic insufficiency, HSCT
Cartilage-hair hypoplasia	HSCT
Barth syndrome	Antibiotic prophylaxis, G-CSF
Cyclic neutropenia	G-CSF. Antibiotic prophylaxis
Idiopathic neutropenia of prematurity (precursors diverted towards erythroid differentiation to compensate for anemia of prematurity)	Supportive care
Inborn Errors of Metabolism	
Organic acidemias (decrease in neutrophil precursors)	Supportive care
Glycogen storage disease type 1b	Supportive care
Increased destruction	
Bacterial or fungal sepsis (increased tissue migration; marrow suppression in severe cases)	Antibiotic and supportive care
Necrotizing enterocolitis (neutrophils move to intestines and peritoneum)	Antibiotic, supportive care surgery if needed
Anti-neutrophil antibody-mediated disorders such as neonatal autoimmune neutropenia, and autoimmune neutropenia of infancy	IVIG or steroids
Alloimmune neutropenia associated with anti-HNA-1b antibodies (antigen present on neutrophil precursors)	IVIG
Drug-induced neutropenia (β-lactam antibiotics, thiazides, ranitidine, acyclovir, etc.)	Remove offending drug
Cyclic neutropenia	G-CSF. Antibiotic prophylaxis
Idiopathic neutropenia of prematurity (blood precursors pushed towards erythroid differentiation, so as to compensate for anemia of prematurity)	Supportive care
Pseudoneutropenia (benign condition): The circulating neutrophil pool is smaller than marginated pool	None
Hemophagocytic lymphohistocytosis (HLH)	Most likely primary HLH. Regimen of HLH therapy, HSCT if no response

Abbreviations: G-CSF, granulocyte-colony stimulating factor; IVIG, intravenous immunoglobulin birth and neutropenia may last for 1–9 weeks. G-CSF treatment helps in immediate and marked rise in neutrophil counts, but its use is not routinely indicated, the treatment decisions are based on duration and severity and of neutropenia.

HOW TO USE RECOMBINANT G-CSF?

G-CSF is given by the subcutaneous route but can be given intravenously, the usual starting dose is 5–10 µg/kg/day. In many cases a rise in ANC will occur after 24–48 hours. If not the dose may be increased in increments of 10 µg/kg at weekly intervals. If no response by 2–3 weeks, it should be stopped. Short term G-CSF treatment is well tolerated, even in neonates. But there are adverse effects of long term use-splenic rupture, risk of malignancy and myelodysplasia.

Other modalities such as intravenous immunoglobulin (IVIG) have also been tried in neonatal neutropenia. It is usually used for infants with autoimmune and alloimmune neutropenia. IVIG acts by mobilizing neutrophils from marrow storage pools, and binding to some circulating antibodies. Steroids have some efficacy in autoimmune neutropenia but generally ineffective in alloimmune neutropenia. Exchange transfusions are not effective in treating immune-mediated neutropenias.

Granulocyte transfusions have been used and current guidelines accept them as a modality of treatment. Though evidence based trials do not exist to support their routine use. If used then guidelines[33] suggest avoiding G-CSF or steroids in the donor to mobilize the granulocytes. This has to be irradiated prior to giving to the newborn.

PREVENTION

All care must be taken to screen mothers and provide for intrapartum antimicrobial prophylaxis for perinatal group B *Streptococcus* (GBS) disease, this is important to prevent newborn mortality and morbidity from GBS. All efforts to prevent nosocomial infections in nurseries is essential.

CONCLUSION

Neutropenia is a commonly faced condition in NICU, especially in premature and critically ill neonates. In a neonate, neutropenia is defined as a neutrophil concentration less than 1,000/µL and severe neutropenia by a count less than 500/µL.

The most common causes are sepsis, maternal hypertension, hemolytic disease, twin-twin transfusion, and alloimmunization.

In infants with severe (ANC <500/µL) and persistent (>5–7 days) neutropenia, detailed clinical and laboratory evaluation is indicated. Initial lab testing should include CBC, careful examination of the peripheral blood film, a complete blood count on the mother with a note on her blood neutrophil concentration, if mother's neutrophil count is normal, maternal neutrophil antigen typing and an antineutrophil antibody screen. In presence of prolonged, refractory or unusual neutropenia, a bone marrow biopsy can be useful.

After establishing the cause of neutropenia, appropriate and prompt treatment should be given, which may include use of growth factors. In unwell neonates with neutropenia, sepsis should be considered as foremost differential and a presumptive course of antibiotics should be started pending the culture reports.

KEY POINTS

- Neutropenia in newborns is very common, may be seen in 8–50% of NICU admissions.
- Neutropenia may be because of common causes such as maternal hypertension, sepsis and alloimmunization or may be because of rare immunodeficiency syndromes.
- A careful assessment helps in to establish the diagnosis.
- Prompt and appropriate treatment should be started to prevent life-threatening events.

REFERENCES

1. Barak Y, Leibovitz E, Mogilner B, et al. The in vivo effect of recombinant human granulocyte-colony stimulating factor in neutropenic neonates with sepsis. Eur J Pediatr. 1997;156:643-6.
2. Ishii E, Masuyama T, Yamaguchi H, et al. Production and expression of granulocyte- and macrophage-colony-stimulating factors in newborns: their roles in leukocytosis at birth. Acta Haematol. 1995;94:23-31.
3. Manroe BL, Weinberg AG, Rosenfeld CR, et al. The neonatal blood count in health and disease. I. Reference values for neutrophilic cells. J Pediatr. 1979;95:89-98.
4. Mouzinho A, Rosenfeld CR, Sanchez PJ, et al. Revised reference ranges for circulating neutrophils in very-low-birth-weight neonates. Pediatrics. 1994;94:7682.
5. Zipursky A, Palko J, Milner R, et al. The hematology of bacterial infections in premature infants. Pediatrics. 1976;57:839-53.
6. Christensen RD, Calhoun DA, Rimsza LM. A practical approach to evaluating and treating neutropenia in the neonatal intensive care unit. Clin Perinatol. 2000;27:577-601.
7. Christensen RD, Harper TE, Rothstein G. Granulocyte-macrophage progenitor cells in term and preterm neonates. J Pediatr. 1986;109:1047-51.
8. Levine DH, Madyastha PR. Isoimmune neonatal neutropenia. Am J Perinatol. 1986;3:231-3.
9. Minchinton RM, McGrath KM. Alloimmune neonatal neutropenia: a neglected diagnosis? Med J Aust. 1987;147:139-41.
10. Maheshwari A, Christensen RD, Calhoun DA. Immune neutropenia in the neonate. Adv Pediatr. 2002;49:317-39.
11. Kameoka J, Funato T, Miura T, et al. Autoimmune neutropenia in pregnant women causing neonatal neutropenia. Br J Haematol. 2001;114:198-200.
12. Neiman AR, Lee LA, Weston WL, et al. Cutaneous manifestations of neonatal lupus without heart block: characteristics of mothers and children enrolled in a national registry. J Pediatr. 2000;137:674-80.
13. Lalezari P, Khorshidi M, Petrosova M. Autoimmune neutropenia of infancy. J Pediatr. 1986;109:764-9.
14. Conway LT, Clay ME, Kline WE, et al. Natural history of primary autoimmune neutropenia in infancy. Pediatrics. 1987;79:728-33.

15. Bruin MC, von dem Borne AE, Tamminga RY, et al. Neutrophil antibody specificity in different types of childhood autoimmune neutropenia. Blood. 1999;94:1797-1802.
16. Calhoun DA, Rimsza LM, Burchfield DJ, et al. Congenital autoimmune neutropenia in two premature neonates. Pediatrics. 2001;108:181-4.
17. Koenig JM, Christensen RD. The mechanism responsible for diminished neutrophil production in neonates delivered of women with pregnancy-induced hypertension. Am J Obstet Gynecol. 1991;165:467-73.
18. Kostman-R. Infantile genetic agranulocytosis. A review with presentation of ten new cases. Acta Paediatr Scand. 1975;64: 362-8.
19. Dale DC, Person RE, Bolyard AA, et al. Mutations in the gene encoding neutrophil elastase in congenital and cyclic neutropenia. Blood. 2000;96:23172-328.
20. Benson KF, Li FQ, Person RE, et al. Mutations associated with neutropenia in dogs and humans disrupt intracellular transport of neutrophil elastase. Nat Genet. 2003;35:90-6.
21. Aprikyan AA, Kutyavin T, Stein S, et al. Cellular and molecular abnormalities in severe congenital neutropenia predisposing to leukemia. ExpHematol. 2003;31:372-81.
22. Kuijpers TW, Maianski NA, Tool AT, et al. Apoptotic neutrophils in the circulation of patients with glycogen storage disease type 1b (GSD1b). Blood. 2003;101:5021-4.
23. Bione S, D'Adamo P, Maestrini E, et al. A novel X-linked gene, G4.5. is responsible for Barth syndrome. Nat Genet. 1996;12:385-9.
24. Imai K, Nonoyama S, Ochs HD. *WASP* (Wiskott-Aldrich syndrome protein) gene mutations and phenotype. Curr Opin Allergy Clin Immunol. 2003;3:427-36.
25. Makitie O, Pukkala E, Kaitila I. Increased mortality in cartilage-hair hypoplasia. Arch Dis Child. 2001;84:65-7.
26. Nakashima E, Mabuchi A, Kashimada K, et al. RMRP mutations in Japanese patients with cartilage-hair hypoplasia. Am J Med Genet. 2003;123A:253-6.
27. Cannistra SA, Griffin JD. Regulation of the production and function of granulocytes and monocytes. Semin Hematol. 1988;25(3):173-88.
28. Rivera-Matos IR, Rakita RM, Mariscalco MM, Elder FF, Dreyer SA, Cleary TG. Leukocyte adhesion deficiency mimicking Hirschsprung disease. J Pediatr. 1995;127(5):755-7.
29. Burgess AW, Metcalf D. The nature and action of granulocyte-macrophage colony stimulating factors. Blood. 1980;56(6): 947-58.
30. Calhoun DA, Christensen RD. Human developmental biology of granulocyte colony-stimulating factor. Clin Perinatol. 2000;27 (3):559-76.
31. Ahmad A, Laborada G, Bussel J, Nesin M. Comparison of recombinant granulocyte colonystimulating factor, recombinant human granulocyte-macrophage colony-stimulating factor and placebo for treatment of septic preterm infants. Pediatr Infect Dis J. 2002;21(11):1061-5.
32. Zeidler C, Welte K, Barak Y, et al. Stem cell transplantation in patients with severe congenital neutropenia without evidence of leukemic transformation. Blood. 2000;95:1195-8.
33. *http://www.transfusionguidelines.org.uk/document-library/documents/position-statement-granulocyte-therapy/download-file/Position%20Statement%20on%20Granulocyte%20Therapy%20February%202014.pdf. (Accessed 5 march 2016)*

SECTION 6

Fetal and Neonatal Malignancy

Section Editors

Girish Chinnaswamy, Arpita Bhattacharya

CHAPTER

30

Cancers in Infants

Akanksha Chichra, Purna Kurkure

INTRODUCTION

Cancers in infants have unique clinical, biological and epidemiological features, which may help us in better understanding of the mechanisms of carcinogenesis. Malignancies of infancy represent 10% of all cancer that is diagnosed among children younger than 15 years of age.[1]

SPECIAL FEATURES

Cancer in infants presents a unique situation to study cancer etiology. The process of oncogenesis in infants is closely related to embryogenesis.[2] Various possible causes have been suggested in this age group including genetic susceptibility, intrauterine and postnatal environmental exposures. Familial cases of Wilms' tumor and retinoblastoma occur at an earlier age. Some genetic syndromes, like Down syndrome (DS) are associated with increased risk of cancer. Evidence suggests that the cause of cancer in infants is related to an acquired or constitutional abnormality of cancer predisposing genes, which are critical during embryogenesis. The fact that some fetal and neonatal malignant tumors manifesting in the first few months of life can spontaneously regress or differentiate supports the role of oncogenes in the modulation of oncogenesis. In a seminal paper in 1971, Alfred Knudson took the idea of multiple hits an important step further.[3] Knudson analyzed 48 cases of retinoblastoma for the occurrence of bilateral or unilateral tumors and the presence of a family history of the disease. Using Poisson statistics, he showed that the distribution observed was consistent with retinoblastoma being caused by two mutations. In familial cases, one hit was inherited whereas the other one was acquired later; in sporadic tumors, both changes were somatic with a similar mutation rate for both hits. The Knudson model explained why multiple tumors occurred in both eyes in inherited cases, but only unilaterally in sporadic occurrences.

FETAL ORIGINS OF CANCER

There is now evidence that chromosome translocations are often the first or initiating events in leukemia, occurring prenatally during fetal development. This evidence comes from two sources—identical twin infants or children with concordant acute lymphoblastic leukemia (ALL)[4] and retrospective scrutiny of neonatal blood spots or Guthrie cards. Polymerase chain reaction (PCR) tests for specific fusion genes, designed for each patient, can detect as few as 1–20 leukemic cells in a blood spot. The presence of the same fusion gene sequence in a neonatal blood spot as is in the patient's leukemic cells at diagnosis[5,6] provides unequivocal evidence that leukemia has been initiated prenatally, probably by formation of the fusion gene itself. The conclusions from Guthrie card studies are that leukemia is fetal in origin in all cases of infant leukemia [with fusions of the mixed-lineage leukemia (MLL) gene], in most cases of the common form of childhood ALL (with TEL-AML1), and in about half of cases of childhood acute myeloblastic leukemia (with translocation of chromosomes 8 and 21).

Children at High Risk for Cancer

Children with predisposition to malignancy include:

- Those with various hereditary cutaneous and neurocutaneous syndromes
- Hereditary or acquired gastrointestinal syndromes
- Chromosomal abnormalities
- Immunodeficiency syndromes
- Congenital malformations
- Survivors of prior cancer.

EPIDEMIOLOGY

The distribution of cancers in infancy varies significantly from that in later childhood. The most common cancers in infants in the United States are:

- Neuroblastoma
- Leukemia
- Brain tumor
- Retinoblastoma.

In the developing countries like India, retinoblastoma is the top ranking tumor in this age group.

CHALLENGES IN MANAGEMENT OF INFANTILE CANCERS

Management of infantile cancers has unique challenges.

Chemotherapy Dosing in Infants

Young children differ significantly in the way their bodies handle drugs. At birth all mechanism of drug elimination are reduced as compared to older children. Both hepatic drug metabolism and renal elimination are as low as 10% of adult values in neonates with the preterm being at the extreme end.[7] This means that children less than 1 year of age would need a 25% lower dose/m^2 to achieve similar serum concentrations. Most of the drugs are calculated based on body weight in infants rather than body surface area as in older children.

Venous Access

Treatment of pediatric malignancies is becoming progressively more complex, implying the adoption of multimodal therapies. A reliable, long-lasting venous access represents one of the critical requirements for the success of these treatments. In infants, treatment can be delivered only through central venous access devices, like Hickman catheters or chemotherapy ports. This places an additional financial burden in the management of these patients.

Nutritional Issues

Cancer and treatment of cancer can have adverse effects on food intake, absorption and metabolism, all of which can result in malnutrition. Malnutrition can affect tolerance of therapy and hence overall outcomes. Malnutrition is of concern particularly in infants as they have limited reserves of energy. In an infant who is not taking orally, a nutritional care plan needs to be instituted right away. If the child is unable to take orally, nasogastric or G tube feedings should be started. Total parenteral nutrition (TPN) should be used for infants who are unable to ingest or absorb calories enterally.

PAIN ASSESSMENT AND MANAGEMENT

Infants with cancer experience pain due to multiple procedures and therapeutic protocols. Effective pain management in infants is usually suboptimal. Assessing pain in infants remains one of the most difficult challenges facing clinicians. The most well-validated pain scoring systems are based on multiple indicators of behavior, physiological parameters and other indicators of pain.

Pain management needs to be multidimensional involving both pharmacological and nonpharmacological strategies.

Pharmacologic agents include opioid analgesics, sedatives, nonsteroidal anti-inflammatory drugs (NSAIDs), local anesthetics and sucrose.

Vaccination in Children with Cancer

The safe and effective usage of vaccines has always been a major challenge in children with compromised immune functions. The main concerns include the safety of vaccines in the immunosuppressed state and the ability of the child to mount and sustain an adequate response. The immune responses to vaccines are influenced by the timing of the vaccines in relation to the chemotherapy, the underlying cancer in the child and the type of chemotherapy being given.

In infants specifically the primary immunization gets interrupted and many of them have to be revaccinated after completion of treatment.

Primary responses to vaccines are more likely to be adversely affected than secondary booster responses, an issue particularly relevant to infants.

Live vaccines are usually withheld for a minimum of 3 months after immunosuppressive therapy. The main concern for inactivated vaccines is whether sustainable and protective responses will result. Vaccination during the maintenance phase of chemotherapy is preferred with boosters advisable after 3 months of completion of therapy.

COMMON HEMATOLYMPHOID AND SOLID TUMORS IN INFANTS

Leukemias

The leukemias as a group represent the most common type of cancer after neuroblastoma, comprising 17% of all cases. As with older children, ALL is the most frequently occurring leukemia.

The two most important forms of infantile leukemias are:
- Infant acute lymphoblastic leukemia
- Leukemia in infants with Down syndrome.

Infant Acute Lymphoblastic Leukemia

Acute lymphoblastic leukemia (ALL) in infants accounts for about 4% of childhood ALL and differs from ALL in older children with respect to immunophenotypic, cytogenetic and molecular genetic features. Compared with ALL in older children, ALL in infants has a dismal outcome because rearrangements of the *MLL* gene occur in about 80% of these patients, leading to an aggressive high risk leukemia. With most recent therapies, about 50% long-term event-free survival is achieved, but early bone marrow relapse remains a major problem.

Infants with ALL have a higher leukocyte count and an increased incidence of hepatosplenomegaly and central nervous system (CNS) involvement than older children with ALL. The median white blood count (WBC) in infant ALL is about 100×10^9/L. About 15% of infants with ALL have CNS involvement and about 13% of male infants have testis involvement. The mediastinum is enlarged in less than 5% of patients.[8]

About two-thirds of infant ALL is characterized by a very immature CD10-negative B-lineage precursor ALL (proB ALL).

Infant ALL cells are more likely to express myeloid-associated antigens. These data suggest that infant ALL arises from an immature precursor cell that is not fully committed to lymphoid differentiation. Intraclonal switch from B-lineage to monocytic-lineage leukemia has been described in infants.[9]

Age less than 6 months and the presence of MLL rearrangements have been found to be poor prognostic factors.

Infant ALL cells are more sensitive than cells from older children with ALL to ara-C (cytarabine) and 2-CdA (2-chlorodeoxyadenosine or cladribine).[10]

Acute Megakaryoblastic Leukemia in Down Syndrome

Children with DS have a tenfold to twentyfold increased risk of developing acute leukemias.[11] About 10% of newborns with DS develop transient myeloproliferative disease (TMD) and 20% of infants with TMD go on to develop acute megakaryoblastic leukemias (AMKLs).

Transient Myeloproliferative Disease

This is an entity unique to infants with DS and is characterized by presence of clonal blasts in peripheral smear similar to those in AMKL. Usually the course of transient myeloproliferative disease (TMD) is uncomplicated and by definition there is spontaneous resolution within 3 months of life. In some cases, the blasts can infiltrate organs like liver, heart and skin and produce symptoms. Intervention is required only for symptomatic cases usually in the form of short course of low-dose cytarabine.

Acute Megakaryoblastic Leukemia

Acute megakaryoblastic leukemia is a subtype of acute myeloid leukemias (AMLs), which is usually rare in children but accounts for 62–86% of AML in children with DS.[12] Another unique feature of this acute leukemia in this population is the higher than usual survival rate of 70–90%.[13] This favorable response of AML in DS children can be partly attributed to the increased sensitivity of the blasts to cytarabine.

Both the blasts of TMD and AMKL have somatic mutations in GATA1, which is the focus of research.[14]

Solid Tumors in Infants

Multidisciplinary approach is key to success in the management of pediatric solid tumors. With inputs of a pediatric oncologist, surgeon, radiotherapist, diagnostic specialists and supportive care services.

Some of the general guidelines in the management of a child with cancer are as follows:

- The general clinical status of the child (performance status) should be evaluated to determine the child's ability to undergo various diagnostic and therapeutic procedures
- Assessment of the extent of disease (staging).
- Complete treatment strategy planning including time and site of biopsy
- Histopathological confirmation of diagnosis with reference to known prognostic factors
- Institution of therapy in sequence as per the strategy decided before
- Monitoring the progress of treatment, side effects of therapy and results
- Supportive services in form of rehabilitation, psychosocial support to the child and parents
- Long-term follow-up with respect to disease activity as well as late effects of therapy.

NEUROBLASTOMA

Neuroblastoma is the most common malignancy in infancy and 40% of neuroblastomas are diagnosed in the 1st year of life.

The natural history of these tumors in infancy follows a more benign clinical course usually, but subsets of infants with adverse biological characteristics behave like older children.

Stage 4-Special

Stage 4-special (4S) tumors are by definition in the infantile age group. They are defined as a localized primary tumor with dissemination limited to skin, liver, and/or bone marrow in absence of cortical bone involvement. Marrow involvement should be minimal (i.e. <10% of total nucleated cells identified as malignant by bone biopsy or by bone marrow aspirate).

More extensive bone marrow involvement would be considered stage 4 disease.

Stage 4S neuroblastoma is a special tumor, which accounts for 7–10% of all neuroblastoma and is associated with excellent prognosis.[15,16] One of its main features is that it may undergo spontaneous regression. In young infants and neonates, the tumor may progress causing massive hepatomegaly, renal obstruction and coagulopathy that can lead to serious complications and death. Symptomatic patients often need urgent intervention with chemotherapy or radiotherapy to survive as early intervention is associated with a better outcome.[17]

Spontaneous Regression

Neuroblastoma is known to show the highest rate of spontaneous regression among malignant tumors.[18] Besides the well-known spontaneous regression in stage 4S disease,[19,20] the high incidence of neuroblastic remnants found during autopsies of newborns suggested for the first time that localized lesions may undergo a similar process.[21,22] In the 1990s, screening studies reported a twofold to threefold higher incidence of neuroblastoma in areas with screening programs.[23,24] This so-called overdiagnosis was explained by spontaneous regression and supports the hypothesis of spontaneous regression in nonstage 4S neuroblastoma.

CLINICAL FEATURES

Infants usually have tumors arising equally from thoracic and adrenal sites. Depending on the site of involvement they can present with superior vena cava syndrome, abdominal lump, pain, neurological deficit or paraneoplastic syndrome.

The paraneoplastic syndromes associated with neuroblastoma include:

- Opsomyoclonus also known as dancing eye-dancing feet syndrome characterized by nystagmus and ataxia
- Secretory diarrhea in tumors that secrete VIPs (vasoactive intestinal peptides).

Infants presenting with paraneoplastic syndromes paradoxically do better and have a better tumor prognosis.

Infants can also present with hypertension, usually more due to renal artery compression by the tumor rather than release of catecholamines.

RISK STRATIFICATION

The important prognostic factors based on which the Children's Oncology Group (COG) risk groups have been devised include:

- *Age*: Infants have good prognosis
- *International neuroblastoma staging system (INSS) stage*: Even higher stage 3 and 4 disease with favorable biological features have good prognosis in this age group
- Pathological classification of pretreatment tumors based on amount of Schwannian stromal component, degree of differentiation, mitosis-karyorrhexis index (MKI) and age in two broad categories of favorable and unfavorable histology
- *NMYC amplification status*: NMYC amplified tumors are relatively rare in infants. NMYC amplification overtakes all other features and categorizes tumor as high-risk
- *DNA ploidy*: Hyperdiploidy with DNA index more than 1.16 indicative of gain of whole chromosome. These tumors express high level of tropomyosin receptor kinase A (TrkA) neurotrophin receptor and may undergo spontaneous maturation and have good prognosis.

Based on these factors patients are divided into three risk categories—low, intermediate and high. Infants usually have low-risk disease, those with stage 3, 4 and NMYC nonamplified will fall in intermediate risk category and any stage tumor with NMYC amplification is considered high risk and have a poor prognosis similar to older children.

RISK-BASED TREATMENT

The treatment of neuroblastoma has evolved over the past 60 years. Generally, treatment is based on whether the tumor is low, intermediate or high risk **(Figs 30.1 and 30.2)**.

- *Low-risk tumors*: The approach is either observation or resection. 5-year overall survival (OS) was 97% in a large COG study.[25]
- *Intermediate-risk tumors*: Chemotherapy is often given before definitive resection. The duration of chemotherapy is based on response to therapy. In recent studies, select patients have been observed without undergoing chemotherapy or attempted resection. The 3-year OS rate for intermediate-risk patients was about 96% in a large COG study,[26] and thus, the current trend is to decrease chemotherapy to diminish side effects.
- *High-risk tumors*: The intensive multimodality approach consists of induction chemotherapy, followed by consolidation with surgery and hematopoietic stem cell transplantation followed by radiation therapy to any residual disease, and treatment of minimal residual disease using differentiation therapy, and immunotherapy, resulting in survival rates of 30–50%.

Treatment of Stage 4S Tumors

The options for treating are:

- Observation for children who are asymptomatic and have favorable biology
- Chemotherapy for symptomatic infants or those with unfavorable biology.

BRAIN TUMORS

Central nervous system malignancies comprised 13% of infant cancer with an incidence rate of nearly 30 per million infants. Astrocytomas and other gliomas (combined) accounted for half of the CNS malignancies followed by primitive neuroectodermal tumors (PNETs) medulloblastomas and ependymomas **(Figs 30.3 to 30.6)**.

There have been significant changes in the management of pediatric brain tumors due to advances in neuroimaging, neurosurgery, radiotherapy techniques and better supportive care.

Designing protocols for infants is a challenge as some techniques cannot be used in this age group and there is a very fine line between successful treatment and catastrophic outcome.[27]

Clinical Features

The most common presentation in this age group is macrocrania, which is seen in more than 50% of the cases. About 40% of children will have symptoms of raised intracranial pressure, seizures are seen in 5–25% of infants. Some of the other common symptoms include failure to thrive, irritability and delayed milestones.[27]

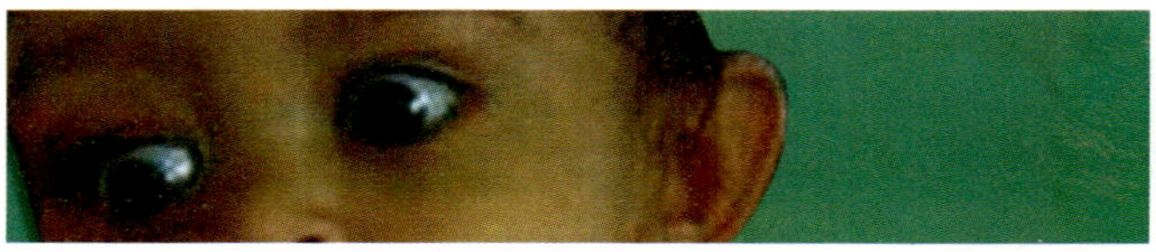

Figure 30.1 Infantile neuroblastoma child with orbital proptosis at diagnosis

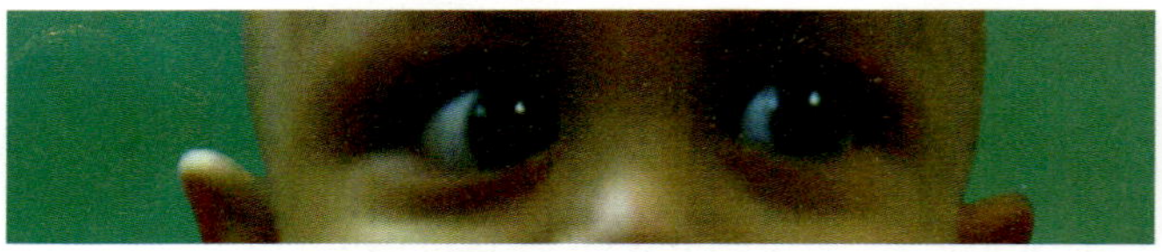

Figure 30.2 Post-treatment

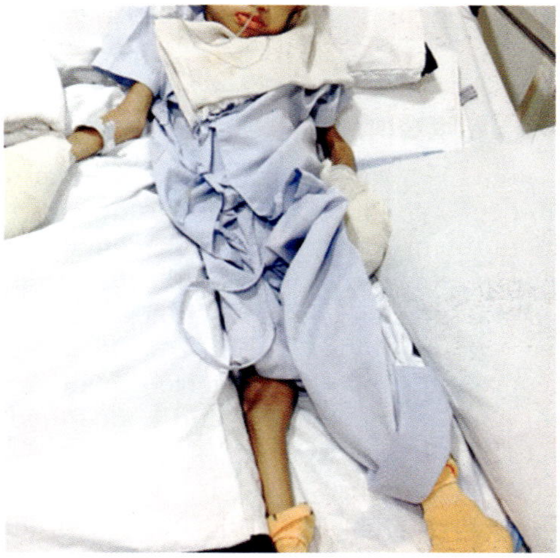

Figure 30.3 Child with hypothalamic tumor presenting with diencephalic syndrome

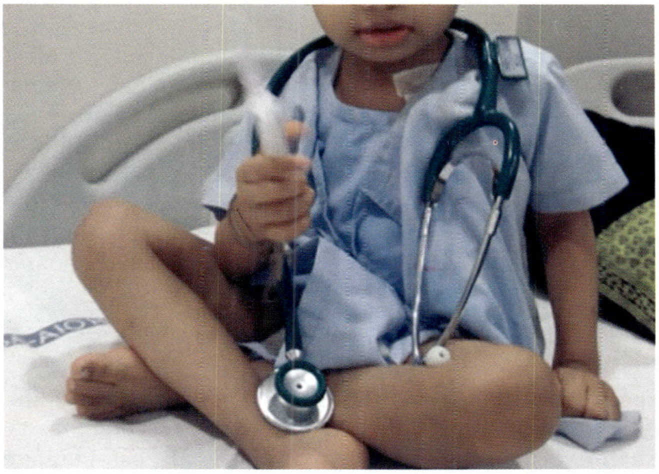

Figure 30.4 On treatment

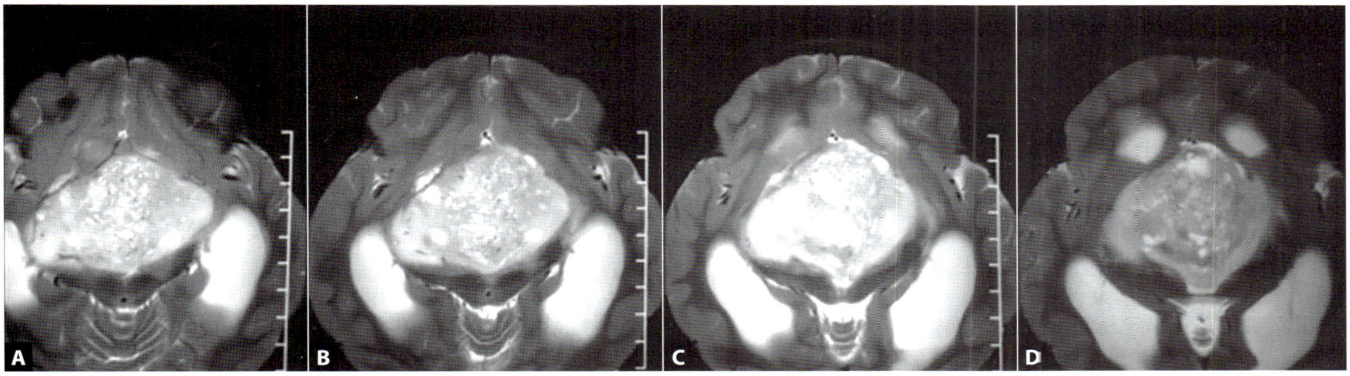

Figures 30.5A to D MRI brain of child at presentation

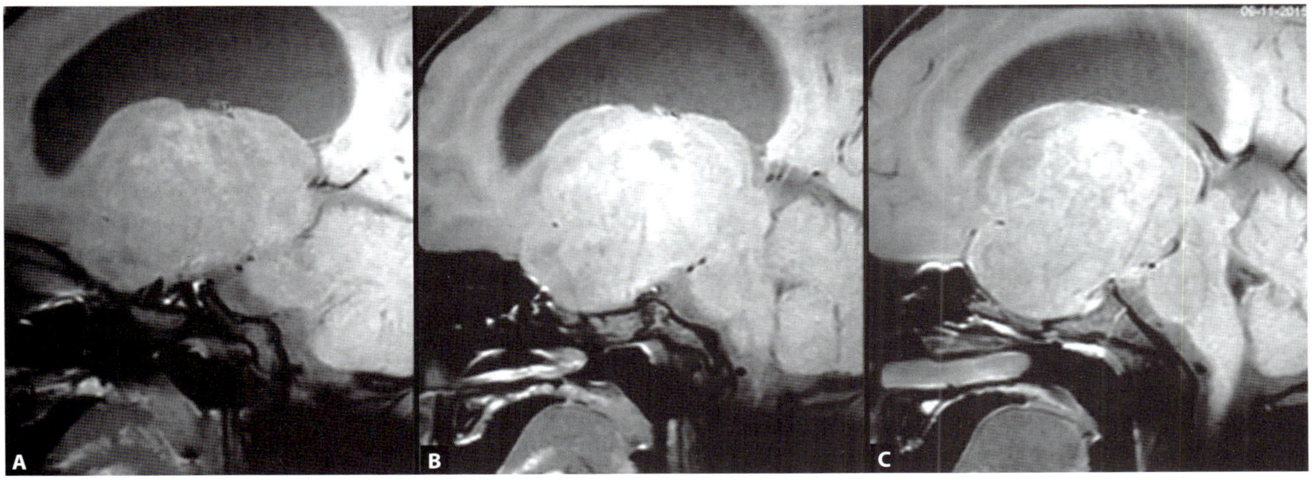

Figures 30.6A to C MRI brain at presentation

Low-grade Gliomas

This is the most common type of CNS tumor in infancy. Most of these tumors arise in the supratentorial midline location, usually in the hypothalamic region and the optic pathway and are not amenable to surgery. They can present with failure to thrive and abnormal movements of eyes.

This subgroup has a poorer outcome due to inability to remove the tumor surgically. Infants with diencephalic syndrome (failure to thrive, etc.) also tend to have a poorer prognosis.

EPENDYMOMA

The clinical features in infants are similar to older age group. A higher propensity to disseminate has been seen in infants. Surgery is the mainstay of treatment and postoperative chemotherapy has been tried in this group of patients with the aim of deferring radiotherapy until the age of 3 years. The results of postoperative chemotherapy have been disappointing.[28]

MEDULLOBLASTOMA

Medulloblastoma is an embryonal tumor of the posterior fossa. Since medulloblastoma occurs most often in the midline of cerebellum at the level of the fourth ventricle, children present frequently with symptoms and signs of obstructive hydrocephalus and cerebellar dysfunction over a period of 2–6 months. This tumor has a high propensity to spread in the subarachnoid space.

The management of medulloblastoma includes surgery followed by adjuvant craniospinal radiotherapy and chemotherapy.

In the late 1980s, the Pediatric Oncology Group used prolonged postoperative chemotherapy in an attempt to delay radiation in infants and young children with malignant brain tumors—including medulloblastoma.[29] Most of the children did badly because of an early relapse.

A subsequent generation of protocols was developed in an attempt to avoid radiation, through intensification of chemotherapy with or without the use of autologous bone marrow transplant. Some of the trials have shown good outcomes for a subset of children with favorable prognostic factors, like desmoplastic histology and nonmetastatic disease.[30-32]

ATYPICAL TERATOID OR RHABDOID TUMOR

Atypical teratoid or rhabdoid tumor is a malignant embryonal tumor containing rhabdoid cells and often additional, disparate components of small embryonal, mesenchymal and epithelial cells. They were described as a distinct entity only in the 1980s. Most of the cases occur in the first 2 years of life with a mean age at diagnosis of 7 months and 94% of affected children are less than 5 years of age.[33,34]

The outcome of this tumor is dismal. Many strategies have been tried, like surgery followed by intensive chemotherapy and even autologous stem cell transplant with uncertain results.[35]

RETINOBLASTOMA

Retinoblastoma is a rare cancer of the eye that occurs in infancy and early childhood. Retinoblastoma accounts for about 12% of infant cancer.[1] Retinoblastoma was the first tumor to draw attention to the genetic etiology of cancer. Despite good understanding of its etiology, mortality from extraocular retinoblastoma is about 70%. In countries with resource constraints where most affected children live, large number of patients present late and hence tend to have extraocular disease.

The most common presentation is leukocoria followed by strabismus. Retinoblastoma may be nonheritable (60%) or heritable (40%), the latter by autosomal-dominant transmission with high penetrance (90%).

Knudson devised the "two hit hypothesis" by recognizing that hereditary retinoblastoma was diagnosed at a younger age than unilateral nonfamilial retinoblastoma. This theory suggested that there are two rate-limiting events in the initiation, two somatic events in nonheritable retinoblastoma or one somatic event after a first intrauterine mutation in heritable variant.[3] Based on retinoblastoma, the concept of tumor suppressor genes was conceived.

The incidence of second primary cancers in patients with familial retinoblastoma is high. The relative risk (RR) for an individual with a germline RB1 mutation to develop other tumor types is 37, if they have been treated with external beam radiotherapy for retinoblastoma and 5 if never treated with radiation.[36]

The treatment depends on whether it is intraocular or extraocular, the stage of the tumor and involves focal therapies, like laser, photocoagulation, cryotherapy for small tumors. Enucleation, chemotherapy and external beam radiotherapy are required for large and/or extraocular tumors.

SCREENING FOR CANCERS IN INFANTS: IS THERE ANY ROLE?

Retinoblastoma is the most common childhood eye cancer. Early detection and prompt treatment can give cure rates up to 95% for intraocular tumors, but extraocular disease carries a very high mortality. Regular screening of newborns by funduscopic examination during routine well baby clinic visit leads to early detection of tumors as has been shown in studies,[37,38] and increases the chances of saving the eye and vision.

Screening infants for neuroblastoma leads to an increase in incidence of early-stage neuroblastoma. There is no concurrent decrease in incidence in screened children of advanced-stage disease, which typically does poorly, or of incidence in children older than 1 year. The cases identified by screening almost exclusively have biologically favorable features.

Based on evidence from large trials in Japan and Québec city, Canada, screening infants for neuroblastoma results in overdiagnosis (diagnosis of some neuroblastomas detectable by mass screening that would not have been clinically diagnosed later). This leads to unnecessary diagnostic and therapeutic procedures with consequent physical and psychological morbidity.

BALANCING CURE AND QUALITY OF LIFE

With nearly three quarters of children with cancer surviving, the long-term quality of life of survivors and the late complications of therapy are an important area of research. Infancy is a sensitive age group as the neurocognitive and neuropsychological sequelae of cancer treatment are maximum in a developing young brain. Also, implications of intensive treatment on physiologically immature organ systems need to be kept in mind.

These children need to be followed up in a dedicated childhood cancer survivor clinics where not only are they screened for organ dysfunctions due to treatment but are also screened for neuropsychological sequelae and given guidance for the same.

CONCLUSION AND KEY POINTS

- Cancer in infants constitute 10% of all cancers in children younger than 15 years of age.
- Infantile cancers are unique clinically and biologically from older children and give us an opportunity to study the mechanism of carcinogenesis.
- Infantile cancers are challenging to treat due to issues of venous access, chemotherapy drug dosing and the different way in which infants metabolize drugs.
- The common tumors in this age are Neuroblastoma, leukemia, brain tumors and retinoblastoma.
- In each category of tumors their are special subsets seen specifically in infants, such as Neuroblastoma stage 4S, MLL rearrangements in ALL.
- Infancy is a sensitive age group as the neurocognitive and neuropsychological sequelae of cancer treatment are maximum in a developing young brain.
- These children need to be followed up in dedicated survivor clinics for early recognition of late side effects.

REFERENCES

1. Howlader N, Noone AM, Krapcho M, Garshell J, Miller D, Altekruse SF, et al. SEER Cancer Statistics Review, 1975-2012, National Cancer Institute. Bethesda, MD. [online] Available *from seer.cancer.gov/csr/1975_2013/*. [Accessed August, 2016].
2. Dreyer Z, Indelicate DJ, Reaman GH, Bleyer WA. Infants and adolescents with cancer: special considerations. In: Pizzo P, Poplack D (Eds). Principles and Practices of Pediatric Oncology, 6th edition. Philadelphia, PA, USA: Lippincott-Raven Publishers; 2011. pp. 446-66.
3. Knudson AG Jr. Mutation and cancer: statistical study of retinoblastoma. Proc Natl Acad Sci USA. 1971;68(4):820-3.
4. Ford AM, Ridge SA, Cabrera ME, Mahmoud H, Steel CM, Chan LC, et al. In utero rearrangements in the trithorax-related oncogene in infant leukaemias. Nature. 1993;363(6427):358-60.
5. Gale KB, Ford AM, Repp R, Borkhardt A, Keller C, Eden OB, et al. Backtracking leukemia to birth: identification of clonotypic gene fusion sequences in neonatal blood spots. Proc Natl Acad Sci USA. 1997;94(25):13950-4.
6. Wiemels JL, Ford AM, Van Wering ER, Postma A, Greaves M. Protracted and variable latency of acute lymphoblastic leukemia after *TEL-AML1* gene fusion in utero. Blood. 1999;94(3):1057-62.
7. Chen N, Aleksa K, Woodland C, Rieder M, Koren G. Ontogeny of drug elimination by the human kidney. Pediatr Nephrol. 2006;21(2):160-8.
8. Pieters R. Biology and treatment of infant leukemias. In: C Pui (Ed). Treatment of Acute Leukemias: New Directions for Clinical Research. Humana Press, Totowa (NJ); 2003. pp. 61-73.
9. Ridge SA, Cabrera ME, Ford AM, Tapia S, Risueño C, Labra S, et al. Rapid intraclonal switch of lineage dominance in congenital leukaemia with a *MLL* gene rearrangement. Leukemia. 1995;9(12):2023-6.
10. Ramakers-van Woerden NL, Beverloo HB, Veerman AJ, Camitta BM, Loonen AH, van Wering ER, et al. In vitro drug-resistance profile in infant acute lymphoblastic leukemia in relation to age, MLL rearrangements and immunophenotype. Leukemia. 2004;18(3):521-9.
11. Hasle H, Clemmensen IH, Mikkelsen M. Risks of leukaemia and solid tumours in individuals with Down's syndrome. Lancet. 2000;355(9199):165-9.
12. Lange BJ, Kobrinsky N, Barnard DR, Arthur DC, Buckley JD, Howells WB, et al. Distinctive demography, biology, and outcome of acute myeloid leukemia and myelodysplastic syndrome in children with Down syndrome: Children's Cancer Group Studies 2861 and 2891. Blood. 1998;91(2):608-15.
13. Creutzig U, Reinhardt D, Diekamp S, Dworzak M, Stary J, Zimmermann M. AML patients with Down syndrome have a high cure rate with AML-BFM therapy with reduced dose intensity. Leukemia. 2005;19(8):1355-60.
14. Ge Y, Jensen TL, Stout ML, Flatley RM, Grohar PJ, Ravindranath Y, et al. The role of cytidine deaminase and GATA1 mutations in the increased cytosine arabinoside sensitivity of Down syndrome myeloblasts and leukemia cell lines. Cancer Res. 2004;64(2):728-35.
15. Nickerson HJ, Matthay KK, Seeger RC, Brodeur GM, Shimada H, Perez C, et al. Favorable biology and outcome of stage IV-S neuroblastoma with supportive care or minimal therapy: a Children's Cancer Group Study. J Clin Oncol. 2000;18(3):477-86.
16. Katzenstein HM, Bowman LC, Brodeur GM, Thorner PS, Joshi VV, Smith EI, et al. Prognostic significance of age, MYCN oncogene amplification, tumor cell ploidy, and histology in 110 infants with stage D(S) neuroblastoma: the pediatric oncology group experience: a pediatric oncology group study. J Clin Oncol. 1998;16(6):2007-17.
17. De Bernardi B, Gerrard M, Boni L, Rubie H, Cañete A, Di Cataldo A, et al. Excellent outcome with reduced treatment for infants with disseminated neuroblastoma without *MYCN* gene amplification. J Clin Oncol. 2009;27(7):1034-40.
18. Everson TC, Cole WH. Spontaneous regression of malignant disease. J Am Med Assoc. 1959;169(15):1758-9.
19. Evans AE, D'Angio GJ, Randolph J. A proposed staging for children with neuroblastoma. Children's Cancer Study Group A. Cancer. 1971;27(2):374-8.

20. D'Angio GJ, Evans AE, Koop CE. Special pattern of widespread neuroblastoma with a favourable prognosis. Lancet. 1971;1(7708):1046-9.
21. Beckwith JB, Perrin EV. In situ neuroblastomas: a contribution to the natural history of neural crest tumors. Am J Pathol. 1963;43:1089-104.
22. Guin GH, Gilbert EF, Jones B. Incidental neuroblastoma in infants. Am J Clin Pathol. 1969;51(1):126-36.
23. Bessho F, Hashizume K, Nakajo T, Kamoshita S. Mass screening in Japan increased the detection of infants with neuroblastoma without a decrease in cases in older children. J Pediatr. 1991;119(2):237-41.
24. Woods WG, Tuchmann M, Bernstein M, Lemieux B. Screening infants for neuroblastoma does not reduce the incidence of poor-prognosis disease. Med Pediatr Oncol. 1998;31:450-4.
25. Strother DR, London WB, Schmidt ML, Brodeur GM, Shimada H, Thorner P, et al. Outcome after surgery alone or with restricted use of chemotherapy for patients with low-risk neuroblastoma: results of Children's Oncology Group study P9641. J Clin Oncol. 2012;30(15):1842-8.
26. Baker DL, Schmidt ML, Cohn SL, Maris JM, London WB, Buxton A, et al. Outcome after reduced chemotherapy for intermediate-risk neuroblastoma. N Engl J Med. 2010;363(14):1313-23.
27. Larouche V, Huang A, Bartels U, Bouffet E. Tumors of the central nervous system in the first year of life. Pediatr Blood Cancer. 2007;49 (7 Suppl):1074-82.
28. Geyer JR, Sposto R, Jennings M, Boyett JM, Axtell RA, Breiger D, et al. Multiagent chemotherapy and deferred radiotherapy in infants with malignant brain tumors: a report from the Children's Cancer Group. J Clin Oncol. 2005;23(30):7621-31.
29. Duffner PK, Horowitz ME, Krischer JP, Friedman HS, Burger PC, Cohen ME, et al. Postoperative chemotherapy and delayed radiation in children less than three years of age with malignant brain tumors. N Engl J Med. 1993;328(24):1725-31.
30. Rutkowski S, Bode U, Deinlein F, Ottensmeier H, Warmuth-Metz M, Soerensen N, et al. Treatment of early childhood medulloblastoma by postoperative chemotherapy alone. N Engl J Med. 2005;352(10):978-86.
31. Grill J, Sainte-Rose C, Jouvet A, Gentet JC, Lejars O, Frappaz D, et al. Treatment of medulloblastoma with postoperative chemotherapy alone: an SFOP prospective trial in young children. Lancet Oncol. 2005;6(8):573-80.
32. Geyer JR, Sposto R, Jennings M, Boyett JM, Axtell RA, Breiger D, et al. Multiagent chemotherapy and deferred radiotherapy in infants with malignant brain tumors: a report from the Children's Cancer Group. J Clin Oncol. 2005;23(30):7621-31.
33. Kleihues P, Sobin LH. World Health Organization classification of tumors. Cancer. 2000;88(12):2887.
34. Packer RJ, Biegel JA, Blaney S, Finlay J, Geyer JR, Heideman R, et al. Atypical teratoid/rhabdoid tumor of the central nervous system: report on workshop. J Pediatr Hematol Oncol. 2002;24(5):337-42.
35. Gardner S, Diez B, Green A, Horn B, Kellie S, Knopp E, et al. Intensive induction chemotherapy followed by high-dose chemotherapy with autologous stem cell rescue (ASCR) in young children newly diagnosed with central nervous system (CNS) atypical teratoid rhabdoid tumors (ATT/RT)— The "Head Start" regimens. Neuro Oncology. 2004;6:455.
36. Wong FL, Boice JD Jr, Abramson DH, Tarone RE, Kleinerman RA, Stovall M, et al. Cancer incidence after retinoblastoma. Radiation dose and sarcoma risk. JAMA. 1997;278(15):1262-7.
37. Abramson DH, Beaverson K, Sangani P, Vora RA, Lee TC, Hochberg HM, et al. Screening for retinoblastoma: presenting signs as prognosticators of patient and ocular survival. Pediatrics. 2003;112(6 Pt 1):1248-55.
38. Rothschild PR, Lévy D, Savignoni A, Lumbroso-Le Rouic L, Aerts I, Gauthier-Villars M, et al. Familial retinoblastoma: fundus screening schedule impact and guideline proposal. A retrospective study. Eye (Lond). 2011;25(12):1555-61.

CHAPTER

31

Neonatal Leukemia

Anirban Das, Akanksha Chichra, Anupama S Borker

INTRODUCTION

Leukemia is an infrequent cancer in the neonatal period.[1] Solid tumors, including neuroblastoma, outnumber hematological malignancies in this age group.[2] However, it remains the second most common malignancy in neonates.[3] Acute myeloid leukemia (AML) is more frequent than acute lymphoblastic leukemia (ALL).[2,3] A tumoral syndrome with hepatosplenomegaly and skin nodules (leukemia cutis) is frequent. The central nervous system (CNS) and lungs are important sites of extrahematopoietic involvement. High total leukocyte counts and presence of rearrangements of the mixed lineage leukemia (MLL) gene are other unique features. Overall the prognosis in this age group remains poor despite intensive therapy.[1-3]

The term "neonatal leukemia" is often used interchangeably with "congenital leukemia". The following diagnostic criteria have been proposed, viz. (1) presentation in the first 4 weeks of life, (2) proliferation of immature myeloid, lymphoid or erythroid cells, (3) infiltration of these cells into nonhematopoietic tissues and, (4) the absence of other diseases which might explain this proliferation.[4,5]

EPIDEMIOLOGY

Neonatal leukemia accounts for less than 1% of all childhood leukemia.[2] Estimated incidence varies between 1 and 5 cases per million live births.[1] It is the leading cause of death from a malignancy in newborns.[3,6] In a retrospective study of leukemia during the first 3 months of life in Northern England, the incidence of acute leukemia was $8.6/10^6$ live births per year.[7] A higher frequency of AML (56–64%) than ALL (21–38%) has been reported in two large series of neonates with congenital leukemia.[3,5,8] Literature from India and South Asia remains confined to case reports and small series.[9-13]

ETIOLOGY AND PATHOGENESIS

The biological differences in leukemia in neonates and infants led to the identification of several risk factors **(Box 31.1)**. Identical twins have a high concordance rate for leukemia. Neonatal leukemia has been reported in association with Down, Turner, Klippel-Feil and Ellis-van Creveld syndromes as well as several trisomy disorders (trisomy 1, 8, 9, 13 and 19).[2,3] Epidemiological studies have correlated a decreasing incidence of low-birth-weight babies and an increased incidence of large-for-date newborns, to an increased incidence of infant ALL and AML.[14] A higher level of insulin-like growth factors, which may result in large-for-date babies, has been postulated to contribute to leukemogenesis.[3] Marcotte et al. have recently reported an increased risk of childhood ALL after prelabor cesarean delivery but not for emergency cesarean delivery, which was attributed to a maladaptive immune activation due to absence of stress response before birth.[15]

Maternal alcohol and marijuana use during pregnancy have been correlated with increased risk of infant leukemia.[2,3] The amount of maternal consumption of food containing DNA topoisomerase II inhibitors was correlated to the risk of developing MLL-rearranged AML.[16,17]

The link between MLL-rearrangement and neonatal or infant leukemia is quite strong.[1-3,5] The MLL gene located at 11q23 codes for a large histone methyltransferase that binds DNA and positively regulates gene transcription, including homeobox (HOX) genes.[18-20]

Box 31.1 Putative associations for the development of neonatal leukemia

- *Chromosomal aberrations*: Trisomy 21 and others (1, 8, 9, 13, and 19)
- *Congenital syndromes*: Ellis-van Creveld, Klippel-Feil
- Identical twin with leukemia
- Large–for-date babies
- Prelabor elective cesarean section
- Maternal alcohol consumption in pregnancy
- Maternal marijuana use in pregnancy
- Maternal exposure to topoisomerase II inhibitors (flavonoids)

6 SECTION Fetal and Neonatal Malignancy

CLINICAL FEATURES

Leukemia in neonates can present with a wide range of signs and symptoms. Antenatal ultrasound can detect hepatosplenomegaly, hydrops, and polyhydramnios as the initial presenting signs. Leukemia has been diagnosed in fetuses with Down syndrome (DS) as early as in the 33rd week of gestation.[3,21] Noonan syndrome (NS) can present with a similar MPD in utero.[22] Diagnosis is established by cord blood sampling.

Leukemia is an important cause of stillbirth.[3] The involved fetuses are often hydropic and macerated with enlarged and edematous placentae. Autopsy reveals leukemic infiltration in multiple organs. Extensive vascular involvement of the placenta by leukemic cells is attributed to cause fetal death.[23]

The unique presentation of neonatal leukemia is with nodular cutaneous infiltrates (leukemia cutis) described as a "blueberry muffin" baby **(Fig. 31.1)**.[2,3] They are also the initial presenting sign in about 50% of neonates, particularly those with AML-M5. It might be the initial clinical manifestation of disease and precede other signs of leukemia by up to 4 months. It may follow a waxing and waning course. In a cohort of Dutch neonates with congenital leukemia, the prevalence of leukemic skin infiltrates was 63.5%.[5] Leukemia in DS might present with a self-limiting vesicular pustular eruption, different from the typical "blueberry muffin" nodular infiltrates, which also harbor immature cells.[2,3]

Hepatosplenomegaly is a common finding in neonatal leukemia. Lymphadenopathy is observed less frequently.[5] CNS involvement is frequent.[2,3,5] A bulging fontanelle is the sign of meningeal leukemic infiltration or an intracranial bleed secondary to thrombocytopenia. Respiratory distress can be attributed to pulmonary hemorrhage and/or extensive leukemic infiltration complicated by atelectasis. Sepsis, pneumonia, and other infections are often the result of neutropenia. Cardiac failure might develop with nonimmune hydrops secondary to severe anemia. Hyperviscosity and leukostasis might compromise CNS, cardiac and pulmonary functions.

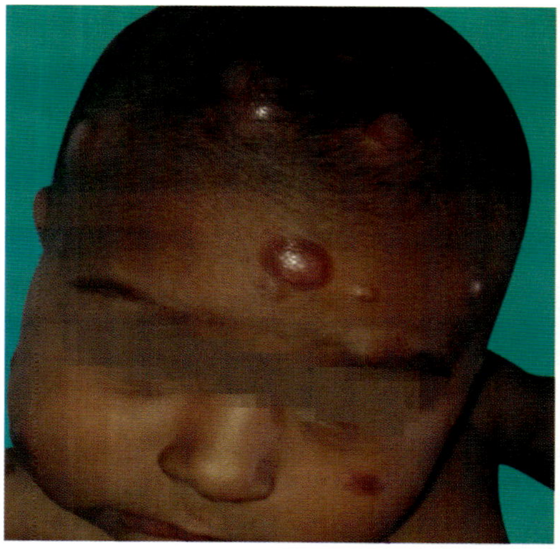

Figure 31.1 The baby presented on day 20 of life with generalized purplish skin nodules ("blueberry muffin" appearance), pallor and hepatosplenomegaly. Acute leukemia is one of the important differentials to consider in such cases

INVESTIGATIONS

Anemia, thrombocytopenia, leukocytosis or leukopenia with neutropenia and presence of blasts in the peripheral smear clinch the diagnosis. Hyperleukocytosis is present in a majority of the patients with a median leukocyte count of 104×10^9/L.[5] Bone marrow aspiration and biopsy need to be performed; however, it needs expertise to perform the procedure in a potentially sick neonate. Immunophenotyping from the bone marrow or even the peripheral blood sample helps distinguish AML from ALL. Acute leukemia of ambiguous lineage (ALAL) is commonly diagnosed in newborns based on the immunophenotyping criteria.[8] Cytogenetic studies help characterize the leukemia. Fluorescent in situ hybridization (FISH) helps in rapid diagnosis of MLL rearrangements.[1]

DIFFERENTIAL DIAGNOSES

Neonatal leukemia needs to be differentiated from leukemoid reactions secondary to sepsis, hemolysis and hypoxia. Hepatosplenomegaly with anemia, thrombocytopenia and leukocytosis can occur in intrauterine infections, including toxoplasmosis, rubella, cytomegalovirus, herpes, syphilis and human immunodeficiency virus (HIV). Differential diagnoses of cutaneous nodules in the neonate include congenital infections, neuroblastoma, rhabdomyosarcoma and histiocytosis.[2,3,5] Hepatic involvement with enlargement, fibrosis and multiple nodules of the liver, mimicking stage 4S neuroblastoma, has been described in AML-M7.[24] A list of common differential diagnoses is provided in **Box 31.2**.

MANAGEMENT AND OUTCOMES FOR MAJOR SUBTYPES OF NEONATAL LEUKEMIA

Neonatal leukemia can be broadly classified and studied under the following heads:

- AML in neonates without DS
- ALL in neonates

Box 31.2 Differential diagnoses for neonatal leukemia

- *Intrauterine infections*: Toxoplasmosis, *cytomegalovirus*, rubella, herpes, syphilis and HIV
- *Postnatal infections*: Severe bacterial sepsis
- *Hematological disorders*: Blood group incompatibilities, twin-to-twin transfusion syndrome, alpha-thalassemia, Diamond-Blackfan anemia, congenital dyserythropoietic anemia
- *Other malignancies*: Neuroblastoma, congenital rhabdomyosarcoma
- *Histiocytic disorders*: Langerhans cell histiocytosis, juvenile xanthogranuloma, hemophagocytic lymphohistiocytosis

Abbreviation: HIV, human immunodeficiency virus

- ALAL in newborns
- Transient abnormal myelopoiesis (TAM) in DS
- Juvenile myelomonocytic leukemia (JMML) and the myeloproliferative disease (MPD) in Noonan syndrome (NS).

Acute Myeloid Leukemia in Neonates without Down Syndrome

Acute myeloid leukemia (AML) accounts for 75% of acute leukemia in the neonates. The common French-American-British (FAB) subtypes include M5 (50%), M4 (20%), M7 and M6. MLL rearrangements are reported in 25–40%.[2,3] Most frequently described ones are t(11;19)(q23;p13) and t(9;11)(p21;q23).[1] MLL-rearranged AML is correlated with the morphological subtypes acute myelomonoblastic leukemia (M4) and monoblastic leukemia (M5). These blasts demonstrate positivity for CD13, CD14, CD15 and CD33. Patients often present with high tumor load, which includes organomegaly in a high white blood cell (WBC) count and CNS involvement.[1,3,5,8] Patients with a t(6;11)(q27;q23) have higher median WBC counts than other MLL-rearranged AML.

In acute megakaryocytic leukemia (M7), immunophenotyping reveals positivity for platelet-associated antigens (CD36, CD41a, b, CD61). Bilateral periosteal reaction, osteolysis, myelofibrosis, liver and lymph nodal fibrosis are frequent. The presence of t(1;22)(p13;q13) translocation (20%) and RBM15-MKL1 fusion are reported, the former with better prognosis.[1,2,3,8]

Treatment of neonatal AML is based on anthracyclines and cytarabine with overall survival (OS) of 30%. Relapse rates are high (50%).[1]

Self-limiting forms of AML are described in neonates especially in cases of aleukemic leukemia cutis and in the absence of MLL rearrangement. Association with hemophagocytosis, t(8;16)(p11;p13) translocation and MYST3-CREBBP rearrangement, and a specific gene-expression profile has been described for some of these spontaneous remissions.[1] Pediatric t(8;16)(p11;p13) AML is a rare clinical entity associated with the FAB M4/M5 subtype and disruption of the MOZ (MYST3) and CBP (CREBBP) genes on chromosomes 8p11 and 16p13, respectively.[25,26] It is associated with spontaneous remissions. It has been recommended that in congenital AML, the presence of a MOZ-CBP fusion should be assayed at diagnosis. If detected and negativity of MRD achieved after induction, then close observation without further consolidation chemotherapy can be considered for such cases.[25,26]

Acute Lymphoblastic Leukemia in Neonates

Acute lymphoblastic leukemia (ALL) in infants is more often associated with a higher tumor load at diagnosis, a rearrangement in the MLL gene, and very immature B-cell phenotype (pro-B ALL) without CD10 expression **(Fig. 31.2)**. Neonatal ALL cells are more resistant to several standard chemotherapeutic agents and have been reported to have a very poor prognosis. Infants less than or equal to 3 months have 5-year event-free survival (EFS) of 42%.[1-3,5,8]

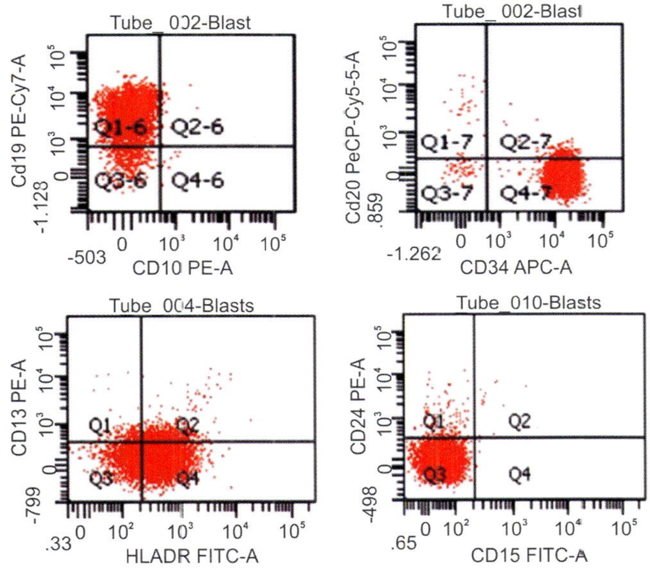

Figure 31.2 Flow cytometry in neonatal acute lymphoblastic leukemia (ALL) often reveals expression of CD34, CD38, CD19 and CD9, with CD10 being negative, suggestive of a pro-B immunophenotype

Linden et al. reported the outcome of 30 patients with congenital ALL treated with the interfant-99 protocol in 2009[27] with 2-year EFS of 20%. Hematopoietic stem-cell transplantation might have a role in therapy, since a high-risk group of infants younger than 6 months with MLL-rearranged ALL had better survival after receiving a transplant.[28]

Acute Leukemia of Ambiguous Lineage in Newborns

Acute leukemia of ambiguous lineage (ALAL) including biphenotypic, bilineal and acute undifferentiated leukemia according to the World Health Organization (WHO) classification is a rare affecting both adults and children (including neonates) with a male predominance. In a series of 145 cases of perinatal leukemia, 10 cases (7%) of ALAL were reported.[3] Lineage switch from myeloid to lymphoid is attributed to selection of an initially occult clone following therapy targeting the dominant clone. About 93% have abnormal karyotypes, the most common being t(v;11q23). Most have a high WBC count and poor outcomes, even with HSCT.[29]

Transient Abnormal Myelopoiesis in Neonates with Down Syndrome

Transient abnormal myelopoiesis seen in 5–10% of children with DS is characterized by clonally proliferated circulating blasts with megakaryoblastic or erythroblastic features, along with dyserythropoiesis and megakaryopoiesis. All children harbor an acquired truncating GATA1 mutation, identical in type to those seen in myeloid leukemia of DS (ML-DS). Bone marrow examination is not helpful as the circulating blast count often exceeds the marrow count. Indeed there is strong evidence that the cell of origin is a fetal liver hematopoietic stem or progenitor, not a bone marrow cell.[1-3,30]

Klusmann et al.[30] reported a median age at diagnosis of 3 days, ranging from 0 day to 65 days. Most of the patients presented with hepatosplenomegaly, pleural or pericardial effusions, or ascites. MLL gene rearrangements were the most frequent single abnormality. The estimated 5-year OS and EFS for the whole group were 85 ± 3% and 63 ± 4%, respectively. Presence of additional cytogenetic aberrations was not a marker of adverse prognosis. Multivariate analysis revealed a correlation between high WBC count, ascites, preterm delivery, bleeding diatheses, failure of spontaneous remission and the occurrence of early death.[30]

Although spontaneous resolution is seen in TAM, mortality due to progressive hepatic fibrosis or cardiorespiratory failure is known. High-risk features include conjugated hyperbilirubinemia, hepatomegaly and raised transaminases, high white cell count and cardiorespiratory compromise; megakaryoblasts can infiltrate the pericardial and pleural cavities. Treatment with low-dose cytarabine (0.5–1.5 mg/kg for 5–12 days) has been used with good results. Monitoring is required because some infants with TAM will later develop AML.

Juvenile Myelomonocytic Leukemia and the Myeloproliferative Disorder of Noonan Syndrome

Juvenile myelomonocytic leukemia is a rare leukemia of early childhood that is associated with genetic abnormalities of the RAS pathway. Median age at presentation is 2 years. Approximately 90% of patients carry either somatic or germ line mutations of PTPN-11, K-RAS, N-RAS, CBL, or NF1 in their leukemic cells. Allogeneic HSCT remains the therapy of choice for most patients with JMML, curing more than 50% of affected children.[31]

A JMML-like condition with spontaneous regression occurs in infants with NS, with the reported incidence as high as 10%, secondary to germline mutations in PTPN11.[32,33] Most cases of NS/MPD resolve spontaneously and progression to AML is exceptional. Fatal progressive disease occurs in 10%. These infants with NS very often also have cardiac anomalies and life-threatening or even fatal complications at least in part caused by leukocytosis and tissue invasion by monocytes, and immature granulocytes may develop in a certain proportion of them. Mild cytoreductive therapy, such as 6-mercaptopurine is recommended.[31]

CONCLUSION

Supportive care measures including hydration, prophylaxis for tumor lysis, antibiotics and transfusion support are important in managing neonates with leukemia. Cytoreduction might be warranted for symptomatic leukostasis as well as large organomegaly interfering with vital functions. Recognition of TAM in DS and NS/MPD is important for prognostication. Despite the current guarded prognosis for several variants of neonatal leukemia, high-intensity multiagent chemotherapy with HSCT can cure a proportion of these patients.

KEY POINTS

- Neonatal leukemia accounts for less than 1% of all childhood leukemia with incidence of 1–5 cases per million live births
- Neonatal leukemia can present with antenatal hydrops and stillbirth
- Presentation with cutaneous skin nodules (leukemia cutis or the "blueberry muffin" appearance) is characteristic in neonates
- Hepatosplenomegaly, lack of lymphadenopathy, involvement of CNS and extramedullary involvement including the lungs are important clinical features
- AML, M4 and M5 subtypes are common and present with high counts, extramedullary disease and MLL rearrangements. Treatment is based on anthracyclines and cytarabine. OS is 30%
- Acute megakaryoblastic leukemia (M7) without associated DS is characterized by t(1;22); osteolysis, liver, and marrow fibrosis might have better outcome in the presence of this translocation
- Neonatal ALL is characterized by a CD10 negative pro-B immunophenotype, high total counts and MLL rearrangement
- TAM in DS secondary to GATA1 mutations is usually self-limiting and has excellent outcomes. However, low-dose cytarabine therapy may be needed
- Neonates with the NS develop a self-limiting MPD resembling JMML secondary to mutations in PTPN11 in the RAS pathway.

REFERENCES

1. Orbach D, Sarnacki S, Brisse HJ, Gauthier-Villars M, Jarreau PH, Tsatsaris V, et al. Neonatal cancer. Lancet Oncol. 2013;14(13):e609-20.
2. Sande JE, Arceci RJ, Lampkin BC. Congenital and neonatal leukemia. Semin Perinatol. 1999;23(4):274-85.
3. Isaacs H Jr. Fetal and neonatal leukemia. J Pediatr Hematol Oncol. 2003;25(5):348-61.
4. Resnik KS, Brod BB. Leukemia cutis in congenital leukemia. Analysis and review of the world literature with report of an additional case. Arch Dermatol. 1993;129(10):1301-6.
5. Bresters D, Reus AC, Veerman AJ, van Wering ER, van der Does-van den Berg A, Kaspers GJ. Congenital leukaemia: the Dutch experience and review of the literature. Br J Haematol. 2002;117(3):513-24.
6. Reaman G, Zeltzer P, Bleyer WA, Amendola B, Level C, Sather H, et al. Acute lymphoblastic leukemia in infants less than one year of age: a cumulative experience of the Children's Cancer Study Group. J Clin Oncol. 1985;3(11):1513-21.
7. Bajwa RP, Skinner R, Windebank KP, Reid MM. Demographic study of leukaemia presenting within the first 3 months of

life in the Northern Health Region of England. J Clin Pathol. 2004;57(2):186-8.
8. van der Linden MH, Creemers S, Pieters R. Diagnosis and management of neonatal leukaemia. Semin Fetal Neonatal Med. 2012;17(4):192-5.
9. Mathur NB, Joshi N, Singh T, Singh M. Congenital acute megakaryocytic leukemia. Indian J Med Paediatr Oncol. 2011;32(3):165-7.
10. Shah MD, Sane SY, Mehta BC, Desai MS, Punjawani D, Gundewar VD, et al. Congenital leukemia (a case report). J Postgrad Med. 1984;30(4):247-9.
11. Narayan S, Sharma S, Chandra J, Kulshreshtha R. Clinico-hematological profile of congenital leukemia. Indian J Pediatr. 2004;71(10):927-8.
12. Raj A, Talukdar S, Das S, Gogoi PK, Das D, Bhattacharya J. Congenital leukemia. Indian J Hematol Blood Transfus. 2014;30(Suppl 1):159-61.
13. Dasgupta MK, Nayek N. Congenital leukemia cutis. Indian Pediatr. 2001;38(11):1315.
14. Hjalgrim LL, Westergaard T, Rostgaard K, Schmiegelow K, Melbye M, Hjalgrim H, et al. Birth weight as a risk factor for childhood leukemia: a meta-analysis of 18 epidemiologic studies. Am J Epidemiol. 2003;158(8):724-35.
15. Marcotte EL, Thomopoulos TP, Infante-Rivard C, Clavel J, Petridou ET, Schüz J, et al. Caesarean delivery and risk of childhood leukaemia: a pooled analysis from the Childhood Leukemia International Consortium (CLIC). Lancet Haematol. 2016;3(4):e176-85.
16. Ross JA. Dietary flavonoids and the MLL gene: A pathway to infant leukemia? Proc Natl Acad Sci USA. 2000;97(9):4411-3.
17. Spector LG, Davies SM, Robison LL, Hilden JM, Roesler M, Ross JA. Birth characteristics, maternal reproductive history, and the risk of infant leukemia: a report from the Children's Oncology Group. Cancer Epidemiol Biomarkers Prev. 2007;16(1):128-34.
18. Slany RK. The molecular biology of mixed lineage leukemia. Haematologica. 2009;94(7):984-93.
19. de Boer J, Walf-Vorderwülbecke V, Williams O. In focus: MLL-rearranged leukemia. Leukemia. 2013;27(6):1224-8.
20. Balgobind BV, Zwaan CM, Pieters R, Van den Heuvel-Eibrink MM. The heterogeneity of pediatric MLL-rearranged acute myeloid leukemia. Leukemia. 2011;25(8):1239-48.
21. Puumala SE, Ross JA, Olshan AF, Robison LL, Smith FO, Spector LG. Reproductive history, infertility treatment, and the risk of acute leukemia in children with Down syndrome: a report from the Children's Oncology Group. Cancer. 2007;110(9):2067-74.
22. Choong K, Freedman MH, Chitayat D, Kelly EN, Taylor G, Zipursky A. Juvenile myelomonocytic leukemia and Noonan syndrome. J Pediatr Hematol Oncol. 1999;2(6)1:523-7.
23. Gray ES, Balch NJ, Kohler H, Thompson WD, Simpson JG. Congenital leukaemia: an unusual cause of stillbirth. Arch Dis Child. 1986;61(10):1001-6.
24. Kawasaki Y, Makimoto M, Nomura K, Hoshino A, Hamashima T, Hiwatari M, et al. Neonatal acute megakaryoblastic leukemia mimicking congenital neuroblastoma. Clin Case Rep. 2015;3(3):145-9.
25. Daifu T, Kato I, Kozuki K, Umeda K, Hiramatsu H, Watanabe K, et al. The clinical utility of genetic testing for t(8;16)(p11;p13) in congenital acute myeloid leukemia. J Pediatr Hematol Oncol. 2014;36(5):e325-7.
26. Coenen EA, Zwaan CM, Reinhardt D, Harrison CJ, Haas OA, de Haas V, et al. Pediatric acute myeloid leukemia with t(8;16)(p11;p13), a distinct clinical and biological entity: a collaborative study by the International-Berlin-Frankfurt-Munster AML-study group. Blood. 2013;122(15):2704-13.
27. van der Linden MH, Valsecchi MG, De Lorenzo P, Möricke A, Janka G, Leblanc TM, et al. Outcome of congenital acute lymphoblastic leukemia treated on the Interfant-99 protocol. Blood. 2009;114(18):3764-8.
28. Mann G, Attarbaschi A, Schrappe M, De Lorenzo P, Peters C, Hann I, et al. Improved outcome with hematopoietic stem cell transplantation in a poor prognostic subgroup of infants with mixed-lineage-leukemia (MLL)-rearranged acute lymphoblastic leukemia: results from the Interfant-99 Study. Blood. 2010;116(15):2644-50.
29. Manola KN. Cytogenetic abnormalities in acute leukaemia of ambiguous lineage: an overview. Br J Haematol. 2013;163(1):24-39.
30. Klusmann JH, Creutzig U, Zimmermann M, Dworzak M, Jorch N, Langebrake C, et al. Treatment and prognostic impact of transient leukemia in neonates with Down syndrome. Blood. 2008;111(6):2991-8.
31. Niemeyer CM. RAS diseases in children. Haematologica. 2014;99(11):1653-62.
32. Roberts AE, Allanson JE, Tartaglia M, Gelb BD. Noonan syndrome. Lancet. 2013;381(9863):333-42.
33. Edwards JJ, Martinelli S, Pannone L, Lo IF, Shi L, Edelmann L, et al. A PTPN11 allele encoding a catalytically impaired SHP2 protein in a patient with a Noonan syndrome phenotype. Am J Med Genet A. 2014;164A(9):2351-5.

CHAPTER 32

Neonatal Liver Tumor

Sajid Qureshi

INTRODUCTION

Neonatal liver tumors (NLTs) are rare heterogeneous group of neoplasm, comprising of benign, malignant and metastatic tumors **(Table 32.1)**. The distribution of these tumors is different from those seen in older children. The most common benign tumors include vascular tumor and hamartoma; hepatoblastoma and neuroblastoma are the most common primary and secondary malignant tumor, respectively.

EPIDEMIOLOGY

The exact incidence of NLT is not known, however, they comprise approximately 5% of all neonatal tumors.[1] Amongst the entire childhood liver tumor, less than 10% occur in neonates.[2]

BENIGN NEONATAL LIVER TUMORS

Infantile hepatic hemangioma (IHH) is the most common benign liver tumor in neonates followed by mesenchymal hamartoma (MH). Rarely focal nodular hyperplasia (FNH) or adenoma may be seen.

Table 32.1 Neonatal liver tumors

Benign	*Malignant*	*Metastatic*
Infantile hemangioma *Focal* *Multifocal* *Diffuse*	**Hepatoblastoma**	**Neuroblastoma**
Mesenchymal hamartoma	Hepatic sarcoma *Embryonal sarcoma* *Angiosarcoma* *Rhabdomyosarcoma*	Leukemia
Focal nodular hyperplasia	Choriocarcinoma	Renal tumors
Teratoma	Rhabdoid tumor	Yolk sac tumors
Adenoma	Hepatocellular carcinoma	Rhabdoid tumors

Note: Common tumors highlighted in bold

INFANTILE HEPATIC HEMANGIOMA

Infantile hepatic hemangioma represents a clinically diverse spectrum of benign hepatic tumors comprising 60% of all NLT.[3] The relative rarity coupled with the lack of knowledge of the pathogenesis of these tumors has resulted in origin of varied terminology. In one classification, small (<2 cm), multiple lesions were classified as hemangiomas, whereas larger (2–15 cm) lesions, usually isolated, were identified as hemangioendotheliomas.[4] In another classification, the term "infantile hepatic hemangioendothelioma" (IHHE) was used and the lesions were divided into two subtypes: Type 1 IHHE and type 2 IHHE.[5] The type 1 IHHE is the more common subtype while the type 2 IHHE comprises less than 5% of vascular lesions of the liver and was considered to be premalignant with the potential to transform into angiosarcoma.[5,6] In addition to the above terminologies, IHH have also been confused with other lesions, like hepatic arteriovenous malformations, epithelioid hemangioendothelioma.[3] This uncertainty has made the diagnosis and therapy of IHHs with little rationale to choose among observation, medical, surgical management or radiological interventions.[7-10] To circumvent this problem, a novel systematic classification scheme encompassing clinical presentation, radiographic appearance, pathologic features, physiologic behavior, and natural history along with a therapeutic algorithm was proposed by the Children's Hospital, Boston.[3] Based on this classification, IHH are divided into three subtypes: Focal, multifocal and diffuse; with each category having a distinctive imaging, pathologic and physiologic features. An IHH registry was created and the classification scheme was validated.[11]

Focal Infantile Hepatic Hemangioma

Most focal lesions are asymptomatic and detected antenatally on routine prenatal ultrasonography (USG). These lesions

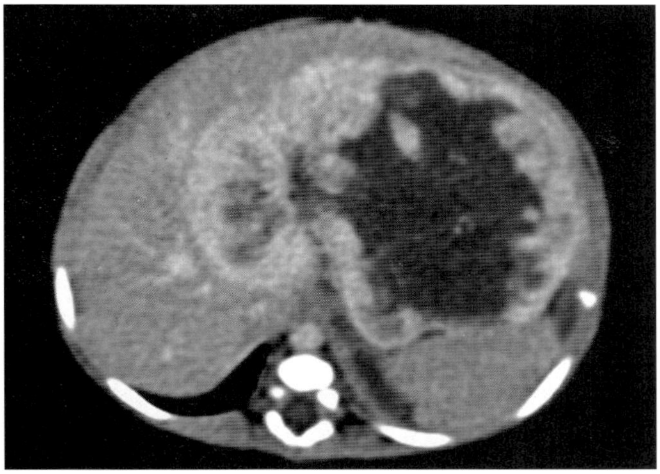

Figure 32.1 Computed tomogram (CT) showing focal infantile hepatic hemangioma (IHH) with centripetal enhancement and central hypodensity

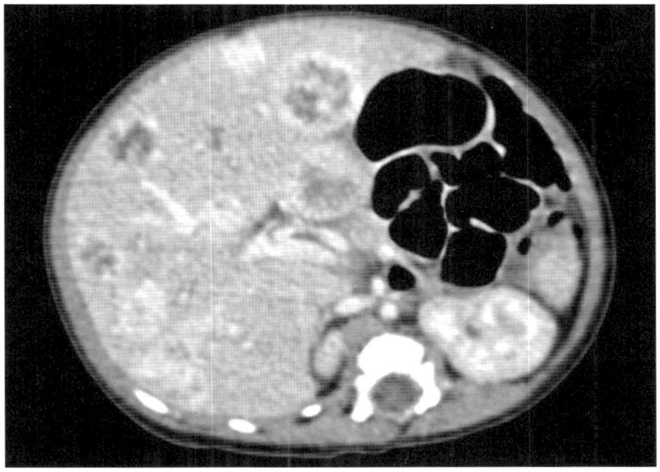

Figure 32.2 Computed tomogram (CT) showing multifocal infantile hepatic hemangioma (IHH)

have an equal sex distribution and are less commonly associated with accompanying cutaneous infantile hemangioma.[12-14] As with cutaneous rapidly involuting congenital hemangioma (RICH), focal IHH does not stain positive for glucose transporter-1 (Glut-1) protein, a marker for hemangiomas of infancy in all stages of their life cycle.[15] Due to these similarities with cutaneous RICH, focal IHH is considered as their hepatic equivalent.[3]

Ultrasonography reveals well-circumscribed high-flow vascular mass. Some focal IHH may have presence of high-flow shunts, which may result in high-output cardiac failure.[3] On magnetic resonance imaging (MRI), focal IHH appears as a well-defined, solitary lesion hypointense on T1 and hyperintense on T2-weighted images. Characteristically, they demonstrate centripetal enhancement and central hypodensity due to necrosis, thrombosis or intralesional hemorrhage on both computed tomography (CT) and MRI **(Fig. 32.1)**.[7]

Asymptomatic focal hepatic hemangioma (HH) is observed with follow-up USG to document regression.[16]

Medical therapy or embolization of high-flow shunts to improve heart failure is required in symptomatic patients.[3,11,16]. Resection or hepatic transplantation is rarely indicated.[3]

Multifocal Infantile Hepatic Hemangioma

Multifocal IHH is not detectable at birth but appear within the 1st week of life.[3] They often come to clinical attention while screening for visceral hemangioma based on the presence of multiple cutaneous infantile hemangiomas (usually 5 or more).[13] Unlike focal lesions, multifocal lesions demonstrate Glut-1 immunoreactivity and have a predictable course, like cutaneous infantile hemangioma, marked by rapid postnatal growth (0–12 months) followed by slow involution (1–5 years).[3,15]

On MRI, they appear as homogenously enhancing spherical lesions, hypointense on T1 and hyperintense on T2-weighted images and separated by normal intervening liver parenchyma. On CT, these lesions are hypodense with uniform or centripetal enhancement **(Fig. 32.2)**. A subset of patients with multifocal IHH will have high-flow shunting vessels resulting in high output cardiac failure. Hypothyroidism also occurs in some patients with multifocal lesions.[3,11,16]

Asymptomatic patients without shunts or hypothyroidism do not require therapy and are observed with follow-up USG to document regression. Propranolol is the first-line pharmacologic agent for symptomatic lesions.[7-19] It is effective both in decreasing or stopping the growth of lesions and in inducing more rapid involution. Propranolol is well tolerated and has an excellent safety profile. The initial doses range from 1 mg/kg/day to 3 mg/kg/day. Treatment is maintained for several months followed by gradual weaning. For complicated cases, corticosteroid and propranolol may be combined because of their perceived synergistic effect. In rare cases, multiagent therapy combining corticosteroid, low-dose vincristine and propranolol is used.[16] Embolization of symptomatic shunts to improve heart failure can be a life saving temporary measure until systemic treatment can take effect.[10] In absence of interventional radiologist, hepatic artery ligation can be used.[19] Presence of congestive cardiac failure is a risk factor for mortality in multifocal IHH, which is reported to be 9% in a recent analysis.[20]

Diffuse Infantile Hepatic Hemangioma

Unlike focal or multifocal IHH, diffuse lesions have a more serious clinical course. The massive liver enlargement causes abdominal compartment syndrome, respiratory distress and multiorgan failure.[3,11,16] Additionally, patients have severe acquired hypothyroidism due to the overproduction of type 3 iodothyronine deiodinase that converts thyroxine into an inactive form.[21] Hypothyroidism of this degree can result in permanent neurologic damage and decrease cardiac output due to impaired contractility.[22] High output cardiac failure is seen less commonly, however, hepatic decompensation may develop due to massive liver involvement.[3,11,16]

Similar to multifocal IHH, the diffuse lesions are also associated with cutaneous hemangiomas and Glut-1 immunoreactivity.[3,13,15] Imaging reveals extensive replacement of the hepatic parenchyma with innumerable centripetal enhancing lesions.[3,11] Management of diffuse IHH includes multimodal therapy consisting of propranolol, corticosteroids and low-dose vincristine.[3] Hypothyroidism correction often requires higher doses of thyroid hormone and usually resolves with resolution of the hemangiomas.[3] Abdominal compartment syndrome may require a decompressive laparotomy. However, these patients respond poorly to medical management and may benefit with liver transplantation.[3,8,9] In general, diffuse IHH has high likelihood of mortality up to 38% and presence of abdominal compartment syndrome is a risk factor for mortality.[20]

Mesenchymal Hamartoma

Mesenchymal hamartoma (MH) is the second most common benign liver tumor in children and constitutes 23% of all NLT.[1] The pathogenesis of MH is poorly understood, however, cytogenetic studies have suggested that it may be a neoplasm rather than a hamartoma. Other hypotheses suggested include developmental abnormalities within the biliary ductal plate; toxic insult resulting in the activation of sinusoidal fat storing cells (Ito cells).[23] Mesenchymal stem villous hyperplasia of placenta has also been associated with MH.[24] MH is composed of both solid (stromal) and cystic components and microscopically, show presence of mesenchymal and epithelial components. The cysts are lined by endothelium or bile duct epithelium and are surrounded by fibrous or myxoid stroma containing bile ducts and multiple vessels, particularly portal vein branches.[23]

Mesenchymal hamartoma usually present postnatally as an asymptomatic palpable mass, however, they can be detected prenatally especially in last trimester.[25] The liver functions are normal though serum AFP can be slightly raised.[26] Radiological imaging shows MH as consisting of mixed solid and cystic areas. Cysts are often multiloculated of variable sizes. The solid component, septa, and the peripheral rim may enhance in CT scans **(Fig. 32.3)** while on MRI low-signal intensity is seen on T1-sequences and variable intensity on T2-sequences.[27]

Distinguishing MH from other malignant lesions can be challenging especially in cases where the serum AFP is elevated. A biopsy is often required in these situations.[28,29]

The standard of care for MH is surgical resection with negative margins.[23] Liver transplantation may have to be considered for unresectable tumors.[23] Surgery is recommended even though they may undergo spontaneous

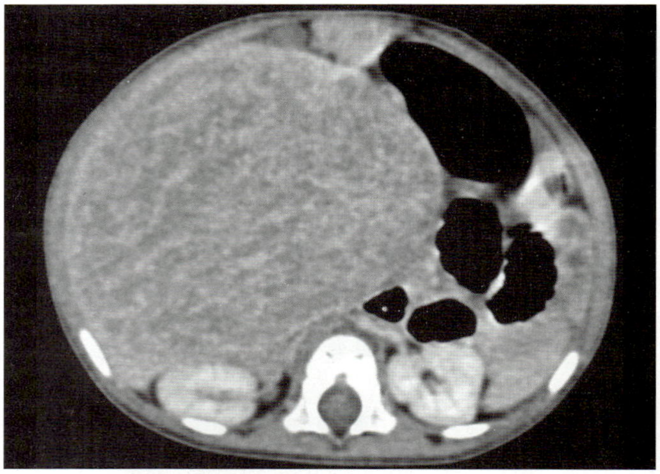

Figure 32.3 Computed tomogram (CT) showing mesenchymal hamartoma (MH)

regression due to the possibility of transformation into undifferentiated embryonal sarcoma (UES).[26,30] The role of chemotherapy or radiotherapy is not well defined in MH.[23]

Focal Nodular Hyperplasia

Focal nodular hyperplasia of the liver is a rare benign lesion, usually seen in older children between 2 years and 5 years of age rather than neonates.[31] Classical CT features include lesion enhanced when compared with normal liver and a hyperintense central scar. Microscopically, the cells are practically identical to the surrounding hepatocytes. Small lesions may be asymptomatic and can be followed up closely with imaging when there is no doubt regarding diagnosis, however, biopsy or resection may be necessary to establish the diagnosis especially in symptomatic patients.[31]

Hepatic Teratoma

True hepatic teratomas although very rare occur most often in the neonates.[31] They are typically cystic and contain mature or immature elements. These tumors usually lack malignant components. Serum AFP may be markedly elevated in these patients. Surgical excision results in cure.

MALIGNANT NEONATAL LIVER TUMORS

Hepatoblastoma is the most common malignant liver tumor in neonates. Rarely other tumors like sarcomas (UES or rhabdomyosarcoma), rhabdoid tumor and angiosarcomas have been reported.

Hepatoblastoma

Hepatoblastoma typically occurs in children less than 4 years of age with a median age at diagnosis of 18 months. Congenital hepatoblastoma diagnosed in the 1st month

Table 32.2 The International Society of Pediatric Oncology Liver Tumor Study Group (SIOPEL) classification of hepatoblastoma

Type	*Subtype*
Epithelial type (55%)	Fetal (30%) Mixed embryonal/fetal (20%) Macrotrabecular (3%) Small cell undifferentiated (2%)
Mixed epithelial and mesenchymal (45%)	Without teratoid features With teratoid features
Not otherwise specified (NOS)	

of life is rare and was initially considered disease that is more aggressive with poor outcomes.[32] However, a recent review of 79 patients (largest series till date) with congenital hepatoblastoma noted better outcomes than reported earlier and suggested management similar to older age patients.[33] Although hepatoblastoma has various syndromic associations, congenital hepatoblastoma has been associated with Beckwith-Wiedemann syndrome.[33] Low-birth-weight is associated with hepatoblastoma; however, it does not increase the likelihood of congenital hepatoblastoma.[33]

Hepatoblastoma is derived from undifferentiated embryonal tissue. The International Society of Pediatric Oncology Liver Tumor Study Group (SIOPEL) classification of pathological types of hepatoblastoma is given in **Table 32.2**.[34] The pure fetal variant of hepatoblastoma carries a favorable prognosis and small cell undifferentiated subtype of hepatoblastoma has a very poor prognosis.[35,36] Although there is no relationship between the age and predominant cell type in hepatoblastoma, pure fetal histology was initially considered associated with congenital hepatoblastoma and with atypical metastases to the brain, placenta and bone presumably due to the distinct fetal circulation.[32] However, this association was not shown in the later study and could be fortuitous.[33]

Prenatal diagnosis of hepatoblastoma by routine ultrasound is rare; however, hydramnios and fetal hydrops with antenatal and postnatal death have been reported.[32] Mechanical compression during labor can result in tumor rupture with fatal intra-abdominal hemorrhage.[1,2] Generally, the classic postnatal presentation is a palpable abdominal mass. The distinctive abnormal laboratory finding is elevated AFP. This has to be differentiated from the physiological elevation in neonates **(Table 32.3)**.

Table 32.3 Nomogram for alpha-fetoprotein (AFP) value references in infants

Age (days)	*AFP mean (ng/mL)*	*AFP 95.5% interval (ng/mL)*
0	41,687 9	9,120–190,546
1	36,391	7,943–165,959
2	31,769	6,950–144,544
3	27,733	6,026–125,893
4	24,210	5,297–109,648
5	21,135	4,624–96,605
6	18,450	4,037–84,334
7	16,107	3,524–73,621
8–14	9,333	1,480–58,887
15–21	3,631	575–22,910
22–28	1,396	316–6,310
29–45	417	30–5,754
46–60	178	16–1,995
61–90	80	6–1,045
91–120	36	3–417
121–150	20	2–216
151–180	13	1.25–129
181–720	8	0.8–87

Some congenital hepatoblastoma and small cell undifferentiated histological type may present with low or normal levels of AFP.[32,33,36] The imaging features of hepatoblastoma are not characteristic and calcification, vascular invasion, multifocality and large size are frequently seen **(Fig. 32.4)**.

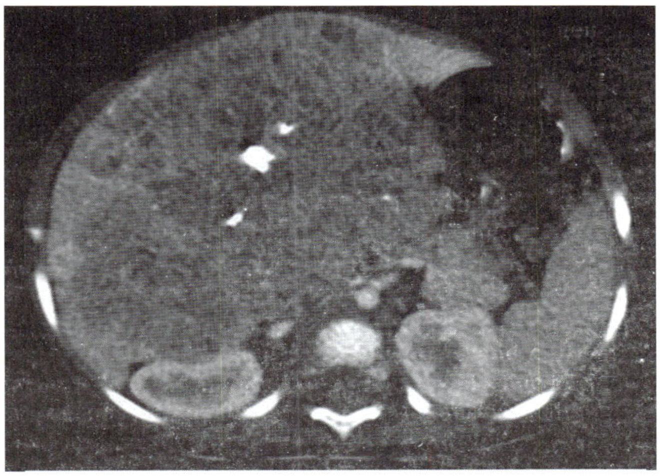

Figure 32.4 Computed tomogram (CT) showing pretreatment extent (PRETEXT) 3 hepatoblastoma

Biopsy is usually recommended for achieving tissue diagnosis especially in presence of normal AFP level and presence of equivocal radiological features. Metastatic workup includes CT scan of thorax. Due to the fetal circulation, metastasis may bypass liver to brain, bone and placental sites hence they are to be ruled out in metastatic workup.[32,33]

The pretreatment evaluation system of tumor extension (PRETEXT) was developed by the SIOPEL, which defines the tumor extension before any therapeutic intervention.[37] This system divides the liver into four sectors, an anterior and a posterior sector on the right and a medial and a lateral sector on the left. The patients are assigned to two broad categories of risk stratification: standard risk and high risk, which depend upon PRETEXT group and biologic variables. Standard risk tumors are PRETEXT I, II, or III. SIOPEL high-risk tumors are PRETEXT IV, or any tumor with metastasis (m), ingrowth of the vena cava (v), the portal vein (p) or contiguous extrahepatic disease (e), and tumors that fail to express AFP with AFP less than 100 at diagnosis. The Children's Oncology Group (COG) adopted a different system based mostly on surgical findings.[38]

Surgery with complete excision of the tumor is the mainstay of treatment; however, the timing of surgery varies among various groups. SIOPEL recommends surgery after neoadjuvant chemotherapy.[39] Depending on the risk stratification single agent cisplatin or a combination with doxorubicin and carboplatin is used.[40] Cisplatin is considered as gold standard for hepatoblastoma with response rate of more than 80%. Chemotherapy in congenital hepatoblastoma has to be offered carefully due to dose restrictions. The advantages of chemotherapy include regression in tumor size and the PRETEXT group thereby resections become easier and initial unresectable tumors may become resectable.[40] COG protocol recommend upfront tumor resection for PRETEXT I and II tumors if resection is feasible. If the resection margins are negative and the histology is of pure fetal type no adjuvant chemotherapy is offered.[35] Liver transplant is an option for unresectable disease, and should be planned at the outset so that patient can be referred to transplant unit. Liver transplants in infants are technically challenging and require lifelong immunosuppression.[41]

Undifferentiated Embryonal Sarcoma

Undifferentiated embryonal sarcoma of the liver is a rare childhood hepatic tumor that occurs more frequently in older children but has also been described in neonates.[31,42] Malignant transformation from MH or a solitary liver cyst to UES has been reported.[30] It is generally considered a highly invasive malignant tumor with lung, peritoneum and pleura as the typical sites for distant metastasis. Survival has improved in recent multimodal approaches, designed for patients with soft tissue sarcomas at other sites, including multiagent chemotherapy and delayed surgery.[43]

Infantile Choriocarcinoma of the Liver

It is a very rare tumor and its origin as primary fetal tumor or metastasis from a choriocarcinoma in the placenta of the mother is not clear.[2] Most have metastasis to maternal organs and elevated beta-human chorionic gonadotropin (HCG) and AFP levels. Infantile choriocarcinoma responds to chemotherapy with cisplatin, etoposide and bleomycin combination and resection may be possible.[44]

Malignant Rhabdoid Tumor

Malignant rhabdoid tumor (MRT) is primarily seen in kidneys; however, it has been reported in other sites including central nervous system, liver and in soft tissues.[31] Presentation with spontaneous tumor rupture is seen in 17% of patients, which is much more frequent than rupture in any other hepatic malignancy.[45] The AFP is usually within normal range and a biopsy is required for diagnosis. Various combinations chemotherapies have been used with limited success. The average survival rates of these children ranged from 5 days to 5 months. There are only a few reports of children achieving long-term survival with different therapeutic regimens.[46]

Angiosarcoma

Hepatic angiosarcoma is a rare and high-grade malignant liver tumor in older children.[47] Malignant transformation of diffuse IHH to angiosarcoma has been reported.[31] Early metastatic disease to the lungs is commonly seen. Prognosis is poor, even after multiagent chemotherapy, surgical resection, radiation and liver transplantation.[48]

METASTATIC LIVER LESION

Neuroblastoma

Neuroblastoma is the most common extracranial solid tumor in children, accounting for 6–10% of all childhood cancers. Approximately 60% have metastatic disease at presentation and the common sites for metastasis are bone marrow, bone and liver. Stage 4S or MS neuroblastoma is a distinctive entity representing 7–10% of all neuroblastoma. It is defined as disease in less than 18 months child with a localized primary adrenal or extra-adrenal tumor and metastasis restricted to the liver, skin, and bone marrow involvement less than 10% with no cortical bone involvement.[49] Although, it is associated with survival rates of 70–90% due to the possibility of regression and spontaneous tumor maturation, some of these neonates may present with extensive and diffuse liver involvement that can cause respiratory compromise and symptoms of abdominal compartment syndrome with decreased venous return, renal impairment and coagulation disorders secondary to extensive hepatic infiltration. Chemotherapy and liver radiation have been advocated; however, surgical management by abdominal decompression may be necessary in patients with progressive disease and life-threatening symptoms.[50]

RECENT ADVANCES

Propranolol, a beta blocker, has shown impressive results with cutaneous hemangioma recently. Due to these results its use was extended for visceral hemangiomas. Following its success and excellent safety profile, propranolol has become the first-line pharmacologic agent for functional or life-threatening hemangiomas, including multifocal or diffuse HH with associated hypothyroidism and/or cardiac failure.[17,18] The mechanism of action includes cessation and rapid involution of the lesions.[51] The dose range from 1 mg/kg/day to 3 mg/kg/day and the treatment can be continued for a year or maximal response.

INDIAN DATA

Benign Liver Tumors

The current practice at our center is high-quality imaging and tumor marker assessment at presentation for all liver tumors. In presence of classic radiological feature of a vascular tumor, medical therapy is initiated with propranolol at 1–3 mg/kg/day. USG assessment is performed at regular intervals to guide the response to therapy. Propranolol can be continued until 6 months to 1 year depending on the clinical response. In absence of any response or progression, surgery is contemplated. In case of equivocal radiological findings or abnormal serum AFP levels, biopsy is recommended. We have recently published our experience of management of benign liver tumors in children.[52] Conservative treatment for IHH was effective in 50% of the patients in our series; however, in the remaining conservative treatment failed and surgery was performed. Overall, surgery was required in two-thirds of our patients with benign liver tumors. Our study confirmed that surgical excision could be performed safely with minimal blood loss. Nonanatomical resection does not compromise the oncological outcomes and whenever feasible can be performed without any added morbidity.

Malignant Liver Tumors

Our approach to malignant liver tumors includes initial serum AFP assessment in addition to high-quality imaging. The decision for a biopsy is mostly based on AFP levels; however, we have liberal indications for a biopsy especially in presence of discordant tumor burden and AFP level. The SIOPEL protocol is presently followed in our institution for hepatoblastoma and based on the staging and risk stratification, cisplatin-based chemotherapy followed by surgical resection is performed. Although we have very limited experience with congenital hepatoblastoma, we have recently published our findings with multifocal and unifocal hepatoblastoma.[53] Apart from hepatoblastoma, we have managed a few patients with MRT **(Fig. 32.5)** and UES. Stage 4S neuroblastomas with liver infiltration were managed with chemotherapy and occasional radiotherapy; however, we have never encountered patients who did not respond to these measures and required decompressive laparotomy. There were two patients, however, who had a rapid fulminant course before initiation of therapy due to late presentation.

CONCLUSION

Neonatal liver tumors are very rare. The most common benign tumor is infantile hepatic hemangioma, the nomenclature and therapy of which are very well defined now. Their treatment may range from observation to medical or surgical interventions. Hepatoblastoma and metastases from neuroblastoma are the other common malignant tumors. Neonatal hepatoblastomas are managed on similar principles as for childhood hepatoblastoma with appropriate

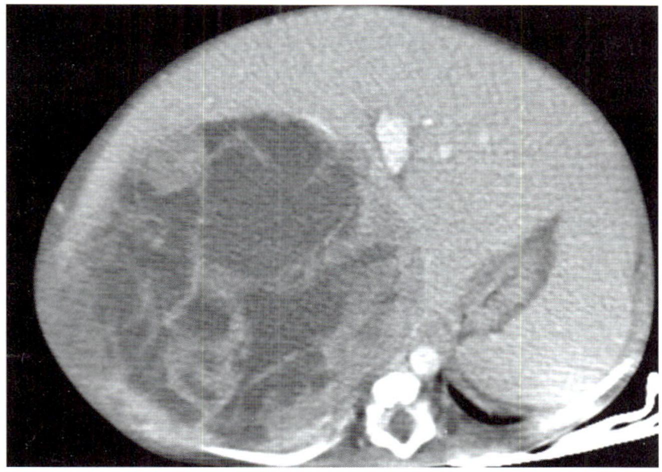

Figure 32.5 Computed tomogram (CT) showing extrarenal rhabdoid tumor of the liver

chemotherapy dosage modifications. Neuroblastoma metastases may be part of stage 4S disease which is usually associated with favorable outcome, however, hepatic decompensation secondary to extensive infiltration require aggressive treatment.

KEY POINTS

- IHH is the most common benign tumor of neonates
- The subtype of hemangioma (focal, multifocal and diffuse) guides the best modality of treatment
- Asymptomatic lesion can be observed and medical management with propranolol is effective in symptomatic patients
- Surgical resection with negative margins is the preferred treatment for MH
- Surgery is recommended since there is a possibility of transformation into UES
- Congenital hepatoblastoma is managed on similar lines as hepatoblastoma in old age children with appropriate chemotherapy dose adjustment
- Treatment consists of initial cisplatin-based chemotherapy as per risk stratification followed by surgery.

REFERENCES

1. Isaacs H Jr. Fetal and neonatal hepatic tumors. J Pediatr Surg. 2007;42(11):1797-803.
2. von Schweinitz D. Neonatal liver tumours. Semin Neonatol. 2003;8(5):403-10.
3. Christison-Lagay ER, Burrows PE, Alomari A, Dubois J, Kozakewich HP, Lane TS, et al. Hepatic hemangiomas: subtype classification and development of a clinical practice algorithm and registry. J Pediatr Surg. 2007;42(1):62-7.
4. Regier TS, Ramji FG. Pediatric hepatic hemangioma. Radiographics. 2004;24(6):1719-24.
5. Makin E, Davenport M. Fetal and neonatal liver tumours. Early Hum Dev. 2010;86(10):637-42.

6. Kirchner SG, Heller RM, Kasselberg AG, Greene HL. Infantile hepatic hemangioendothelioma with subsequent malignant degeneration. Pediatr Radiol. 1981;11(1):42-5.
7. Kassarjian A, Zurakowski D, Dubois J, Paltiel HJ, Fishman SJ, Burrows PE. Infantile hepatic hemangiomas: clinical and imaging findings and their correlation with therapy. Am J Roentgenol. 2004;182(3):785-95.
8. Kasahara M, Kiuchi T, Haga H, Uemoto S, Uryuhara K, Fujimoto Y, et al. Monosegmental living-donor liver transplantation for infantile hepatic hemangioendothelioma. J Pediatr Surg. 2003;38(7):1108-11.
9. Walsh R, Harrington J, Beneck D, Ozkaynak MF. Congenital infantile hepatic hemangioendothelioma type II treated with orthotopic liver transplantation. J Pediatr Hematol Oncol. 2004;26(2):121-3.
10. Warmann S, Bertram H, Kardorff R, Sasse M, Hausdorf G, Fuchs J. Interventional treatment of infantile hepatic hemangioendothelioma. J Pediatr Surg. 2003;38(8):1177-81.
11. Kulungowski AM, Alomari AI, Chawla A, Christison-Lagay ER, Fishman SJ. Lessons from a liver hemangioma registry: subtype classification. J Pediatr Surg. 2012;47(1):165-70.
12. Boon LM, Enjolras O, Mulliken JB. Congenital hemangioma: evidence of accelerated involution. J Pediatr. 1996;128(3):329-35.
13. Horii KA, Drolet BA, Frieden IJ, Baselga E, Chamlin SL, Haggstrom AN, et al. Prospective study of the frequency of hepatic hemangiomas in infants with multiple cutaneous infantile hemangiomas. Pediatr Dermatol. 2011;28(3):245-53.
14. Mulliken JB, Enjolras O. Congenital hemangiomas and infantile hemangioma: missing links. J Am Acad Dermatol. 2004;50(6):875-82.
15. Hernández F, Navarro M, Encinas JL, López Gutiérrez JC, López Santamaría M, Leal N, et al. The role of GLUT1 immunostaining in the diagnosis and classification of liver vascular tumors in children. J Pediatr Surg. 2005;40(5):801-4.
16. Belinda HD, Fishman SJ, Azizkhan RG. Hepatic vascular tumors. Semin Pediatr Surg. 2014;23(4):168-72.
17. Mhanna A, Franklin WH, Mancini AJ. Hepatic infantile hemangiomas treated with oral propranolol—a case series. Pediatr Dermatol. 2011;28(1):39-45.
18. Léauté-Labrèze C, Dumas de la Roque E, Hubiche T, Boralevi F, Thambo JB, Taïeb A. Propranolol for severe hemangiomas of infancy. N Engl J Med. 2008;358(24):2649-51.
19. Davenport M, Hansen L, Heaton ND, Howard ER. Hemangioendothelioma of the liver in infants. J Pediatr Surg. 1995;30(1):44-8.
20. Rialon KL, Murillo R, Fevurly RD, Kulungowski AM, Christison-Lagay ER, Zurakowski D, et al. Risk factors for mortality in patients with multifocal and diffuse hepatic hemangiomas. J Pediatr Surg. 2015;50(5):837-41.
21. Huang SA, Tu HM, Harney JW, Venihaki M, Butte AJ, Kozakewich HP, et al. Severe hypothyroidism caused by type 3 iodothyronine deiodinase in infantile hemangiomas. N Engl J Med. 2000;343(3):185-9.
22. LaFranchi S. Congenital hypothyroidism: etiologies, diagnosis and management. Thyroid. 1999;9(7):735-40.
23. Stringer MD, Alizai NK. Mesenchymal hamartoma of the liver: a systematic review. J Pediatr Surg. 2005;40(11):1681-90.
24. Kitano Y, Ruchelli E, Weiner S, Adzick NS. Hepatic mesenchymal hamartoma associated with mesenchymal stem villous hyperplasia of the placenta. Fetal Diagn Ther. 2000;15(3):134-8.
25. Dickinson JE, Knowles S, Phillips JM. Prenatal diagnosis of hepatic mesenchymal hamartoma. Prenat Diagn. 1999;19(1):81-4.
26. Boman F, Bossard C, Fabre M, Diab N, Bonnevalle M, Boccon-Gibod L. Mesenchymal hamartomas of the liver may be associated with increased serum alpha foetoprotein concentrations and mimic hepatoblastomas. Eur J Pediatr Surg. 2004;14(1):63-6.
27. Anil G, Fortier M, Low Y. Cystic hepatic mesenchymal hamartoma: the role of radiology in diagnosis and perioperative management. Br J Radiol. 2011;84(1001):e91-4.
28. Millard J, Fraser N, Stewart RJ. Mesenchymal hamartoma of the liver: is biopsy always necessary? Pediatr Surg Int. 2006;22(7):622-5.
29. Kenney IJ, Hendry GM, Mackinlay GA. Spontaneous regression of mesenchymal hamartoma: observations using ultrasound. J Clin Ultrasound. 1986;14(1):72-6.
30. Begueret H, Trouette H, Vielh P, Laurent C, MacGrogan G, Delsol M, et al. Hepatic undifferentiated embryonal sarcoma: malignant evolution of mesenchymal hamartoma? Study of one case with immunohistochemical and flow cytometric emphasis. J Hepatol. 2001;34(1):178-9.
31. Meyers RL. Tumors of the liver in children. Surg Oncol. 2007;16(3):195-203.
32. Ammann RA, Plaschkes J, Leibundgut K. Congenital hepatoblastoma: a distinct entity? Med Pediatr Oncol. 1999;32(6):466-8.
33. Trobaugh-Lotrario AD, Chaiyachati BH, Meyers RL, Häberle B, Tomlinson GE, Katzenstein HM, et al. Outcomes for patients with congenital hepatoblastoma. Pediatr Blood Cancer. 2013;60(11):1817-25.
34. Zimmerman A, Lopez-Terrada D. Pathology of pediatric liver tumors. In: Zimmerman A (Ed). Pediatric Liver Tumors. Berlin Heidelberg, Germany: Springer-Verlag; 2011. pp. 83-94.
35. Malogolowkin MH, Katzenstein HM, Meyers RL, Krailo MD, Rowland JM, Haas J, et al. Complete surgical resection is curative for children with hepatoblastoma with pure fetal histology: a report from the Children's Oncology Group. J Clin Oncol. 2011;29(24):3301-6.
36. Trobaugh-Lotrario AD, Tomlinson GE, Finegold MJ, Gore L, Feusner JH. Small cell undifferentiated variant of hepatoblastoma: adverse clinical and molecular features similar to rhabdoid tumors. Pediatr Blood Cancer. 2009;52(3): 328-34.
37. Roebuck DJ, Aronson D, Clapuyt P, Czauderna P, de Ville de Goyet J, Gauthier F, et al. 2005 PRETEXT: a revised staging system for primary malignant liver tumours of childhood developed by the SIOPEL group. Pediatr Radiol. 2007;37(2):123-32.
38. Meyers RL, Katzenstein HM, Malogolowkin MH. Predictive value of staging systems in hepatoblastoma. J Clin Oncol. 2007;25(6):737-8.
39. Czauderna P, Otte JB, Aronson DC, Gauthier F, Mackinlay G, Roebuck D, et al. Guidelines for surgical treatment of hepatoblastoma in the modern era—recommendations from the Childhood Liver Tumour Strategy Group of the International Society of Paediatric Oncology (SIOPEL). Eur J Cancer. 2005;41(7):1031-6.
40. Perilongo G, Malogolowkin M, Feusner J. Hepatoblastoma clinical research: lessons learned and future challenges. Pediatr Blood Cancer. 2012;59(5):818-21.
41. Stringer MD. The role of liver transplantation in the management of paediatric liver tumours. Ann R Coll Surg Engl. 2007;89(1):12-21.
42. Ismail H, Dembowska-Bagińska B, Broniszczak D, Kaliciński P, Maruszewski P, Kluge P, et al. Treatment of undifferentiated embryonal sarcoma of the liver in children--single center experience. J Pediatr Surg. 2013;48(11):2202-6.

43. Bisogno G, Pilz T, Perilongo G, Ferrari A, Harms D, Ninfo V, et al. Undifferentiated sarcoma of the liver in childhood: a curable disease. Cancer. 2002;94(1):252-7.
44. Blohm ME, Calaminus G, Gnekow AK, Heidemann PH, Bolkenius M, Weinel P, et al. Disseminated choriocarcinoma in infancy is curable by chemotherapy and delayed tumour resection. Eur J Cancer. 2001;37(1):72-8.
45. Trobaugh-Lotrario AD, Finegold MJ, Feusner JH. Rhabdoid tumors of the liver: rare, aggressive, and poorly responsive to standard cytotoxic chemotherapy. Pediatr Blood Cancer. 2011;57(3):423-8.
46. Jayaram A, Finegold MJ, Parham DM, Jasty R. Successful management of rhabdoid tumor of the liver. J Pediatr Hematol Oncol. 2007;29(6):406-8.
47. Awan S, Davenport M, Portmann B, Howard ER. Angiosarcoma of liver in children. J Pediatr Surg. 1996;31(12):1729-32.
48. Ferrari A, Casanova M, Bisogno G, Cecchetto G, Meazza C, Gandola L, et al. Malignant vascular tumors in children and adolescents: a report from the Italian and German Soft Tissue Sarcoma Cooperative Group. Med Pediatr Oncol. 2002; 39(2):109-14.
49. Iehara T, Hiyama E, Tajiri T, Yoneda A, Hamazaki M, Fukuzawa M, et al. Is the prognosis of stage 4s neuroblastoma in patients 12 months of age and older really excellent? Eur J Cancer. 2012;48(11):1707-12.
50. Mabrut JY, Dubois R, Pelizzo G, Floret D, Frappaz D, Chappuis JP. Abdominal expansion using a polytetrafluoroethylene prosthesis in the treatment of Pepper syndrome. Pediatr Surg Int. 2000;16(3):219-21.
51. Chim H, Armijo BS, Miller E. Gliniak C, Serret MA, Gosain AK. Propranolol induces regression of hemangioma cells through HIF-1α-mediated inhibition of VEGF-A. Ann Surg. 2012;256(1):146-56.
52. Qureshi SS, Bhagat M, Kembhavi S, Vora T, Ramadwar M, Chinnaswamy G, et al. Benign liver tumors in children: outcomes after resection. Pediatr Surg Int. 2015;31(12): 1145-9.
53. Qureshi SS, Bhagat M, Kembhavi S, Vora T, Ramadwar M, Talole S. PRETEXT II-III multifocal hepatoblastoma: significance of resection of satellite lesions irrespective of their disappearance after chemotherapy. Pediatr Surg Int. 2015;31(6):573-9.

CHAPTER 33

Neuroblastoma

Arpita Bhattacharya, Dipshikha Maiti

INTRODUCTION

Neuroblastoma, originally described by Virchow in 1863, is a developmental tumor arising from the primordial neural crest cells, which are the precursors of the sympathetic nervous system. Neuroblastoma is the third most common childhood cancer after leukemia and brain tumors, and the most common solid extracranial tumor. It is the most common malignancy in the neonatal period and infancy.[1,2] Neuroblastoma is an enigma because of its extensive biological heterogeneity and varying behavior ranging from spontaneous regression to cases of highly-aggressive metastatic disease unresponsive to standard or investigational anticancer treatment. Neuroblastomas in children less than 18 months of age often have a favorable prognosis. Some of these children with specific patterns of metastases, designated as stage 4S disease have a high likelihood of undergoing spontaneous regression even without treatment.[3,4]

EPIDEMIOLOGY

Neuroblastoma constitutes around 6–10% of all childhood cancers. Age-standardized incidence rate of neuroblastoma has been reported variously as 7–12 per million. Males have a slightly higher incidence than females with a male-to-female ratio of 1.2:1.[5] Median age at diagnosis is around 19 months. Around 40% of patients are diagnosed in infancy, 35% are aged 1–2 years, and 25% are older than 2 years when diagnosed. Stage 4s neuroblastoma represents approximately 7–10% of all neuroblastoma cases.[1,6]

PATHOGENESIS

The biological heterogeneity of neuroblastoma can at least partly be explained by its genetic heterogeneity. Genetic and molecular markers are now important tools that are routinely incorporated into therapeutic decision making. The most significant genetic defects are briefly described here.

PLOIDY (TUMOR CELL DNA CONTENT)

According to their DNA index, neuroblastomas can be broadly grouped into two groups: near-diploid or near tetraploid (DNA index ~ 1 or ~ 2), and those with a near-triploid (DNA index ~1.5). Tumor ploidy is often used to risk stratify infants with stage 4 or 4S disease. Hyperdiploid DNA index is often associated with favorable outcome.[7,8]

MYCN Oncogene Amplification

The *MYCN* oncogene is located on chromosome 2p24. *MYCN* amplification occurs in approximately 22% of primary neuroblastomas. It is consistently associated with metastatic disease, rapid tumor progression and poor prognosis. It is also associated with other unfavorable prognostic factors like unfavorable histology, 1p deletion and diploidy.[9]

Chromosome 1p36 Loss

Deletion of chromosome 1p has been detected in approximately 35% neuroblastomas. *CHD5* is proposed as one of the tumor suppressor genes residing in this region. Low *CHD5* expression is significantly associated with unfavorable biology and outcome.[10] Deletion of chromosome 1p sequences is more common in high-stage tumors and is often associated with *MYCN* amplification. Other tumor suppressor genes located in chromosome 1p that are believed to be potentially associated with neuroblastoma are KIF1BB and miR34a.[11]

Unbalanced Chromosome 17q Gain

Unbalanced gain of chromosome 17q is the most common genetic aberration seen in neuroblastomas, occurring in over 50% of neuroblastomas. Unbalanced chromosome 17q gain is an independent parameter for poor outcome, whereas whole-chromosome 17 gain was associated with good prognosis.[12]

Chromosome 11q Loss

Deletions of the long arm of chromosome 11 have been identified in 35–40% of neuroblastomas. Chromosome 11q deletions are often associated with aggressive tumors, even in absence of *MYCN* amplification and with intact chromosome 1p. Recently, tumor suppressor genes, *CADM1* has been delineated as presumptive causative candidate in chromosome 11q loss.[13]

FAMILIAL NEUROBLASTOMA AND GENETIC SUSCEPTIBILITY

Familial neuroblastoma is a rare entity occurring in 1–2% patients. Familial cases often present with multiple or multifocal tumors and at a younger age than sporadic cases, consistent with Knudson's two-hit hypothesis.

Germline mutations in the *anaplastic lymphoma kinase (ALK)* and *paired-like homeobox 2B (PHOX2B)* genes were identified in familial neuroblastoma cases. *ALK* is a member of the tyrosine kinase family and mutations result in constitutive activation of the gene.[14]

PATHOLOGY

Neuroblastoma belongs to the category of "small, round blue cell tumor". Neuroblastic layer (NBL) arises from neuroblasts, which are small round cells with scant cytoplasm, dark nuclei and small indistinct nucleoli. Sometimes cells form typical clusters termed Homer-Wright rosettes. International Neuroblastoma Pathology Classification (INPC) was established in 1999 to standardize the morphologic classification of neuroblastic tumors. This classification system incorporates age, presence or absence of Schwannian stroma, degree of differentiation and mitosis-karyorrhexis index (MKI) to classify tumors as with favorable or unfavorable histology. It classifies neuroblastic tumors into four different categories:

1. Neuroblastoma (Schwannian stroma poor).
2. Ganglioneuroblastoma (stroma rich).
3. Ganglioneuroma (stroma dominant).
4. Ganglioneuroblastoma (nodular composite).

Favorable histological characteristics include low or intermediate MKI and differentiating or partially differentiating tumor in children less than 18 months, or low MKI differentiating tumor in children 18 months to 5 years.[15,16]

CLINICAL PRESENTATION

Neuroblastomas may be incidentally discovered during imaging for other reasons, e.g. antenatal ultrasound or chest radiograph for pneumonia. Fetal neuroblastoma has been seen in antenatal scans as early as 19 weeks with mean age at discovery of 36 weeks.[17]

Neuroblastoma is the most common malignancy in the neonatal period and infancy (30–50%) **(Figs 33.1A and B)**. This tumor has very good prognosis. It is almost always adrenal in origin (90%), usually stages 1, 2, or 4S. Despite metastatic spread, these tumors usually have favorable behavior and survival rate more than 90%.

Though up to 40% of infants with neuroblastoma may recover without any active treatment, life-threatening issues may arise especially in neonates due to respiratory, renal, gastrointestinal impairment, or due to coagulopathy secondary to massive liver enlargement.

In children more than 18 months, neuroblastoma has a wide spectrum of clinical features depending on the site and extent of the primary tumor and the presence of distant metastases. Most primary tumors occur in the abdomen (60%) followed by thoracic and cervical regions. In 1% cases, the primary tumor may not be found. The usual clinical manifestation is abdominal distension. Children may present with a palpable abdominal mass which may be an incidental finding in an otherwise healthy child or in a child clearly unwell from metastatic tumor. Less often, subcutaneous bluish, nontender, "blueberry muffin" nodules may be seen. Metastatic involvement of the periorbital bones and soft tissues results in ecchymosed orbital proptosis described as "raccoon eyes". Bone marrow involvement may lead to symptoms such as weight loss, anemia, fever and irritability. Massive hepatic metastases can cause increased intra-abdominal pressure ("Pepper syndrome") and severe respiratory compromise **(Fig. 33.2)**. Paraspinal tumors may

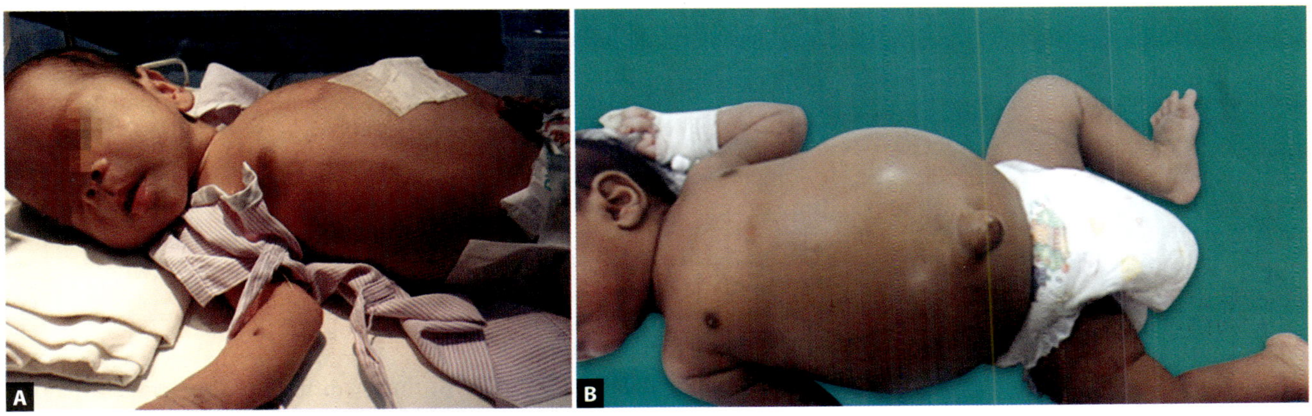

Figures 33.1A and B Infants with neuroblastoma. Note the large umbilical hernia in B

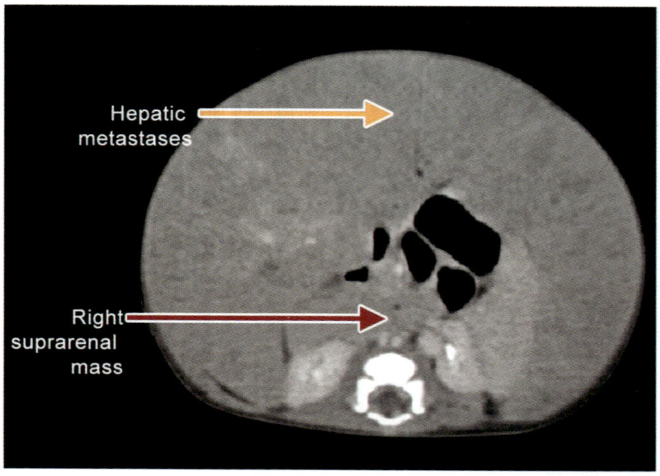

Figure 33.2 Computed tomography (CT) scan of abdomen showing right adrenal primary tumor and massive hepatomegaly from hepatic metastases

extend to the neural foramina and cause compression of nerve roots leading to paraplegia and bladder-bowel dysfunction. Horner syndrome (unilateral ptosis, miosis and anhidrosis) may be seen in case of high thoracic or cervical masses. In less than 2% of cases, neuroblastomas can present with paraneoplastic syndromes, the most common ones being opsoclonus-myoclonus-ataxia syndrome or watery diarrhea from tumor production of vasoactive intestinal peptide.[1]

Staging

The International Neuroblastoma Staging System (INSS) was framed from a consensus international group meeting in 1986 and was revised in 1993 for staging of neuroblastomas.[18] This is a system based on operative findings, and thus unsuitable for pretreatment staging and risk assessment **(Table 33.1)**.

Stage 1: Localized tumor, no lymph node involvement.

Stage 2: Localized tumors, ipsilateral lymph node involvement.

Stage 3: Unresectable tumors which extend across the midline and/or contralateral nodes.

Stage 4: All patients diagnosed more than or equal to 12 months of age with distant disease (lymph nodes, bones, bone marrow, liver and other organs).

Stage 4S ("S" standing for special stage): Age <1 year with metastases restricted to the liver, skin, and/or bone marrow (<10% of tumor in the marrow), in whom the primary tumor is localized (INSS 1 or 2).

In 1971, Evans et al. first described this subset of advanced stage neuroblastoma with favorable prognosis and a high rate of spontaneous regression despite widespread disease.[19]

The International Neuroblastoma Risk Group (INRG) classification system was developed to facilitate the assessment of pretreatment risk classification independent of surgical resection **(Tables 33.2 and 33.3)**. This is based on clinical criteria and image defined risk factors (IDRFs).[20]

Table 33.1 International Neuroblastoma Staging System (INSS)

Stage	*Description*
1	Localized tumor, complete gross excision; negative representative regional lymph nodes
2A	Localized tumor, incomplete gross excision; identifiable lymph nodes negative (ipsi- and contralateral)
2B	Localized tumor, complete or incomplete gross excision; ipsilateral positive regional lymph nodes, contralateral negative lymph nodes
3	Unresectable tumor infiltrating across the midline, with or without regional lymph node involvement or midline tumor with bilateral extension by infiltration or by lymph node involvement
4	Any primary tumor with dissemination to distal lymph nodes, conrtical bone, bone marrow, liver, or other organs (except as defined in stage 4S)
4S	Localized primary tumor, as defined for stage 1 or 2, with dissemination to liver, skin, or bone marrow. Only applies in infants <1 year of age

Source: Modified from Kushner[4]

Table 33.2 International Neuroblastoma Risk Group Staging System

Stage	*Description*
L1	Localized tumor not involving vital structures as defined by the list of image-defined risk factors and confined to one body compartment
L2	Locoregional tumor with presence of one or more image-defined risk factors
M	Distant metastatic disease (except stage MS)
MS	Metastatic disease in children younger than 18 months with metastases confined to skin, liver, and/or bone marrow

Locoregional tumors are staged L1 or L2 depending whether or not one or more of the 20 IDRFs are present. Metastatic tumors are designated M.

A special category MS is reserved for infants less than 18 months whose tumor metastases are confined to liver, skin and/or bone marrow.

PROGNOSTIC FACTORS

Neuroblastoma is remarkable in its diverse clinical behavior with some tumors regressing or maturing, whereas others progress incessantly despite intensive multimodality treatment. INRG has developed a consensus approach to pretreatment risk stratification based on stage, age, histologic category, grade of tumor differentiation, the status of the *MYCN* oncogene, chromosome 11q status and DNA ploidy.[21]

Table 33.3 International Neuroblastoma Risk Grouping (INRG) of neuroblastoma

INRG stage	*Age (months)*	*Histologic category*	*Grade of tumor differentiation*	*11q*				*Pretreatment risk group*
				MYCN	*Aberration*	*Ploidy*		
L1/L2		GN maturing; GNB intermixed					A	Very low
L1		Any, except GN maturing or GNB intermixed		NA			B	Very low
				Amp			K	High
L2	<18	Any, except GN maturing or GNB intermixed		NA	No		D	Low
					Yes		G	Intermediate
	≥18	GNB nodular; neuroblastoma	Differentiating	NA	No		E	Low
					Yes			
			Poorly differentiated or undifferentiated	NA			H	Intermediate
				Amp			N	High
M	<18			NA		Hyperdiploid	F	Low
	<12			NA		Diploid	I	Intermediate
	12 to <18			NA		Diploid	J	Intermediate
	<18			Amp			O	High
	≥18						P	High
MS	<18				No		C	Very low
				NA	Yes		Q	High
				Amp			R	High

Abbreviations: GN, ganglioneuroma; GNB, ganglioneuroblastoma

Staging is perhaps the best established prognostic factor for neuroblastomas.

Stage 4S INSS or MS INRG diseases have excellent outcome with an overall survival probability of 85–92%.[22,23] Factors associated with a poor prognosis in stage 4S tumors include age less than 2 months at diagnosis, biochemical markers such as raised serum lactate dehydrogenase (LDH), ferritin or neuron-specific enolase (NSE) levels, genetic markers such as N-myc amplification and tumor diploidy.[19,22]

DIAGNOSIS

Imaging in children with neuroblastoma:

- Chest or abdominal radiographs
- Abdominal ultrasound or computed tomography (CT) scan
- Magnetic resonance imaging (MRI)
- Metaiodobenzylguanidine (^{123}I-MIBG) scan
- 2-deoxy-2-[fluorine-18]fluoro-D-glucose (^{18}F-FDG) positron emission tomography (PET) computed tomography (CT) scan.

Other investigations:

- Bilateral bone marrow aspirates and biopsies
- Urinary catecholamines metabolites [vanillylmandelic acid (VMA), HMA and dopamine] (urinary catecholamines may be absent in some prenatally detected or infantile cases probably because of the small size of the tumor).[24]

X-rays may reveal paravertebral or retroperitoneal shadows with calcification in about 30% cases. On ultrasonography (USG), neuroblastomas appear as heterogeneous solid lesions, mostly echogenic. Metastatic involvement or invasion of the liver can be detected with USG. Both CT and MRI can accurately assess the location and the size of the primary tumor, the vascular encasement and tumor resectability. Epidural extension and leptomeningeal dissemination in neuroblastoma are better assessed with MRI.[25]

Metaiodobenzylguanidine scan is particularly helpful in primary tumor identification and metastatic surveillance. MIBG may be performed with ^{131}I or ^{123}I. MIBG is an analog of catecholamine precursors and is concentrated in neuroblastic cells. MIBG scan has high sensitivity (88%) and specificity (99%) in detecting primary tumor and metastates in more than 90% of patients.[26]

The ^{18}F-FDG PET is being evaluated as a staging tool in neuroblastoma, and may better delineate disease extent in thorax, abdomen and pelvis.[27] However, ^{131}I MIBG is more likely to detect bone and bone marrow metastases.

MANAGEMENT

Patients with stage 4S/MS disease without life- or organ-threatening symptoms or adverse genetic features can be safely observed for spontaneous regression. Patients with life-threatening symptoms, most commonly due to rapidly expanding intra-abdominal disease usually need treatment with chemotherapy (such as carboplatin-etoposide combination). This regimen has been proved to be associated with a high response rate in symptomatic infants with stage 4S disease.[28]

Management of older children with neuroblastoma depends on the risk category. Chemotherapy is the main modality of therapy in intermediate or high-risk disease, but is also used in patients with low-risk disease for relief of symptoms or in case of vital organ involvement. Chemotherapy usually includes a combination of alkylating agent, platinum compounds, topoisomerase II inhibitors and vincristine. High-risk tumors require surgery, radiotherapy, chemotherapy, and often consolidation with autologous stem cell transplantations. Even with aggressive treatment, the 3-year event-free survival rate is less than15% in high-risk disease.

SCREENING

Japan had initiated a nationwide mass-screening program for neuroblastoma in 6-month-old infants in 1973 using urinary measurements of urine VMA and homovanillic acid (HVA) levels. Unfortunately, the significance of mass screening for neuroblastoma as a public health measure could not be confirmed by subsequent epidemiologic analyses. It did not alter the incidence of tumors in older children nor did it improve cure rates. Similar screening studies in Germany (infants aged 1 year) and Canada (infants aged 3 weeks to 6 months) did not show any reduction in mortality due to neuroblastoma.[29] These results suggest that the tumors discovered at urinary screening were those likely to remain occult, to regress, or to mature. Consequently, screening for NBL has recently been discontinued in Japan.[30] Universal screening for neuroblastoma is thus not indicated but targeted screening of infants at risk of hereditary neuroblastoma with germline ALK or PHOX2B mutations may be appropriate.

KEY POINTS

- Neuroblastoma is a clinically and biologically diverse disease
- Age at diagnosis, stage, histological features/differentiation and presence/absence of N-MYC amplification determine outcome
- Infants with neuroblastoma often require little or no treatment
- In older children, a multimodal approach including chemotherapy, surgery, high dose therapy with autologous stem cell rescue, radiotherapy and differentiation therapy is required
- Newer therapeutic modalities like anti-GD2 antibody may change the outcome neuroblastoma in older children.

REFERENCES

1. Brodeur GM, Maris JM. Neuroblastoma. In: Pizzo PA, Poplack DG (Eds). Principles and Practice of Pediatric Oncology. Philadelphia, USA: Lippincott, Williams & Wilkins; 2010. pp. 786-822.
2. Maris JM, Hogarty MD, Bagatell R, Cohn SL. Neuroblastoma. Lancet. 2007;369(9579):2106-20.
3. Diede SJ. Spontaneous regression of metastatic cancer: learning from neuroblastoma. Nat Rev Cancer. 2014;14(2):71-2.
4. Matthay KK. Stage 4S neuroblastoma: what makes it special? J Clin Oncol. 1998;16(6):2003-6.
5. Stiller CA, Parkin DM. International variations in the incidence of neuroblastoma. Int J Cancer. 1992;52(4):538-43.
6. National Cancer Institute. SEER pediatric monograph. National Cancer Institute. [online] Available from *www-seer.ims.nci.nih.gov/Publications/PedMono/sympathetic.pdf.* [Accessed September, 2016].
7. Brodeur GM. Neuroblastoma: biological insights into a clinical enigma. Nat Rev Cancer. 2003;3(3):203-16.
8. George RE, London WB, Cohn SL, Maris JM, Kretschmar C, Diller L, et al. Hyperdiploidy plus nonamplified MYCN confers a favorable prognosis in children 12 to 18 months old with disseminated neuroblastoma: a Pediatric Oncology Group study. J Clin Oncol. 2005;23(27):6466-73.
9. Brodeur GM, Seeger RC, Schwab M, Varmus HE, Bishop JM. Amplification of N-myc in untreated human neuroblastomas correlates with advanced disease stage. Science. 1984;224(4653): 1121-4.
10. Fujita T, Igarashi J, Okawa ER, Gotoh T, Manne J, Kolla V, et al. CHD5, a tumor suppressor gene deleted from 1p36.31 in neuroblastomas. J Natl Cancer Inst. 2008;100(13):940-9.
11. Munirajan AK, Ando K, Mukai A, Takahashi M, Suenaga Y, Ohira M, et al. KIF1B beta functions as a haploinsufficient tumor suppressor gene mapped to chromosome 1p36.2 by inducing apoptotic cell death. J Biol Chem. 2008;283(36):24426-34.
12. Bown N, Cotterill S, Lastowska M, O'Neill S, Pearson AD, Plantaz D, et al. Gain of chromosome arm 17q and adverse outcome in patients with neuroblastoma. N Engl J Med. 1999;340(25):1954-61.
13. Michels E, Hoebeeck J, De Preter K, Schramm A, Brichard B, De Paepe A, et al. CADM1 is a strong neuroblastoma candidate gene that maps within a 3.72 Mb critical region of loss on 11q23. BMC Cancer. 2008;8:173.
14. Mossé YP, Laudenslager M, Longo L, Cole KA, Wood A, Attiyeh EF, et al. Identification of ALK as a major familial neuroblastoma predisposition gene. Nature. 2008;455(7215):930-5.
15. Shimada H, Ambros IM, Dehner LP, Hata J, Joshi VV Roald B. Terminology and morphologic criteria of neuroblastic tumors recommendations by the International Neuroblastoma Pathology Committee. Cancer. 1999;86(2):349-63.
16. Shimada H, Ambros IM, Dehner LP, Hata J, Joshi VV, Roald B, et al. The International Neuroblastoma Pathology Classification (the Shimada system). Cancer. 1999;86(2):364-72.
17. Houlihan C, Jampolsky M, Shilad A, Prinicipe D. Prenatal diagnosis of neuroblastoma with sonography and magnetic resonance imaging. J Ultrasound Med. 2004;23(4):547-50.
18. Brodeur GM, Pritchard J, Berthold F, Carlsen NL, Castel V, Castelberry RP, et al. Revisions of the international criteria for neuroblastoma diagnosis, staging, and response to treatment. J Clin Oncol. 1993;11(8):1466-77.
19. Evans AE, D'Angio GJ, Randolph J. A proposed staging for children with neuroblastoma. Children's Cancer Study Group A. Cancer. 1971;27(2):374-8.
20. Monclair T, Brodeur GM, Ambros PF, Brisse HJ, Cecchetto G, Holmes K, et al. The International Neuroblastoma Risk Group (INRG) staging system: an INRG Task Force report. J Clin Oncol. 2009;27(2):298-303.

21. Cohn SL, Pearson AD, London WB, Monclair T, Ambros PF, Brodeur GM, et al. The International Neuroblastoma Risk Group (INRG) classification system: an INRG Task Force report. J Clin Oncol. 2009;27(2):289-97.
22. Katzenstein HM, Bowman LC, Brodeur GM, Thorner PS, Joshi VV, Smith EI, et al. Prognostic significance of age, MYCN oncogene amplification, tumor cell ploidy, and histology in 110 infants with stage D(S) neuroblastoma: the pediatric oncology group experience—a pediatric oncology group study. J Clin Oncol. 1998;16(6):2007-17.
23. Nickerson HJ, Matthay KK, Seeger RC, Brodeur GM, Shimada H, Perez C, et al. Favorable biology and outcome of stage IV-S neuroblastoma with supportive care or minimal therapy: a Children's Cancer Group study. J Clin Oncol. 2000;18(3):477-86.
24. Sauvat F, Sarnacki S, Brisse H, Medioni J, Rubie H, Aigrain Y, et al. Outcome of suprarenal localized masses diagnosed during the perinatal period: a retrospective multicenter study. Cancer. 2002;94(9):2474-80.
25. Siegel MJ, Ishwaran H, Fletcher BD, Meyer JS, Hoffer FA, Jaramillo D, et al. Staging of neuroblastoma at imaging: report of the radiology diagnostic oncology group. Radiology. 2002;223(1):168-75.
26. Frappaz D, Combaret V, Desuzinges C, Bouffet E, Bailly C, Favrot MC, et al. Can MIBG scan replace the need for bone marrow assessment at diagnosis and reassessment in stage 4 neuroblastomas? Bull Cancer. 2004;91(7-8):E253-60.
27. Sharp SE, Shulkin BL, Gelfand MJ, Salisbury S, Furman WL. 123I-MIBG scintigraphy and ^{18}F-FDG PET in neuroblastoma. J Nucl Med. 2009;50(8):1237-43.
28. Schleiermacher G, Rubie H, Hartmann O, Bergeron C, Chastagner P, Mechinaud F, et al. Treatment of stage 4S neuroblastoma—report of 10 years' experience of the French Society of Paediatric Oncology (SFOP). Br J Cancer. 2003;89(3):470-6.
29. Tsubono Y, Hisamichi S. A halt to neuroblastoma screening in Japan. N Engl J Med. 2004;350(19):2010-1.
30. Okazaki T, Kohno S, Mimaya J, Hasegawa S, Urushihara N, Yoshida A, et al. Neuroblastoma detected by mass screening: the Tumor Board's role in its treatment. Pediatr Surg Int. 2004;20(1):27-32.

CHAPTER

34

Renal Tumors in Neonates

Julius Xavier Scott, Latha M Sneha

INTRODUCTION

The incidence of abdominal mass in the neonatal period is approximately 1 in 1,000 live births. The organs or systems of origin are 55% renal, 15% from gastrointestinal (GIT), 15% genital tract, 10% retroperitoneal and 5% involve the liver, spleen and biliary tract.[1] Some of the common nonmalignant renal conditions that a neonatologist or pediatrician should be aware of when a newborn presents with abdominal mass are hydronephrosis, multicystic dysplasia, polycystic kidney, renal vein thrombosis and adrenal hemorrhage. The incidence of neonatal tumors is 1 in 15,000 live births, accounting for only 2% of the pediatric malignancies.[2] Renal tumors comprise 7% of the neonatal malignancies.[3] Mesoblastic nephroma (MN) and Wilms' tumor are the most common tumors of neonatal period. The other renal tumors that would be described in detail in this article are:

- Malignant rhabdoid tumor
- Clear cell sarcoma
- Ossifying renal tumor of infancy
- Nephroblastomatosis
- Cystic nephromas and cystic partially differentiated nephromas (CPDNs).

OVERVIEW OF THE COMMON RENAL TUMORS

The staging criteria for the renal tumors as per the International Society of Paediatric Oncology (SIOP) is given in **Table 34.1**.

Table 34.1 The International Society of Paediatric Oncology (SIOP) staging criteria for renal tumors[4]

Stage	*Description*
I	Tumor limited to the kidney, complete excision
II	Tumor extending outside the kidney, complete excision Invasion beyond the capsule, perirenal or perihilar Invasion of the regional lymph nodes Invasion of extrarenal vessels Invasion of ureter
III	Tumor extending outside the kidney, incomplete excision Preoperative or perioperative biopsy Preoperative or perioperative rupture Peritoneal metastases or penetration Invasion of para-aortic lymph nodes Tumor thrombi at resection margin
IV	Distant metastases
V	Bilateral renal tumors

Fifteen percent of the neonatal renal tumors are detected antenatally, 50% of them are identified during routine postnatal check-ups, when they present with an abdominal mass or while being evaluated for hypertension, hyper-reninism, hydrops fetalis, vomiting, lethargy, pallor, hematuria and failure to thrive.[5,6] Investigations may reveal anemia, hypercalcemia and bone marrow involvement.

Ultrasound abdomen is the initial investigation to identify the renal mass and computed tomography or magnetic resonance imaging (CT or MRI) imaging helps to define the lesion, identify the metastasis and decide about the future plan. In specific cases like Wilms' tumor, where lung is the site of metastasis, X-ray or CT chest is included in the initial evaluation. In malignant rhabdoid tumor, brain imaging is done to rule out primary central nervous system (CNS) lesion. In clear cell sarcoma, whole body positron emission tomography (PET), CT or bone scan are recommended to identify bony metastases.

In uncomplicated, low-grade tumors, primary radical nephroureterectomy is the only treatment. In high-grade tumors, surgery and chemotherapy are preferred.

As MN is the most common tumor in the neonatal period and majority of them behave like benign tumors, the outcomes is generally very good and even the aggressive types have been found to have good response to surgery and adjuvant chemotherapy.

Ten percent of the Wilms' tumor have been found to be associated with congenital syndromes, like sporadic aniridia,

Table 34.2 Congenital syndromes and their risk of renal malignancies

Syndromes	*Associated features*	*Risk of malignancy*
Denys-Drash syndrome	Gonadal dysgenesis *Nephropathy*: Diffuse mesangial sclerosis Wilms' tumor	50–100%
Beckwith-Wiedemann syndrome (BWS)	Congenital exomphalos Macroglossia Gigantism Hemihypertrophy Genitourinary abnormalities Wilms' tumor Adrenocortical neoplasia	7.5%
WAGR syndrome	Wilms' tumor Aniridia Genitourinary malformations Mental retardation	50%
Simpson-Golabi-Behmel syndrome	Over growth syndrome Congenital diaphragmatic hernia Craniofacial—hypertelorism, large mouth, large tongue, upturned broad nose Skeletal and cardiac abnormalities Renal abnormalities—multicystic dysplastic kidneys Single umbilical artery Wilms' tumor Hepatoblastoma	10%

Abbreviation: WAGR, Wilms tumor-aniridia syndrome, aniridia-Wilms' tumor syndrome

Denys-Drash syndrome, Beckwith-Wiedemann syndrome (BWS), WAGR syndrome and Simpson-Golabi-Behmel syndrome.[7] The associated features and the risk of developing tumors in these congenital syndromes are given in **Table 34.2**.

The incidence of end-stage renal failure is 36% in WAGR and 74% in Denys-Drash syndrome and 90% in bilateral tumors in WAGR syndrome.[8] Identification of syndromes should lead to screening for Wilms' and other embryonic tumors. When the risk of developing tumors is more than 5% in any associated syndromes, these infants should be subjected to screening—clinical and ultrasound evaluation every 3 months till they are 5 years of age and 7 years of age in case of BWS.[5]

The characteristics of individual renal tumors are given below:

MESOBLASTIC NEPHROMA

First described in 1967, MN is a mesenchymal tumor with low malignant potential. It is the most common renal tumor accounting for 54–66% of renal tumors found in the neonatal period and the first 3 months of life.[9] With a slight male preponderance (male : female, 1.5 : 1) they are usually unilateral. A palpable abdominal mass is the most common presentation, while evaluation for hydrops fetalis, hypertension, hematuria, hyper-reninism might lead to the diagnosis in others.[10] Imaging studies reveal a typical solid lesion extending from the normal renal parenchyma in most of the cases and within the parenchyma in some cases. Though the lesion might be found to extend to the renal vessels or inferior vena cava, it usually does not invade them.[11] Stage IV or V tumors are exceptionally rare and majority of the MNs are low-stage tumors with 82% of stage I or II and 8.5% of stage III.[9]

Table 34.3 Characteristics of classical and cellular types of mesoblastic nephromas

Classical type	*Cellular type*
• Bland spindle cells • Few mitoses • Absence of necrosis • Infiltrative edge • No identifiable genetic marker • Benign nature	• Accounts for 50% of the cases • Presentation at older age group than classical type • High mitotic index • Hypercellularity • Necrosis and hemorrhage • Atypical growth pattern • Invasion of adjacent structures • *ETV6-NTRK3* gene fusion associated with translocation t(12:15), (p13:q25) • More aggressive in nature

Histological Classification

Mesoblastic nephromas is histologically classified into three types: (1) classical, (2) mixed and (3) cellular. All the variants are generally benign in nature and composed of spindled cell bundles of immature renal stromal cells. MNs are easily distinguished from the Wilms' tumor by the absence of renal blastema and metanephric elements and they characteristically infiltrate the kidney rather than forming the pseudo capsules in Wilms' tumor.

The characteristic features of the histological subtypes are given in **Table 34.3**.

Occasionally the mixed and cellular types have been found to be more aggressive and metastases to lung, brain, liver, heart and bone have been reported.[12] The presence of translocation has not been found to correlate with relapse rate or outcome.[13] Core biopsy of the lesion would not help in differentiating it from the stromal component of Wilms' tumor.

Radical nephroureterectomy is the main stay of treatment. Due to the infiltrative growth pattern of MNs, invading the renal parenchyma, renal capsule and perirenal tissues, local or partial resection of MNs is discouraged and higher incidence of local recurrence has been reported in positive resected margins.[14] Postoperative chemotherapy is reserved for aggressive tumors.

The outcome is generally good with an event-free survival (EFS) of 94% and overall survival (OS) rate of 96%. An EFS of 100% was noted in children under 3 months of age at diagnosis against 83% seen in older children. Furtwaengler et al. has reported death or relapses only in patients with cellular subtypes.[14]

WILMS' TUMOR

Accounting for 20% of cases, Wilms' tumor is the second most common neonatal renal tumor.[6] Generally a sporadic condition, family history is noted in 1% cases. With equal male and female preponderance, Wilms' tumor has a clinical presentation similar to MNs with 50% of them presenting as palpable abdominal masses and 16% diagnosed antenatally and rest while evaluating for polyhydramnios, hydrops fetalis and other congenital syndromes.[6] Imaging studies showing a tumor thrombus in inferior vena cava or renal vein or an associated pulmonary lesions strongly supports the diagnosis of Wilms' tumor against MNs. The predominant morphological type is the classical triphasic with tubules, blastema and stroma. The presence or absence of anaplasia determines the favorable or unfavorable histology. The pathology has been found to be favorable in majority of the neonatal Wilms' tumors. The majority of Wilms' tumor is low-stage tumors with 80% of stage I or II. Loss of heterozygosity (LOH) at 11p, 16q and 1p has been found to be associated with increased risk of relapse and hence this group of tumors needs chemotherapy in addition to the primary nephrectomy.[15]

Treatment

Primary radical nephroureterectomy is the treatment of choice in low-risk cases. The need for postoperative chemotherapy in unilateral Wilms' tumor is rare in neonatal period. The associated nephropathy seen in some syndromes makes nephron sparing surgery an ideal option in such children. The incidence of end-stage renal failure is 36% in WAGR and 74% in Denys-Drash syndrome and 90% in bilateral tumors in WAGR syndrome. Hence, in cases of synchronous bilateral tumors at presentation or identification of syndromes with high-risk of metachronous tumors, nephron-sparing surgery is attempted after a period of preoperative chemotherapy to preserve as much renal function as possible.[5] For bilateral Wilms' tumor, 6 weeks of chemotherapy with vincristine, actinomycin D, doxorubicin at 50% dose reduction, followed by surgery and further chemotherapy according to the histology and staging are recommended.[5]

Neonatal Wilms' tumor also has a very good prognosis with EFS of 86% and OS of 93%.

MALIGNANT RHABDOID TUMOR OF THE KIDNEY

First described in 1978, malignant rhabdoid tumor of the kidney (MRTK) is a very aggressive renal tumor and commonly presents with stage III or IV disease. But it is very rare accounting for 11% of renal tumors and primarily occurs in the neonatal period and infancy.[16]

Abdominal mass is the most common presentation, but in 9% of cases metastatic disease presentation is seen.[6] Metastases to lung, abdomen, lymph nodes, liver, bone, skin and brain have been reported.

Imaging studies shows characteristic curvilinear calcifications around tumor lobules and subcapsular fluid collections, which are rarely seen in other renal tumors.[17] Due to the close association between malignant rhabdoid tumor of kidney with brain tumors and primitive neuroectodermal tumor (PNET), early imaging of brain is warranted. Histologically rhabdoid tumors might resemble rhabdomyosarcoma but immunohistochemistry reveals no skeletal muscle markers or myoblastic differentiation.

Deletions at chromosome locus 22q11.1, which contains the gene *SMARCB1/INI1*, a tumor suppressor gene, has been frequently identified in MRTKs.[18] Germline mutations have been identified in one-third of patients with rhabdoid tumors.[19] Germline mutations are associated with other tumors like rhabdoid tumors of brain, schwannomas and meningiomas.[20]

Treatment includes radical nephroureterectomy combined with chemotherapy and radiotherapy. The chemoresistance and early onset of local and distant metastases contributes to the poor outcomes. The OS rates in neonates are 8.7%.[6]

CLEAR CELL SARCOMA OF THE KIDNEY

Described as the bone metastasis tumor of the kidney, due to its classical metastasis to bones, clear cell sarcoma of the kidney (CCSK) accounts for only 3% of the neonatal renal tumors. It is more commonly found in older children and 30% of them are stage IV disease at presentation.[6] Apart from bone metastasis, lymph node metastases have been the most common at presentation followed by lung and liver involvement.[21] There is a male predominance (male : female, 2 : 1). Typical presentation is abdominal mass and in view of the aggressive nature of the disease, bone scan is essential after the histological confirmation.

The classical histology is cords and nests of medium-sized cells separated by clear intercellular matrix and surrounded by thin fibrovascular septa.[21]

Treatment is primary surgery followed by chemotherapy and radiotherapy. The outcome of neonatal CCSKA has been found to be higher than in older children. EFS of 49% and OS 51% were reported in a study of infants up to 7 months of age.[9]

OSSIFYING RENAL TUMOR OF INFANCY

Rare tumor, first described in 1980, it has a predilection for the upper poles of left kidney. Gross hematuria is the most common presentation and there is an increased male predominance 3:1. X-rays show a 2–3 cm calcified mass in the kidney and ultrasound will reveal an echogenic mass. Histologically, they are composed of osteoblasts, spindle cells with an osteoid core.[5]

Nephrectomy is the commonly practiced treatment, though some recommend nephron-sparing surgery due to the benign nature of the lesion. Recurrences have been reported after partial resections and hence partial resection is not recommended.[22] Excellent outcomes in all cases have made chemotherapy unnecessary.

NEPHROBLASTOMATOSIS

It is the persistence of metanephric blastema beyond 36 weeks of gestation. Nephroblastomatosis and nephrogenic rests within the kidney are considered as precursors of Wilms' tumor and other renal tumors.[23] It is seen in 20–50% of Wilms' tumor nephrectomy specimens and also found in association with BWS and aniridia. Depending upon the distribution, it is classified into perilobular, intralobular and panlobular. Biopsies may be indistinguishable from Wilms' tumor and the edge of the specimen should be looked into for the invasive margin of Wilms' tumor against a distinct margin of nephroblastomatosis.[5]

Incidental finding of nephroblastomatosis in the neonatal period necessitates close observation as there is no need for prophylactic treatment when it is premalignant. Diffusion-weighted MRI can identify the changes within the lesions that signify the onset of malignant transformation, long before the growth of the lesion is identified.[5]

Increase in the size of the lesion or changes in the diffusion coefficient on MRI warrants chemotherapy with vincristine alone or with actinomycin D. If the lesion is chemorefractory and continues to grow, cis-Retinoic acid is the choice to stall the growth.[24]

MISCELLANEOUS RENAL TUMORS

Cystic renal tumors form a spectrum with cystic nephroma at the benign end, cystic partially differentiated nephroma in the intermediate region and Wilms' tumor with multicystic areas at the malignant end.

Cystic Nephroma

Initially considered as lesion of developmental origin, multilocular cystic renal tumor's malignant potential was identified by Boggs and Kimmelstiel in 1956.[25] It is a rare, benign renal neoplasm that is purely cystic and is lined by epithelium and fibrous septa that contains mature tubules. It is associated with pleuropulmonary blastoma in a small number of cases.[5] Painless abdominal mass is the common presentation. It is a well-circumscribed mass with thick fibrous capsule, contains multiple fluid filled noncommunicating loculi separated by thin translucent septa. No solid components is seen. It is difficult to distinguish from malignant cystic lesions clinically and radiologically. Histologically, they are cystic lesions with thin walled septations and septations lined by differentiated cells and no blastemal or embryonic elements within the septa unlike in CPDN. Radical nephrectomy is curative but spillage or rupture has lead to local recurrence. Generally, the outcome is excellent.[5]

Cystic Partially Differentiated Nephroma

It is a multilocular cystic neoplasm composed of epithelial and stromal elements along with nephroblastomatous tissue. It has a male predominance 2:1 and is a low-grade malignant tumor. Painless abdominal mass is the most common presentation and sudden progressive enlargement with hematuria has also been reported.[26] Ultrasonography shows the hypoechoic cysts delineated by hyperechoic septae.[27] CPDN is a well-circumscribed solitary mass with multiseptated fluid filled loculi surrounded by thick fibrous capsule, occupying the entire renal pole.

Histologically, the cysts are lined by hobnail-shaped eosinophilic cells and septa contain epithelial structures resembling mature renal tubules, blastema and with or without embryonal stromal The presence or absence of blastemal element in the septal walls distinguishes the CPDN from cystic nephroma. Joshi and Beckwith had subclassified CPDN into grade I and II based on the content of mature septal elements. Grade I has more than 50% mature elements and grade II less than 50% mature elements in septa.[28] Due to the potential of the blastemal elements for aggressive behavior, simple nephrectomy is the best option of treatment and has an excellent prognosis. Incomplete resection have resulted in recurrence but metastasis has not been reported.[29]

Intrarenal Neuroblastoma

Intrarenal neuroblastoma typically results from direct renal invasion of an adrenal neuroblastoma through the renal capsule or lymphatic perivascular spread but true intrarenal neuroblastoma is rare. It is proposed that the sequestered adrenal rests during fetal life or intrarenal sympathetic ganglia might be the cause. Though most of the neuroblastomas in infants are of adrenal origin, intrarenal neuroblastoma has been rarely reported.[30,31] A high proportion of intrarenal neuroblastoma has been found to be of unfavorable histology due to higher incidence of anaplasia when compared to the adrenal origin.[32]

Renal Primitive Neuroectodermal Tumor

Primitive neuroectodermal tumor is of neural crest origin mostly presenting as bone or soft tissue masses. Renal PNET was reported by Mor et al.[33] The presenting symptoms and clinical signs are similar to other renal tumors. The diagnosis in made only postoperatively, based on histopathology and immunohistochemical stains. Renal PNET is more aggressive

6 SECTION Fetal and Neonatal Malignancy

than PNET arising from other sites. Around 50% of them present with distant metastases to regional lymph nodes, lungs and liver. They also have a high tendency for early local recurrence. Treatment is radical nephrectomy and chemotherapy as per Ewing's protocol.

To conclude, though the neonatal renal tumors are rare, neonatologists and the pediatricians who are the primary physicians should be able to identify the association of renal malignancies with the recognized syndromes and the diagnosis of the syndromes should lead to the screening for malignancies. In view of the rarity of the tumors and the high risk of toxicity in this vulnerable population, treatment should always be managed by multidisciplinary team. Early diagnosis, initiation of proper treatment plan incorporating multicentric clinical trials at national and international levels concentrating on decreasing the morbidity should be initiated at the earliest for achieving the best outcomes in this fragile population.

CONCLUSION

Due to the rarity of the renal tumors and need to recognize the distinct features of different tumors, neonatologists and pediatricians should be referring these babies to a tertiary care center with a multispecialty care inclusive of pathologist, genetics, pediatric oncology, radiation oncologist and pediatric surgeons.

Early recognition and appropriate treatment are the keystones for improved survival rates.

KEY POINTS

- Neonatal renal tumors are rare, accounting for only 7% neonatal malignancies
- Survival is generally excellent for majority of the tumor groups in this age group
- Multidisciplinary approach is essential for the appropriate and adequate management of renal tumors.

REFERENCES

1. Marshall ZS, Donald BS. Abdominal masses in the newborn. Pediatr Rev. 1989;11:172-9.
2. Moore SW, Satgé D, Sasco AJ, Zimmermann A, Plaschkes J. The epidemiology of neonatal tumours. Report of an international working group. Pediatr Surg Int. 2003;19(7):509-19.
3. Makin E, Davenport M. Fetal and neonatal liver tumours. Early Hum Dev. 2010;86(10):637-42.
4. Vujanić GM, Sandstedt B, Harms D, Kelsey A, Leuschner I, de Kraker J. Revised International Society of Paediatric Oncology (SIOP) working classification of renal tumors of childhood. Med Pediatr Oncol. 2002;38(2):79-82.
5. Powis M. Neonatal renal tumours. Early Hum Dev. 2010;86(10):607-12.
6. Isaacs H Jr. Fetal and neonatal renal tumors. J Pediatr Surg. 2008;43(9):1587-95.
7. Alessandri JL, Cuillier F, Ramful D, Ernould S, Robin S, de Napoli-Cocci S, et al. Perlman syndrome: report, prenatal findings and review. Am J Med Genet A. 2008;146A(19):2532-7.
8. Breslow NE, Collins AJ, Ritchey ML, Grigoriev YA, Peterson SM, Green DM. End stage renal disease in patients with Wilms tumor: results from the National Wilms Tumor Study Group and the United States Renal Data System. J Urol. 2005;174(5):1972-5.
9. van den Heuvel-Eibrink MM, Grundy P, Graf N, Pritchard-Jones K, Bergeron C, Patte C, et al. Characteristics and survival of 750 children diagnosed with a renal tumor in the first seven months of life: A collaborative study by the SIOP/GPOH/SFOP, NWTSG, and UKCCSG Wilms tumor study groups. Pediatr Blood Cancer. 2008;50(6):1130-4.
10. Malone PS, Duffy PG, Ransley PG, Risdon RA, Cook T, Taylor M. Congenital mesoblastic nephroma, renin production, and hypertension. J Pediatr Surg. 1989;24(6):599-600.
11. Riccabona M. Imaging of renal tumours in infancy and childhood. Eur Radiol. 2003;13(Suppl 4):L116-29.
12. Steinfeld AD, Crowley CA, O'Shea PA, Tefft M. Recurrent and metastatic mesoblastic nephroma in infancy. J Clin Oncol. 1984;2(8):956-60.
13. Anderson J, Gibson S, Sebire NJ. Expression of ETV6-NTRK in classical, cellular and mixed subtypes of congenital mesoblastic nephroma. Histopathology. 2006;48(6):748-53.
14. Furtwaengler R, Reinhard H, Leuschner I, Schenk JP, Goebel U, Claviez A, et al. Mesoblastic nephroma—a report from the Gesellschaft fur Pädiatrische Onkologie und Hämatologie (GPOH). Cancer. 2006;106(10):2275-83.
15. Grundy P, Telzerow P, Moksness J, Breslow NE. Clinicopathologic correlates of loss of heterozygosity in Wilms' tumor: a preliminary analysis. Med Pediatr Oncol. 1996;27(5):429-33.
16. Beckwith JB, Palmer NF. Histopathology and prognosis of Wilms tumors: results from the First National Wilms' Tumor Study. Cancer. 1978;41(5):1937-48.
17. Agrons GA, Kingsman KD, Wagner BJ, Sotelo-Avila C. Rhabdoid tumour of the kidney in children: a comparative study of 21 cases. Am J Roentgenol. 1997;168(2):447-51.
18. Biegel JA, Zhou JY, Rorke LB, Stenstrom C, Wainwright LM, Fogelgren B. Germ-line and acquired mutations of INI1 in atypical teratoid and rhabdoid tumors. Cancer Res. 1999;59(1):74-9.
19. Loeb DM, Hill DA, Dome JS. Complete response of recurrent cellular congenital mesoblastic nephroma to chemotherapy. J Pediatr Hematol Oncol. 2002;24(6):478-81.
20. Thompson PA, Chintagumpala M. Renal and hepatic tumors in the neonatal period. Semin fetal Neonatal Med. 2012;17(4):216-21.
21. Argani P, Perlman EJ, Breslow NE, Browning NG, Green DM, D'Angio GJ, et al. Clear cell sarcoma of the kidney: a review of 351 cases from the National Wilms Tumor Study Group Pathology Center. Am J Surg Pathol. 2000;24(1):4-18.
22. Charles AK, Berry PJ, Joyce MR, Keen CE. Ossifying renal tumor of infancy. Pediatr Pathol Lab Med. 1997;17(2):332-4.
23. Beckwith JB, Kiviat NB, Bonadio JF. Nephrogenic rests, nephroblastomatosis, and the pathogenesis of Wilms' tumor. Pediatr Pathol. 1990;10(1-2):1-36.
24. Witt O, Hämmerling S, Stockklausner C, Schenk JP, Günther P, Behnisch W, et al. 13-cis retinoic acid treatment of a patient with chemotherapy refractory nephroblastomatosis. J Pediatr Hematol Oncol. 2009;31(4):296-9.
25. Boggs LK, Kimmelstiel P. Benign multilocular cystic nephroma: report of two cases of so-called multilocular cyst of the kidney. J Urol. 1956;76(5):530-41.
26. Joshi VV, Banerjee AK, Yadav K, Pathak IC. Cystic partially differenciated nephroblastoma: a clinicopathologic entity

in the spectrum of infantile renal neoplasia. Cancer. 1977;40(2):789-95.

27. Wilkinson C, Palit V, Bardapure M, Thomas J, Browning AJ, Gill K, et al. Adult multilocular cystic nephroma: Report of six cases with clinical, radiopathologic correlation and review of literature. Urol Ann. 2013;5(1):13-7.
28. Joshi VV, Beckwith JB. Multilocular cyst of the kidney (cystic nephroma) and cystic partially differentiated nephroblastoma. Terminology and criteria for diagnosis. Cancer. 1989;64(2):466-79.
29. Kumar VR, Rajamani G, Raman ML. Cystic partially differentiated nephroblastoma with ureteric extension. Indian J Pathol Microbiol. 2010;53(4):831-2.
30. Garnier S, Maillet O, Haouy S, Saguintaah M, Serre I, Galifer RB, et al. Prenatal intrarenal neuroblastoma mimicking a mesoblastic nephroma: a case report J Pediatr Surg. 2012; 47(8):e21-3.
31. Lall A, Bajpai M, Gupta DK. Intrarenalneuroblastoma—a diagnostic dilemma: A report of three cases. Indian J Urol. 2001;17:170-2.
32. Shanmugapriya S, Chadaga H, Joseph S, Panicker VK, Rajendran S. "Intra abdominal round cell tumour of childhood a dilemma of site and origin". Sri Ramachandra Journal of Medicine. 2009;2(2).
33. Mor Y, Nass D, Raviv G, Neumann Y, Nativ O, Goldwasser B, et al. Malignant peripheral primitive neuroectodermal tumour (PNET) of the kidney. Med Pediatr Oncol. 1994; 23(5):437-40.

CHAPTER

35

Neonatal Soft Tissue Sarcomas

Venkatraman Radhakrishnan

INTRODUCTION

Soft tissue sarcomas (STSs) are a heterogeneous group of malignant disorders arising from mesenchymal tissue like muscle, fat, fibrous tissue, peripheral nerves and skin. These tumors are extremely rare in the neonatal period (first 28 days of life). The true incidence of neonatal STS is not known. Data from surveillance, epidemiology and end research (SEER) database in United States of America indicate that STS accounted for 8% of all tumors in children less than 1 year of age and ranked 5th among the most commonly seen cancers in infants.[1,2] The management of neonatal STS is challenging because of the toxicity and tolerability of treatment modalities like surgery, radiotherapy and chemotherapy.

APPROACH TO A NEONATE WITH SOFT TISSUE SWELLING

Majority of the soft tissue swellings in the neonatal period are benign.[1,2] Therefore, it requires a very high degree of clinical suspicion to diagnose STS in the neonatal period. While taking the history it is important to ascertain if the swelling was detected in antenatal ultrasound scans and if the mother was exposed to any carcinogens during her pregnancy. The time of onset of the swelling and the rapidity of the growth need to be ascertained. History of birth trauma should be asked to rule out hematomas. The appearance of the swelling after vaccination with bacillus Calmette-Guérin (BCG) or hepatitis B could indicate an inflammatory lymph node enlargement. Physical examination of the swelling should include assessment of tenderness, consistency, mobility, plane of swelling, neurovascular deficits and any swelling elsewhere **(Fig. 35.1)**.

Enlargement of draining lymph nodes should be ascertained. Abdomen should be palpated to look for organomegaly or presence of mass. Neuroblastoma is the most common solid tumor seen in infancy, it commonly presents as an abdominal mass. However, patients with metastatic neuroblastoma can present with soft tissue swellings that can mimic STS.[1,2]

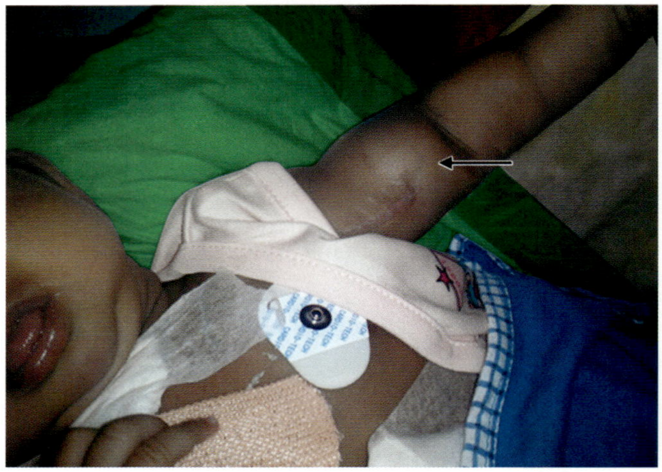

Figure 35.1 Soft tissue swelling in the left biceps muscles of a neonate with synovial sarcoma

Prior to doing a biopsy, it is mandatory to do a complete blood count and a differential count, this is because acute leukemias can present with cutaneous nodules and soft tissue swelling. A bone marrow aspiration and biopsy should be performed if there is a suspicion of leukemia or if the soft tissue swelling is a malignant tumor of embryonal origin like rhabdomyosarcoma or Ewing's sarcoma. Magnetic resonance imaging (MRI) or computed tomographic (CT) scan of the tumor is required to define its size, location, surgical resectability and relationship to surrounding structures including blood vessels and nerves **(Fig. 35.2)**.

A chest X-ray and ultrasound of abdomen and pelvis should be obtained for evaluation of metastatic disease. Biopsy of the tumor is required to establish the diagnosis of STS **(Fig. 35.3)**. Doppler ultrasound of the tumor should be done prior to the biopsy to exclude a vascular tumor, thereby avoiding the complication of bleeding. The biopsy can be core needle or incisional biopsy for large tumors or an excisional biopsy for smaller tumors. The biopsy should be performed by a trained surgical oncologist or pediatric

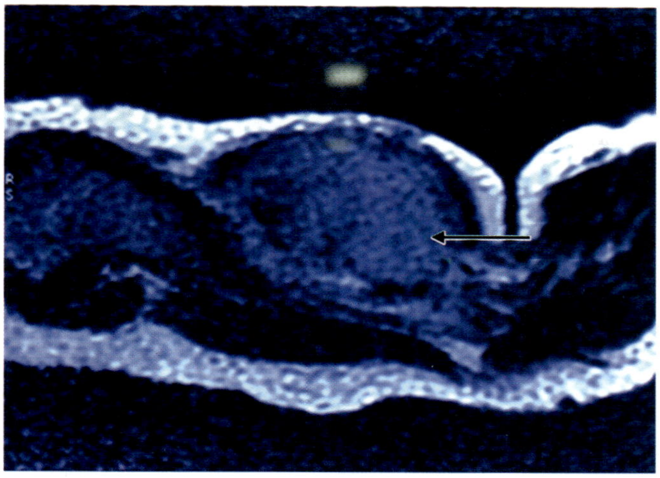

Figure 35.2 Magnetic resonance imaging (MRI) showing mass in left biceps muscle in a neonate with synovial sarcoma

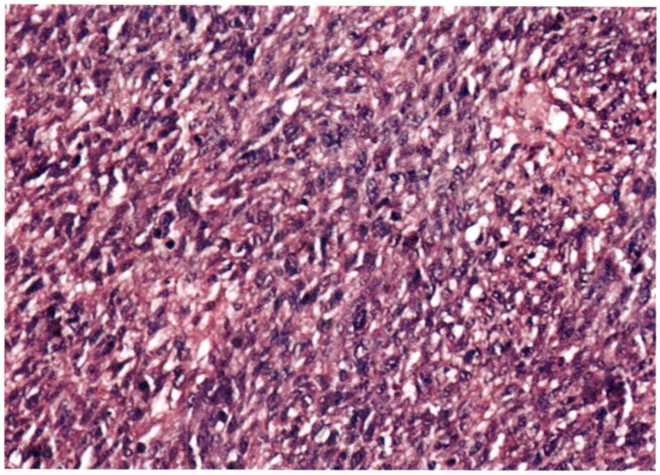

Figure 35.3 Sheets of atypical spindle cells with increased mitoses seen in a neonate with high-grade sarcoma (H&E 20X)

Table 35.1 Initial immunohistochemical panel for the evaluation of pleomorphic spindle cell neoplasm

Immunohistochemistry (IHC) stain	Pleomorphic neoplasm
Pan keratin positive	Pleomorphic carcinoma
S100 positive	Melanoma
Lymphoid marker positive	Lymphoma/follicular dendritic tumor
Vimentin positive, keratin negative, S100 negative, lymphoid negative	Sarcoma

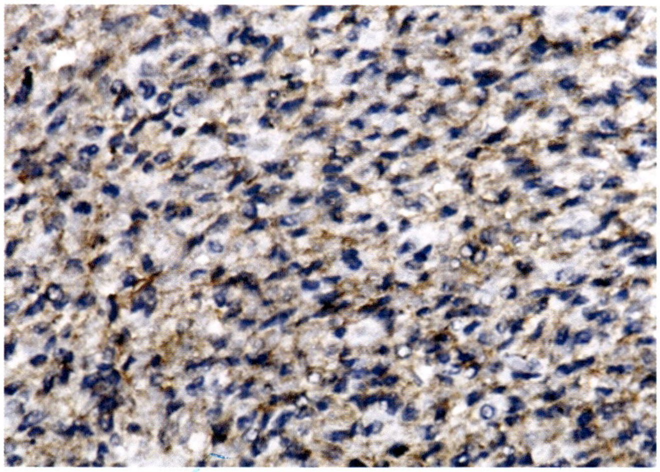

Figure 35.4 Tumor cells show membrane positivity for cluster of differentiation 99 (CD99) (DAB 400X)

surgeon, so that future surgical excision is not compromised. Immunohistochemistry (IHC) is required to distinguish between common soft tissue neoplasms and other neonatal malignancies **(Table 35.1) (Fig. 35.4)**.

Immunohistochemistry is also needed to differentiate the various forms of STS **(Table 35.2)**. STS can like Ewing's sarcoma and synovial sarcoma appear histologically as small round blue cell tumors and can be differentiated from other small round tumors using IHC **(Table 35.3)**. When IHC is noncontributory cytogenetic and molecular testing is required to confirm the diagnosis **(Table 35.4)**.

COMMON SOFT TISSUE NEOPLASMS

A retrospective review conducted by Children's Cancer Group (CCG) in United States identified 32 neonatal STS treated between 1971 and 1991.[3] STS was twice as common in boys as girls (21/32 vs 11/32). The common histological types were fibrosarcoma (12/32), rhabdomyosarcomas (RMSs) (11/32) and non-RMS (9/32). The tumors were commonly seen in head and neck (34%), extremities (28%) and trunk (32%). The overall survival rate in this study was 59%.

Rhabdomyosarcoma

Rhabdomyosarcoma is the most common mesenchymal tumor of childhood. The tumor cells are high grade and resemble embryonal skeletal muscle. RMS is an aggressive tumor with high propensity to metastasis. The prognosis depends on site, histology and stage. Less than 5% of all RMS arise in infants and congenital RMS have also been reported in the literature. RMS in neonates is most commonly seen in head and neck, genitourinary or extremity regions. The symptoms depend on the site of origin of the tumor. RMS rapidly increase in size and are commonly misdiagnosed as vascular tumors. Neonatal RMS has been associated with increased involvement of skin and brain. Evaluation of the patient should include a biopsy or excision of the mass if possible, bone marrow aspiration and biopsy, CT scan of the chest, abdomen and pelvis and the involved site. Histologically, RMS is classified as embryonal or alveolar. Embryonal RMS is seen in younger children and is associated with a better prognosis than alveolar RMS, which tends to occur in older children and usually presents as an extremity tumor. Alveolar RMS is associated with t(2;5) translocation and embryonal RMS is associated with allelic loss in

Table 35.2 Differential diagnosis of nonpleomorphic spindle cell sarcoma

STS	*S100*	*Desmin*	*Actins*	*EMA*	*HMB-45*
Synovial sarcoma	±	–	–	+	–
Malignant peripheral nerve sheath tumor (MPNST)	+/(–)	–	–	+	–
Leiomyosarcoma (LMS)	–	+	+	–/(+)	–
Fibrosarcoma	–	–	–/(+)	–	–
Clear cell sarcoma	+	–	–	–	+

Abbreviations: EMA, epithelial membrane antigen; STS, soft tissue sarcoma; HMB, β-hydroxy-β-methylbutyrate
Keys: –/+: positive in 30% of tumors. +: positive in more than 70%. –: negative in more than 70%. +/(–): between 50% and 70% positive, often weekly. –/(+): positive in up to 30%.

Table 35.3 Immunoprofile of small round cell tumors of soft tissue

Markers	*Ewing's sarcoma*	*RMS*	*SS*	*ES*	*Leukemia lymphoma*
Lymphoid marker (CD45, CD79a, CD19 and CD3 TdT)	–	–	–	–	+
CD99	+	–	+	–	+/–
FLI-1	+	–	–	–	+/–
Cytokeratin/EMA	–/(+)	–	+/(–)	+/+	–
Desmin	–	+	–	–	–
Myogenin	–	+	–	–	–
S100	–/(+)	–	–/+	–	–
CD34	–	–	–	+/–	–

Abbreviations: RMS, rhabdomyosarcoma; SS, synovial sarcoma; ES, epithelioid sarcoma; EMA, epithelial membrane antigen
Keys: –/+: positive in 30% of tumors; +: positive in more than 70%; –: negative in more than 70%; +/(–): between 50% and 70% positive, often weekly; –/(+): positive in up to 30%.

Table 35.4 Cytogenetic abnormalities seen in soft tissue sarcomas

Soft tissue sarcoma	*Translocation*	*Fusion transcripts*
Alveolar rhabdomyosarcoma	t(2;13)(q35;q14) t(1;13)(p36;q14)	PAX3-FKHR PAX7-FKHR
Ewing's family of tumors	t(11;22)(q24;q12) t(21;22)(q22:q12)	EWS-FLI1 EWS-ERG1
Synovial sarcoma	t(X;18)(p11;q11)	SYT-SSX1 or SSX2 or SSX4
Clear cell sarcoma	t(12;22)(q13;q12)	EWS-ATF1
Dermatofibrosarcoma	t(17;22)(q22;q13)	COL1A1-PDGFB
Infantile fibrosarcoma	t(12;15)(p13;q25)	ETV6-NTRK3
Myxoid liposarcoma	t(12;16)(q13;p11)	TLS-CHOP
Extraskeletal myxoid liposarcoma	t(9;22)(q22;q12)	EWS-CHN

chromosome 11p15. These cytogenetic abnormalities can be used to diagnose RMS if the histopathology is inconclusive.

Outcomes in neonatal RMS have been poor due to the inability to deliver adequate doses of chemotherapy and radiotherapy and aggressive nature of the disease. More than half the patients have metastatic disease at presentation. Patients with complete surgical excision with negative margins have the best prognosis.

Rhabdomyosarcoma requires multimodality management with chemotherapy, surgery and radiotherapy. Patients are first given neoadjuvant chemotherapy with 3 weekly vincristine, actinomycin-D and cyclophosphamide (VAC) and weekly vincristine for 2–3 months. The tumor is then reassessed for local treatment with either surgery or radiotherapy depending on location and resectability without any significant morbidity. Adjuvant chemotherapy is continued after local treatment for up to 45 weeks duration. Patients with localized tumors in head and neck region (nonparameningeal) and genitourinary region (vagina and uterus) have better prognosis compared to tumors in other sites. Chemotoxicity is more common in infants. Chemotherapy doses in infants are calculated according to body weight and not according to body surface area as done in older children. The chemotherapy is usually administered at 50–75% of the calculated dose to reduce morbidity and mortality. It is prudent to avoid anthracyclines like doxorubicin and ifosfamide in neonates due to significant cardiotoxicity and nephrotoxicity associated with these agents respectively. These agents can be added once the child crosses 3 months of age. Radiotherapy is an integral part of RMS treatment. However, significant long-term toxicities preclude its use in infants. Radiotherapy may be avoided in infants with completely resected tumors. If radiotherapy needs to be given then it should be delayed as long as possible, provided the tumor is responding to chemotherapy.

Fibrosarcoma

Fibrosarcoma arise from connective tissue. Neonatal fibrosarcomas are histologically similar to adult fibrosarcomas. However, unlike adult fibrosarcomas the neonatal fibrosarcomas have excellent prognosis. They are much more common in the first 6 months of life than in later infancy. The 5 years disease-free survival with this condition has been reported to be more than 80%. Majority of the tumors present as limb swelling. Histologically, they are aggressive tumors composed of spindle shaped cells that are reactive to vimentin. The most common differential diagnosis for neonatal fibrosarcomas is fibromatosis. Fibromatosis is benign but locally aggressive tumors, which histologically resemble fibrosarcomas. Surgical resection is the definitive treatment for fibrosarcomas. These tumors have a high local recurrence rate of up to 50%. Local recurrences can be managed with repeat surgical resection. The role of adjuvant chemotherapy in neonatal fibrosarcoma is not clear. Neoadjuvant chemotherapy may be used to downstage inoperable tumors or reduce the size of tumors if upfront surgery will be mutilating. Commonly used chemotherapeutic agents in RMS like vincristine, actinomycin-D, adriamycin, cyclophosphamide have been tried. There are few reports of use of radiotherapy for downstaging tumors.[1,2] Palliative chemotherapy is indicated in patients with metastatic disease.

Lipoblastoma and Liposarcoma

These tumors arise from adipose tissue. Lipoblastomas are benign tumors more commonly seen in children less than 3 years than in adults. Liposarcomas are more commonly seen in adults. Histologically, it is not possible to differentiate between lipoblastomas and liposarcomas, the only feature that distinguishes liposarcoma from lipoblastomas is the propensity of liposarcoma to metastasis unlike lipoblastoma. Histologically, the myxoid liposarcoma is the most common variant seen in infants, other variants like well-differentiated, round cell and pleomorphic have not been described in infants. Myxoid liposarcoma has the t(12;16) chromosomal translocation unlike lipoblastoma which is associated with chromosome 8 deletions. Surgery is the definitive treatment for liposarcomas and lipoblastoma. The role of chemotherapy and radiotherapy in this condition is not well-established.

Other Nonrhabdomyosarcoma Soft Tissue Tumors

Leiomyosarcomas are STSs arising from smooth muscle. They are rare in children and mostly occur in neonates. The most common site is small intestine and these children present with intestinal obstruction or perforation. Surgical resection is the treatment of choice and there is no role for chemotherapy or radiotherapy. Leiomyosarcoma in neonates have better prognosis than adults as they are detected in an early stage due to symptoms. Synovial sarcomas, malignant peripheral nerve sheath tumors, osteosarcoma, epithelioid sarcoma and alveolar soft part sarcoma have been rarely seen in neonates.[4,5]

KEY MESSAGE

Neonatal STS are rare and require high degree of suspicion for diagnosis. The histology and stage of the STS will determine the treatment modalities and prognosis.

CONCLUSION

Neonatal STS are a heterogeneous group of tumors whose outcomes and response to treatment are different compared to histologically similar tumors in older children and adults. Surgery is the primary modality of treatment in neonatal STS and uses of chemotherapy and radiotherapy are limited due to their increased toxicity in the neonatal period.

REFERENCES

1. Ferrari A, Orbach D, Sultan I, Casanova M, Bisogno G. Neonatal soft tissue sarcomas. Semin Fetal Neonatal Med. 2012;17(4):231-8.
2. Palumbo JS, Zwerdling T. Soft tissue sarcomas of infancy. Semin Perinatol. 1999;23(4):299-309.
3. Dillon PW, Whalen TV, Azizkhan RG, Haase GM, Coran AG, King DR, et al. Neonatal soft tissue sarcomas: the influence of pathology on treatment and survival. Children's Cancer Group Surgical Committee. J Pediatr Surg. 1995;30(7):1038-41.
4. Radhakrishnan V, Joel A, Sundersingh S, Raja A. Synovial Sarcoma in a Neonate. Indian Pediatr. 2016;53(4):345-6.
5. Desandes E, Guissou S, Ducassou S, Lacour B. Neonatal Solid Tumors: Incidence and Survival in France. Pediatr Blood Cancer. 2016;63(8):1375-80.

CHAPTER 36

Fetal and Neonatal Germ Cell Tumors

Maya Prasad

INTRODUCTION

Germ cell tumors (GCTs) are the most common tumors diagnosed in the neonatal and perinatal period. GCTs account for nearly 35–40% of all tumors in the 1st month of life. Approximately 95% of these tumors are benign teratomas and occur at extragonadal sites, such as sacrococcygeal, retroperitoneal, mediastinal and cervical regions.[1] A small percentage of these tumors may contain yolk sac element, either alone or in combination with the teratoma component.[2] The rate of malignancy in sacrococcygeal teratoma (SCT) is higher with later presentation (usually beyond the neonatal period) or with delayed treatment of a lesion initially noted in the neonatal period. Although most tumors in the perinatal period are benign, they can cause complications such as hydrops fetalis and premature delivery, leading to a disproportionately high morbidity (and occasional mortality). Fortunately, the use of antenatal diagnostic techniques and fetal surgical interventions, when appropriate, has helped reduce the mortality and morbidity of perinatal tumors.[1-3]

EPIDEMIOLOGY

In the newborn period, the majority of GCT is extragonadal as compared to the rest of childhood when gonadal sites are more common. Neonatal GCTs are also much more frequent in females than males (female : male = 3 : 1), which is again a reversal of the ratio seen during the rest of childhood and adulthood.

The estimated incidence of SCT is 1 per 35,000–40,000 live births.[1] Since most perinatal GCTs have a benign histology, they are not included in the surveillance, epidemiology, and end results (SEERs) data, and we do not have accurate epidemiological data in this subset of tumors.[4] Data from India is also lacking with very few institutional case series and case reports. One retrospective case series of pediatric GCTs had 12 patients who presented in the neonatal period. Of these, 11 were diagnosed to have SCT (M : F = 4 : 7) and one to have retroperitoneal teratoma. The female preponderance in neonates was striking since older patients were predominantly male.[5]

ETIOLOGY AND PATHOGENESIS

The most accepted theory regarding the etiology of GCTs is that they arise from defects in germline development.[1,2,6] Defects in migration of pluripotent germ cells from the yolk sac to the embryo along the gonadal ridge during the 4th–5th weeks of embryogenesis result in persistence of ectopic gem cells. This explains the typical location of GCTs along the midline from the cervical region to the coccyx. Reactivation of pluripotency genes such as OCT3/4 and NANOG have been postulated to contribute to malignant potential in GCTs. Other theories explaining the etiology of teratomas include origin from the primitive node of embryo around week 3 of embryogenesis, or as a result of incomplete twinning.[2,6] Erasure of maternal and paternal imprinting patterns have also been implicated in gonadal and extragonadal GCTs.[1]

As with other tumors, there have been several advances in the understanding of the biology of GCTs. Studies using comparative genomic hybridization have shown that most teratomas, especially those in prepubertal children without yolk sac component, have normal genetic profiles. However, even in young children with yolk sac tumors (YSTs), there is an increased frequency of changes such as loss of chromosomes 1p, 6q and 18q as well as gains of chromosomes 1q, 3p and 20q.[7,8]

CLINICAL PRESENTATION

The clinical presentation of GCT in neonates depends on the site of tumor. The most common site of GCT in the perinatal period is SCT in 30–40%. Other frequent sites for neonatal GCT include head and neck (13%), intracranial (13%), oropharynx and nasopharynx (7.5%) and cardiac (7.5%). Less common presentations include fetus-in-fetu (FIF) (5%), orbital, mediastinal and gastric (3% each) and facial tumors (1%).[2]

The more important sites of occurrence of neonatal GCT are described in brief below:

Sacrococcygeal Teratoma

Sacrococcygeal teratomas are the most common form of perinatal GCTs, and account for around 35–40% with a marked female preponderance of around 4 : 1.[2] Typically, SCTs present as masses arising from the sacrococcygeal region **(Figs 36.1 to 36.3)**.

These tumors may have variable extension into the presacral space. SCTs usually present as isolated lesions, but may be associated with other congenital anomalies. These associated malformations include genitourinary malformations (hypospadias and vesicoureteric reflux), congenital heart disease, central nervous system malformations (anencephaly, spina bifida, Dandy-Walker malformation), congenital dislocation of hip and esophageal atresia.[9,10] Although these associated malformations are rare, there needs to be a high index of suspicion in cases of SCT and antenatal as well as postnatal screening is warranted. SCTs are highly-vascular tumors and when associated with rapid growth can lead to the development of high output cardiac failure and hydrops fetalis. When untreated, mortality in these cases is nearly 100%.[11,12] Even in antenatally diagnosed cases of hydrops fetalis who undergo fetal intervention, mortality approaches 50%.[13] Infants without these extreme complications are still likely to encounter morbidity such as prematurity, bleeding from the highly vascular tumor site and need for intensive care. Untreated, large and longstanding tumors may cause lower limb weakness, urinary obstruction, constipation, abdominal mass and failure to thrive.[14]

Sacrococcygeal teratomas have been conventionally classified by Altman et al. into four types[15] **(Figs 36.4A to D)**.

1. *Type I*: These are the most common type of tumors that are predominantly external with a minimal presacral component
2. *Type II*: These tumors are external but have a significant intrapelvic component
3. *Type III*: These tumors are external but pelvic with significant extension into the abdomen
4. *Type IV*: These tumors are entirely presacral or internal.

This classification has implications for prognosis as well as treatment. In his original publication, Altman noted that older infants with SCT tended to have higher rates of malignant component.

Head and Neck Germ Cell Tumors

This group includes a spectrum of lesions arising from the cervicofacial region including the nasopharynx, oropharynx, hypopharynx, larynx and other head and neck sites. Some craniofacial and cervical lesions can be life-threatening and often present during the fetal or perinatal period. Large tumors of neck and palate may be noted on routine antenatal scans either due to the mass itself or due to polyhydramnios caused by obstructed swallowing. Some of these tumors may cause respiratory obstruction and may require either fetal therapy or immediate postpartum airway management. Apart from antenatal ultrasound, computed tomography (CT) scan or magnetic resonance imaging (MRI) scan may be required to delineate the accurate extent of the tumor.[16]

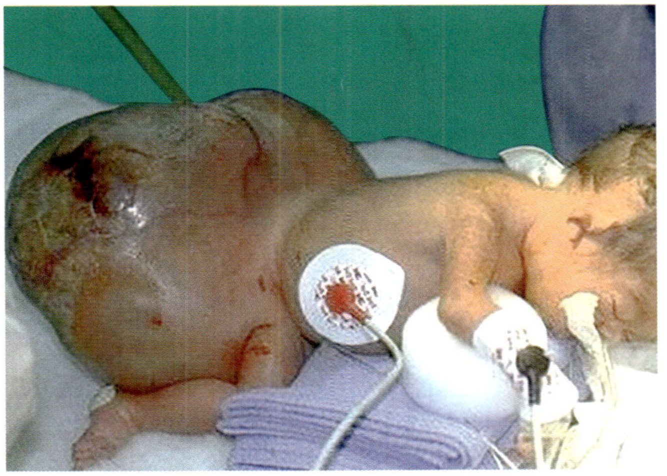

Figure 36.1 A large sacrococcygeal teratoma in a neonate

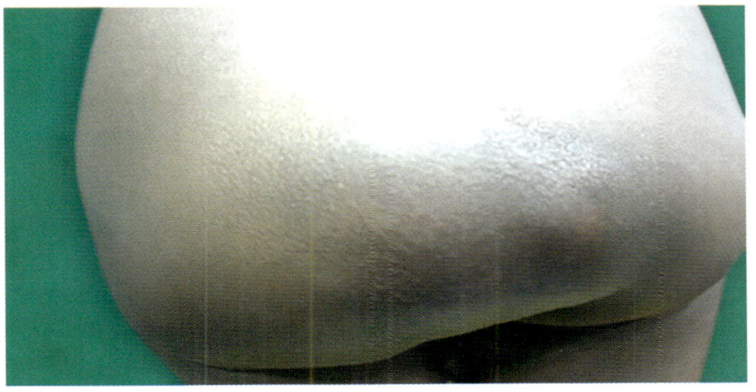

Figure 36.2 Sacrococcygeal teratoma in an older infant

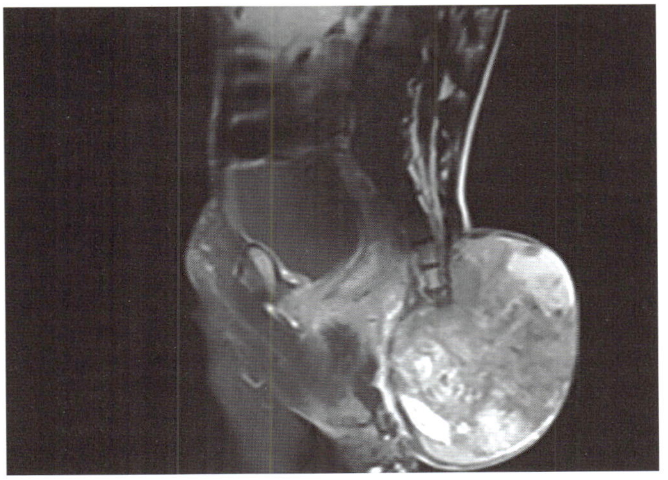

Figure 36.3 Magnetic resonance imaging (MRI) scan of sacrococcygeal teratoma (SCT) showing a large external component

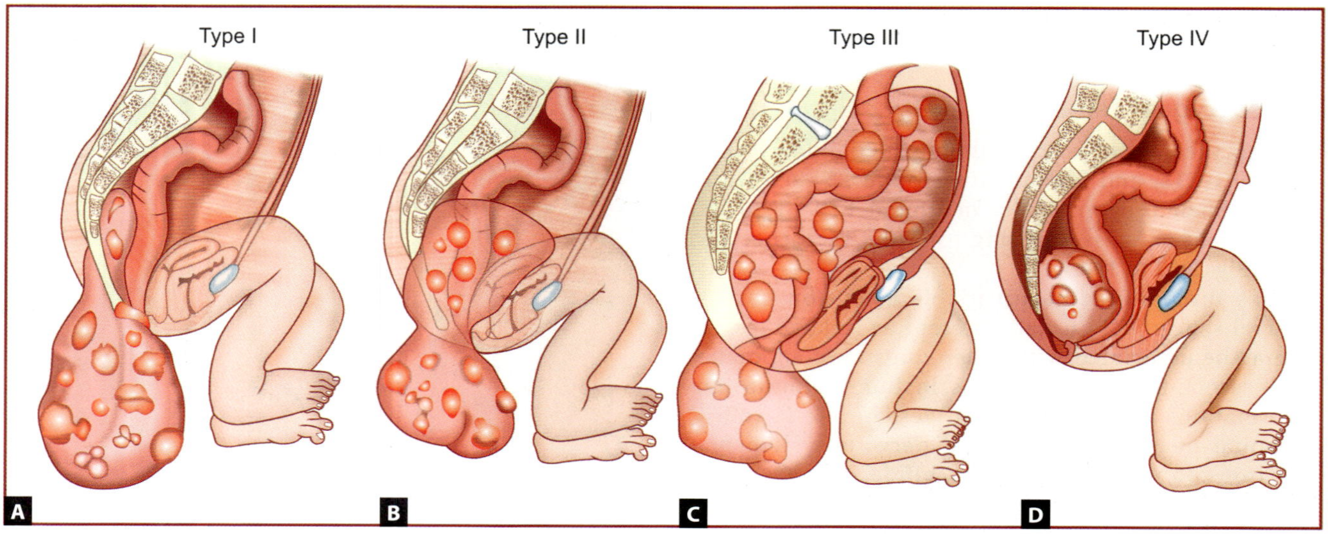

Figures 36.4A to D Altman classification of sacrococcygeal teratoma (SCT)
Source: Adapted from reference 15.

Mediastinal Germ Cell Tumors

The mediastinum is the second most common site of perinatally diagnosed GCTs, the most common site being anterior mediastinum. Other less common areas within the thoracic cavity include the posterior mediastinum, intracardiac and pericardial cavity. Mediastinal GCTs can be seen at any age, from the fetal or newborn period to adolescents. Symptoms due to such lesions are often related to the size of tumor. Large tumors and pericardial or intracardiac tumors can present with hydrops fetalis or airway compression, necessitating antenatal intervention.[17] Delay in the diagnosis of such tumors can be fatal.[18] Other lesions may be noted on routine antenatal scans and even smaller lesions may present in infancy with dyspnea and cough. Apart from ultrasound scans, local CT scans and MRI scans as well as fetal echocardiography may be required to delineate the extent of tumors.

Abdominal Germ Cell Tumors

The abdomen is a less common site for GCTs in the perinatal period when compared to older children. The retroperitoneum and stomach as well as other abdominal viscera may be affected. The retroperitoneum or pelvic region accounts for around 5% of perinatal GCTs and is also the most common site for FIF malformations.[19] Large retroperitoneal lesions often present with an abdominal mass or with gastrointestinal complaints such as constipation and feeding difficulties. Smaller masses may also be detected later in life. Ultrasound and MRI scans help in diagnosis and planning the management. Gastric teratomas are rare, predominantly exogastric lesions, which present with abdominal distension and respiratory distress. Endogastric lesions grow into the lumen and cause gastric outlet obstruction. Abdominal X-rays, ultrasound and CT scans help in diagnosis and delineation of extent.[20,21] Despite the rarity and severity of presentation, gastric teratomas often have an excellent prognosis and surgical excision is curative.

Intracranial Germ Cell Tumors

Brain is a rare site for GCTs. However, intracranial GCTs are the most common brain tumors in young infants, accounting for up to 50% at this age, and most frequently arising from the pineal gland. Large tumors may present with variable degrees of hydrocephalus. Patients often present in the postnatal period with symptoms of increased intracranial tension. Although teratoma is the predominant histology in neonates, the incidence of malignancy increases with age. Further details will be dealt within the chapter on neonatal brain tumors.

Gonadal Germ Cell Tumor

Unlike in older children and adolescents, gonads are a rare site for GCTs in the neonates. However, testicular and ovarian teratomas are well described in literature. Teratoma is the most common benign testicular tumor in neonates, and mature teratomas are the most common ovarian tumors.[6] Ovarian tumors are often diagnosed on routine antenatal scans. Predominantly cystic tumors (dermoids) can be managed by excision alone. Solid tumors often have an immature component and may require salpingo-oophorectomy and/or chemotherapy.[22]

HISTOLOGY

The predominant histologic subtype among fetal or neonatal GCTs is teratoma, followed by YST. Pure YSTs are rarely seen;

a yolk sac component is seen within roughly 5% of neonatal teratomas. In a large series of neonatal GCTs, teratomas of the sacrococcygeal region had the highest incidence of YST.[2] Choriocarcinoma and embryonal carcinoma are other rarely seen histologies. Germinoma or seminoma is not seen in neonates. Teratomas can be either mature or immature. Mature teratomas often contain differentiated adult type tissue from the ectoderm or other germ layers. They are often cystic. Immature teratomas contain a mixture of adult type tissue with embryonal type tissue in varying proportions. Immature teratomas are often graded, based on the amount of embryonal type tissue present with grade 3 immature teratomas considered to have the worst prognosis.[23]

Choriocarcinomas, although rare, deserve special mention because of their aggressive presentation and poor prognosis. They are considered a variant of gestational trophoblastic disease arising from the placenta. This tumor is known to metastasize to multiple organs such as lung, liver, brain and skin, and neonates and young infants present with severe anemia, failure to thrive, hepatomegaly, seizures, respiratory distress and hemoptysis.[24] Markedly elevated β-human chorionic gonadotropin (β-hCG) levels should raise suspicion of this disease, which is rapidly fatal if left untreated. Treatment is multiagent chemotherapy with cisplatin or carboplatin and etoposide, often with methotrexate, followed by surgical resection if there is active residual tumor.[25]

Fetus-in-Fetu

This term is used to describe the inclusion of one fetus inside another.[1] Understandably, this is a rare condition, and the exact origins are still debated. Theories include a well-differentiated teratoma [as in the World Health Organization (WHO) classification], or the inclusion of a parasitic monochorionic, monozygotic twin inside another.[26] Often FIF and teratoma may coexist. The retroperitoneum is the most common site for FIF, but it has also been described in other abdominal and thoracic sites.[27,28] These masses are usually noted on antenatal scans, but there are anecdotal reports where the discovery was made later in life. Surgical resection is often curative, but a few cases of malignant recurrence have been reported. It is recommended to monitor serial values of serum alfa-fetoprotein (AFP) following resection.[1]

DIAGNOSIS AND WORKUP IN FETAL AND NEONATAL GERM CELL TUMORS

Antenatal Diagnosis

In today's world, routine fetal anomaly screening programs allow for prenatal diagnosis in many cases. Large masses such as SCTs, mediastinal and cervical tumors can be picked up on the "anomaly scans" done around 20 weeks of gestation, while polyhydramnios may indicate obstruction to swallowing caused by large cervicofacial tumors. Hydrops fetalis can be noted as a consequence of rapidly growing, highly vascular tumors or intracardiac or pericardiac tumors. Once abnormality is detected on antenatal ultrasound, further evaluation with CT or MRI scans or fetal ultrasound with Doppler evaluation (depending on the site of tumor) may be used to document the extent of the tumor as well as identifying serious fetal complications, and planning fetal therapy, if required.[10] In SCTs, MRI can characterize the intrapelvic and abdominal extent of the tumors more accurately and provide more information on compression of adjacent organs, which in turn helps with accurate prenatal counseling and improved preoperative planning for surgical resection. Serial ultrasound scans should be done in order to monitor tumor size, amniotic fluid volume and the status of the fetus, and to plan early delivery if warranted.

Postnatal Diagnosis

In cases where antenatal scans were not performed, or have failed to detect tumors, diagnosis of neonatal GCTs is often made on immediate postnatal examination. Clinical examination may reveal visible protruding mass as with SCT and abdominal tumors. Some neonates may be asymptomatic and instead present in early infancy with abdominal distension, constipation, urinary obstruction (abdominal tumors), respiratory distress and cough (mediastinal tumors), or signs of increased intracranial tension, macrocephaly and hydrocephalus (intracranial tumors).[2]

In all suspected cases, extensive local imaging is warranted to delineate the extent of disease, the effect on surrounding structures and to plan further management. Imaging in mediastinal and sacrococcygeal tumors should include a MRI of local spine to look for intraspinal extension **(Box 36.1)**.

Sacrococcygeal teratomas and mediastinal teratomas are known to be rarely associated with other congenital anomalies, so a careful physical examination should look for these as well.

Tumor Markers

As in older children, serum levels of tumor markers such as AFP and β-hCG are useful in the diagnosis and surveillance of neonatal GCTs.

Serum alpha fetoprotein: High levels of AFP are commonly associated with YST histology and some embryonal carcinomas. Serial monitoring of AFP may be useful in the few cases of neonatal YST (or immature teratoma) who receive chemotherapy, and also to monitor for postoperative recurrence or residual tumor (postoperative half-life 5–7 days). However, AFP levels need to be interpreted with caution in the neonatal period and early infancy. This is because AFP is normally synthesized by the fetal liver and yolk sac, and is normally elevated at birth. Levels of AFP progressively decline in the 1st year of life, and it is recommended to use the age-related nomogram in children less than 2 years of age.[29] **Table 36.1** roughly indicates the normal age-appropriate values of AFP.

Box 36.1 Evaluation of a suspected germ cell tumor in a neonate

Evaluation of suspected germ cell tumor

- *Abnormal mass noted on antenatal ultrasound:* Further evaluation as below
- Imaging:
  - *Antenatal*: CECT or MRI of involved area. Fetal echocardiography or Doppler, if cardiac mass
  - *Postnatal*: Ultrasound of the involved site
  - CECT of the involved site and chest
  - MRI in cases with suspected intraspinal extension (tumors in the mediastinum and sacrococcygeal region)
  - Echocardiography
  - Serial evaluation in antenatal cases and selected postnatally detected cases
  - Imaging for suspected associated congenital anomalies
- *Tumor markers*: AFP (to be adjusted for age)
  B-hCG
  Serial evaluation postexcision (see text)
- *Pathology*: Not mandatory prior to upfront resection

Abbreviations: CECT, contrast-enhanced computed tomography; AFP, alfa-fetoprotein; hCG, human chorionic gonadotropin; MRI, magnetic resonance imagining

Table 36.1 Normal range of serum alfa-fetoprotein (AFP) values in normal term babies

Age (in days)	*Mean AFP (ng/mL)*	*AFP 95% range (ng/mL)*
0	41,687	9,120–190,546
1	36,391	7,943–165,959
2	31,769	6,950–144,544
3	27,733	6,026–125,893
4	24,210	5,297–109,648
5	21,135	4,624–96,605
6	18,450	4,037–84,334
7	16,107	3,524–73,621
8–14	9,333	1,480–58,887
15–21	3,631	575–22,910
22–28	1,396	316–6,310
29–45	417	30–5,754
46–60	178	16–1,995
61–90	80	6 – 1,045
91–120	36	3–417
121–150	20	2–216
151–180	13	1.25–129
181–720	8	0.8–87

Source: Adapted from reference 29.

Other reasons for elevated AFP in the neonates and young infants include liver tumors such as hepatoblastoma, omphalocele and neural tube defects.

- β-hCG is significantly elevated in infantile choriocarcinoma, and like other tumor markers, can be used for the initial diagnosis in a clinically suspected case, as well as to monitor response to treatment and to detect residual or recurrent tumor.
- Lactate dehydrogenase-1 (LDH-1) may be elevated in endodermal sinus tumor, YST, dysgerminoma and choriocarcinoma, but it is often elevated in nonmalignant conditions as well, thus limiting its use.

MANAGEMENT OF FETAL AND NEONATAL GERM CELL TUMORS

This section will focus on management of the major subsets of neonatal GCTs, namely SCT, head and neck GCTs and mediastinal GCTs. The management of less frequent tumors has been briefly described in the respective sections. The management of intracranial GCT will be dealt within the chapter on neonatal brain tumors.

Surgery is the backbone in the treatment of fetal and neonatal GCTs. As most tumors are benign, chemotherapy is indicated in very few cases.

Fetal Interventions

As described in earlier sections, there are some scenarios where urgent intervention is needed during intrauterine or fetal life. These include high output cardiac failure and hydrops fetalis in highly vascular and rapidly growing tumors, and respiratory or esophageal obstruction in cervicofacial and mediastinal tumors. Once an anomaly is detected on routine antenatal ultrasound, appropriate prenatal imaging such as fetal MRI and high-definition ultrasound is critical to assess the degree of involvement of surrounding structures, and to decide on the possible need for emergent fetal or perinatal intervention to secure adequate airway access. Rapid access to the airway after birth can be extremely challenging even at well-equipped centers. The strategy of "ex utero intrapartum treatment" (EXIT) is being increasingly adopted at specialized fetal surgery centers. This procedure is based on maintaining uteroplacental gas exchange for a prolonged period of time through intensive inhibition of the uterine contractility, allowing access to the fetal airway in a controlled and secure manner. During this period, the fetus is under uteroplacental support, and the procedure may provide time to resect the tumor before the placental circulation is interrupted. EXIT has been used in cervical and thoracic tumors as well as benign processes such as congenital high airway obstruction syndrome (CHAOS), unilateral pulmonary agenesis and congenital diaphragmatic hernia (CDH). As expected, this highly specialized procedure requires a multidisciplinary team of anesthesiologists, fetal or pediatric surgeons, neonatologists or oncologists, maternal fetal medicine specialists and trained nursing staff at a fetal treatment center.[30-32] In certain cases, complete removal of the tumor can be carried out in staged process to minimize morbidity.[33]

Fetal hydrops is usually considered a potential indicator for fetal intervention. Mortality rates are high, and treatment options are limited. In a fetus that has not attained pulmonary maturity and cannot be delivered, fetal interventions such as laser vessel ablation, interstitial laser ablation +/– vascular coiling, radiofrequency ablation, alcohol sclerosis, cyst drainage, amniodrainage, or vesicoamniotic shunt preoperative embolization can be considered to interrupt the vascular flow.[1,34] Antenatal resection may debulk and devascularize the tumor, thus eliminating the large arteriovenous shunt through the tumor and effectively reversing the hydrops.[2] Fetal surgery should be performed at specialized centers with expertise and infrastructure. In patients who have achieved pulmonary maturity, delivery and standard postnatal resection are recommended. Maternal corticosteroids are usually administered to accelerate pulmonary development in a near-term fetus.

Management in the Neonatal Period

In most neonatal GCTs, surgical excision is the treatment of choice. It is often impossible to achieve microscopic complete resection in these tumors, especially abdominal and mediastinal tumors. As most are mature or immature teratomas, no adjuvant chemotherapy is required except in a few situations which are described in the next section.

Sacrococcygeal Teratoma

In neonates with SCT, complete surgical excision with coccygectomy is the procedure of choice. Most neonatal SCTs have a significant external component (Altman I or II), which can be completely excised in the neonatal period using abdominal and/or perineal approaches to completely mobilize the tumor. In large and vascular lesions, either an open or laparoscopic approach can be used to ligate the medial sacral vessels. Heroic surgery involving resection of major abdominal or neurovascular structures should not be attempted; instead staged procedures may be considered.[33] Rarely, neonates present with metastatic disease and in such cases, it is advisable to plan an initial biopsy, followed by chemotherapy and then a delayed resection, which has been found to have superior outcomes to upfront failed resection.[7] Close follow-up is warranted after surgery, and should include serial AFP levels and rectal examination every 3 months until age 3 years to evaluate for recurrence. Radiological follow-up with ultrasound and/or CT scan may also be required as the recurrence may not be secreting AFP. Recurrent tumors are observed in 10–20% of initially benign tumors and 50% of these are malignant.[35]

Abdominal Germ Cell Tumor

Complete surgical resection is the procedure of choice in abdominal tumors. Abdominal tumors are often adherent to or may compress surrounding vessels and other structures making resection difficult. Accurate radiological studies may aid in preoperative planning and subsequent surgery.

Thoracic or Mediastinal Tumors

The treatment of choice is complete resection, which generally requires a median sternotomy or unilateral thoracotomy depending on the location and size of the tumor. Small lesions may be amenable to video-assisted thoracic surgery (VATS). Due to the location of these tumors, it is essential to identify and preserve the major neurovascular structures.

Abdominal and mediastinal tumors also warrant postoperative monitoring of tumor markers (serum AFP) for tumor recurrence.

Chemotherapy in Neonatal Germ Cell Tumor

Most neonatal GCTs are either mature or immature teratomas not requiring further treatment, and only 5% contain a malignant element, mostly YST. Thus, chemotherapy is rarely needed for GCT in the neonatal period. Very little data is available regarding chemotherapy in neonatal GCTs, and most of the information is extrapolated from older infants and children. The indications for chemotherapy in neonatal GCT include advanced malignant tumors and malignant recurrences in SCT postresection (generally beyond the neonatal period).

Malignant SCTs as well as retroperitoneal and mediastinal GCTs are usually very advanced at diagnosis; two-thirds of patients have locoregional disease and 50% are metastatic. For patients with locally advanced SCTs, mediastinal tumors or large pelvic tumors, tumor biopsy followed by preoperative chemotherapy can facilitate subsequent complete tumor resection and improve patient outcome.[36-38] Platinum-based multiagent regimens with either cisplatin or carboplatin are the cornerstone of treatment, and their introduction has significant improved outcome in malignant GCTs. The standard regimens in pediatric GCTs are PEB (cisplatin, etoposide and bleomycin) and JEB (carboplatin, etoposide and bleomycin), but there is no standard regimen for neonates. Even in a Pediatric Oncology Group or Children's Cancer Group intergroup study with a large proportion of advanced stage disease, the 6-year event-free survival (EFS) using PEB was 83%.[39] Other studies using carboplatin and cisplatin have also shown EFS rates of 75–85% and overall survival (OS) rates of 80–90%.[37,38] However, cisplatin is known to have several immediate and late toxicities, including nephrotoxicity, neurotoxicity and ototoxicity as well as early onset of cardiovascular disease and increased risk of cancer. This is especially true in neonates, in whom most organ functions are immature and very difficult to assess and monitor. A recent systematic review has suggested the use of carboplatin in younger children with low-intermediate risk features, while reserving cisplatin for older children or those with high-risk features. Over the past 25 years, carboplatin has replaced cisplatin in most groups of GCT in the United Kingdom with recent head-to-head comparisons showing equal efficacy.[40]

Mature and immature teratomas are both considered benign lesions and are treated with surgery alone. Surgical excision is safe and effective treatment for 80–100% of children with immature teratoma.[41] A recent collaborative analysis of ovarian immature teratomas in seven pediatric and two adult trials found that although among grade 3 patients, the stage was significantly associated with relapse, the use of adjuvant chemotherapy did not decrease relapses in the pediatric cohort.[42]

It is recommended that if chemotherapy is essential in a neonate, it has to be administered in a pediatric oncology unit with expertise and infrastructure for chemotherapy, supportive care and monitoring or managing the adverse effects in this subset of extremely challenging patients.

OUTCOMES AND PROGNOSTIC FACTORS

Since neonatal GCTs (especially malignant GCTs) are very rare, outcome data need to be extrapolated from larger pediatric studies, which contain all age groups. A large study of over 500 perinatal teratomas found that the survival rate overall was 63%. Survival rates varied considerably from 11% (intracranial) to 100% (gastric). Other sites with favorable prognosis were FIF (96% survival), facial (88%), orbital (85%), cardiac and placental (75%). Sites with intermediate prognosis were mediastinal (69%), sacrococcygeal and cervical (68%) and palatal or nasopharyngeal (56%).[2]

Approximately 2–35% (average 12.5%) of neonates operated for SCT experience recurrence of disease. About 50% have a malignant component at recurrence.

The variables associated with a higher risk of recurrence include the following:[1,36,37,41,43,44]

- Site of tumor (as described above)
- Presence of immature elements (33% recurrence) compared with mature teratoma (10% recurrence)
- Higher grade of immature teratoma (e.g. grade 3)
- Nonremoval of coccyx and spillage of tumor during surgery
- Metastasis and spinal involvement in malignant SCT
- High AFP levels are usually considered adverse prognostic factors, but in the first 6–9 months the normal ranges need to be kept in mind and adjusted for age
- In malignant sacrococcygeal as well as mediastinal tumors, the prognostic effect of incomplete tumor resection is not as significant, if an intensive platinum-based treatment is applied
- No molecular markers of outcome have so far been identified in pediatric GCT.

LATE EFFECTS OF TREATMENT AND FOLLOW-UP

Neonatal SCT is known to result in significant morbidity, either directly or as a consequence of surgical therapy.[1,35] These include:

- *Gastrointestinal side effects:* Constipation, fecal incontinence
- *Genitourinary complications:* Urinary incontinence, neuropathic bladder vesicoureteric reflux and recurrent urinary tract infections
- *Lower extremity neurological sequelae:* Paraparesis
- Psychologically unacceptable cosmetic scars
- Renal and ototoxicity in the rare cases who receive chemotherapy.

Careful postnatal follow-up by a multidisciplinary team is required for timely identification and treatment of complications. In case of identified problems, symptom management, investigational studies including functional evaluations and rehabilitation are warranted.

Surveillance for recurrent disease postresection:

- Clinical evaluation includes per rectal examination every 3 months for the first 3 years
- Serial serum AFP levels—3 monthly until normal values, followed by 3–6 monthly until 3 years of age
- Radiological evaluation in individual cases.

FUTURE DIRECTIONS

Although outcomes in neonatal GCTs are superior to several other pediatric tumors, there are several challenges in the management. One of the major concerns is the extremely young age and fragile nature of neonates, who need to be managed in specialized centers. Clinical and translational research needs to focus on improving outcomes.

- Understanding the biology of disease process and identifying molecular markers of prognosis in order to further refine treatment strategy
- Further improvements in antenatal diagnosis and fetal therapy of emergent situations and complications in perinatal GCTs.

KEY POINTS

- GCTs are the most common tumor seen in newborns. Less than 5% have a malignant component
- Advances in radiology have enabled antenatal diagnosis of the majority of tumors
- Fetal therapy is an option in emergent situations or when potential complications are anticipated, and has helped reduce morbidity and mortality in such cases
- A multidisciplinary team of obstetricians, neonatologists or oncologists, surgeons, anesthesiologists and radiologists is ideally required for the management
- The treatment of choice in the majority is surgical excision followed by observation

- If chemotherapy is needed, a carboplatin-based regimen should be considered to minimize short- and long-term toxicity and needs to be administered at specialized centers
- All patients who undergo excision need to be monitored for long-term sequelae and recurrence.

REFERENCES

1. Frazier AL, Weldon C, Amatruda J. Fetal and neonatal germ cell tumors. Semin Fetal Neonatal Med. 2012;17(4):222-30.
2. Isaacs H Jr. Perinatal (fetal and neonatal) germ cell tumors. J Pediatr Surg. 2004;39(7):1003-13.
3. Sandoval JA, Williams RF. Neonatal Germ Cell Tumors. Curr Pediatr Rev. 2015;11(3):205-15.
4. National Cancer Institute, National Institutes of Health. (2015). Childhood Extracranial Germ Cell Tumors Treatment (PDQ®)—Health Professional Version. General Information about Childhood Extracranial Germ Cell Tumors (GCTs). [online] Available from *www.cancer.gov/types/extracranial-germ-cell/hp/germ-cell-treatment-pdq.* [Accessed September, 2016].
5. Chattopadhyay S, Das S, Sinha SK, Ghosh D, Dutta T. Pediatric germ cell tumors: an overview. Journal of Indian Association of Pediatric Surgeons. 2004;9(2):67.
6. Lakhoo K. Neonatal teratomas. Early Hum Dev. 2010;86(10): 643-7.
7. Göbel U, Schneider DT, Calaminus G, Jürgens H, Spaar HJ, Sternschulte W, et al. Multimodal treatment of malignant sacrococcygeal germ cell tumors: a prospective analysis of 66 patients of the German cooperative protocols MAKEI 83/86 and 89. J Clin Oncol. 2001;19(7):1943-50.
8. Mazumdar M, Bajorin DF, Bacik J, Higgins G, Motzer RJ, Bosl GJ. Predicting outcome to chemotherapy in patients with germ cell tumors: the value of the rate of decline of human chorionic gonadotrophin and alpha-fetoprotein during therapy. J Clin Oncol. 2001;19(9):2534-41.
9. Subbarao P, Bhatnagar V, Mitra DK. The association of sacrococcygeal teratoma with high anorectal and genital malformations. Aust N Z J Surg. 1994;64(3):214-5.
10. Gucciardo L, Uyttebroek A, De Wever I, Renard M, Claus F, Devlieger R, et al. Prenatal assessment and management of sacrococcygeal teratoma. Prenat Diagn. 2011;31(7):678-88.
11. Chisholm CA, Heider AL, Kuller JA, von Allmen D, McMahon MJ, Chescheir NC. Prenatal diagnosis and perinatal management of fetal sacrococcygeal teratoma. Am J Perinatol. 1998;15(8):503-5.
12. Adzick NS. Open fetal surgery for life-threatening fetal anomalies. Semin Fetal Neonatal Med. 2010;15(1):1-8.
13. Swamy R, Embleton N, Hale J. Sacrococcygeal teratoma over two decades: birth prevalence, prenatal diagnosis and clinical outcomes. Prenat Diagn. 2008;28(11):1048-51.
14. Barksdale EM Jr, Obokhare I. Teratomas in infants and children. Curr Opin Pediatr. 2009;21(3):344-9.
15. Altman RP, Randolph JG, Lilly JR. Sacrococcygeal teratoma: American Academy of Pediatrics Surgical Section Survey-1973. J Pediatr Surg. 1974;9(3):389-98.
16. Herman TE, Siegel MJ. Cervical teratoma. J Perinatol. 2008;28(9):649-51.
17. Merchant AM, Hedrick HL, Johnson MP, Wilson RD, Crombleholme TM, Howell LJ, et al. Management of fetal mediastinal teratoma. J Pediatr Surg. 2005;40(1):228-31.
18. Gobbi D, Rubino M, Chiandetti L, Zanon GF, Cecchetto G. Neonatal intrapericardial teratoma: a challenge for the pediatric surgeon. J Pediatr Surg. 2007;42(1):E3-6.
19. Eyssartier E, Harper L, Michel JL, Rivière JP, Vanderbecken S, De Napoli-Cocci S. Rapidly growing mature retroperitoneal teratomas. J Pediatr Hematol Oncol. 2009;31(9):705-6.
20. Saleem SM, Hussain S, Nazir Z. Gastric teratoma—a rare benign tumor of neonates. Ann Trop Paediatr. 2003;23(4):305-8.
21. Sarin YK, Agarwal LD, Jhamaria VN, Goyal RB, Sharma R, Shekhawat NS. Immature gastric teratoma. Indian J Pediatr. 1997;64(6):896-8.
22. De Backer A, Madern GC, Oosterhuis JW, Hakvoort-Cammel FG, Hazebroek FW. Ovarian germ cell tumors in children: a clinical study of 66 patients. Pediatr Blood Cancer. 2006;46(4):459-64.
23. Norris HJ, Zirkin HJ, Benson WL. Immature (malignant) teratoma of the ovary: A clinical and pathologic study of 58 cases. Obstetrical & Gynecological Survey. 1977;32(1):50-2.
24. Blohm ME, Göbel U. Unexplained anaemia and failure to thrive as initial symptoms of infantile choriocarcinoma: a review. Eur J Pediatr. 2004;163(1):1-6.
25. Johnson EJ, Crofton PM, O'Neill JM, Wilkinson AG, McKenzie KJ, Munro FD, et al. Infantile choriocarcinoma treated with chemotherapy alone. Med Pediatr Oncol. 2003;41(6):550-7.
26. Scully RE, Young RH, Clement PB. Tumors of the ovary, maldeveloped gonads, fallopian tube, and broad ligament. Atlas of tumor pathology, 3rd series, fascicle 23. Washington, DC: Armed Forces Institute of Pathology; 1998. p. 81.
27. Escobar MA, Rossman JE, Caty MG. Fetus-in-fetu: report of a case and a review of the literature. J Pediatr Surg. 2008;43(5):943-6.
28. Hopkins KL, Dickson PK, Ball TI, Ricketts RR, O'Shea PA, Abramowsky CR. Fetus-in-fetu with malignant recurrence. J Pediatr Surg. 1997;32(10):1476-9.
29. Blohm ME, Vesterling- Hörner D, Calaminus G, Göbel U. Alpha 1-fetoprotein (AFP) reference values in infants up to 2 years of age. Pediatr Hematol Oncol. 1998;15(2):135-42.
30. Laje P, Howell LJ, Johnson MP, Hedrick HL, Flake AW, Adzick NS. Perinatal management of congenital oropharyngeal tumors: the ex utero intrapartum treatment (EXIT) approach. J Pediatr Surg. 2013;48(10):2005-10.
31. Hirose S, Harrison MR, Farmer DL, Lee H, Nobuhara KK. The ex utero intrapartum treatment procedure: Looking back at the EXIT. J Pediatr Surg. 2004;39(3):375-80.
32. Taghavi K, Beasley S. The ex utero intrapartum treatment (EXIT) procedure: application of a new therapeutic paradigm. J Paediatr Child Health. 2013;49(9):E420-7.
33. Azizkhan RG, Haase GM, Applebaum H, Dillon PW, Coran AG, King PA, et al. Diagnosis, management, and outcome of cervicofacial teratomas in neonates: a Childrens Cancer Group study. J Pediatr Surg. 1995;30(2):312-6.
34. Van Mieghem T, Al-Ibrahim A, Deprest J, Lewi L, Langer JC, Baud D, et al. Minimally invasive therapy for fetal sacrococcygeal teratoma: case series and systematic review of the literature. Ultrasound Obstet Gynecol. 2014;43(6):611-9.
35. Rescorla FJ. Pediatric germ cell tumors. Semin Pediatr Surg. 2012;21(1):51-60.
36. Mann JR, Raafat F, Robinson K, Imeson J, Gornall P, Sokal M, et al. The United Kingdom Children's Cancer Study Group's second germ cell tumor study: carboplatin, etoposide, and bleomycin are effective treatment for children with malignant extracranial germ cell tumors, with acceptable toxicity. J Clin Oncol. 2000;18(22):3809-18.

37. Calaminus G, Schneider DT, Bökkerink JP, Gadner H, Harms D, Willers R, et al. Prognostic value of tumor size, metastases, extension into bone, and increased tumor marker in children with malignant sacrococcygeal germ cell tumors: a prospective evaluation of 71 patients treated in the German cooperative protocols Maligne Keimzelltumoren (MAKEI) 83/86 and MAKEI 89. J Clin Oncol. 2003;21(5):781-6.
38. Rescorla F, Billmire D, Stolar C, Vinocur C, Colombani P, Cullen J, et al. The effect of cisplatin dose and surgical resection in children with malignant germ cell tumors at the sacrococcygeal region: a pediatric intergroup trial (POG 9049/CCG 8882). J Pediatr Surg. 2001;36(1):12-7.
39. Billmire D, Vinocur C, Rescorla F, Colombani P, Cushing B, Hawkins E, et al. Malignant retroperitoneal and abdominal germ cell tumors: an intergroup study. J Pediatr Surg. 2003;38(3):315-8.
40. Shaikh F, Nathan PC, Hale J, Uleryk E, Frazier L. Is there a role for carboplatin in the treatment of malignant germ cell tumors? A systematic review of adult and pediatric trials. Pediatr Blood Cancer. 2013;60(4):587-92.
41. Marina N, London WB, Frazier AL, Lauer S, Rescorla F, Cushing B, et al. Prognostic factors in children with extragonadal malignant germ cell tumors: a pediatric intergroup study. J Clin Oncol. 2006;24(16):2544-8.
42. Pashankar F, Hale JP, Dang H, Krailo M, Brady WE, Rodriguez-Galindo C, et al. Is adjuvant chemotherapy indicated in ovarian immature teratomas? A combined data analysis from the Malignant Germ Cell Tumor International Collaborative. Cancer. 2016;122(2):230-7.
43. Frazier AL, Hale JP, Rodriguez-Galindo C, Dang H, Olson T, Murray MJ, et al. Revised risk classification for pediatric extracranial germ cell tumors based on 25 years of clinical trial data from the United Kingdom and United States. J Clin Oncol. 2015;33(2)195:201.
44. De Backer A, Madern GC, Hakvoort-Cammel FG, Haentjens P, Oosterhuis JW, Hazebroek FW. Study of the factors associated with recurrence in children with sacrococcygeal teratoma. J Pediatr Surg. 2006;41(1):173-81.

CHAPTER

37

Retinoblastoma and its Prenatal Screening

Ashwin Mallipatna, Swathi Shetty, Prathima Radhakrishnan

INTRODUCTION

Retinoblastoma is a cancer of the eye that affects children under the age of 5 years, caused by mutations in the *RB1* gene.[1,2] Mutations in both *RB1* alleles within the precursor retinal cell are essential with one mutation that may be germline or somatic and the second one that is always somatic. Mutations in the *RB1* gene cause retinoblastoma. Mutations in both *RB1* alleles within the precursor retinal cell are considered essential to cause disease. Identification of the *RB1* germline status of a patient allows differentiation between sporadic and heritable retinoblastoma variants. Application of this knowledge is crucial for assessing short-term (risk of additional tumors in the same eye and other eye) and long-term (risk of nonocular malignant tumors) prognosis and offering cost effective surveillance strategies.[3]

Prenatal screening for retinoblastoma requires a sound understanding of the clinical and genetic aspects of the disease. Genetic testing and genetic counseling are essential components of care for all children diagnosed with the disease. This will rely on accurate interpretation of the available clinical and molecular data. The American Joint Committee on Cancer (AJCC) has acknowledged the importance of detecting this heritable trait and has introduced the letter "H" to denote a heritable trait of all cancers, starting with retinoblastoma.[3a] In this chapter we discuss the clinically relevant aspects of the genetics of the disease and then understand the intricacies of its prenatal testing.

INHERITANCE PATTERN

Retinoblastoma is inherited in a dominant manner. Not every individual who inherits the germline mutation is affected, though. Half of all affected children are estimated to be heritable and carry a germline *RB1* mutation.[1] Each child born to a person with a germline *RB1* mutation has a 50% statistical risk of inheriting the mutation, as is characteristic of dominant inheritance. However, about 90% of persons with a germline *RB1* mutation are thought to develop retinoblastoma (60% multifocal, 30% unifocal) and the remaining 10% remain unaffected carriers. About 10% of children with unilateral or bilateral retinoblastoma have a positive family history.

Knudson first proposed the "two-hit" hypothesis whereby two complementary mutational events are required for the development of retinoblastoma.[4] Inheritable retinoblastoma, the first "hit", or mutation is a germline mutation and present in all cells of the affected child. The second mutation usually occurs in multiple retinal progenitor cells resulting in multifocal or bilateral retinoblastoma. In sporadic (nonheritable) retinoblastoma, there is no germline mutation and both mutations occur somatically in a single retinal progenitor cell causing unifocal (unilateral) retinoblastoma.

CLINICAL FEATURES

The age of diagnosis is earlier in heritable retinoblastoma at an average age of 15 months whereas nonheritable cases usually present later with an average age of 24 months.[2] It is assumed that all children with bilateral involvement of retinoblastoma have a germline mutation, even if genetic testing is unable to identify the mutation (which occurs in approximately 5% of cases). In addition, a germline *RB1* mutation is present in about 15% of children with unilateral retinoblastoma.

The most common signs of presentation are a white pupil (leukocoria) and strabismus.[2] Clinical signs of advanced intraocular disease include secondary neovascular, glaucoma or massive tumor necrosis and intraocular hemorrhage.[5] More advanced tumors could undergo extensive intraocular necrosis leading to an aseptic orbital cellulitis. The tumor appears as a white-yellow lesion arising from the retina. Calcification is a pathognomonic feature of larger tumors and is of diagnostic value when detected by ultrasonography or radiological imaging. In each affected eye, tumors can occur as a single lesion or in multiples (multifocal). Each lesion can produce "seeds" that disseminate into the vitreous or subretinal spaces. An exudative retinal detachment allows the tumor to seed into the subretinal space. The morphology of seeds in the vitreous can be described as dust, clouds or pearl-like spheres.[6,7] These could extend into the anterior chamber.

An invasive tumor may break Bruch's membrane and spread into the predominantly vascular choroid, potentially allowing tumor cells to metastasize via a hematogenous route.[8] Alternatively, the tumor might spread via the lamina cribrosa into the optic nerve, allowing the tumor to access cerebrospinal fluid and the central nervous system. Tumor extending spreading through sclera can metastasize through lymphatics.

With timely detection, more than 95% of those affected can survive if a multidisciplinary team provides coordinated and collaborative treatment between specialized centers with appropriate expertise, up-to-date protocols and modern equipment.[9] The treatments may involve surgery (enucleation), chemotherapy (intravenous, intra-arterial, periocular or intraocular), focal therapies (laser and cryotherapy) and radiation (brachytherapy and external beam radiation). Treatment prioritizes patient survival and then at preserving the eyeball and optimizing visual function.

Distinct Clinical Features of Heritable Retinoblastoma

Children with germline mutations usually present with bilateral retinoblastoma. All children with a positive family history of retinoblastoma are considered to have heritable retinoblastoma.

13q Deletion Syndrome

It is estimated that 5–6% of all children with retinoblastoma have an interstitial chromosome deletion or translocation of region 13q14.[10] Such children may demonstrate dysmorphic features, developmental delay and psychomotor retardation. The degree of severity correlates with the size of the chromosomal deletion and involvement of contiguous genes. Some of the characteristic facial features associated with this syndrome include thickened and anteverted earlobes, high and broad forehead, prominent philtrum, short nose and thick everted lower lip.[11] Testing for chromosome deletions and translocations is typically performed using karyotype and/or chromosomal microarray. With use of karyotyping and chromosomal microarray in genetic testing for children with mental retardation, 13q deletion syndrome may be identified prior to the diagnosis of retinoblastoma. These children should be followed with frequent eye exams as recommended for all children with heritable retinoblastoma.

Trilateral Retinoblastoma

Occurrence of a primitive neuroectodermal tumor (or a pinealoblastoma) known to occur in the setting of heritable retinoblastoma has been termed as "trilateral" retinoblastoma.[12,13] These tumors may be located in the pineal gland or suprasellar or parasellar region. The chance of developing trilateral retinoblastoma is less than 0.5% for children with unilateral retinoblastoma, 5–13% for bilateral retinoblastoma and 5–15% for familial bilateral retinoblastoma.[14] Unfortunately the survival for children with trilateral retinoblastoma is poor. Screening recommendations for intracranial malignancies include gadolinium-enhanced magnetic resonance imaging every 6 months until the age of 4.5 years for children with heritable form of retinoblastoma.[15]

Second Malignant Neoplasms

The risk of other (nonocular) malignancies in individuals with heritable retinoblastoma significantly increases over their lifespan. The most common second cancers include osteosarcoma, soft tissue sarcoma, melanoma and epithelial cancers. Some studies suggest those with familial retinoblastoma have a greater risk for second cancers compared to those with a de novo *RB1* mutation.[16] Individuals with heritable disease who received external beam radiation therapy have a further increased risk of developing malignancies, especially in the radiation field. Avoiding exposure to DNA-damaging agents such as tobacco, ultraviolet (UV)-radiation, and X-ray is recommended for individuals with heritable retinoblastoma.

Retinoma or Retinocytoma

A retinoma is a rare, benign variant of retinoblastoma also caused by mutations in the *RB1* gene.[17] Studies have shown that retinoma is a precursor of retinoblastoma. On occasion, retinoma may undergo malignant transformation.[18] In contrast to retinoblastoma, retinomas diagnosed in childhood or adulthood are usually asymptomatic.

RB1 Gene and Function

The *RB1* gene is a tumor suppressor gene that regulates cell cycle. Located on the long arm of chromosome 13, the gene consists of 27 exons dispersed over 200 kb of genomic DNA.[19] The retinoblastoma protein regulates the cell cycle by acting as a transcriptional repressor by targeting the E2F transcription factors. Dividing cells are therefore prevented from entering the S phase of mitosis and proceed to unregulated cycles of mitosis.

RB1 Gene Mutations

Mutations in the *RB1* gene result in a loss of function that inactivates the RB1 protein. The retinoblastoma protein is frequently inactivated by deletions and nonsense mutations.[20] To date, many *RB1* gene mutations have been identified that cause heritable retinoblastoma.[21,22] Although suspected hotspots have been identified, they account for only 40% of the mutations. The rest of the mutations are scattered throughout the entire gene, most frequently in exons 9, 10, 14, 17, 18, 20 and 23. Children with splicing mutations are often diagnosed at a later age than children with frame shift, nonsense or missense mutations. Most *RB1* germline mutations are highly penetrant. The penetrance, or chance to develop retinoblastoma with a typical "null" germline mutation, is 90% or higher. However, in a few families, the penetrance is much lower than 90% with high proportion of unilateral retinoblastoma (reduced expressivity) or carriers (no tumors at all, incomplete penetrance).[23] Mutations associated with low penetrance are typically missense mutations or mutations in the promoter region that produce a low level of retinoblastoma protein rather than total absence of protein.[20]

RB1+/+ MYCNA Tumors

A rare and genetically unique form of retinoblastoma was discovered in which both alleles of the *RB1* gene were normal, and instead expression of the *MYCN* gene was considerably amplified.[24] This form of tumor is clinically indistinguishable from *RB1* mutated tumors. It has exclusively been discovered in 1–3% of children with unilateral retinoblastoma, especially in those under the age of 12 months. Histopathology of these tumors seems to demonstrate undifferentiated cells with large, prominent, multiple nucleoli, and necrosis, apoptosis and little calcification. The histopathology feature of this form of retinoblastoma resembles that of other MYCN amplified tumors such as neuroblastoma. The characteristics of this type of tumor strongly suggest nonhereditary disease, without risk for retinoblastoma in the other eye, for other malignant cancers throughout life and risk of familial transmission.

Genetic Testing

A meticulous and comprehensive approach can detect about 95% of the *RB1* mutations.[25] Identification of the *RB1* mutation reduces overall health care expenditures by identifying those children who are at risk for additional intraocular tumors (ipsilateral or contralateral eye), trilateral retinoblastoma or second malignant tumors, thereby sparing relatives who test negative for the *RB1* germline mutation from unnecessary screening evaluations.[22] According to the AJCC, it is recommended that genetic testing be conducted in a certified laboratory with demonstrated high sensitivity (percentage of all tested samples in which the mutations are found, resulting in a useful report) and turnaround time to identify *RB1* mutations.[9] The cost of testing is becoming more affordable with advances in genetic testing technology such as next generation sequencing (Aravind BMC central).

The one retinoblastoma world website (http://1rbw.org) aims to list all genetic testing laboratories that perform retinoblastoma testing, including their contact information, test sensitivity and relevant information about their processes. As of January 2016, there were two centers in India with more that can be added voluntarily in the future.

Indications for Testing

A clinical diagnosis of retinoblastoma in a child whose germline *RB1* status is not already known is an indication for testing. A child with bilateral disease, with trilateral retinoblastoma, and those with a family history almost certainly carry a germline *RB1* gene mutation, making them at risk for developing second malignant neoplasms. Genetic testing may detect at risk members of the family who may harbor the *RB1* mutation, including possibility of prenatal testing to the parents. Children with unilateral disease without any family history require genetic testing to determine their risk for additional intraocular tumors (ipsilateral or contralateral eye), trilateral retinoblastoma or second malignant tumors.

Genetic Counseling

Genetic counseling is essential to educate the family (and when older, the patients themselves) about the heritability of retinoblastoma, genetic testing, risks of future malignancies, recurrence risks for relatives and reproductive options. Genetic counseling should occur soon after the initial diagnosis and again when a survivor enters reproductive age or prior to planning a family.

Prenatal Screening for Retinoblastoma

Studies have shown that the parents perceived risk of retinoblastoma in their offspring influences their decision to have children in the future.[26] When the familial *RB1* germline mutation is known, options for testing an embryo or fetus including preimplantation genetic diagnosis (PGD) and prenatal diagnosis (PND) can be discussed with parents of an affected child as well as adult survivors of retinoblastoma. PGD is performed by testing an embryo for the presence of the *RB1* mutation following *in vitro* fertilization (IVF). It is important to note that de novo *RB1* mutations have occurred in children conceived by IVF.[27]

Prenatal diagnosis with chorionic villus sampling (at 11–15 weeks gestation) or amniocentesis (after 16 weeks gestation) may be used to determine whether a fetus is affected to either plan for surveillance or make decisions regarding continuing the pregnancy. These procedures are associated with a small risk of miscarriage. It is important to rule out contamination of fetal tissue with the mother's tissue, which could occur during sampling.

If the mutation is identified prenatally, ultrasound scans and fetal magnetic resonance imaging may identify large intraocular tumors.[28] A mid trimester ultrasound scan of the fetus includes evaluation of the fetal eyes in axial and coronal planes. With large intraocular tumors, gross tumor location, size, extension and calcifications can be assessed. Doppler imaging may be used to differentiate tumor vascularization from hemorrhage.

Preterm delivery may be considered to allow for early treatment of tumors or early ocular examination.[9] If PND is not performed, cord blood or an infant s peripheral blood may be used for testing after delivery. When test results are not yet available, at risk children should have ocular evaluation soon after delivery.

CONCLUSION

Retinoblastoma is initiated by mutations in both alleles of the RB1 gene. About half of the patients may carry a constitutional RB1 gene mutation. Prenatal screening for retinoblastoma would allow us to detect children with cancer earlier. When the familial RB1 germline mutation is known, preimplantation genetic diagnosis (PGD) and prenatal diagnosis (PND) become possible. This chapter discusses the genetics of retinoblastoma and its application for prenatal diagnosis.

REFERENCES

1. Gallie BL, Soliman SE. Retinoblastoma. In: Lambert SR, Lyons CJ (Eds.) Taylor and Hoyt's Pediatric Ophthalmology and Strabismus, 5th edition. London, UK: Elsevier; 2016. pp. 424-41.
2. Marr BP, Singh AD. Retinoblastoma: Evaluation and diagnosis. In: Singh AD, Damato B (Eds). Clinical Ophthalmic Oncology: Retinal Tumors, 2nd edition. New York, NY, USA: Springer; 2015. pp. 1-11.
3. Noorani HZ, Khan HN, Gallie BL, Detsky AS. Cost comparison of molecular versus conventional screening of relatives at risk for retinoblastoma. Am J Hum Genet. 1996;59(2):301-7.

3a. Mallipatna AC, Gallie BL, Chévez-Barrios P, Lumbroso-Le Rouic L, Chantada G, Doz F, Munier FL, Albert DM, Català-Mora J, Desjardins LG, Suzuki S, Carroll WL, Finger PT. Retinoblastoma. In: Amin MB, Edge SB, Greene FL, et al (Eds.). AJCC Cancer Staging Manual, 8th edn, New York, USA: Springer; 2017. pp. 819-31.

4. Knudson AG Jr. Mutation and cancer: statistical study of retinoblastoma. Proc Natl Acad Sci USA. 1971;68(4):820-3.
5. Murphree AL. Intraocular retinoblastoma: the case for a new group classification. In: Singh AD (Ed). Ophthalmic Oncology: Ophthalmology Clinics of North America. Philadelphia, PA, USA: Elsevier-Saunders; 2005. pp. 41-53.
6. Munier FL. Classification and management of seeds in retinoblastoma. Ellsworth Lecture Ghent August 24th, 2013. Ophthalmic Genet. 2014;35(4):193-207|.
7. Francis JH, Abramson DH, Gaillard MC, Marr BP, Beck-Popovic M, Munier FL. The classification of vitreous seeds in retinoblastoma and response to intravitreal melphalan. Ophthalmology. 2015;122(6):1173-9.
8. Chantada GL, Dunkel IJ, de Dávila MT, Abramson DH. Retinoblastoma patients with high risk ocular pathological features: who needs adjuvant therapy? Br J Ophthalmol. 2004;88(8):1069-73.
9. Gallie B. Canadian guidelines for retinoblastoma care. Can J Ophthalmol. 2009;44(6):639-42.
10. Bojinova RI, Schorderet DF, Addor MC, Gaide AC, Thonney F, Pescia G, et al. Further delineation of the facial 13q14 deletion syndrome in 13 retinoblastoma patients. Ophthalmic Genet. 2001;22(1):11-8.
11. Baud O, Cormier-Daire V, Lyonnet S, Desjardins L, Turleau C, Doz F. Dysmorphic phenotype and neurological impairment in 22 retinoblastoma patients with constitutional cytogenetic 13q deletion. Clin Genet. 1999;55(6):478-82.
12. Bader JL, Meadows AT, Zimmerman LE, Rorke LB, Voute PA, Champion LA, et al. Bilateral retinoblastoma with ectopic intracranial retinoblastoma: trilateral retinoblastoma. Cancer Genet Cytogenet. 1982;5(3):203-13.
13. Jurkiewicz E, Pakula- Kościesza I, Rutynowska O, Nowak K. Trilateral retinoblastoma: an institutional experience and review of the literature. Childs Nerv Syst. 2010;26(1):129-32.
14. Kivelä T. Trilateral retinoblastoma: a meta-analysis of hereditary retinoblastoma associated with primary ectopic intracranial retinoblastoma. J Clin Oncol. 1999;17(6):1829-37.
15. Singh AD, Shields CL, Shields JA. New insights into trilateral retinoblastoma. Cancer. 1999;86(1):3-5.
16. Kleinerman RA, Yu CL, Little MP, Li Y, Abramson D, Seddon J, et al. Variation of second cancer risk by family history of retinoblastoma among long-term survivors. J Clin Oncol. 2012;30(9):950-7.
17. Dimaras H, Khetan V, Halliday W, Orlic M, Prigoda NL, Piovesan B, et al. Loss of RB1 induces non-proliferative retinoma: increasing genomic instability correlates with progression to retinoblastoma. Hum Mol Genet. 2008;17(10):1363-72.
18. Singh AD, Santos CM, Shields CL, Shields JA, Eagle RC Jr. Observations on 17 patients with retinocytoma. Arch Ophthalmol. 2000;118(2):199-205.
19. Hong FD, Huang HJ, To H, Young LJ, Oro A, Bookstein R, et al. Structure of the human retinoblastoma gene. Proc Natl Acad Sci U S A. 1989;86(14):5502-6.
20. Valverde JR, Alonso J, Palacios I, Pestaña A. RB1 gene mutation up-date, a meta-analysis based on 932 reported mutations available in a searchable database. BMC Genet. 2005;6:53.
21. Lohmann DR, Brandt B, Höpping W, Passarge E, Horsthemke B. The spectrum of RB1 germ-line mutations in hereditary retinoblastoma. Am J Hum Genet. 1996;58(5):940-9.
22. Richter S, Vandezande K, Chen N, Zhang K, Sutherland J, Anderson J, et al. Sensitive and efficient detection of RB1 gene mutations enhances care for families with retinoblastoma. Am J Hum Genet. 2003;72(2):253-69.
23. Ahmad NN, Melo MB, Singh AD, Donoso LA, Shields JA. A possible hot spot in exon 21 of the retinoblastoma gene predisposing to a low penetrant retinoblastoma phenotype? Ophthalmic Genet. 1999;20(4):225-31.
24. Rushlow DE, Mol BM, Kennett JY, Yee S, Pajovic S, Thériault BL, et al. Characterisation of retinoblastomas without RB1 mutations: genomic, gene expression, and clinical studies. Lancet Oncol. 2013;14(4):327-34.
25. Lohmann DR, Gallie BL. Retinoblastoma. In: Pagon RA, Adam MP, Ardinger HH (Eds). Gene Reviews (R). Seattle (WA): University of Washington, Seattle, University of Washington, Seattle; All rights reserved. 2013.
26. Dommering CJ, Garvelink MM, Moll AC, van Dijk J, Imhof SM, Meijers-Heijboer H, et al. Reproductive behavior of individuals with increased risk of having a child with retinoblastoma. Clin Genet. 2012;81(3):216-23.
27. Barbosa RH, Vargas FR, Lucena E, Bonvicino CR, Seuánez HN. Constitutive RB1 mutation in a child conceived by in vitro fertilization: implications for genetic counseling. BMC Med Genet. 2009;10:75.
28. Paquette LB, Miller D, Jackson HA, Lee T, Randolph L, Murphree AL, et al. In utero detection of retinoblastoma with fetal magnetic resonance and ultrasound: initial experience. AJP Rep. 2012;2(1):55-62.

CHAPTER

38

Pharmacology of Anticancer Drugs in Neonate

Saroj P Panda

INTRODUCTION

In last several decades, pediatric cancer treatment has advanced remarkably with the improvement in multimodal treatment strategies. Approximately 80% of newly diagnosed cancer patients less than 15 years of age can be cured. Despite a remarkable improvement in management of pediatric cancer, determination of appropriate chemotherapeutic regimen in neonates and very young infant poses a significant dilemma. There is limited published data on the pharmacokinetic and pharmacodynamic of antineoplastic agents in this patient population. Rapidly changing developmental physiologic processes (ontogeny) can lead to varying levels of medication exposure and clearance, which may potentially cause devastating consequences. Most pronounced are the pharmacokinetic changes occurring in first few months of life. Little is known regarding specific alterations in the pharmacology of antineoplastic agents in neonates, but the knowledge of general changes in absorption, distribution, metabolism, and elimination of drugs in pediatric age group can be extrapolated to this population.

ABSORPTION

The majority of chemotherapeutic drugs are administered intravenously. In a few patients, oral administration is used. Gastrointestinal absorption depends on gastric acid production, gastric pH, pepsin secretion, gastric emptying time, intestinal transit time, gastrointestinal enzymatic activity and the chemical characteristics of the drug. Secretion of both gastric acid and pepsin is significantly decreased in infancy, lowest pH occurring within the first 10 days and increasing between 10 days and 30 days of life (Kearns and Reed, 1989). As a result of this, increased absorption of drugs related to state of ionization of weak acids (e.g. methotrexate) can be expected. Gastric emptying time and intestinal motility are delayed in the neonatal period (Heimann et al. 1980). Since both methotrexate and 6-mercaptopurine are water soluble, changes in biliary function and biliary composition are less important. Infants up to 4 months of age have low activity of amylase and other pancreatic enzymes (Lebenthal et al. 1983). Thus, drugs which require pancreatic enzyme secretions for hydrolysis may demonstrate unreliable absorption.

DISTRIBUTION

During early developmental period, issues related to drug distribution which need to be considered are differences in body composition (e.g. total body water, extracellular water, body fat) and altered drug binding to various plasma and tissue proteins. The approximate total body water is 87% and 75% of body weight in premature and full-term neonates, respectively. It falls to 60% at 1 year and 55% by adulthood (Friis-Hansen et al. 1971). Similarly, extracellular water content falls from 45% of total body water in the full-term neonate to 20% in the adult. The clinical implications of these shifts in body composition have not been fully defined. For water-soluble drugs volume of distribution is larger due to the large extracellular water component. Lipid soluble drugs also have relatively larger volume distribution in infants as compared to older children due to the relatively higher amount of body fat. During first few months of life total body fat increases, at later ages a relative decrease occurs.

There are several physiologic variables, which can produce both quantitative as well as qualitative differences in plasma protein binding of drugs **(Table 38.1)**.

Many drugs have been found to be less bound to serum proteins in the neonate than in adults (Stewart and Hampton et al. 1987). Albumin, the major drug binding protein in plasma, binds primarily acidic drugs. Basic drugs bind more avidly to alpha-1 acid glycoprotein and lipoprotein than to albumin. Alterations in protein binding of drugs may lead to an increase in the unbound fraction (presumably the pharmacologically active constituent), and thus an increased pharmacologic or toxic response. Plasma protein levels generally approach adult values by 1 year of age. Though clinical importance of protein binding of antineoplastic agents has not yet been well defined, differences in serum albumin concentrations have

Table 38.1 Physiological variables potentially altering plasma protein binding of drugs*

Parameter	*Neonate*	*Infant*	*Child*
Total protein	↓	↓	≈
Plasma albumin	↓	≈	≈
Fetal albumin	+	–	–
Plasma globulin	↓	↓	≈
Unconjugated bilirubin	↑	≈	≈
Free fatty acids	↑	≈	≈
Blood pH	↓	≈	≈
Alpha-1 acid glycoprotein	↑	NA	≈

Keys: ↓, decreased relative to adult values; ↑, elevated relative to adult values; ≈, same as adult values; +, present; –, absent; NA, not available. *Relative to adult values.

been found recently to alter the plasma protein binding of etoposide, teniposide, vincristine, doxorubicin (Stewart et al. 1989, Boos et al. 1995, Urien et al. 2011).

METABOLISM

Human organs playing important role in drug metabolism include liver, lungs, kidney and gastrointestinal tract. Liver is probably the most important site for metabolism of cytostatic drugs. Liver volume and hepatic blood flow determine the amount of drug that can be metabolized. Younger children have a relative high liver volume, and liver volume has a close relation with body surface area and hepatic blood flow.

Drug metabolism can be separated into two phases. Phase I reactions are those which involve biotransformation of a molecule to more water soluble and often inactive metabolites. Phase II reactions involve conjugation of a drug or phase I metabolite with endogenous molecules (e.g. glucuronic acid, sulfate) rendering them more water soluble.

Phase I reactions are often catalyzed by the mixed-function oxidase system and typically involve substrate oxidation. Concentrations of the various forms of cytochrome P-450 and cytochrome P-450 reductase are important determinants for the rate of metabolism. There appears to be a gradual increase in enzyme activity with age, from birth to 5 weeks (Aranda et al. 1974). The activity of some P-450 enzymes is absent at birth (e.g. mephenytoin hydroxylase), while the quantity and activity of other enzymes approximates 20–70% of adult values (Pelkonen et al. 1973). A number of antineoplastic agents require bioactivation for cytotoxic effects (e.g. cyclophosphamide, ifosfamide) or inactivation (e.g. daunorubicin, vincristine and fluorouracil). Decrease in metabolic activity may result in either inability to form the active moiety or prolongation of cytotoxic activity depending on the drug type. Examples of phase II reaction include glucuronic acid conjugation, glutathione conjugation, sulfation and acetylation. Not all glucuronidases appear to be under the same developmental regulation. There is a nonuniform variation during the process of development.

RENAL EXCRETION

Kidney represents a primary route of elimination for many antineoplastic agents. Renal elimination is dependent on glomerular filtration, tubular secretion and renal blood flow. There is evidence of morphologic and functional tubular immaturity at birth. Tubular function appears to be fully developed by 7 months of age (Siegel and Moran et al. 1981). Renal blood flow increases with age as a result of an increase in cardiac output and a decrease in peripheral vascular resistance to attain adult rates by 5 months of age (Besunder et al. 1988). Glomerular filtration rate (GFR) is approximately 40 mL/minute/1.73 m^2 for a term infant at birth, which reaches the adult values by 2.5–5 months of age (Milsap and Szefler et al. 1986). The clinical implications for maturation of GFR become apparent when considering drugs that are primarily eliminated by glomerular filtration (e.g. methotrexate, platinum compounds). Chemotherapeutic agents that depend on renal function for elimination will be cleared more slowly in neonates and consequently will have lower plasma clearance with an increased risk of toxicity.

CONCLUSION

Children are not "small adults". Because of developing physiological processes, children differ from adults in each of the four pharmacokinetic stages. These differences lead to varying levels of medication exposure and clearance. Whether dosing should be based on body surface area (as is the practice in adult patients) or on body weight is another complicating factor. Although reduced doses are recommended for infants and very young children, inconsistencies exist between tumor types and clinical protocols as to the magnitude of the dose reductions employed. Existing data in infant patient populations in many cases do not suggest marked differences in pharmacokinetics compared with older children, but information is currently available only on a limited number of drugs (Veal et al. 2012). As many currently used antineoplastic agents are likely to be important in the treatment of infants and young children in the foreseeable future, it would seem advantageous for appropriately planned population pharmacokinetic studies to be carried out in this patient population.

KEY MESSAGE

Children differ from adults in all four pharmacokinetic stages which can lead to varying levels of medication exposure and clearance.

BIBLIOGRAPHY

1. Björkman S. Prediction of cytochrome P450-mediated hepatic drug clearance in neonates, infants and children: how accurate are available scaling methods? Clin Pharmacokinet. 2006;45(1):1-11.
2. Cole M, Boddy AV, Kearns P, Teh KH, Price L, Parry A, et al. Potential clinical impact of taking multiple blood samples for research studies in paediatric oncology: how much do we really know? Pediatr Blood Cancer. 2006;46(7):723-7.
3. Howlader N, Noone AM, Krapcho M, Miller D, Bishop K, Altekruse SF. (2016). SEER Cancer Statistics Review (CSR) 1975-2013. [online] Available from seer.cancer.gov/csr/1975_2013/. [Accessed September, 2016].
4. Kearns GL, Abdel-Rahman SM, Alander SW, Blowey DL, Leeder JS, Kauffman RE. Developmental pharmacology—drug disposition, action, and therapy in infants and children. N Engl J Med. 2003;349(12):1157-67.
5. McLeod HL, Relling MV, Crom WR, Silverstein K, Groom S, Rodman JH, et al. Disposition of antineoplastic agents in the very young child. Br J Cancer Suppl. 1992;18:S23-9.
6. Rhodin MM, Anderson BJ, Peters AM, Coulthard MG, Wilkins B, Cole M, et al. Human renal function maturation: a quantitative description using weight and postmenstrual age. Pediatr Nephrol. 2009;24(1):67-76.
7. Sharkey I, Boddy AV, Wallace H, Mycroft J, Hollis R, Picton S. Body surface area estimation in children using weight alone: application in paediatric oncology. Br J Cancer. 2001;85(1): 23-8.
8. Van den Berg H, van den Anker JN, Beijnen JH. Cytostatic drugs in infants: a review on pharmacokinetic data in infants. Cancer Treat Rev. 2012;38(1):3-26.
9. Veal GJ, Boddy AV. Chemotherapy in newborns and preterm babies. Semin Fetal Neonatal Med. 2012;17(4):243-8.
10. Veal GJ, Cole M, Errington J, Pearson AD, Gerrard M, Whyman G, et al. Pharmacokinetics of carboplatin and etoposide in infant neuroblastoma patients. Cancer Chemother Pharmacol. 2010;65(6):1057-66.

CHAPTER

39 Challenges in Neonatal Malignancies

Nirav Thacker, Shripad D Banavali

INTRODUCTION

Children are most vulnerable during the neonatal period with 45% of all under-five deaths occurring in the first 28 days of life.[1] With pediatric oncology still being in its infancy in developing countries, neonatal oncology has not even reached its fetal stage. Tumors in newborn period are uncommon, but not rare enough to be neglected. Although a few tumors are exclusive to neonates, most behave differently to their counterparts in older children. Genetic factors probably are an important cause of neonatal cancers, and other congenital abnormalities are frequently present in these children. Unfamiliarity with neonatal tumors can cause delay in diagnosis, unnecessary aggressive treatment in nonthreatening tumor or a well-intentioned observation in a sinister tumor.

EPIDEMIOLOGY

Neonatal tumors are uncommon with incidence of one in every 12,500–27,500 live births. There is considerable variation in incidence of reported neonatal tumors with maximum incidence in Japanese population and lowest incidence amongst blacks in USA (Stage, 2003). Male to Female ratio is unity in most of the cases with exception of teratoma (Gurney, Severson, Davis and Robison, 1995). Nearly 50% of neonatal tumors present on the 1st day of life (Weitzman and Grant, 1997).

Though benign neonatal tumors are relatively more common; malignant tumors are a rarity comprising only 2% of childhood malignancies. Although neonatal tumors differ in distribution from their childhood counterparts, almost all childhood tumors are known to occur in neonates. As per available literature, teratoma tops the list of neonatal tumors (benign and malignant), followed by neuroblastoma which is the most common malignant tumor. Mesenchymal tumors, renal tumors, central nervous system (CNS) tumors and leukemia add to the list of neonatal tumors **(Table 39.1)**. Leukemia is leading cause of death from tumors in 1st month of life, fortunately having a lower incidence.[2]

Table 39.1 Distribution of neonatal tumors

Tumor	*Neonates (Barson, 1980)*	*Neonates (Las Heras and Isaacs, 1980)*
Teratoma	24%	40%
Neuroblastoma	23%	12%
Mesenchymal	8%	9%
Renal	7%	5%
Central nervous system (CNS)	6%	2%
Leukemia	6%	12%

CHALLENGES IN NEONATAL MALIGNANCIES

Gaps in Epidemiology

Effective management of any disease is dependent on the accuracy and amount of epidemiological details available for the disease. Knowledge of incidence, prevalence, age, sex distribution, natural history of the disease is essential for planning its therapy.

The actual prevalence of neonatal tumors is difficult to estimate owing to small numbers and considerable heterogeneity in its reporting with respect to site of origin and pathological nature of the tumor. The data is even scantier in developing countries as seen in the **Table 39.2**. Almost all studies have a bias of being hospital based. To add to this problem, there is also variable reporting of tumors occurring in stillborn and in those dying in the neonatal period. A crystal clear picture is improbable and pending prospective registry-based studies, epidemiology is more of an art trying to make sense of missing pieces to complete the picture.

Obstetric and Perinatal Challenges

Parents, who have family history of predisposition syndromes or family history of cancer, should get a referral to genetic clinic for counseling and also get a good sonography or magnetic

Year	Author	Country	Number
1978	Barson	UK	270
1982	Gale et al.	USA	22
1985	Isaacs	USA	110
1986	Pinter and Hock	Hungary	141 (+ infants)
1987	Las Heras	USA	42
1987	Campbell et al.	Canada	102
1988	Davis et al.	Scotland	51
1989	Crom et al.	USA	34
1989	Plaschkes et al.	Switzerland	39
1990	Mur	Argentina	51
1992	Werb et al.	Australia	46
1992	Teinturier et al.	France	75
1994	Borch et al.	Denmark	76
1994	Parkes et al.	UK	149 (+ leukemia)
1995	Moore et al.	South Africa	60
1995	Xue H	USA	35
1996	Plaschkes	International, SIOP	192
1996	Chakova	Bulgaria	30
1998	Zhou	China	15
2000	Halperin	USA	23
2002	Rao	UK	83
2002	Hadley	South Africa	42

Table 39.2 Number of neonatal cancer cases from various countries

Abbreviation: SIOP, International Society of Pediatric Oncology

resonance imaging (MRI) evaluation done during antenatal check-ups. Since there is some data to show association of *in vitro* fertilization (IVF) and increased coincidence of tumors, like brain tumors, retinoblastoma and Wilms' tumor, children conceived through IVF should also be included in this list.

How best to diagnose and treat these neonates when the diagnosis is made during prenatal check-up is still not clear. Most of fetal tumors can be diagnosed prenatally either on routine ultrasound or as a result of complications such as polyhydramnios, hydrops or intrauterine fetal death. Differentiating benign from malignant is not easy on ultrasonography as neither rapid increase in size nor increased vascularity is suggestive of malignancy. Prenatal biopsy comes with its associated risks and very little clinical benefit for distinguishing benign from malignant.[3] Amniocentesis for karyotype is not very helpful except for genetic testing as most fetal tumors are not frequently aneuploid. Prenatally detected mass would need serial follow-up with imaging.

Antenatally treatment options would include therapeutic amnioreduction, open fetal surgery especially in cases of sacrococcygeal teratoma. A planned preterm delivery would be needed in specific cases. Vaginal delivery would be avoided in large tumors with risk of shoulder dystocia or tumor rupture. Large head, neck and thoracic tumors would need EXIT (ex-utero intrapartum treatment) at delivery.[4]

To summarize, all congenital tumors are high-risk pregnancies and deliveries, which would require planning with a large multidisciplinary team including fetomaternal specialist, obstetricians, radiologists, neonatologists, pediatric surgeons and oncologists whose availability is limited in a developing country setup.

Challenging Pathology

Neonatal tumors pose several questions to pathologists, as normal developing tissues and nonmalignant lesions might show characteristics that mimic neoplasia.[5] Also the histological features reflecting malignancy might not correlate with its clinical behavior.[6] For example, the mitotic index might not as relevant or must be increased to reach a value appropriate for prognosis as in neuroblastoma. Congenital fibrosarcoma, which is malignant by histological criteria but nonaggressive clinically and relatively benign course of neonatal teratomas with immature elements further, highlights the clinicohistological disparity in neonates. This is further complicated by difficulty of obtaining sufficient viable tissue for diagnosis.

Association with Congenital Abnormalities

There is a significant association of congenital anomalies with neonatal tumors, which occur in approximately 15% of neonates with tumor. Registry data from Australia showed a nearly 4.5 times higher prevalence of congenital malformations in neonates with tumor as compared to controls.[7] Teratomas may be associated with not only regional but also distal congenital abnormalities. This further complicates the management of neonates, which needs to encompass a comprehensive plan for the patient as a whole rather than in isolation for either condition.

Neonatal tumors might also be related to chromosomal abnormalities, particularly Down's syndrome, which has been associated with increased incidence of leukemia, retroperitoneal teratomas, and also other congenital malformations. Treatment of neonatal tumors thus necessitates a stronger and wider multidisciplinary approach, which would only be available at a few centers.

WHICH TUMORS TO TREAT?

Malignant or benign nature of tumor does not always guide treatment strategy in neonates. A well-intentioned observation in a benign tumor could become life-threatening, whereas administration of toxic chemotherapy in a malignant tumor (e.g. neuroblastoma stage IVS) could be overkill. Some benign tumors merely by their location and size (e.g. cervical or cardiac teratoma) may warrant emergent management, while some may have a potential toward malignancy. A thorough knowledge of the tumor and its behavior is a must while planning treatment, which can be guided by some extent by the four clinical groupings recognized by Plaschkes (Plaschkes J, 1996) **(Table 39.3)**.

Table 39.3 Clinical groups of neonatal tumors

• Benign tumors	• Life-threatening because of size and location (e.g. cervical teratoma) • Have a known tendency toward malignant transformation (sacrococcygeal teratoma, giant nevus) • Benign tumors, not life-threatening or tending toward malignant transformation (mesoblastic nephroma)
• Tumors demonstrating local invasiveness but no metastatic potential	• Congenital fibrosarcoma, fibromatoses
• Malignant tumors	• Behave more like those occurring in older children • Behave better than expected (hepatoblastoma, neuroblastoma) • Behave worse than expected (congenital alveolar rhabdomyosarcoma, leukemia) • Demonstrate unpredictable or uncertain behavior
• Extremely rare tumors	• Carcinoma, lymphoma, Hodgkin disease, Kaposi sarcoma

CHALLENGES IN TREATMENT

Neonatal cancer raises diagnostic, therapeutic and ethical issues, and management requires a multidisciplinary approach. They are commonly sensitive to same therapeutic agents as their counterparts in older children. However, the neonate's rapid growth and significantly different physiology make delivering the same therapy more challenging. A delicate balance between therapy and long-term side effects need to be maintained. Also supportive care needed is unique in this age-group and is as important as other therapy, if not more.

Neonatal Intensive Care Unit and Nursing Care

Care of a neonate with malignancy adds a unique challenge to an already complex supportive care. A neonate with cancer should have an individualized care plan to help the nurse in the assessment, therapy administration and evaluation of care. The pediatric oncology team should work in concert with neonatal intensive care unit (NICU) nurse caring for the neonate. The oncology nurse can provide specific inputs to the NICU staff about care of the neonate with a malignancy with special emphasis on the care of venous access devices and management of the side effects of chemotherapy.

Despite the complexity of the care required by the neonate with cancer, attention must be given to providing this infant with developmentally appropriate support. Careful attention to the environment and to the routine care provided is important in assuring that an already fragile infant is not overwhelmed with inappropriate stimulation. Care plans should address developmental issues, such as positioning, non-nutritive sucking, facilitating self-comforting behaviors, and providing appropriate levels and types of stimulation.

Chemotherapeutic Challenges

The unique and rapidly changing differences in drug absorption, distribution, metabolism, and excretion in this age group complicate the use of chemotherapy in neonates as a result of which chemotherapy use in neonates is also associated with higher incidence of immediate complications such as infections.[8] A number of intrinsic neonatal factors such as higher total body water, lower body fat, differential drug binding of fetal albumin and immature neonatal kidneys and immature neonatal liver make drug dosing difficult with unpredictable drug levels.[9] There is hardly any pharmacokinetics or pharmacodynamic data available for most chemotherapy drugs in neonates, and dosing guidelines often are extrapolated from data in older children, which in turn are sometimes extrapolated from adults. The side effects of chemotherapy toxicity may be subtle in neonates and difficult to distinguish from other physiologic problems.

This is considerable disparity in practically all aspects of drug absorption, distribution, metabolism, and excretion between the neonate and older child or adult, which are continually changing as the baby grows. Drug distribution in neonates is distinctive, as, total body water constitutes 80% of body weight in them as compared to 50–55% in older children and adults. Extracellular water is 45% of body weight at birth and falls to 20% by 3 years of age. For chemotherapeutic agents that distribute in water, administering drugs as a dose per kilogram may have unpredictable consequences. On the other hand, total body and extracellular water are virtually constant over age when calculated as liters per square meter of body surface area. It is, therefore, reasonable to expect more standard concentration of drug in a water volume of distribution if surface area is used to calculate dose.

For drugs dependent on gastrointestinal absorption and hepatic activation or metabolism, one must be aware of the slow gastric emptying time, relatively high gastric pH, absent or lower functioning of hepatic enzymatic pathways, and lower binding of drugs by plasma proteins in the neonate. These factors may result in unexpectedly elevated tissue concentrations of chemotherapeutic agents unless adjustments are made in dosing.[10,11] The glomerular filtration rate is low at birth and changes rapidly during early growth and development. The ability of the newborn kidney to concentrate and acidify urine is restricted. Urinary pH is lower in the newborn than the older child. Drugs that are more soluble in alkaline urine, such as methotrexate, may be less well excreted.[8] Drugs that are not extensively metabolized owing to immaturity of hepatic enzymes depend mainly on renal function for excretion and have a higher risk of exaggerated pharmacological effects and toxicities.

Based on findings of pharmacokinetic studies of several antineoplastic drugs in young children,[10] it is advisable to give drugs such as anthracyclines, vincristine, cisplatin and actinomycin at reduced doses probably weight based, whereas antimetabolites such as methotrexate, mercaptopurine, thioguanine, etoposide and teniposide need standard BSA-based dosing.

Surgical Challenges

The surgical management of neonatal tumors is closely interlinked to the details of metabolic homeostasis. The newborn requires close monitoring of physiologic support in view of a very minimal margin for error. Fluid management and caloric intake are of vital importance. The liver glycogen stores in the infant are readily depleted and gluconeogenesis is inefficient as a means to replenish required amounts of glucose. Hypocalcemia may occur due to transient deficient parathyroid hormone during the first few days of life or due to elevated corticosteroid levels. Temperature regulation requires avoidance of heat loss during diagnostic studies or in the operating room.[12]

Radiotherapy Challenges

Because of the immaturity of major organs, the neonate is even more vulnerable than the young child to the major long-term toxicity of radiation therapy. The acute morbidity resulting in gastrointestinal toxicity, bone-marrow depression, and skin reactions is usually reversible and is not treatment-limiting, but the profound long-term effects on the brain, lung, liver, kidney and bone, are not preventable and are usually irreversible.[13] This major treatment problem is particularly observed in babies with brain tumors. There is no documented case of a newborn who received therapeutic doses of radiation to the brain and survived, but young children who have been treated and survived have a very high incidence of mental retardation. It is difficult to differentiate the morbidity of radiation therapy from that produced by the tumor itself, the surgery, or the effects of chemotherapy on the developing nervous system, nonetheless most therapeutic protocols for brain tumors in the young consist of high-dose chemotherapy in an attempt to delay or even avoid radiation therapy. However, the use of restricted field, low-dose radiation therapy under specific circumstances may be life-saving.

PROBLEMS SPECIFIC TO DEVELOPING COUNTRIES

In addition to the challenges highlighted above, developing countries face certain unique challenges.

Bigger Public Health Issues

Prematurity, birth asphyxia and infections still account for nearly 80% of neonatal deaths in India.[14] Thus pushing neonatal malignancies down the triage list of the public health planning.

LACK OF ADEQUATE EXPERTISE, EQUIPMENT AND INFRASTRUCTURE

The number of neonatologists and tertiary care neonatal units are still grossly inadequate to handle the burden of preterm, low-birth-weight and other high-risk neonates, thus making handling neonatal tumors even more challenging in terms of resource and infrastructure. There is no concept of having a pharmacologist attached to clinical units, who can monitor the drug levels and guide in proper dosing in neonates, so as to avoid both under and overdosing. On the other hand, the paucity of oncologists in developing countries makes the situation even more complex. There is no specialized environment for neonatal surgery.

Treatment Refusal and Abandonment

Considering the fact that there is excessive parental stress when a neonatal cancer is diagnosed, these parents require proper counseling at the start of therapy and at various steps thereafter. Such expert genetic and social counseling is not available in developing countries. Thus, in developing countries where treatment refusal and abandonment is a significant problem already in pediatric oncology, it is much more amplified in neonatology.

CONCLUSION

Management of prenatal and neonatal cancers requires extension of the usual multidisciplinary pediatric oncology team to include obstetricians and neonatologists. Although neonatal cancers are rare, a significant percentage of these patients can be successfully treated and cured with minimal long-term complications. However, management of neonates is quite demanding with respect to time of both parents and physicians, finances, and available infrastructure. Therefore, the proposed treatment and the risks involved should be discussed in detail with the parents before it is implemented. Initial intensive treatment using chemotherapy might be justified in some cases; however, palliative care is also sometimes the most worthwhile option (Orbach D et al., 2013).

KEY MESSAGE

Tumors in newborn period are uncommon, but not rare enough to be neglected. The most common among them are teratoma, neuroblastoma, mesenchymal tumors, renal tumors, CNS tumors and leukemia. Parents with strong family history of predisposition syndromes should get a ante-natal referral to genetic clinic for counseling evaluation. There is a significant association of congenital anomalies with neonatal tumors. There are many challenges in the treatment of neonatal malignancies including making a proper diagnosis, delivery of effective therapy, and maintaining a delicate balance between therapy and long-term side effects. Neonates with malignancy should ideally be treated in a center which has an NICU and appropriate nursing care available. It is important to know which tumors to treat and which to observe. The unique and rapidly changing differences in drug absorption, distribution, metabolism, and excretion in this age group complicate the use of chemotherapy in neonates. The unique and rapidly changing differences in drug absorption, distribution, metabolism, and excretion in this age group complicate the use of chemotherapy in neonates. The surgical management demands particular attention to the details of metabolic homeostasis. Though radiotherapy in full doses is nearly never given in neonates, the use of restricted field, low-dose radiation therapy under specific circumstances may be life-saving. These challenges are further multiplied in a developing country setting because of lack of adequately trained manpower as well as inadequate infrastructure, further decreasing the outcomes and making palliative care many-times the most worthwhile option.

REFERENCES

1. Black RE, Cousens S, Johnson HL, Lawn JE, Rudan I, Bassani DG, et al. Global, regional, and national causes of child mortality in 2008: a systematic analysis. Lancet. 2010;375(9730):1969-87.
2. Bader JL, Miller RW. US cancer incidence and mortality in the first year of life. Am J Dis Child. 1979;133(2):157-9.
3. Kamil D, Tepelmann J, Berg C, Heep A, Axt-Fliedner R, Gembruch U, et al. Spectrum and outcome of prenatally diagnosed fetal tumors. Ultrasound Obstet Gynecol. 2008;31(3): 296-302.
4. Lazar DA, Olutoye OO, Moise KJ Jr, Ivey RT, Johnson A, Ayres N, et al. Ex-utero intrapartum treatment procedure for giant neck masses--fetal and maternal outcomes. J Pediatr Surg. 2011;46(5):817-22.
5. Batcup G. Cancer in the very young child--pitfalls and problems for the pathologist. Br J Cancer Suppl. 1992;18:S5-7.
6. Moore SW, Satgé D, Sasco AJ, Zimmermann A, Plaschkes J. The epidemiology of neonatal tumours. Report of an international working group. Pediatr Surg Int. 2003;19(7):509-19.
7. Altmann AE, Halliday JL, Giles GG. Associations between congenital malformations and childhood cancer. A register-based case-control study. Br J Cancer. 1998;78(9):1244-9.
8. Siegel SE, Moran RG. Problems in the chemotherapy of cancer in the neonate. Am J Pediatr Hematol Oncol. 1981;3(3):287-96.
9. Fernandez KS. Solid tumors in the neonatal period. NeoReviews. 2014;15(2):e56-68.
10. McLeod HL, Relling MV, Crom WR, Rivera GK, Crist WM, Evans WE, et al. Disposition of antineoplastic agents in the very young child. Br J Cancer Suppl. 1992;18:S23-9.
11. Hutson JR, Weitzman S, Schechter T, Arceci RJ, Kim RB, Finkelstein Y. Pharmacokinetic and pharmacogenetic determinants and considerations in chemotherapy selection and dosing in infants. Expert Opin Drug Metab Toxicol. 2012;8(6):709-22.
12. de Lorimier AA, Harrison MR. Surgical treatment of tumors in the newborn. Am J Pediatr Hematol Oncol. 1981;3(3):271-7.
13. Littman P, D'Angio GJ. Radiation therapy in the neonate. Am J Pediatr Hematol Oncol. 1981;3(3):279-85.
14. Bassani DG, Kumar R, Awasthi S, Morris SK, Paul VK, Shet A, et al. Causes of neonatal and child mortality in India : a nationally representative mortality survey. Lancet. 2010;376(9755):1853-60.

SECTION 7

Blood Transfusion (Component Therapy) and Supportive Therapy

Section Editors

Anand Deshpande, Avneet Kaur

injury (TRALI). RBC transfusions have also been studied to be associated with an increased risk of death, necrotizing enterocolitis (NEC), extension of intraventricular hemorrhage (IVH), or transient increase in respiratory support; however, high quality evidence for a causal relationship with any of these adverse events is lacking.[3-5] These potential complications underscore the need to carefully evaluate a neonate's ability to deliver oxygen to tissues prior to ordering a nonemergent transfusion, and to document benefit following the transfusion.

Indications for Packed Red Blood Cell Transfusion

Anemia

Anemia occurs when the RBC mass does not adequately meet the oxygen demands of the tissue, which in turn is dependent on cardiac output and arterial oxygen content. Hemoglobin concentration, arterial oxygen saturation and oxygen carrying capacity of hemoglobin predict the arterial oxygen content. Thus, by increasing the hemoglobin concentration the oxygen supply to tissues can be increased, which is the complication of anemia.

The criterion for PRBC transfusion is dependent on whether it is acute or chronic anemia, the clinical signs due to inadequate oxygen delivery like increasing heart rate, acidosis, and apnea and the degree of respiratory support needed. Although conventionally target hemoglobin and hematocrit (Hct) have been used as clinical indicators for RBC transfusion.

Acute Blood Loss

Immediate treatment for neonates with acute blood loss is fluid resuscitation followed by assessment of status and decision of need for PRBC transfusion. Indications for a RBC transfusion in acute blood loss are:

- More than 20% blood loss
- 10–20% blood loss with signs of poor oxygen delivery, such as tachycardia, persistent acidosis
- Ongoing hemorrhage.

Chronic Anemia

Physiological anemia presenting as gradual fall in hemoglobin after birth occurs in all neonates due to decreased production of erythropoietin. In preterm babies, this anemia is more severe and occurs much earlier than term neonates and is called as anemia of prematurity. Other causes for increased anemia in preterm are repeated phlebotomy losses, lower blood volumes and reduced lifespan of RBCs as compared to full-term infants.

British Committee for Standards in Haematology Transfusion Task Force, 2004[6] have suggested the threshold for transfusions in infants less than 4 months **(Table 40.1)**. Roseff et al. have suggested some more threshold for transfusion based on clinical and respiratory status of neonates **(Box 40.1)**.[7]

Table 40.1 Selected guidelines from the United Kingdom and United States of America

The British Committee for Standards in Haematology Transfusion Task Force (BCSH), 2004 has issued the following suggested transfusion thresholds for infants under 4 months of age[6]

Transfusion of red blood cells	*Level*
Anemia in first 24 hours	Hb 12 g/dL hematocrit count (Hct 0.36)
Cumulative blood loss in 1 week in a neonate requiring intensive care	10% blood volume
Neonate receiving intensive care	Hb 12 g/dL
Acute blood loss	10%
Chronic oxygen dependency	Hb 11 g/dL
Late anemia, stable infant	Hb 7 g/dL

Box 40.1 The guidelines from Roseff et al. (USA, 2002)[7]

Guidelines for transfusion of RBCs in patients less than 4 months of age

1. Hct <20% with low reticulocyte count and symptoms of anemia.*
2. Hct <30% with an infant:
   - On <35% hood O_2
   - On O_2 by nasal cannula
   - On continuous positive airway pressure and/or intermittent mandatory ventilation with mechanical ventilation with mean airway pressure <6 cm H_2O
   - With *significant* apnea or bradycardia†
   - With *significant* tachycardia or tachypnea‡
   - With *low weight gain*§
3. Hct <35% with an infant:
   - On >35% hood O_2
   - On continuous positive airway pressure/intermittent mandatory ventilation with mean airway pressure ≥6–8 cm H_2O
4. Hct <45% with an infant:
   - On ECMO
   - With congenital cyanotic heart disease

* Tachycardia, tachypnea, poor feeding

† More than six episodes in 12 hours or two episodes in 24 hours requiring bag and mask ventilation while receiving therapeutic doses of methylxanthines

‡ Heart rate >180 beats/min for 24 hours; respiratory rate >80 breaths min for 24 hours

§ Gain of <10 g/day observed over 4 days while receiving ≥100 kcal/kg/day

Abbreviations: Hct, hematocrit; ECMO, extracorporeal membrane oxygenation

EVIDENCE FOR THRESHOLD OF TRANSFUSION

Based on hemoglobin and Hct values, RBC transfusion is administered universally in neonates, children and adults. However, the threshold levels of hemoglobin for deciding need of transfusions have changed over time. Recently, a more restrictive approach has emerged due to concerns of risk of transmission of infections associated with blood transfusions. This has reduced the transfusion rates in newborns but whether this strategy is better than liberal approach is not clear from the present evidence.

A meta-analysis including four major trials with 614 neonates done in 2011 compared low versus high targets thresholds in neonates.[8] It revealed that Infants in the low threshold group received fewer transfusions. There was no difference in the rate of mortality between the groups and there was no difference in the composite outcome of death and serious morbidity at the time of discharge, defined as severe retinopathy of prematurity (ROP), bronchopulmonary dysplasia (BPD), or brain injury on ultrasound [risk ratio (RR) = 1.07; 95% confidence interval (CI) = 0.96–1.2].

The premature infants in need of transfusion (PINT) study also showed no difference between the low and high-target Hct groups at 18–21 months corrected age in the composite outcome of death or neurodevelopment impairment, defined as cerebral palsy, significant visual and hearing impairment, and Bayley Scales of Infant Development-II (BSID-II) mental development index (MDI) score less than 70.[9] However, another small trial by Bell et al. (Iowa trial) showed that restrictive threshold group had high apneas and more grade 4 IVH and periventricular leukomalacia.[10] Bell concluded that "the drive to eliminate transfusions by tolerating moderate-to-severe iatrogenic anemia should be halted until more information is available".[11]

Prerequisite and Dose of Transfusion

Ideally, samples from both mother and neonate should be tested prior to transfusion for blood group and for any atypical red cell antibodies. Neonate's serum may contain transplacentally acquired maternal immunoglobulin G (IgG) anti-A and/or anti-B. The preferred blood is the newborn's ABO and Rh group, and it should be compatible with any ABO or atypical red cell antibody present in the maternal serum. In exchange, transfusions for Rh-incompatibility, if the mother's and the baby's blood groups are the same, use Rh-negative blood of baby's ABO group. In case mother's and baby's blood group is not compatible, use group O-and Rh-negative blood for exchange transfusion.[12] All hospitals must have facility for provision of urgent uncross-matched group O Rh-negative blood in case of a perinatal emergency.

Conventionally, 10–20 mL/kg is the volume of blood given in neonates.[13] Rates of 7–10 mL/kg/hour are usually tolerated in neonates without cardiac failure. However, in babies with cardiac failure rate should be 2 mL/kg/hour. Another approach is to calculate the volume of blood transfused by target Hct selection using this formula:

$$\text{Volume of PRBC} = \frac{\text{Blood volume (mL/kg)} \times (\text{desired} - \text{actual Hct})}{\text{Hct of transfused RBC}}$$

Each transfusion of 10 mL/kg of body weight should increase hemoglobin level by 3 g/dL.

Age of Blood to be Used

Previously, it was a routine practice to use fresh PRBCs due to: (1) increased level of potassium in stored red blood cells and (2) reduced 2, 3-diphosphoglycerate (DPG) in stored blood. However, these factors come to play when neonates require large volume transfusions (20 mL/kg). A recent study showed that use of fresh RBCs compared with standard blood bank practice did not improve outcome from major neonatal morbidities like NEC, ROP, BPD, IVH in premature very low-birth-weight (VLBW) infants requiring transfusions. Thus, the present strategy is to assign a fresh unit of RBC to a neonate and multiple aliquots from same unit can be prepared and used till blood bank get norms and as and when neonate requires, rather than newer bags from various donors. This reduces the chances of side effects to neonates due to multiple donor exposure.

Granulocyte Transfusion

Neonates are prone to sepsis and infections due to poor immune response, functional and quantitative deficiency of neutrophils and low complements levels. Preterm babies further have lower immunoglobulin levels, prolonged and invasive environment in neonatal intensive care unit (NICU), which further increases the risk of sepsis. In spite of use of good antibiotics and antifungals, neonatal sepsis carry high mortality.

INDICATIONS

Neonates with severe sepsis, who are worsening despite antibiotics and who have severe neutropenia for more than 24 hours may benefit from intravenous immune globulin (IVIG), granulocyte transfusion, granulocyte-colony stimulating factor (G-CSF). However, which of these therapies is better is not clear from the currently available evidence.

DOSE AND DURATION OF THERAPY

The suggested dose is 1–2 × 10^9 granulocytes/kg. The component must be ABO compatible with the recipient (as it is heavily contaminated with red cells), RhD compatible (RhD negative for RhD negative females) and irradiated to a minimum dose of 25 Gy prior to administration. It should also be CMV seronegative, if appropriate. The optimal duration of therapy is unclear but two or more daily infusions of an appropriate dose have been associated with improved outcome.

PREPARATION

Granulocyte concentrates are obtained by centrifugation of refrigerated whole blood units. To obtain adequate doses, the donor needs to be preconditioned with steroids or G-CSF. These have to be then stored unagitated at room temperature and should be administered within 12 hours of preparation. If stored for more than 8–12 hours it is associated with marked loss of function.

Platelet Transfusions

Thrombocytopenia is a common abnormality in sick neonates affecting 20–35% of those admitted to NICUs.[14,15] Approximately 75% of these neonates have mild-to-moderate thrombocytopenia defined as a platelet count of 50–150 $\times 10^9$/L, and 25% have platelet counts less than 50 $\times 10^9$/L, a level which is thought to increase the bleeding risk.

Indications

Indications of platelet transfusion can be therapeutic or prophylactic.

Therapeutic: They are ordered to treat bleeding neonate irrespective of level of preexisting hemorrhage.

Prophylactic: Rationale behind use of prophylactic platelet transfusions is that low platelets carry a risk of intracranial hemorrhage. The cut-offs of prophylactic transfusion vary from unit-to-unit owing to lack of strong evidence.

Platelet Transfusion Practices

For neonatal thrombocytopenia, platelet transfusions remain the mainstay of treatment. There has been lack of agreement across the world regarding threshold of platelet transfusion owing to lack of evidence from robust clinical trials. Around 9% of babies admitted to NICU in a center in US received platelet transfusion where the criteria were liberal. In a recent survey done to compare transfusion practices in North America versus Europe, the transfusion thresholds chosen by European neonatologists were substantially lower than that chosen by North American neonatologists.[16,17]

Is There a Relationship between Low Platelets and Increased Bleeding

Combination of low platelets and their dysfunction has been proposed as one of the major reason of increased risk of IVH in preterm babies. Several studies have shown an association between thrombocytopenia and increased IVH although it does not establish causality.

Majority of the newborn who have IVH hemorrhage have normal or slightly decreased platelets at time of bleed indicating that there are other factors like cardiovascular instability and vascular fragility that are involved in pathogenesis apart from low platelets only.

Multiple studies have tried to look into this matter. A recent large prospective cross-sectional observational study (PlaNet-1) was carried out to know the incidence of severe thrombocytopenia and major hemorrhages. In the study, 9% of the babies have severe hemorrhages and 87% of those with severe hemorrhages were babies with gestational age less than 28 weeks. Of the babies with severe hemorrhages, majority of them had normal or minimally decreased platelet count at time of hemorrhage. The strongest predictors of hemorrhage were gestational age less than 28 weeks, postnatal age less than 10 days and diagnosis of NEC.[18]

Cut-off for Platelet Transfusion

Despite the frequent occurrence of thrombocytopenia in NICU (incidence) and frequent administration of platelets for thrombocytopenia, not many studies have looked into what should be the ideal cut-off for platelet count to be transfused.

EVIDENCE

Levels at which platelets should be transfused in an individual baby are variable because of lack of good quality studies. Till date there is only one randomized controlled trial (RCT) by Andrew et al.[19] in which he examined the effect of prophylactic platelet transfusion in premature babies with mild thrombocytopenia (50 – 150 $\times 10^9$/L) in 1st week of life. They found no difference in frequency or severity of IVHs when platelet count was maintained above 150 $\times 10^9$/L or was allowed to fall till 60 $\times 10^9$/L. Conclusions of the study were that in nonbleeding premature babies if platelet count is more than 60 $\times 10^9$/L than giving platelet transfusion does not help. Study did not answer that withholding platelet transfusion in stable premature babies with platelet count less than 60 $\times 10^9$/L will lead to increase risk of intracranial bleeding.

In retrospective review, Murray and colleagues looked into outcomes of babies who received platelet transfusion at threshold of 30 $\times 10^9$/L in case they are clinically stable or between 30 $\times 10^9$/L–50 $\times 10^9$/L in case they are clinically unstable or had previous hemorrhage.[20] No major hemorrhages were observed in the group of severely thrombocytopenic infants suggesting that a cut-off of 30 $\times$ 10^9/L in clinically stable premature babies is an acceptable cut-off but the results need to be analyzed with caution owing to the retrospective nature of study. Many recent retrospective reviews have tried to analyze the appropriate cut-off of platelet transfusion in premature neonates but no clear cut-off has been decided. PlaNet-2 study[21] is a multicentric RCT ongoing in Europe that is comparing restrictive versus liberal transfusion (50 vs 25 $\times 10^9$/L). Results are awaited. Below is the guidelines mentioned in a recent review article in clinics in perinatology. They are more of expert recommendations rather than truly evidence based.

Platelet Count versus Mass

Platelet mass is the product of platelet count (per microliter) and mean platelet volume. Recently many investigators believe that platelet mass may be a better indicator of platelet transfusion and may be it can decrease the number of transfusions. In a study conducted in two Intermountain Healthcare NICUs, platelet count-based guidelines were used for 1 year and then switched to platelet mass-guided transfusion guidelines. Fewer transfusions were administered to neonates during the period of time using platelet mass-guided transfusions, and no differences were found in bleeding outcomes.[22] This approach needs to be tested in prospective randomized controlled settings before guidelines on basis of platelet mass can be formed **(Table 40.2)**.

Guidelines for platelet transfusion are described in **Table 40.2**.

TYPES OF PLATELETS AVAILABLE

Random Donor Platelet

Each unit of a random donor pool is obtained from a single whole blood unit. Multiple such units from many donors can be pooled together or each such unit can be given separately. PRBC is separated from the platelet rich plasma, which is then respun at a higher speed to make a concentrated platelet button.

Single Donor Platelet

Single donor platelet (SDP) units are obtained by a process called plateletpheresis. Here, from a single donor itself multiple platelet units are separated. This is achieved by returning RBCs and platelet poor plasma to donor's circulation after plateletpheresis. The procedure is repeated 4–6 times, yielding 4–6 units of platelets from one individual. It is especially useful to prevent alloimmunization in multiply transfused patients. Both SDPs and random donor platelets (RDPs) are irradiated. It is more cost-effective to screen the larger SDP units for bacterial contamination than to screen individual random donor units.

The concentration of platelets is more in SDP than in RDP, with SDP having a platelet concentration of 3×10^{11} per unit and RDP having a concentration of 0.5×10^{10} per unit. In newborns, RDP are normally adequate to treat thrombocytopenia. Only if thrombocytopenia is prolonged and severe, SDP are needed.

Dose of Platelet Concentrate

Despite so many differences in the cut-off used for prophylactic platelet transfusion in neonates with thrombocytopenia, most agree that dose should be 10–15 mL/kg of a CMV-safe standard platelet suspension derived from a RDP unit (whole-blood-derived) or from a plateletpheresis unit. Volume reduction is not routinely recommended. Try to use one donor in one random unit to restrict number of donor exposure.

Table 40.2 Recommended level of platelets at which platelet concentrate should be given

Platelet count ($\times 10^9$/L)	*Guidelines for platelet transfusions*
<30	Transfuse all
30–50	Transfuse if • Very low-birth-weight babies in first 7 days of life • Clinically unstable • Coexisting coagulopathy • Grade III or IV intraventricular hemorrhage • Before surgery
50–100	Transfuse in case of active bleeding, neonatal alloimmune thrombocytopenia with intraventricular hemorrhage

SIDE EFFECTS

Concerns of CMV Infection

Ideal should be to obtain platelets from donors without detectable levels of CMV antibodies. Still the rate of CMV infection following transfusion with CMV-negative platelets is 1–4% owing to an intrinsic false-negative rate of the test for antibody to CMV, a low-antibody titer, or transient viremia quenching the circulating antibody.[23] Since majority of the adult population is having CMV antibodies, this becomes a limiting factor. Alternative is to do leukocyte reduction, although the comparable safety provided against CMV infection is controversial.

Transfusion-associated Graft versus Host Disease

It is caused by contaminating T-lymphocytes in platelet concentrates. Transfusion-associated graft versus host disease (TA-GVHD) presents between 8 days and 10 days after a transfusion and is characterized by rash, diarrhea, elevated hepatic transaminases, hyperbilirubinemia and pancytopenia. TA-GVHD is also characterized by an extremely high mortality rate (>90%). Exposure of platelets to 2,500 cGy of gamma irradiation before transfusion effectively prevents GVHD.

INDICATIONS OF IRRADIATED CELLULAR PRODUCTS

Definitely indicated in cases of suspected or confirmed underlying immunodeficiency (e.g. DiGeorge syndrome, Wiskott-Aldrich syndrome), intrauterine or exchange transfusions, or blood transfusions from a first- or second-degree relative or a human leukocyte antigen (HLA)-matched donor.

FUTURE DIRECTIONS

Nowadays although platelets are being transfused based on count or mass, evidence does suggest that factors other than the degree of thrombocytopenia determine the bleeding risk. Larger studies are needed to better characterize the platelet function and hemostatic profile of preterm babies and there is a need to develop and validate test that incorporate both function and count to evaluate hemostasis like platelet function analyzer (PFA-100).

KEY POINTS

- Transfusion of various components is integral in managing sick neonates in NICU.

- We should try to restrict transfusions as far as possible owing to side effects associated with them.
- Keep your unit guidelines based on best literature and follow them.
- Try to make satellite bags from single unit to avoid number of donor exposures.

REFERENCES

1. Ohls RJ. Transfusions in the preterm neonates. Neo Rev. 2007;8:377-86.
2. Rohde JM, Dimcheff DE, Blumberg N, Saint S, Langa KM, Kuhn L, et al. Health care-associated infection after red blood cell transfusion: a systematic review and meta-analysis. JAMA. 2014;311(13):1317-26.
3. dos Santos AM, Guinsburg R, de Almeida MF, Procianoy RS, Leone CR, Marba ST, et al. Red blood cell transfusions are independently associated with intra-hospital mortality in very low birth weight preterm infants. J Pediatr. 2011;159(3): 371-6.
4. Baer VL, Lambert DK, Henry E, Snow GL, Christensen RD. Red blood cell transfusion of preterm neonates with a Grade 1 intraventricular hemorrhage is associated with extension to a Grade 3 or 4 hemorrhage. Transfusion. 2011;51(9):1933-9.
5. Rashid N, Al-Sufayan F, Seshia MM, Baier RJ. Post transfusion lung injury in the neonatal population. J Perinatol. 2013;33(4):292-6.
6. British Committee for Standards in Haematology (BCSH). [online] Available from www.bcshguidelines.com. [Accessed October, 2016].
7. Roseff SD, Luban NL, Manno CS. Guidelines for assessing appropriateness of pediatric transfusion. Transfusion. 2002;42(11):1398-412.
8. Whyte R, Kirpalani H. Low versus high haemoglobin concentration threshold for blood transfusion for preventing morbidity and mortality in very low birth weight infants. Cochrane Database Syst Rev. 2011;(11):CD000512.
9. Kirpalani H, Whyte RK, Andersen C, Asztalos EV, Heddle N, Blajchman MA, et al. The Premature Infants in Need of Transfusion (PINT) study: A randomized, controlled trial of a restrictive (low) versus liberal (high) transfusion threshold for extremely low birth weight infants. J Pediatr. 2006;149(3):301-7.
10. Bell EF, Strauss RG, Widness JA, Mahoney LT, Mock DM, Seward VJ, et al. Randomized trial of liberal versus restrictive guidelines for red blood cell transfusion in preterm infants. Pediatrics. 2005;115(6):1685-91.
11. Bell EF. Transfusion thresholds for preterm infants: how low should we go? J Pediatr. 2006;149(3):287-9.
12. Chatterjee K, Sen A. Step-by-Step Blood Transfusion Services, 1st edition. New Delhi, India: Jaypee Brothers Medical Publishers Pvt Ltd; 2006. pp. 238-300.
13. Paul DA, Leef KH, Locke RG, Stefano JL. Transfusion volume in infants with very low birth weight: a randomized trial of 10 versus 20 mL/kg. J Pediatr Hematol Oncol. 2002;24(1):43-6.
14. Engelfriet CP, Reesink HW, Klein HG, Murphy MF, Pamphilon D, Devereux S, et al. International forum: granulocyte transfusions. Vox Sang. 2000;79(1):59-66.
15. Castle V, Andrew M, Kelton J, Giron D, Johnston M, Carter C, et al. Frequency and mechanism of neonatal thrombocytopenia. J Pediatr. 1986;108(5 Pt 1):749-55.
16. Josephson CD, Su LL, Christensen RD, Hillyer CD, Castillejo MI, Emory MR, et al. Platelet transfusion practices among neonatologists in the United States and Canada: results of a survey. Pediatrics. 2009;123(1):278-85.
17. Cremer M, Sola-Visner M, Roll S, Josephson CD, Yilmaz Z, Bührer C, et al. Platelet transfusions in neonates: practices in the United States vary significantly from those in Austria, Germany, and Switzerland. Transfusion. 2011;51(12):2634-41.
18. Stanworth SJ, Clarke P, Watts T, Ballard S, Choo L, Morris T, et al. Prospective, observational study of outcomes in neonates with severe thrombocytopenia. Pediatrics. 2009;124(5):e826-34.
19. Andrew M, Vegh P, Caco C, Kirpalani H, Jefferies A, Ohlsson A, et al. A randomized, controlled trial of platelet transfusions in thrombocytopenic premature infants. J Pediatr. 1993;123(2):285-91.
20. Murray NA, Howarth LJ, McCloy MP, Letsky EA, Roberts IA. Platelet transfusion in the management of severe thrombocytopenia in neonatal intensive care unit patients. Transfus Med. 2002;12(1):35-41.
21. Curley A, Venkatesh V, Stanworth S, Clarke P, Watts T, New H, et al. Platelets for neonatal transfusion— study 2: a randomised controlled trial to compare two different platelet count thresholds for prophylactic platelet transfusion to preterm neonates. Neonatology. 2014;106(2):102-6.
22. Gerday E, Baer VL, Lambert DK, Paul DA, Sola-Visner MC, Pysher TJ, et al. Testing platelet mass versus platelet count to guide platelet transfusions in the neonatal intensive care unit. Transfusion. 2009;49(10):2034-9.
23. Miller WJ, McCullough J, Balfour HH Jr, Haake RJ, Ramsay NK, Goldman A, et al. Prevention of cytomegalovirus infection following bone marrow transplantation: a randomized trial of blood product screening. Bone Marrow Transplant. 1991;7(3):227-34.

CHAPTER

41

Plasma and its Derivatives

Vivek Choudhury

INTRODUCTION

Neonates receiving intensive care are often transfused with blood products despite a lack of supporting evidence. Extremely low-birth-weight newborns remain the most heavily transfused group of patients with about 85% of them receiving a transfusion by the end of their hospital stay.[1] Use of blood products in neonates needs to be strictly regulated to avoid the inherent risks associated with transfusion.

Fresh frozen plasma (FFP), a blood component, has also been used frequently in neonates despite evidence for its use with most neonatal surveys reporting that almost half of FFP transfusions are used prophylactically.[2]

COAGULATION SYSTEM IN NEONATES

Coagulation system in neonates differs from the adult coagulation system in various ways. The activity of most coagulation factors is approximately 50% the adult levels at birth reaching adult levels by 6 months of age. This difference is more so for the vitamin K-dependent clotting factors, which are reduced further in preterm infants. The levels of components of the anticoagulant system (antithrombin, protein S, protein C) are also significantly lower at birth compared with adults. Fibrinogen levels in neonates are similar to adult ranges.[3]

Hemostasis in any individual is achieved with the complex interplay of vascular endothelium, platelets, waterfall coagulation cascade, anticoagulation mechanisms and the fibrinolytic system. A routine "coagulation" screen measures a component of these pathways and usually consists of an activated partial thromboplastin time (aPTT), prothrombin time (PT), fibrinogen levels and platelet count.

Few studies have looked into the reference ranges in the neonatal population. The study by Andrew et al.[4] reported results in term infants. With a similar methodology, a subsequent study assessed the clotting function in neonates from 30 weeks to 36 weeks gestation.[5] More recently, studies by Christensen et al.[6] sought to report the reference ranges for extreme preterms and infants below 34 weeks gestation. The results of all these studies across various gestations are shown in **Table 41.1**.

The results of standard coagulation tests in neonates would therefore vary from that of adult ranges. Therefore, the results should not be interpreted in isolation, but alongside reference ranges based on gestational age and postnatal age of the infant as well as review of bleeding history and other hemostatic markers, such as platelet count. Moreover, these tests have significant limitations as predictors of bleeding in any patient group, including neonates and the use of plasma or its derivatives has little effect on correcting the abnormal coagulation tests when mild and moderate results are noted.[7] FFP transfusions have been used prophylactically in neonates to prevent intraventricular hemorrhage in preterms or as a plasma expander but there is no evidence to support its effectiveness. On the contrary, a large randomized control trial (Northern Neonatal Nursing Initiative Trial Group) evaluating use of plasma to prevent intraventricular hemorrhage in preterm infants failed to show any benefit.[8]

Table 41.1 Reference ranges of common coagulation tests in neonates*

	<28 weeks	*28–34 weeks*	*30–36 weeks*	*Term infants*
PT (Sec), 95th percentile	>21	>21	>16	>16
aPTT (Sec), 95th percentile	>64	>57	>55	>55
Fibrinogen levels (g/dL), 5–95th percentile	0.71–5.35	0.87–4.70	2.25–3.41	1.50–3.73

Abbreviations: aPTT, activated partial thromboplastin time; PT, prothrombin time

*Reference ranges based on studies by Andrew et al. and Christensen et al.

Therefore, in clinical practice, prophylactic use of FFP in neonates with abnormal coagulation tests should be discouraged as they have poor predictive ability for bleeding. An appropriate transfusion policy is one that emphasizes its use in the event of clinical bleeding.[3]

PLASMA AND ITS DERIVATIVES

Fresh Frozen Plasma

Plasma that is recovered from whole blood or plasmapheresis from healthy human donors and frozen within a specific period of time after collection is referred as FFP.

Hemostasis efficacy and side effect profile are equivalent irrespective of whether FFP is prepared from units of whole blood or from plasmapheresis. The time to freezing after collection determines whether the product becomes FFP (frozen within 6–8 hours of collection) or F24 plasma (frozen within 24 hours of collection). Both products can be stored at -30°C or colder, and both are equivalent, although slightly lower factor VIII and factor V levels are present in F24 plasma. The term "frozen plasma" (FP) is used to encompass both these products and can be stored up to 12 months. To reduce the risk of complications associated with plasma transfusions, it is preferred that these products should be pathogen reduced. There are presently two methods of inactivating pathogens in plasma either treatment with methylene blue and light (MBFFP) or solvent detergent (SDFFP).[9] Pathogen-reduced plasma is currently not available in India.

Fresh frozen plasma can be used after thawing. Immediately after being thawed, the standard FFP contains near normal levels of many plasma proteins, including procoagulant and inhibitory components of the coagulation cascades, acute phase proteins, immunoglobulins and albumin. Once thawed, FFP should be used immediately but can be stored for up to 24 hours at 4°C.[9]

Cryoprecipitate

Cryoprecipitate is the cryoglobulin fraction prepared from FFP by thawing at 2–4°C. Undissolved cryoprecipitate is collected by centrifugation and resuspended in a reduced volume of plasma. It contains about 80–100 U of factor VIII in 10–25 mL of plasma, 300 mg of fibrinogen, von Willebrand factor and varying amounts of factor XIII.[9]

Cryoprecipitate can be stored for 12 months at –18°C or lower. Thawed cryoprecipitate can be stored for 6 hours at 2–6°C.

Other derivatives of plasma like prothrombin complex concentrates (PCCs) or activated factor VII are used very infrequently in neonates.

PLASMA TRANSFUSION GUIDELINES IN NEONATES

Transfusion guidelines in neonates are based on low level of evidence and as such there is dearth of recommendations from major societies. In 2004, the British Committee for Standards in Hematology updated its document on transfusion guidelines for neonates and older children and presently remains the basis for recommendations for blood component transfusions in neonates. In this document, the quality of evidence was used to grade the strength of recommendations. Apart from a few conditions where the use of FFP is not supported by results of controlled clinical studies, there was low level of evidence for usually recommended indications for FFP transfusion.[10]

These guidelines highlight that the use of plasma or its derivatives in neonates should be limited to few specific conditions but the lack of robust scientific evidence in the many clinical settings may lead to a wide variety of transfusion practices among neonatologists.

Clinical Use of Fresh Frozen Plasma in Neonates[10]

Use of Fresh Frozen Plasma Indicated

- Hemorrhagic disease of the newborn (HDN) with bleeding: Use FFP along with intravenous vitamin K
- At risk of bleeding (preterm, intubated, previous intraventricular hemorrhage or undergoing invasive procedure) along with significant coagulopathy (e.g. PT or aPTT > 1.5 times the normal)
- Bleeding neonates with abnormal coagulation tests or undergoing an invasive procedure should receive FFP as well as vitamin K
- Fresh-frozen plasma should only be used to replace single inherited clotting factor deficiencies if individual factor is not available or affordable
- Fresh-frozen plasma is indicated for demonstrable multifactor deficiencies associated with severe bleeding and/or disseminated intravascular coagulation (DIC).

(Shortening of prolonged clotting times is unpredictable and should be checked following administration. Neonates should only receive pathogen-reduced FFP [PRFFP] if available).

Use of Fresh Frozen Plasma Not Indicated

- Fresh-frozen plasma should never be used as a volume replacement in management of neonatal hypotension as it is not shown to be superior to crystalloids or colloids
- Prophylactic use in preterm infants to prevent periventricular hemorrhage (PVH) has been shown to confer no benefit and should therefore be avoided
- Polycythemia in neonates
- No conclusive data to support use of FFP in newborns with T-activation with low anti-T activity [e.g. necrotizing enterocolitis (NEC)]
- Fresh-frozen plasma has not shown to confer clinical benefit when given to neonates with severe sepsis to improve immune function
- No definitive evidence or lack of clinical benefit of use of FFP in DIC with no bleeding or its prophylactic use to prevent DIC and/or reduce transfusion requirements.

Cryoprecipitate

Cryoprecipitate is preferred over FFP because of its small volume while treating bleeding neonates with congenital factor deficiencies. However, it is important to note that cryoprecipitate contains factors VIII, XIII, von Willebrand factor and fibrinogen and as such it cannot be used for treating the more extensive coagulation factor deficiencies.

Use of Cryoprecipitate in Neonates

- Von Willebrand disease (vWD)
- Dysfibrinogenemia or afibrinogenemia
- Factor VIII deficiency
- Factor XIII deficiency.

Plasma and its Derivatives for Neonatal Transfusion: Practice Points

- Use blood group AB plasma or one that's compatible with the recipient's ABO red blood cell antigen for transfusion
- 10–20 mL/kg of FFP to be infused usually
- 5 mL/kg is the usual volume for cryoprecipitate.

ADVERSE EFFECTS WITH PLASMA TRANSFUSION

Complications associated with FFP may slightly differ from that compared with red cells and platelets with only few studies reporting the complications of FFP transfusions. Viral infections (such as HIV, hepatitis B virus, hepatitis C virus, parvovirus B19) have been reported, although these risks remain low with present technologies for screening infections in blood donations. Although anaphylaxis is rare, allergic reactions resulting in urticaria have been reported. Transfusion-related acute lung injury (TRALI) is a serious reaction and reported more commonly with FFP transfusions in comparison to other blood component therapy. Transfusion associated circulatory overload (TACO) is caused by high fluid volume infused within a short time and seems to be underreported following neonatal transfusions.[11]

CONCLUSION

Coagulation abnormalities are seen commonly in neonates and represent a clinically important problem. In comparison to older child or an adult, the coagulation system in neonates shows different levels of clotting factors and functionality. Only few neonatal trials have explored the management of coagulation abnormalities in terms of indications as well as therapeutic targets. An appropriate FFP transfusion strategy in neonates should be one that emphasizes its therapeutic use in the event of clinical bleeding rather than prophylactic use. Further well-designed clinical trials are needed for the development of evidence-based guidelines for plasma transfusions in neonates.

KEY POINTS

- NICUs should implement guidelines for use of FFP to minimize unnecessary transfusions.
- The use of FFP in neonates should be guided by presence of clinical bleeding and results of coagulation tests that are interpreted with appropriate gestational age references.
- Routine coagulation testing in NICU admissions is not indicated as it leads to increased FFP transfusions without evidence of benefit.

REFERENCES

1. Murray NA, Roberts IA. Neonatal transfusion practice. Arch Dis Child Fetal Neonatal Ed. 2004;89(2):F101-7.
2. Stanworth SJ, Grant-Casey J, Lowe D, Laffan M, New H, Murphy MF, et al. The use of fresh-frozen plasma in England: high levels of inappropriate use in adults and children. Transfusion. 2011;51(1):62-70.
3. Pal S, Curley A, Stanworth SJ. Interpretation of clotting tests in the neonate. Arch Dis Child Fetal Neonatal Ed. 2015;100(3):F270-4.
4. Andrew M, Paes B, Milner R, Johnston M, Mitchell L, Tollefsen DM, et al. Development of the human coagulation system in the healthy premature infant. Blood. 1988;72(5):1651-7.
5. Andrew M, Paes B, Milner R, Johnston M, Mitchell L, Tollefsen DM, et al. Development of the human coagulation system in the full-term infant. Blood. 1987;70(1):165-72.
6. Christensen RD, Baer VL, Lambert DK, Henry E, Ilstrup SJ, Bennett ST. Reference intervals for common coagulation tests of preterm infants (CME). Transfusion. 2014;54(3):627-32.
7. Segal JB, Dzik WH; Transfusion Medicine/Hemostasis Clinical Trials Network. Paucity of studies to support that abnormal coagulation test results predict bleeding in the setting of invasive procedures: an evidence-based review. Transfusion. 2005;45(9):1413-25.
8. Randomised trial of prophylactic early fresh-frozen plasma or gelatin or glucose in preterm babies: outcome at 2 years. Northern Neonatal Nursing Initiative Trial Group. Lancet. 1996;348(9022):229-32.
9. Poterjoy BS, Josephson CD. Platelets, frozen plasma, and cryoprecipitate: what is the clinical evidence for their use in the neonatal intensive care unit? Semin Perinatol. 2009;33(1):66-74.
10. Gibson BE, Todd A, Roberts I, Pamphilon D, Rodeck C, Bolton-Maggs P, et al. Transfusion guidelines for neonates and older children. Br J Haematol. 2004;124(4) 433-53.
11. Stainsby D, Jones H, Wells AW, Gibson B, Cohen H; SHOT Steering Group. Adverse outcomes of blood transfusion in children: analysis of UK reports to the serious hazards of transfusion scheme 1996-2005. Br J Haematol. 2008;141(1):73-9.

CHAPTER 42

Technical Aspects of Blood and Blood Components Transfusion including Leukodepletion and Irradiation

Rajesh B Sawant, Anand Deshpande

INTRODUCTION

We have been successful in achieving good quality as well as safety in the various aspects of blood donation, component preparation and their testing. However, the various aspects related to transport and bedside practices of blood administration have remained neglected and not standardized since a long time. The process of transfusion includes pretransfusion blood sampling, the prescription, requesting, collection and administration of blood components to adults, children and neonates. If an assured and unambiguous audit trail is to be achieved in transfusion, it requires complete documentation at every stage of the process. Clear communication between all staffs involved in the transfusion process, including all clinical and laboratory staff and other support staff, is essential. Training and competency assessment is needed at regular intervals for all staff involved in the blood transfusion process.

The Serious Hazards of Transfusion (SHOT) scheme has continually shown that "wrong blood in tube" episodes are a frequently reported transfusion hazard, which are mainly due to human error leading to misidentification of the patient during blood sampling, blood component collection and delivery or administration, and can lead to life-threatening hemolytic transfusion reactions and other significant morbidity. We have attempted to address a few most important and technical aspects related to blood administration in the following section.

SOME TECHNICAL ASPECTS ABOUT THE ADMINISTRATION OF BLOOD AND BLOOD COMPONENTS

Blood or components may be administered safely through a peripheral line or most of the central venous access devices. Problems may occur with some peripherally inserted central catheters (PICCs) with small tubing diameters for blood or platelet administration leading to slow flow rates and clogging. Standard 18–24-gauge ultra-thin needles and catheters are used. But the smaller the gauge, the slower is the flow rate. The 18–20 gauge size is recommended for adults. The 22–24 gauge or larger is recommended for pediatric patients. The vein size and integrity, and the rate of infusion should be considered while deciding, which cannula size is to be used. An infusion set containing an integral filter of 170–200 microns (standard clot screen filter) must be used for whole blood, red cells, platelets, plasma and cryoprecipitate. This filter removes clots and small clumps of debris that may form during collection and storage of the component. When blood is being administered by syringe to small infants or neonates the blood shall be drawn into the syringe via a 170–200 micron filter. The component (particularly red cells and whole blood) should be mixed thoroughly by gentle inversion before use. If multiple blood components need to be administered sequentially through the same set, one must ensure that the components are ABO incompatible. After a red cell component or plasma transfusion, a new blood administration set should be used to transfuse platelets since the red cells/debris trapped in the filter would trap the platelets. Blood administration sets should normally be changed after a maximum of 6 hours. In the massive transfusion setting, the blood administration set may be changed at the discretion of the nurse or doctor administering the blood, i.e. if they become blocked or have been used to transfuse multiple units. Intravenous (IV) fluids should not be infused through the same blood component administration set as the fluid may be incompatible with the blood in line. A lumen of a multilumen central catheter can be used for transfusion while the other lumen or lumina are in use. If drugs need to be administered via the same IV line as a transfusion, the transfusion should be stopped and the line flushed with normal saline. Administer the drug, flush the line with normal saline and then restart the transfusion. This should not result in the transfusion of red cells exceeding 4 hours from the time of their issue. Never add any infusion solution or drug or medication to a blood component as it may lead to hemolysis or clotting. Calcium (e.g. haemaccel/gelofusine) should never be given with blood cell components collected in an anticoagulant containing citrate as they may cause clotting of the infusion line. 5% dextrose in water or hypotonic sodium solutions may cause red cells to hemolyze.

The only fluids that can be given concurrently through the same IV device as a red cell transfusion are ABO compatible plasma, plasma protein fractions, 4% albumin or normal saline.

Infusion Devices

Electronic volumetric pumps are designed to deliver fluids, including blood and components, at specified flow rates. The manufacturer of the pump chosen for transfusion shall be able to demonstrate that the pump does not cause hemolysis or damage to blood components.

If the manufacturer has documented safety of use with red blood cells or other blood components, IV infusion pumps may be used by following the manufacturer's instructions. When an electronic pump is used for transfusion of red cells, the pump tubing shall incorporate a 170–200 micron filter. The use of electronic volumetric pumps may be limited to transfusion to patients via a central venous catheter (including PICC and implanted "ports") where "free-flow" cannot be guaranteed; or transfusion to small pediatric patients—where very slow rates are required.

External pressure devices make it possible to administer a unit of red cell within a few minutes. These should only be used in an emergency situation and with a large gauge venous access needle. The external pressure device should have a gauge to measure the pressure, and should exert the pressure evenly over the entire bag. It should never exceed 300 mm Hg. It must be monitored at all times when in use.

Syringes

If syringes are used for transfusion, incorporating an in-line filter (170–200 micron) is a must. The syringes should have lever-lock connections, should be single use only and should be discarded appropriately. There should be a label attached to the syringe showing date and time of preparation and expiry date and time. Also, it should have identical donor or patient information as the original pack from which the component was drawn. The syringe is filled by drawing fluid from the primary container thereby creating an open system. This creates potential problems of sterility and storage. In addition, when blood is removed from the primary pack, the risk of mislabeling and patient misidentification is increased. As an alternative, the use of T-connectors allows continuous attachment of the syringe to the primary pack. Syringe drivers are devices in which a standard syringe is placed on a housing that depresses the plunger at a given rate. Syringe drivers are useful for transfusion to neonates and for continuous infusion of coagulation factors such as factor VIII or factor IX.

At the end of the transfusion, the empty bag should be discarded according to the hospital policy for disposal of clinical waste. The blood transfusion compatibility report form should be filed in the patient's clinical records.

Warming of Blood

Patients who benefitted from warmed blood include adults and children receiving massive transfusion, infants requiring exchange transfusion and patients with clinically significant high-titer cold agglutinins, active in vitro at 37°C. Blood warmers are indicated when the flow rate more than 50 mL/kg/hour in adults, more than 15 mL/kg/hour in children and for exchange transfusions in infants. When transfusing patients with clinically significant cold agglutinins, warming of blood units is a prerequisite (drugs must not be added to blood under any circumstance in these patients).

Blood warmers must be subjected to regular servicing and used in accordance with the manufacturer's instructions. Blood components must not be warmed by improvisations such as putting the pack into hot water, in a microwave, or on a radiator, as uncontrolled heating can damage the contents of the pack. Red blood cells and plasma exposed to temperatures over 40°C may cause severe transfusion reactions in the recipients.

The patient should be informed in a timely manner before transfusion takes place about the risks and benefits of blood transfusion and the alternatives to transfusion, which are available (e.g. preoperative iron therapy, intraoperative cell salvage and postoperative cell salvage). Patients should be made aware of the importance of the correct blood component transfused and the need to report any adverse events immediately. It is useful to provide a patient information leaflet, which deals with the above issues.

The patient must be positively identified by being asked their full name and date of birth, if they are capable of responding. Either one or two members of staff (depending on hospital policy) must have the responsibility for carrying out the identity check of the patient and the unit of blood at the patient's bedside. Patients undergoing transfusion must wear an identification wristband with their full name, date of birth and patient identification number. The details on the wristband must be checked and be identical with the details on the blood bag. The blood group on the unit must be compatible with the blood group of the patient as indicated on the blood bag label. The blood group may not be identical but it must be compatible and in cases where the blood groups may differ, a specific comment should have been made on the compatibility form to indicate that the blood is compatible. The unit must be checked to ensure it has not passed its expiry date, shows no signs of leakage, unusual color or hemolysis (or clumping or cloudiness in the case of platelet transfusions). The unit must be checked for compliance with any special requirement on the prescription chart, e.g. leukodepleted or gamma irradiated. The person who has carried out the above checks must sign the blood transfusion compatibility form and the prescription chart. If any discrepancy is found during the bedside checks, then the unit should not be transfused to the patient and the transfusion laboratory should be informed immediately. The unit and compatibility form should be returned to the transfusion laboratory.

Start and finish times of each unit should be recorded so that any adverse events can be correctly identified and reported. Before the start of each unit of blood or component and at the end of each transfusion episode, vital signs should be measured and recorded. These observations should be recorded separately from the routine observations so that they are clearly related to the transfusion. Patient's temperature and pulse should be recorded 15 minutes after the start of each unit of blood or component. Visual observation of the patient is the best way of assessing their condition during the transfusion. Further, observations are necessary only if the patient becomes unwell or shows signs of a transfusion reaction. Unconscious patients are more difficult to monitor for signs of a transfusion reaction. Routine observations should continue and transfusion reactions should be considered, if there is a change or deterioration in the patient's condition. It is good practice to avoid transfusing patients out of routine working hours unless clinically essential. Transfusions should take place in clinical areas where patients can be readily observed throughout the procedure and can alert ward staff if they experience any adverse effects.

Documentation

A permanent record of the administration of the blood or components and any relevant observations should be kept in the patient's clinical records. The blood transfusion compatibility report signed by the person checking and administering the transfusion should be kept in the patient's clinical records. The blood transfusion prescription chart and the nursing observations made during the transfusion episode should be retained in the patient's notes. A record of the indication for the transfusion and the impact of the transfusion (i.e. whether the transfusion achieved the desired result) should be kept in the patient's notes. A record of any adverse events occurring during or after the transfusion and the management of those events should also be kept in the patient's notes. The final fate of the blood bag or transfusion episode must be recorded and the transfusion laboratory must have a reporting system in place so that they are adequately informed.

LEUKOCYTE DEPLETION AND GAMMA IRRADIATION OF BLOOD COMPONENTS

Leukocyte Depletion of Cellular Blood Components

Leukocytes are in general not meant for transfusions but are invariably present as contaminants in all blood components and they mediate adverse reactions like febrile nonhemolytic transfusion reactions (FNHTRs), alloimmunization, transmission of infectious diseases [e.g. cytomegalovirus (CMV)], graft-versus-host disease (GVHD), transfusion-related acute lung injury and immunomodulation. Exclusive use of leukodepleted components can decrease alloimmunization, CMV transmission and FNHTRs. Improvement in the extent of WBC reduction has been achievable in RBCs and platelets due to recent advances in filtration as well as apheresis techniques so that components with less than 10^6 contaminating WBCs can be readily available. In addition, studies have examined the importance of the timing of WBC reduction. Cytokines released from WBCs during component storage may either directly or indirectly mediate FNHTRs in transfusion recipients by acting on recipient cells and releasing pyrogens. This can be prevented by prestorage leukodepletion. Blood components should be preferably leukodepleted before storage by the transfusion laboratory. Moreover, poststorage leukodepletion is ineffective and not quality controlled; further supporting the use of prestorage leukodepleted components. In addition, severe hypotension and respiratory distress have been observed after transfusion of components leukodepleted using negatively charged filters at the bedside (i.e. poststorage), further limiting their utility. Interestingly, this reaction may be related to bradykinin release, which is of particular concern in patients on angiotensin-converting enzyme (ACE) inhibitors.

Cellular blood component therapy is associated with side effect of alloimmunization, which can lead to significant patient morbidity. This is particularly so in patients requiring prolonged blood product support such as the leukemia and stem cell transplant patients.

Clinical trials have suggested that leukodepletion of cellular blood products reduces post-transfusion alloimmunization, which is a major factor contributing to reduced efficacy of platelet transfusions as measured by posttransfusion platelet count increments. Alloimmune destruction of platelets is mediated by expression of foreign class I histocompatibility locus antigen (HLA) on these cells but the presence of contaminating leukocytes enhances the immunogenicity of platelet products in transfusion recipients.

When alloimmunized patients require platelet transfusion, platelet components have to be harvested from HLA-compatible donors. Procurement of these HLA-matched platelets is not only logistically complicated and costly, but is also often ineffective at circumventing refractoriness. Prevention of the alloimmunized state would be a more attractive alternative. A variety of clinical studies have confirmed to some extent that removal of leukocytes from cellular blood products might achieve the goal of preventing alloimmunization. However, most studies have used poststorage, bedside filtration methods rather than prestorage techniques, which may be still more effective in preventing this complication, and have focused on patients receiving chemotherapy for acute leukemia.

Prestorage leukodepletion is performed in the blood center using standard operating procedures and quality controls, which should result in less failure of leukodepletion, which occurs in 5% or more of blood components filtered at the bedside. In addition, prestorage leukodepletion will minimize the transfusion of potentially immunogenic white blood cell (WBC) fragments, which accumulate during storage and may not be removed by filtration.

There is controversy as to whether the theoretical benefit of prestorage leukodepletion will be realized in clinical practice and whether the cost of this procedure is justified. At present, the effect of leukocyte reduction on reducing the incidence of platelet alloimmunization in multitransfused leukemia and stem cell transplant patients in our set-up is unknown (not reported). Furthermore, it would be interesting to study if these patients who are already potentially sensitized to foreign HLA antigens by prior pregnancy or transfusion would derive any benefit from prestorage leukodepletion in their response to subsequent platelet transfusions.

Gamma Irradiation of Blood Components

The reason for irradiating blood and blood components is to prevent GVHD by decreasing the number of viable T- lymphocytes. GVHD occurs when viable T-lymphocytes in transfused blood or blood components engraft, multiply, and react against the tissues of the recipient. GVHD may be seen when blood components are transfused to immunocompromised recipients, such as bone marrow transplant patients, patients with malignancies receiving aggressive chemotherapy and persons with congenital immune deficiency syndromes.

While some forms of immune suppression on the part of the recipient usually sets the stage for GVHD in marrow transplant or transfusion recipients, a number of cases of fatal transfusion associated graft-versus-host disease (TA-GVHD) have been described in apparently immunologically normal patients who received directed blood donations from first degree relatives. GVHD may occur more frequently in cases of family member transfusions than in random donor transfusions because family members are more likely to share the same HLA haplotypes than people in the population at large. In many of these cases, it was found that the donors were HLA homozygous for one of the recipient's haplotypes. In such situations, the recipient's lymphocytes do not recognize HLA antigens on the donor's lymphocytes as foreign, and the donor's lymphocytes can survive indefinitely and may react immunologically against the recipient's tissues, which express a heterologous haplotype. This mechanism has been invoked as the cause of postoperative erythroderma, a disease of transfused cardiac surgery patients that is well described in the Japanese literature. The genetic homogeneity of the Japanese population increases the likelihood that donors will be homozygous for an extended HLA haplotype and contributes to the apparent increased risk of the disease in Japan. While less well reported outside Japan, many similar cases have been observed. Second-degree relatives pose a significant risk as well. The risks from directed donor blood have been calculated and rates similar to their predictions now are emerging.

RISK FACTORS ASSOCIATED WITH OCCURRENCE OF TRANSFUSION ASSOCIATED GRAFT-VERSUS-HOST DISEASE

The risk factors for TA-GVHD can be summarized as follows:

- *Viable and immunocompetent lymphocyte content of the component transfused*: Due to the higher numbers of viable and immunocompetent lymphocytes in freshly collected blood, fresh blood has been found to be associated with higher incidence of TA-GVHD. Many reports have confirmed presence of donor lymphocytes (chimerism) in immunocompetent recipients following transfusion of unirradiated blood. The viability of these lymphocytes decreases with storage.
- *Level of immunocompetence in the transfusion recipient*: The risk of TA-GVHD depends mainly on age, level of immunosuppression and history of prior transfusions. Transfusion recipients with lower immune-competence are unable to eliminate donor lymphocytes by allogeneic response and hence are at an increased risk of GVHD. The transfusion-related immunomodulatory effect leads to significant immunosuppression in the recipients of multiple transfusions and thus increases the risk of TA-GVHD after first blood transfusion.
- *HLA disparity*: After transfusion, the immunocompetent lymphocytes from the donor unit are cleared from the recipients circulation by the T-cells and NK cells of the recipient. In transfusions where partial HLA identity between the donor and the recipient exists, the donor lymphocytes escape attack by alloreactive T-cells or NK cells from the recipient and consequently increase the risk of TA-GVHD. The best supporting data for the above occurrence is from Japan where relatively homogeneous population results in higher probability of partial HLA identity contributing to the highest incidence of TA-GVHD. By similar analogy, when the donor is a first or second-degree relative of the patient, and the same blood is intended for transfusion to the patient (directed blood donation), there is an increased possibility of HLA-haploid entity, which may lead to TA-GVHD.

INDICATIONS FOR IRRADIATION OF BLOOD AND BLOOD COMPONENTS

Established Indications

- Intrauterine transfusion recipients
- Neonatal exchange transfusion recipients
- Bone marrow transplant recipients
- Congenital cellular immunodeficiency syndrome patients
- Premature newborns (less than 1,200 g)
- Patients receiving HLA-matched components or directed donations from first or second-degree relatives
- Granulocyte concentrates for transfusion
- Patients with certain solid tumors such as neuroblastoma and glioblastoma
- Patients with Hodgkin's disease or non-Hodgkin's lymphoma.

Indications Under Review

- Solid organ transplant recipients
- Patients with hematologic malignancies such as acute leukemia
- Patients receiving cross-match compatible platelets
- Term newborns on extracorporeal membrane oxygenators.

No Established Indications

- Patients with aplastic anemia not receiving immunosuppressive therapy
- Full-term neonates without other risks

- Patients with acquired immune deficiency syndrome (AIDS) or human immunodeficiency virus (HIV)
- Most patients receiving chemotherapy.

BLOOD AND BLOOD COMPONENTS TO BE IRRADIATED

All cellular blood components should be irradiated before transfusion to recipients who are prone for TA-GVHD. Fresh-frozen plasma, cryoprecipitate and coagulation factor concentrates need not be irradiated since they contain very few viable lymphocytes.

Approximately about 10^3 WBCs are capable of causing TA-GVHD. Methods of producing leukocyte-reduced blood and blood components (including washing, filtration and centrifugation) reduce the number of viable T-lymphocytes, but may not decrease the risk of TA-GVHD as effectively as gamma irradiation.

All leukodepleted blood components to be transfused to susceptible individuals therefore need to be irradiated.

At present, gamma irradiation of blood components is achieved using radioactive isotopes, such as Cesium-137 ($t_{1/2}$ = 30.17 years) or Cobalt-60 ($t_{1/2}$ = 5.27 years).

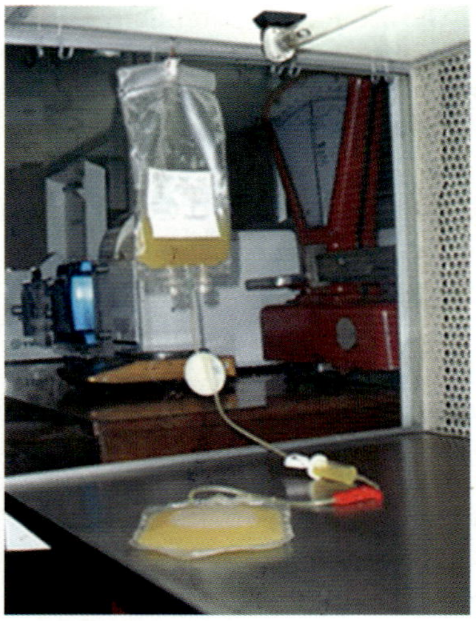

Figure 42.1 Leukodepletion filter for platelets

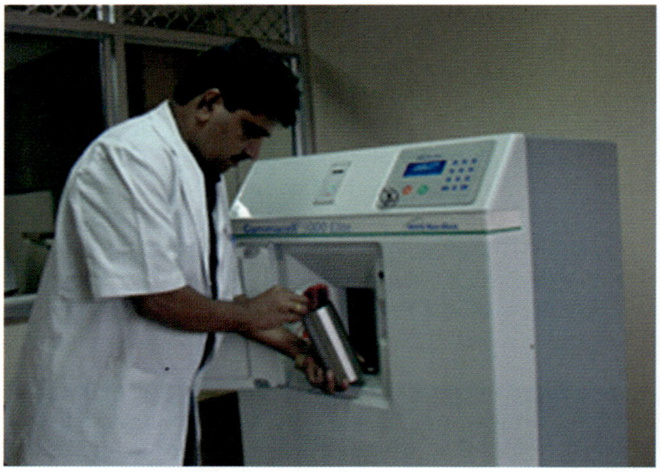

Figure 42.2 Gammacell Elite blood irradiator

Irradiation and WBC Reduction

When used alone, WBC reduction is not completely effective in preventing the development of TA-GVHD. Indeed, there are several reports in the literature about patients who developed TA-GVHD after WBC reduction by filtration. A leukodepleted unit has to be gamma irradiated also for prevention of TA-GVHD in susceptible patients.

Storage of Red Cells after Irradiation

The US Food and Drug Association (FDA) guidelines call for a 28 days maximum storage period for red cells after irradiation, irrespective of the day of storage on which the treatment was performed with the provision that the total storage time cannot exceed that for nonirradiated red cells. The European guidelines recommend irradiation only up to 14th day of the shelf life of red cells and their postirradiation storage for maximum 14 days. Platelets can be irradiated at any point of time during their shelf life and stored postirradiation up to their usual expiry date. In routine practice, blood units are gamma irradiated just prior to their issue for transfusion to the patient.

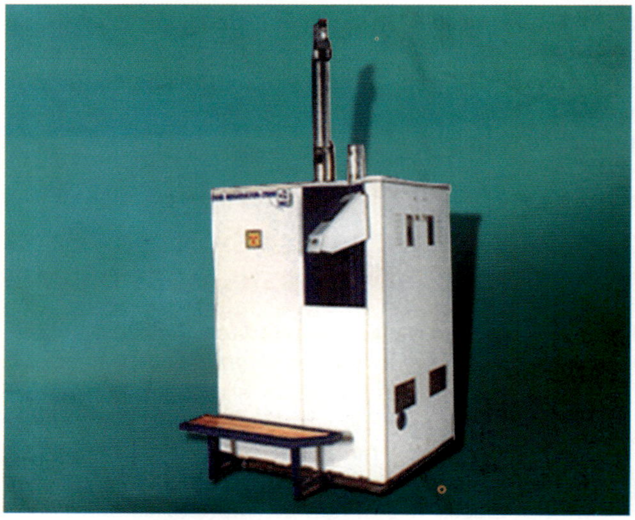

Figure 42.3 Indigenous blood irradiator BI 2000

DOSIMETRY OF BLOOD IRRADIATOR (FIGS 42.1 TO 42.4)

The dose of irradiation delivered should be 2,500 cGy targeted to the central portion of the container and the minimum dose should be 1,500 cGy at any other point. The time required to deliver the dose should be based on the radiation intensity of the source. The decay of the source should be calculated according to manufacturer's instructions. US FDA currently recommends recalibration of the source annually for Cesium-137 and semiannually for Cobalt-60.

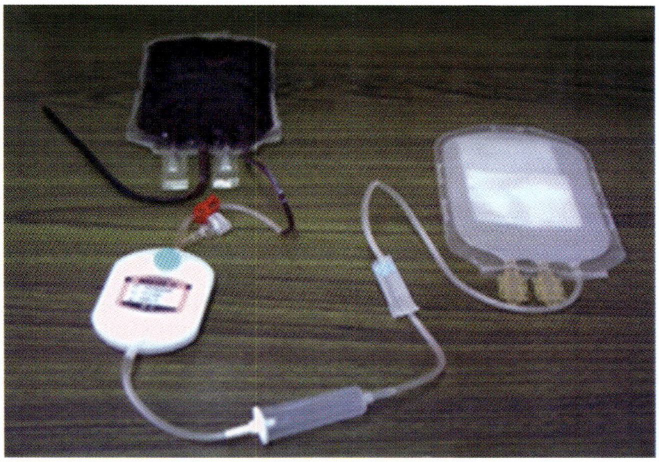

Figure 42.4 Leukodepletion filter for red cell components

The SOP should indicate the maximum number of units of blood or blood components that can be irradiated at one time, which may be dictated by the device manufacturer's procedure and based on the firm's validation data.

At no time should the total irradiation dose exceed 5,000 cGy to any portion of the container.

The irradiation of cellular blood components at the dose of 15 Gy prior to transfusion may be insufficient to prevent TA-GVHD in heavily immunosuppressed patients.

The UK guidelines for blood irradiation state that all parts of the blood bags should receive at least 25 Gy. These guidelines are based on the work of Pelszynski et al. (1994) and Luban and DePalma (1996) who demonstrated that 25 Gy achieves a 5 log depletion of T-cells in a T-cell clonogenic assay.

Indicators

An irradiation indicator should be used with each irradiated batch. There should be procedures for the quality control of the indicator system in use, which should include, but are not limited to storage of indicator, verification that the indicator has not been exposed to unacceptable temperatures, and explanation of expected results for each new lot (comparison with the old lot) and corrective action. There must be documentation of such quality control.

Labeling

The immediate container of blood and blood components that has been irradiated should be permanently labeled as irradiated.

Shelf Life

The outdating period for red blood cell products should not be more than 28 days from the date of irradiation, but should not exceed the expiry date of the original product. The shelf life of platelets need not change after irradiation, since they are not adversely affected by irradiation.

Quality Assurance

The following procedures should be used to validate the irradiation system.

Process Validation

Validation is performed using a dosimetry system. The dosimetry system should provide a dose map. The medium for dosimetry should be one that closely resembles blood, e.g. water or some types of acrylic. Using predetermined parameters, validation should include measuring the amount of irradiation absorbed by the product. Validation should be performed on a fully loaded canister to obtain the maximum and minimum dose of irradiation to which the blood and blood components will be subjected. The process should monitor the temperature of the blood products during the irradiation procedure to ensure that the time the blood products spend out of a controlled environment is limited to prevent the warming of the red cell products above 10 °C and platelet products above 24°C.

Quality Control

Each Day of Use

The timer on the irradiator should be compared visually against a certified stopwatch and the results of the comparison should be documented. If a moving turntable is part of the equipment, a visual check of the turntable should be made to determine that it is rotating. Observations should be documented.

Monthly: If the irradiator in use has a backup timer, the two timers should be checked monthly using a certified stopwatch. Observations should be documented.

Periodically: Periodic check for radiation leakage with a Geiger counter or using a wipe test is a must, though blood irradiators are considered safe.

Record-keeping: Records must document the significant steps in irradiation of each component, including the identification number of the unit, duration of the irradiation procedure, dose of irradiation, date, time, site of irradiation, and the identity of the person performing the irradiation. The quality assurance personnel should review these records periodically.

CONCLUSION

Administering blood components and caring for the transfused patient is a task routinely performed by resident doctors and nurses, and it is associated with a lot of risks. Errors commonly occur in patient identification, sample labeling, documentation, verbal requests and the final bedside checking of blood. Care and monitoring of the transfused patient is also of paramount importance. Training of all concerned staff in procedure of bedside blood administration practices and handling the operational risks of blood transfusion shall go a long way in ensuring transfusion safety in our hospitals.

KEY POINTS

- Decision to transfuse blood components should be communicated to the patient and documented appropriately.
- Accurate patient identification and pre-transfusion sample labeling are critical requirements for ensuring transfusion safety.
- Consent for transfusion is required by standards as well as regulation in many countries.
- Addition of medication to blood components during transfusion is not recommended.
- Warming of blood prior to routine transfusions is not necessary.
- Checking the identity of unconscious/compromised patient prior to any transfusion should be done extra-carefully.
- Ensure that the right patient gets the right amount of transfusion of the right component at the right rate and time.
- Gamma irradiation and leukocyte depletion are special processes to prevent transfusion associated graft versus host disease and leukocyte-mediated adverse effects, respectively.

RECOMMENDED FURTHER READING

Technical Aspects of Blood and Blood Components Transfusion

1. Birch C, Hogan C, Mahoney G. Co-administration of drugs and blood products. Anaesth Intensive Care. 2001:29(2):137-40.
2. Blest A, Roberts M, Murdock J, Watson D, Brunskill S. How often should a red blood cell administration set be changed while a patient is being transfused? A commentary and review of the literature. Transfus Med. 2008;18(2):121-33.
3. Friedman MT, Elbrahim A. Adequacy of physician documentation of red blood cell transfusion and correlation with assessment of transfusion appropriateness. Arch Pathol Lab Med. 2006;130(4):474-9.
4. Serious Hazards of Transfusion (SHOT) scheme (1996-2008). SHOT Annual reports 1996-2008. SHOT office. Manchester. [online] Available from www.shotuk.org/home.htm. [Accessed October, 2016].
5. The administration of blood and blood components and the management of transfused patient. British Committee for Standards in Haematology, Blood Transfusion Task Force. Royal College of Nursing and the Royal College of Surgeons of England. Transfus Med. 1999;9(3):227-38.
6. Watson D, Murdock J, Dorée C, Murphy M, Roberts M, Blest A, et al. Blood transfusion administration-one- or two-person checks: which is the safest method? Transfusion. 2008;48(4):783-9.
7. Yousef HM, Padmore RF, Neurath DD, Rock GA. The effect of patient-controlled analgesia on coadministered red blood cells. Transfusion. 2006;46(3):372-6.

Leukodepletion

1. Andreu G, Dewailly J, Leberre C, Quarre MC, Bidet ML, Tardivel R, et al. Prevention of HLA immunization with leukocyte-poor packed red cells and platelet concentrates obtained by filtration. Blood. 1988;72(3):964-9.
2. Blajchman MA, Bardossy L, Carmen RA, Goldman M, Heddle NM, Singal DP. An animal model of allogeneic donor platelet refractoriness: the effect of the time of leukodepletion. Blood. 1992;79(5):1371-5.
3. Leukocyte reduction and ultraviolet B irradiation of platelets to prevent alloimmunization and refractoriness to platelet transfusions. The Trial to Reduce Alloimmunization to Platelets Study Group. N Engl J Med. 1997;337(26):1861-9.
4. Novotny VM, van Doorn R, Witvliet MD, Claas FH, Brand A. Occurrence of allogeneic HLA and non-HLA antibodies after transfusion of prestorage filtered platelets and red blood cells: a prospective study. Blood. 1995;85(7):1736-41.
5. Oksanen K, Kekomäki R, Ruutu T, Koskimies S, Myllylä G. Prevention of alloimmunization in patients with acute leukemia by use of white cell-reduced blood components: a randomized trial. Transfusion. 1991;31(7):588-94.
6. Schiffer CA, Dutcher JP, Aisner J, Hogge D, Wiernik PH, Reilly JP. A randomized trial of leukocyte-depleted platelet transfusion to modify alloimmunization in patients with leukemia. Blood. 1983;62(4):815-20.
7. Sintnicolaas K, Van Marwijk Kooij M, van Prooijen HC, van Dijk BA, van Putten WL, Claas FH, et al. Leukocyte depletion of random single-donor platelet transfusions does not prevent secondary human leukocyte antigen-alloimmunization and refractoriness: a randomized prospective study. Blood. 1995;85(3):824-8.
8. Sniecinski I, O'Donnell MR, Nowicki B, Hill LR. Prevention of refractoriness and HLA-alloimmunization using filtered blood products. Blood. 1988;71(5):1402-7.
9. Van Marwijk Kooy M, van Prooijen HC, Moes M, Bosma-Stants I, Akkerman JW. Use of leukocyte-depleted platelet concentrates for the prevention of refractoriness and primary HLA alloimmunization: a prospective, randomized trial. Blood. 1991;77(1):201-5.
10. Williamson LM, Wimperis JZ, Williamson P, Copplestone JA, Gooi HC, Morgenstern GR, et al. Bedside filtration of blood products in the prevention of HLA alloimmunization—a prospective, randomized study. Alloimmunisation Study Group. Blood. 1994;83(10):3028-35.

Gamma Irradiation of Blood Components

1. Anderson KC, Goodnough LT, Sayers M, Pisciotto PT, Kurtz SR, Lane TA, et al. Variation in blood component irradiation practice: implications for prevention of transfusion-associated graft-versus-host disease. Blood. 1991;77(10):2096-102.
2. Asai T, Inaba S, Ohto H, Osada K, Suzuki G, Takahashi K, et al. Guidelines for irradiation of blood and blood components to prevent post-transfusion graft-vs.-host disease in Japan. Transfus Med. 2000;10(4):315-20.
3. Chang H, Voralia M, Bali M, Sher GD, Branch DR. Irreversible loss of donor blood leucocyte activation may explain a paucity of transfusion-associated graft-versus-host disease from stored blood. Br J Haematol. 2000;111(1):146-56.
4. Guidelines on gamma irradiation of blood components for the prevention of transfusion-associated graft-versus-host disease. Prepared by the BCSH Blood transfusion task force. Transfus Med. 1996;6:261-71.
5. Kanter MH. Transfusion-associated graft-versus-host disease: do transfusions from second-degree relatives pose a greater risk than those from first-degree relatives? Transfusion. 1992;32(4):323-7.

6. Leitman SF. Dose, dosimetry, and quality improvement of irradiated blood components. Transfusion. 1993;33(6):447-9.
7. Luban NL, DePalma L. Transfusion-associated graft-versus-host disease in the neonate-expanding the spectrum of disease. Transfusion. 1996;36(2):101-3.
8. Moroff G, Luban NL. The irradiation of blood and blood components to prevent graft-versus-host disease: technical issues and guidelines. Transfus Med Rev. 1997;11(1):15-26.
9. Ohto H, Anderson KC. Are guidelines for use of gamma irradiation for the prevention of transfusion-associated graft-versus-host disease adequate for newborns? Transfus Med. 1997;7(2):172-3.
10. Pelszynski MM, Moroff G, Luban NL, Taylor BJ, Quinones RR. Effect of gamma irradiation of red blood cell units on T-cell inactivation as assessed by limiting dilution analysis: implications for preventing transfusion-associated graft-versus-host disease. Blood. 1994;83(6):1683-9.
11. Sakakibara T, Ida T, Mannouji E, Kikuchi T, Tatsuno K, Kawase M, et al. Post-transfusion graft-versus-host disease following open heart surgery; report of six cases. J Cardiovasc Surg (Torino). 1989;30(4):687-91.
12. Thaler M, Shamiss A, Orgad S, Huszar M, Nussinovitch N, Meisel S, et al. The role of blood from HLA-homozygous donors in fatal transfusion-associated graft-versus-host disease after open-heart surgery. N Engl J Med. 1989;321(1):25-8.
13. Wagner FF, Flegel WA. Transfusion associated graft-versus-host disease: risk due to homozygous HLA haplotypes. Transfusion. 1995;35(4):284-91.

CHAPTER 43

Risk of Transfusion in Fetus and Neonate

Sanjeev Chetry, Kumar Ankur, Avijeet Yadav

INTRODUCTION

Fetal and neonatal medicine is a field with many new procedures and techniques. In many fetal and neonatal conditions, transfusions of blood products are life-saving. Currently, most of the protocols used with fetuses and newborns are expert based rather than evidence based.

INTRAUTERINE TRANSFUSION

Fetal anemia is a serious complication of pregnancy that may result from immune-associated conditions with rhesus D (RhD) sensitization being the most common cause. There are also nonimmune etiologic factors of fetal anemia such as parvovirus B19 infection, fetomaternal hemorrhage (FMH), homozygous thalassemia and placental chorioangioma **(Box 43.1)**.[1-4]

Fetal anemia, depending on severity, could cause increased cardiac output, tissue hypoxia, lactic acidosis, fetal hydrops and eventually intrauterine death.

Hemolytic disease of the fetus or newborn (HDFN) secondary to red cell alloimmunization is characterized by severe fetal anemia. However, with introduction of intravenous RhD immunoglobulin (IVIG) prophylaxis in 1968, it has dramatically decreased the incidence of hemolytic disease from 2% to 0.1%. Antibodies to other red cell antigens of the Rh blood group system and antigens of nonrhesus blood group systems (Kell, Duffy, etc.) may also be implicated in HDFN.

Parvovirus B19 infection accounts for about 27% of cases of nonimmune hydrops in anatomically normal fetuses, and fetal anemia usually occurs with infection in the second and third trimesters.[4] Parvovirus B19 causes inhibition of erythropoiesis at the late normoblast stage and also thrombocytopenia.

Box 43.1 Causes of fetal anemia

- Rh-isoimmunization
- Parvovirus B19 infection
- Fetomaternal hemorrhage
- Homozygous thalassemia
- Placental chorioangioma

Fetomaternal hemorrhage is a rare but severe pregnancy complication with an unexpected onset that can lead to severe fetal anemia, hydrops and fetal death (perinatal mortality ranges from 33% to 50%).[5]

Placenta chorioangiomas are benign tumors of the placenta that complicate 1% of pregnancies and may cause fetal anemia, hydrops and fetal death.[2]

EVALUATION OF FETAL ANEMIA

Previously standard evaluation of fetuses at risk of moderate and severe fetal anemia used to be based on invasive procedures such as amniocentesis to evaluate bilirubin levels in the amniotic fluid and cordocentesis for direct determination of fetal blood count.

Nowadays noninvasive evaluation with serial ultrasound monitoring and indirect Coombs maternal titers is included in the standard monitoring of these pregnancies.

Several ultrasound parameters have been evaluated as predictors of fetal anemia, but none of them could reliably distinguish mild from severe anemia with the exception of fetal ascites, which is compatible with advanced disease and severe anemia, i.e. hematocrit (HCT) 15% or hemoglobin (Hb) 5 g/dL.[6-9] Evaluating the peak systolic velocity in the middle cerebral artery (MCA-PSV) is now considered to be the most reliable tool to provide sensitive prediction of the severity of fetal anemia.

MANAGEMENT OF FETAL ANEMIA

Intrauterine transfusion (IUT) for fetuses with severe anemia is the main therapeutic intervention in affected pregnancies and represents one of the greater achievements of fetal therapy associated with survival rates of more than 90% in nonhydropic fetuses.[10]

The aims of IUT are:

- To prevent or treat fetal hydrops before the fetus can be delivered
- To enable the pregnancy to advance to a gestational age that will ensure survival of the neonate (in practice, up to 36–37 weeks) with as few invasive procedures as possible (because of the risk of fetal loss).

Intrauterine transfusion can be done by either intraperitoneal route or intravascular route. William-Liley performed the first IUT via the intraperitoneal route where blood is transfused to the peritoneal cavity of the fetus from where the donor cells were absorbed into the fetal circulation via the subdiaphragmatic lymphatics and thoracic duct. Intraperitoneal technique had an overall perinatal survival rate of 50% and a procedure-related risk of 7.2%.[11]

Rodeck et al. in 1981 first described the technique of intravascular transfusion by needing the umbilical cord with the use of fetoscopy.[12] Since the mid-1980s until now, the standard method for fetal transfusion in most centers is the direct access to fetal circulation by puncturing the umbilical cord under ultrasound guidance. This form of in utero transfusion allows the definite diagnosis of anemia and direct intravascular infusion of packed red cells into the fetal circulation. Intravascular transfusion is clearly advantageous compared with intraperitoneal approach in cases of fetal hydrops where uptake of donor cells into fetal circulation is poor.

Preparation of Packed Red Blood Cells for Intrauterine Transfusion

Red cells preparations for IUT should:

- Be group O or ABO identical with the fetus (if known) and RhD negative
- Cross-match compatible with maternal serum
- Be less than 5-day-old and in citrate phosphate dextrose (CPD) anticoagulant
- Be cytomegalovirus (CMV) seronegative
- Be irradiated to prevent transfusion-associated graft-versus-host disease (TA-GVHD); the red cells are irradiated with 25 Gy
- Have a HCT (packed cell volume, PCV) of up to but not more than 75
- Be in a volume calculated from the formula of Rodeck and Deans (1999):

(Desired PCV-fetal PCV/ donor PCV-desired PCV) × fetoplacental BV; where BV is blood volume.

- Be transfused at a rate of 5–10 mL/minute.

RISK OF INTRAUTERINE TRANSFUSION

Intrauterine transfusion is now considered as a relatively safe procedure in fetal medicine with a perinatal fetal loss rate of 2% and an acceptable complication rate. Transient fetal bradycardia is the most common complication occurring in 8% of the procedures and fetal distress caused by rupture, spasm, hematoma of the umbilical cord, and hemorrhage from the puncture site, volume overload, or chorioamnionitis can lead to the decision of emergency delivery.[10,13,14]

Box 43.2 Complications of intrauterine packed red blood cell (PRBC) transfusion

- Transient fetal bradycardia
- Hematoma of umbilical cord
- Hemorrhage from punctures site
- Volume overload
- Chorioamnionitis
- Iron overload

Iron overload is a long-term effect of both hemolysis and transfusion. It can play a role in neonatal cholestasis and hepatitis **(Box 43.2)**.[15]

INTRAUTERINE PLATELET TRANSFUSION

The practice of intrauterine platelet transfusion (IUPT) for fetal thrombocytopenia is more controversial. Most threatening thrombocytopenia occurs in fetal or neonatal alloimmune thrombocytopenia.

The indication for IUPT is prevention of severe *in-utero* bleeding. In addition, to prevent bleeding from the IUT procedure to correct anemia, it is recommended to correct the platelet count as well in rare cases. In parvovirus B19 infection, 50% of affected fetuses have thrombocytopenia below 50,000/dL, which further decreases after transfusion of red blood cells (RBCs) alone where IUPT may be beneficial to prevent life-threatening bleeding.[16]

Preparation of Platelet for Intrauterine Platelet Transfusion

Platelets for IUPT products are generally obtained by apheresis from selected donors. In cases of nonalloimmune thrombocytopenia, the donors should be HPA-1a and/or HPA-5b negative, in cases of other antagonisms, washed maternal platelets must be used. Leukocytes are removed from the platelets to prevent CMV transmission. After washing, the platelets can be resuspended to the required concentration in AB-citrate plasma in 0.9% NaCl or in platelet additive solution. Irradiation of the product with 25 Gy is done to prevent TA-GVHD and a storage interval less than 24–48 hours after withdrawal to provide a long platelet survival.

Risk of Intrauterine Platelet Transfusion

Platelet transfusions can also be complicated by fetal bradycardia, which is the most common adverse effect.[17]

ADVERSE EFFECTS OF TRANSFUSION IN NEONATES

Despite of recent advances in screening and pathogen inactivation, RBC transfusion is the transplantation of active tissue and cannot be entirely risk-free. The risks of transfusion can be classified as follows **(Table 43.1)**:

Table 43.1 The adverse effects of transfusion in neonates

Transfusion-transmitted infections	*Immunomodulation*	*Transfusion-related injury*	*Volume or electrolyte disturbances*
Viral—Hepatitis B Hepatitis C HIV	Alloimmunization	Transfusion-associated graft-versus-host disease (TA-GVHD)	Volume overload Hyperkalemia
CMV Parasite-malaria Prion-vCJD		Transfusion-related acute lung injury (TRALI)	Hypoglycemia

Abbreviations: CMV, cytomegalovirus; HIV, human immunodeficiency virus; vCJD, variant Creutzfeldt-Jakob disease

- Transfusion-transmitted infections (viral, bacterial, parasitical or prional)
- The adverse effects of leukocytes (including immunomodulation, graft-versus-host disease transfusion-related acute lung injury and alloimmunization)
- Acute volume or electrolyte disturbances
- Blood group incompatibilities (often mistransfusion errors).

Viral Infections

Transmissible diseases can be caused by viruses such as human immunodeficiency virus (HIV), hepatitis B and C viruses (HBV and HCV) and CMV.

Viral infections contaminate platelet products more commonly than RBC products due to a higher temperature used for storage of platelet products. Insensitivity of pathogen testing is an issue, and risk of viral infections with blood transfusions remains real. Risk of post-transfusion hepatitis B or C in India is about 10% in adults despite routine testing because of low-viremia and mutant strain undetectable by routine enzyme-linked immunosorbent assay (ELISA). HIV prevalence among blood donors is different in various parts of the country.

Cytomegalovirus

Transfusion-related CMV infections in newborns were initially identified in the year 1969, and since then, transfusion-associated CMV transmission is a well-known entity. It has been reported that there is a seroconversion rate of 10–30% in preterm newborns transfused with CMV positive blood. Leukodepletion and selection of CMV negative donors decrease the risk of transfusion-transmitted CMV.

Parasites

Plasmodium, trypanosome, and several other parasites may be transmitted through blood depending on the endemicity of the area. Transfusion transmitted malaria is not uncommon in India.

Prions

Variant Creutzfeldt-Jakob disease (vCJD) is an established complication of blood transfusion and has been reported since 2004. Restricted transfusions and avoidance of transfusions, unless essential, are the only ways currently to prevent transmission.

Alloimmunization

Alloimmunization is an uncommon occurrence before the age of 4 months, and is caused by transfusion of blood products, which are mismatched for highly immunogenic antigens.

TRANSFUSION-ASSOCIATED GRAFT VERSUS HOST DISEASE

Newborns are at risk for TA-GVHD, if they have received IUTs, exchange transfusions, or are very small, or immunocompromised. Unchecked donor T-cell proliferation is the cause of TA-GVHD, and it can be effectively prevented by leukoreduction of the transfused blood products. Most centers now γ-irradiate blood to deactivate lymphocytes and prevent graft-versus-host disease. This complication is rare in newborn infants.

Transfusion-related Acute Lung Injury

It refers to noncardiogenic pulmonary edema complicating transfusion therapy. It is a common and under-reported complication occurring after therapy with blood components. It has been associated with all plasma-containing blood products, most commonly whole blood, packed RBCs, fresh-frozen plasma (FFP) and platelets. Transfusion-related acute lung injury is rare in neonate but is the subject of ongoing review.

Allergic Reactions

Allergic reactions are caused by presence of preformed immunoglobulin E antibody against an allergen in the transfused plasma, and are a rare occurrence in newborns. Hemolytic transfusion reactions are also rare in the newborn.

Fluid Overload

Neonates are at increased risk of fluid overload from transfusion because the volume of the blood component issued may exceed the volume that may be transfused safely into neonates. Care should be taken to ensure that in the absence of blood loss, volumes infused do not exceed 10–20 mL/kg.

Metabolic Complications

These complications occur with large volume of transfusions, such as exchange transfusions.

Hyperkalemia

In stored blood, potassium levels tend to be high. It has been seen that after storage for around 42 days, potassium levels may reach 50 mEq/L in a RBC unit. Though small volume transfusions do not have much risk of metabolic disturbances, large volume transfusions may lead to hyperkalemia. Washing PRBCs before reconstituting with FFP before exchange transfusion helps in preventing this complication.

Hypoglycemia

Blood stored in CPD blood has a high content of glucose leading to a rebound rise in insulin release 1–2 hours after transfusion. This may lead to hypoglycemia and routine monitoring is necessary, particularly after exchange transfusion, after 2 and 6 hours to ensure that this complication does not occur.

Acid-base Derangements

Metabolism of citrate in CPD leads to late metabolic alkalosis. Metabolic acidosis is an immediate complication.

CONCLUSION

As blood transfusion is an invasive procedure and carries with it inherent risk of complication, the need for transfusion should be ascertained and strict guidelines should be adhered to reduce the rate as well as complication of transfusion.

KEY POINTS

- Transfusion guidelines in fetuses and newborns are expert based rather than evidence based.
- The average perinatal fetal loss rate following intrauterine transfusion is 2%.
- Transient fetal bradycardia is the most common complication following intrauterine transfusion.
- Neonates are at increased risk of fluid overload from transfusion.
- The need for transfusion should be ascertained and strict guidelines should be adhered to minimize transfusion reaction.

REFERENCES

1. Carr S, Rubin L, Dixon D, Star J, Dailey J. Intrauterine therapy for homozygous alpha-thalassemia. Obstet Gynecol. 1995;85(5):876-9.
2. Haak MC, Oosterhof H, Mouw RJ, Oepkes D, Vandenbussche FP. Pathophysiology and treatment of fetal anemia due to placental chorioangioma. Ultrasound Obstet Gynecol. 1999;14(1):68-70.
3. Van Dongen H, Klumper FJ, Sikkel E, Vandenbussche FP, Oepkes D. Non-invasive tests to predict fetal anemia in Kell-alloimmunized pregnancies. Ultrasound Obstet Gynecol. 2005;25(4):341-5.
4. von Kaisenberg CS, Jonat W. Fetal parvovirus B19 infection. Ultrasound Obstet Gynecol. 2001;18(3):280-8.
5. Giacoia GP. Severe fetomaternal hemorrhage: a review. Obstet Gynecol Surv. 1997;52(6):372-80.
6. Papantoniou N. Is there any role for cordocentesis and amniocentesis in assessment of rhesus disease? Ultrasound Rev Obstet Gynecol. 2004;4(4):239-44.
7. Oepkes D, Seaward PG, Vandenbussche FP, Windrim R, Kingdom J, Beyene J, et al. Doppler ultrasonography versus amniocentesis to predict fetal anemia. N Engl J Med. 2006;355(2):156-64.
8. Whitecar PW, Moise KJ Jr. Sonographic methods to detect fetal anemia in red blood cell alloimmunization. Obstet Gynecol Surv. 2000;55(4):240-50.
9. Bahado-Singh R, Oz U, Deren O, Kovanchi E, Hsu CD, Copel J, et al. Splenic artery Doppler peak systolic velocity predicts severe fetal anemia in rhesus disease. Am J Obstet Gynecol. 2000;182(5):1222-6.
10. Moise KJ Jr. Management of rhesus alloimmunization in pregnancy. Obstet Gynecol. 2008;112:164-76.
11. Frigoletto FD Jr, Umansky I, Birnholz J, Acker D, Easterday CL, Harris GB, et al. Intrauterine fetal transfusion in 365 fetuses during fifteen years. Am J Obstet Gynecol. 1981:139(7):781-90.
12. Rodeck CH, Kemp JR, Holman CA, Whitmore DN, Karnicki J, Austin MA. Direct intravascular fetal blood transfusion by fetoscopy in severe rhesus isoimmunisation. Lancet. 1981;1(8221):625-7.
13. Oepkes D, Adama van Scheltema P. Intrauterine fetal transfusions in the management of fetal anemia and fetal thrombocytopenia. Semin Fetal Neonatal Med. 2007;12(6): 432-8.
14. Weiner CP, Williamson RA, Wenstrom KD, Sipes SL, Widness JA, Grant SS, et al. Management of fetal hemolytic disease by cordocentesis. II. Outcome of treatment. Am J Obstet Gynecol. 1991;165(5 Pt 1):1302-7.
15. Lasker MR, Eddleman K, Toor AH. Neonatal hepatitis and excessive hepatic iron deposition following intrauterine blood transfusion. Am J Perinatol. 1995;12(1):14-7.
16. de Haan TR, van den Akker ES, Porcelijn L, Oepkes D, Kroes AC, Walther FJ. Thrombocytopenia in hydropic fetuses with parvovirus B19 infection: incidence, treatment and correlation with fetal B19 viral load. BJOG. 2008;115(1):76-81.
17. Yazicioglu HF, Hartwig D, von Witzleben- Schürholz E, Neppert J, Gembruch U. Fetal bradycardia following intrauterine platelet transfusion: might elevated levels of donor soluble CD40 ligand play a role? Acta Obstet Gynecol Scand. 2004;83(9):868-9.

CHAPTER 44

Hematological Growth Factors as Supportive Therapy

Satyen K Hemrajani, Anupam Sachdeva

INTRODUCTION

The hematopoietic growth factors are glycoproteins which play an important role in the proliferation, differentiation and survival of hematopoietic stem cells and its progenitor along with this they also help in the activation of functions of many mature cells. These growth factors bind to certain specific surface receptors on the target cell and regulate the diffrentiation of myeloid and erythroid series cells. These growth factors are namely: multicolony-stimulating factor (multi-CSF) [interleukin-3 (IL-3)], granulocyte macrophage colony-stimulating factor (GM-CSF), G-CSF, M-CSF, erythropoietin (EPO), lymphopoietin (IL-7) and megakaryopoietin (IL-11). Committed RBC precursors have EPO receptors that bind to EPO; early granulocyte precursors bind to G-CSF and IL-3 by specific receptors; and G-CSF binds to receptors on slightly more mature, committed granulocyte precursors. Thrombopoietin (TPO) interacts with megakaryocytes and stimulates their numbers and ability to produce greater numbers of platelets. There is functional overlap between these growth factors, and each factor has multiple biological actions.

Of all the hematopoietic growth factors, G-CSF, GM-CSF and erythropoietin have been extensively studied in adult and neonatal clinical trials as supportive therapy for hematological and nonhematological purposes. After finding their potential benefits, stem cell CSF and M-CSF or thrombopoietin are also being studied. TPO mimetics (romiplostim and eltrombopag) have demonstrated efficacy in raising platelet counts in idiopathic thrombocytopenic purpura (ITP) patients. They have been used in both pre- and postsplenectomy patients. There may be a potential role of these and other analogues of these growth factors in the near future.

HISTORY

In the 1960s it was first recognized that normal and leukemic progenitor cells can be cultured and grown in semisolid media in presence of factors known as growth factors.[1,2] These factors came to be known as colony stimulating factors (CSFs) as they could help in formation of colonies of blood cells by bone marrow cells in artificial semisolid medium.[3] In the next decade different types of CSFs were identified based on the various type of colonies of blood cells they could support. This further led to the conclusion that the different blood cells were developing under the effect of exposure of progenitor cells to CSFs having different lineage specificities.[3,4]

The successful cloning of the hematopoietic growth factors and their receptors has provided an incredible array of tools for analysis of the molecular and cellular biology of hematopoiesis, and for the production of recombinant proteins for evaluation of the biology of the various factors *in vivo* and *in vitro*.

GRANULOCYTE-COLONY STIMULATING FACTOR OR GRANULOCYTE-MACROPHAGE COLONY-STIMULATING FACTOR

Amongst the CSFs the factors that affect myeloid cell lines are of two types, i.e. granulocyte colony stimulating factor (G-CSF) and granulocyte-macrophage colony stimulating factors (GM-CSFs). G-CSF are cytokines that stimulate the production of bone marrow neutrophils granulocyte lineage wheras GM-CSF induces growth of multilineage progenitor cells including granulocyte and macrophages.

Myelopoiesis in Neonates

The common progenitor cell for granulocytes is the granulocyte colony-forming unit. The next division of these progenitor cells gives rise to committed stem cells which in turn gives rise to myleoblasts followed by promyelocytes, myelocytes, metamyelocytes, band cells and finally, segmented neutrophils. By definition the proliferative pool consists of promyelocytes and myelocytes, all of which possess the possibility of cell division. The neutrophil storage pool usually indicates the variety of cells that have lost the

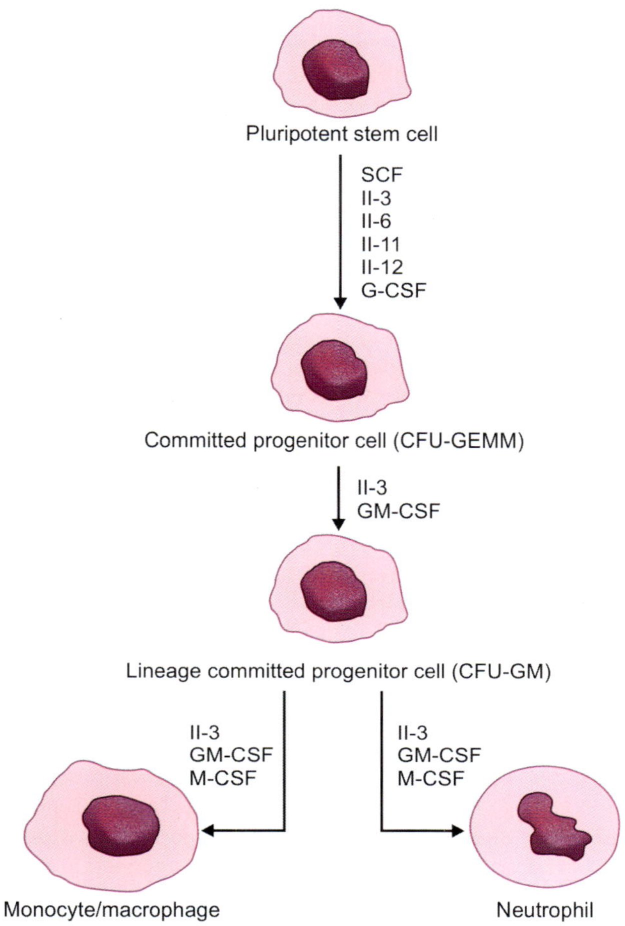

Figure 44.1 Diagrammatic representation of myelopoiesis in a neonate leading to generation of neutrophil or monocyte

Abbreviations: SCF, stem cell factor; CFU-GEMM, colony forming unit-granulocyte-erythrocyte-monocyte-macrophage; CFU-GM, colony forming unit–granulocyte macrophage; M-CSF, macrophage colony-stimulating factors; IL, interleukin

capability of cell division, i.e. band forms, metamyelocytes and segmented neutrophils, before being released into circulation **(Fig. 44.1)**.

The mature neutrophils are present in several different compartment of body such as bone marrow storage pool, circulating and marginated pool and the tissue pool. Approximately, half of the neutrophils that reside in the blood are associated with vascular endothelium, comprising the so called marginated pool.

The number of total white blood cells are quite high during the 1st hour of life and are probably due to demargination from the stress at birth. Circulating neutrophils survive for approximately 8 hours. Those that migrate into the extravascular tissues where they may survive for an additional 24 hours after which apoptosis occurs.

Fetal and Neonatal Myeloid Series: Differences from Adult Myeloid Series

The fetal and neonatal bone marrow contains expanded precursor cell populations, and the basal proliferative rates of these are nearly maximal.[5] The neonate lacks an adequate number of myeloid progenitor cells and has a decreased myeloid proliferative rate, which causes a decreased ability to release and mobilize neutrophils from storage pools.[6] The neutrophil storage pool in neonates is smaller than that of the adult and may rapidly exhaust in face of sepsis, which creates a high demand, which leads to neutropenia in serious infection.[7] During states of increased demand for blood cells, such as bacterial sepsis, quantitative deficiencies in neonatal myeloid progenitor activity and decreased availability of high mature neutrophil effector cells predispose the neonates to a high incidence of infection. This leads to a continuous cascade of events leading to perpetuation of the infection in the absence of adequate cellular immunity leading to serious sepsis and death. The dysregulation of expression and production of hematopoietic cytokines lead to quantitative and qualitative defects in the phagocytes and contributes to infectious complications in neonate **(Table 44.1)**.

Fetal and neonatal neutrophils chemotaxis and phagocytic ability is also decreased because of:

- Diminished L-selectin expression, a molecule important for adhesion of neutrophils to endothelial cells[8]
- Generation of low filamentous F-actin by neutrophils after stimulation, a cytoskeletal contractile element for locomotion of neutrophils[9]

Table 44.1 Pathophysiologic response to bacterial sepsis in adult and neonatal rats

CFU-GM	*Adult rats*	*Neonate*
Myeloid progenitor pool		
At rest (%)	100	10
Sepsis	2–3 fold increase	Decrease
Proliferative rate		
At rest (%)	Low	High
Sepsis	Increase	No change (already maximal)
Neutrophil storage pool		
At rest (%)	100	25
Sepsis	Initial decrease	Decrease
Peripheral neutrophil count during sepsis	Transient neutropenia followed by neutrophilia	Prolonged neutropenia

Source: Adapted from reference 5.
Abbreviation: CFU-GM, colony forming unit-granulocyte macrophage

- Increased fluidity of the neutrophil cell membrane, which also hampers ability of chemotaxis[10]
- Reduced microtubule formations leading to inability of neonatal polymorphonuclear leukocyte (PMNs) to achieve a fully bipolar shape change on stimulation[11]
- Reduced deformability of neutrophils of newborn, especially in immature forms,[12] and
- Delayed transmigration of neutrophils in neonatal rats due to defect in the expression of P-selectin on surface of endothelial cells.[13]

ROLE OF G-CSF AND GM-CSF IN NEONATAL SEPSIS

The G-CSF and GM-CSF are myeloid-specific colony stimulating factors that stimulate the proliferation of myeloid stem cells and progenitor cells, induce the release of mature effector neutrophils from the bone marrow myeloid storage pools, enhance neutrophils effector functions, like phagocytosis, chemotaxis, adherence, migration and deformability and reduced neutrophil apoptosis. G-CSF is a primary regulator of the circulating concentrations of neutrophils even in steady state. The GM-CSF, however, is not playing any role in steady state conditions but may be induced in inflamed tissues to promote neutrophil and macrophage maturation.[14]

The cord blood and peripheral blood of healthy preterm and term neonates are known to have low amount of G-CSF and GM-CSF. They are also influenced by many factors, such as presence of maternal or fetal infection, pre-eclampsia, twin pregnancy, use of antenatal steroids, etc. The G-CSF concentration in healthy term neonate parallels neonatal neutrophil counts in the first few weeks of life. Information regarding normal levels of G-CSF in preterm neonates is inconsistent. Sepsis induces G-CSF concentration in neonates but the levels induced are still lower as compared to those by stimulating adult cells, which explains the defective upregulation of neutrophil production and function during infection.[15]

Preclinical *in vivo* Effects of Myelopoietic Growth Factors in Animal Trials

In a small study on newborn rats, Cairo et al. compared giving G-CSF (5 μg/kg/day) versus placebo to newborn rats for a period of 7 days. He then studied effects of placebo and G-CSF on the blood cells and bone marrow. Results of this trial showed that prophylactic use of G-CSF (5 μg/kg/day) led to an increase in absolute neutrophil counts by 750%, the bone marrow neutrophil storage pools by 100% and increased the colony forming unit of granulocyte macrophage (CFU-GM) and its colonies. No significant changes were seen in the bone marrow neutrophil proliferative pool (NPP), in liver/spleen, CFU-GM colonies, or in the CFU-GM proliferative rate.[16]

In the same trial after 7 days of prophylactic G-CSF, a lethal dose of GBS was given to these animals and subsequently, appropriate antibiotic or placebo was administered by random allocation. In group of animals who received G-CSF and no antibiotics, 40% survived as compared to 100% survival in patients who received both antibiotics and G-CSF. At 72 hours there was a 100% mortality in G-CSF and placebo treated group only, 50% mortality in the antibiotic group and 0% mortality in the G-CSF and antibiotic treated group.[16] The improvement in mortality rate after prophylactic administration of G-CSF presumably occurs secondary to stimulation of myeloid maturation and possible to maturation of the granulocyte function. This effect of single pulse of G-CSF as adjuvant to antibiotic therapy was evaluated by Cairo et al.[17] They found group of animals that received prophylactic G-CSF (given 6 hours before GBS inoculation) with antibiotics had better survival as compared to group that received antibiotics only (70% vs 10%, $p < 0.001$) and in therapy also the G-CSF and antibiotics group had a better survival as compared to animals treated with antibiotics only (91% vs 28%, $p < 0.001$).

The role of GM-CSF in preventing against experimental sepsis was tested in neonatal rats. In this study neonatal rats were treated with either saline or recombinant murine GM-CSF at different doses (0.3, 3, 30, 300, 3,000, 10,000 pg/g) followed by administration of almost lethal dose of *Staphylococcus aureus*. The results of this study revealed that maximum survival was documented when GM-CSF was used in a dose of 30 pg/g (54% vs 10% control, $p < 0.001$), and blood cultures were positive in 26/32 saline treated group versus 5/31 GM-CSF treated animals ($p < 0.001$).[18] The synergistic effect of GM-CSF with antibiotics was studied in animals with the primary outcome being mortality rates in GBS sepsis. In one such trial by Cairo et al., newborn rats were given recombinant GM-CSF alone, placebo only, GM-CSF and antibiotics , or antibiotics only for 7 days and were inoculated with group B *Streptococcus* after a week on 8th day. Both groups of neonatal rats receiving placebo plus antibiotics or GM-CSF plus antibiotics had no significant difference in survival rates (57% vs 59%, p = NS).[19]

In vitro studies of myelopoietic growth factors have documented that use of GM-CSF enhances adult neutrophils oxidative metabolism, increases chemotaxis, promotes phagocytosis, and it induces the expression of surface adhesion glycoproteins resulting in increased neutrophil aggregation.[5,20,21] In cord blood neutrophils, an earlier but less maximal superoxide generation (enhancement of oxidative metabolism) is seen.[22] Similar results were found when G-CSF was used for priming the neutrophils.[23]

CLINICAL TRIALS OF G-CSF

The earliest published report on G-CSF use was by Roberts in 1991 who documented successful correction of persistent neutropenia and associated recurrent infections in a preterm infant following use of G-CSF. This neonate who weighed 654 grams neonate had absolute neutrophil counts (ANCs) of < 1,000 cells/μL. The infant was treated with 10 μg/kg/day of G-CSF and finally discharged in stable condition.[24]

Gillan et al. conducted a randomized, placebo-controlled trial to study the safety, pharmacokinetics and biological efficacy of recombinant human G-CSF in 42 neonates of <3 days of age. G-CSF was administered in doses of 1, 5 or 10 µg/kg/day every 24 hours or 5 or 10 µg/kg/day every 12 hours for 3 days. The results showed it was well tolerated, not associated with recognized acute toxicity and its half-life was 4.4 hours. G-CSF induced a significant increase in ANC within 24 hours, which was sustained for 3 days. Bone marrow (BM) aspirates showed a significant increase in storage pool of neutrophils and increased expression of neutrophil adhesion and aggregation receptor was also found in peripheral neutrophils after the 10 µg/kg/day dose.[25]

In another study, the ability of G-CSF to reverse neutropenia associated with pre-eclampsia and reduce the incidence of sepsis was evaluated. G-CSF was administered in dose of 10 µg/kg/day dose or 5 µg/kg/day to 15 very low-birth weight neonates with neutropenia (ANC < 1,500 cells/mm^3 for 3 days) and their neutrophil counts were compared with matched control (n = 13). The increase in ANC was twofold at 24 hours, fourfold at 72 hours and by 14-fold at 7 days in 10 µg/kg/day. The increase was somewhat less in the 5 µg/kg/day group (twofold at 72 hours and fivefold at 7 days). The reduction of incidence of sepsis was significant in the treated infants as compared to control group (13% vs 54%, $p < 0.05$). However, one should not forget that it was a nonrandomized, nonblinded study, which is a weak evidence.[26]

To test the hypothesis that recombinant G-CSF given prophylactically would reduce the incidence of nosocomial infections; a multicentric, placebo-controlled trial was conducted by Kuhn et al. in 25 neonatal units. The population tested were premature <32 weeks with peripheral blood counts showing <1,500 cells/mm^3 for at least 24 hours in the first 3 weeks of life. Total 200 infants were recruited with 102 receiving G-CSF and 98 were controls. There was a more rapid increase in the ANC after the second dose of G-CSF with a ninefold increase documented as compared to threefold increase in the placebo group. Amongst the two groups survival free of confirmed infection for 4 weeks after treatment was 74/102 in treated group and 66/98 in the placebo group (p = 0.42), which was not clinically significant. There was no difference in the mortality before discharge of both the groups. On secondary analysis, the investigators found that a reduced neutrophil response is small for gestational age (SGA) infants and a better survival at 2 weeks in AGA infants.[27]

Miura et al. conducted a similar trial on 44 preterm neonates (<5 days old) with clinical diagnosis of early onset neonatal sepsis in Brazil. They found that in the treatment group (G-CSF 10 µg/kg/day for 3 days), the ANCs significantly increased but the difference disappeared after 10 days, bone marrow neutrophil storage pool was significantly increased, nosocomial infections were significantly reduced (2/22 in treated group as compared to 9/19 in placebo group, $p < 0.02$) but mortality was not significantly reduced.[28]

In a meta-analysis, Bernstein et al. reported that 73 G-CSF recipients had a lower mortality than 82 infants in the control arm (odds ratio 0.17, 95% CI 0.03-0.70, $p < 0.05$). However, when nonrandomized studies were excluded, the effects did not remain statistically adequate (odds ratio 0.43, 95% CI -0.14–1.23, $p < 0.13$).[29]

The Cochrane review conducted by Carr et al. on the use of G-CSF/GM-CSF in neonatal sepsis identified and included 7 treatment studies (n = 257) and 3 prophylaxis studies (n = 359). They found that in preterm infants with suspected sepsis, use of G-CSF or GM-CSF in addition to antibiotics did not improve survival [typical relative risk of death 0.71 (95% CI 0.38–1.33)]. The subgroup analysis of 97 infants from three treatment studies, who also had neutropenia (<1,700/mm^3) with sepsis at trial entry, showed a significant reduction in mortality by day 14 (RR 0.34, 95% CI = 0.12–0.92; NNT = 6, 95% CI = 3–33). The prophylaxis studies did not demonstrate a reduction in mortality in neonates receiving GM-CSF (RR = 0.59, 95% CI = 0.24–1.44); risk difference = –0.03 (95% CI = –0.08–0.02).[30] However, since 2003 when this review has been conducted, new studies have been done using G-CSF and GM-CSF. These studies, which were not included in the Cochrane and their results, are discussed further below.

A double-blinded randomized, placebo-controlled trial was conducted by Borjianyazdi et al. in 46 preterm neonates (gestation between 30 weeks and 37 weeks) with neutropenia and clinical sepsis within first 10 days of life. They were treated with G-CSF at a dose of 10 µg/kg/day for 5 days. They documented that there was no significant decrease in the mortality in the treatment group but in the same group there was a decrease in blood culture positive sepsis and a decrease in the length of hospital stay (25 + 6 vs 30 + 7 days, p = 0.042) as compared to the no treatment group.[31]

Gathwala et al. conducted trial in Indian settings using G-CSF in 78 preterm (<34 weeks, 1,100–2,500 g) with neutropenia (<1,500 cells/mm^3) in the first 3 weeks of life and having clinical signs of sepsis and blood culture positive. They were administered the drug for 3 days along with antibiotics for 5 days. There was clear selection bias in this study with lack of inclusion of ELBW babies and very preterm babies. They documented a clear and rapid increase in neutrophil counts in the treated group, and as secondary outcome, they documented a decrease in all-cause mortality in the treated group (10% vs 35%, $p < 0.05$).[32]

Russell et al. conducted a prospective, randomized study in four centers across Britain and tested G-CSF in very low-birth-weight (VLBW) neonates with neutropenia (ANC $< 5 \times 10^9$/L) and clinical evidence of sepsis. They received treatment with G-CSF for a maximum of 14 days, along with standard treatment of antibiotics. They documented a trend toward a reduction in duration of ventilation, intensive care, antibiotic use in the treated group. At 6 and 12 months after treatment, there was a significant reduction in the mortality in the treated group (1/13 vs 7/15, $p < 0.038$) but no reduction in deaths during the 42 days study period was documented. Adverse events and oxygenation index were not increased by use of G-CSF.[33]

CLINICAL TRIAL OF GM-CSF

A phase III multicentric, double-blinded, randomized trial was done to see the use of GM-CSF as a prophylactic strategy in VLBW neonates. A total of 264 neonates were enrolled in this study and received either GM-CSF (8 μg/kg/day) or placebo for 21 days. The results showed that the peripheral neutrophil count was significantly increased in the GM-CSF treated group on days 7, 14, 21 and day 28 but there was no difference in the incidence of confirmed nosocomial infection between the two groups (40% vs 39%, p = NS).[34]

The PROGRAMS trial is one of the largest single blind, multicentric (26 centers), randomized controlled trial of GM-CSF as a prophylaxis for sepsis. The study was conducted over 6 years in 26 centers and on 280 neonates <31 weeks and SGA (<10th centile for birth weight). These patients were randomized to receive either GM-CSF 10 μg/kg/day subcutaneously for 5 days or continued on standard management. The results of this trial suggested that the absolute neutrophil count (ANC) in the GM-CSF treated group increased significantly more rapidly in the treated group during the first 11 days. An equally rapid and sustained correction of neutrophil count was observed in the subgroup neutropenic at entry. But, there was no significant difference in the sepsis free survival up to 2nd week (14 day) of onset of trial (93 of 139 treated infants, 105 of 141 control infants; difference –8%, 95% CI –18 to 3). Therefore, GM-CSF does not result in reduction of systemic sepsis, mortality or short-term clinical morbidity.[35]

Subsequently, the same group was able to follow-up these babies for a period of 2 years and then 5 years and they reported the results. After 2 years, the authors found no significant difference in survival without severe disability. At 5 years, they had 74% and 78% follow-up in control and treatment arm. They found no significant differences in cognitive, general health or educational outcomes. There was a suggestion of worse respiratory outcomes in the treatment group at 2 years, reported as increased cough, wheeze without infection and signs of chronic respiratory disease (e.g. Harrison's sulcus), which was replicated at 5 years though this did not reflect in the bronchodilator use or need for hospitalization for respiratory disease.[36,37]

Venkateswaran et al., in a observation study looked at the therapeutic role of GM-CSF, administered this drug in a dose of 5 μg/kg q24h for 5 days to 8 neonates with a gestation of at least 30 weeks and weighing >1,000 g. All these patients had diagnosis of severe infection or NEC and neutropenia (defined as an absolute granulocyte count <3000/mL). All 8 patients survived the septic episode and their neutropenia resolved.[38]

G-CSF OR GM-CSF: WHICH ONE HAS BETTER EFFECT IN NEONATE?

Ahmad et al. looked at a head-to-head comparison of G-CSF versus GM-CSF versus placebo, G-CSF (5 μg/kg intravenously q12h) was compared to GM-CSF (4 μg/kg intravenously q12h) or placebo for the treatment of symptomatic, septic premature neonates in a small study (n = 28 patients). Neonates receiving G-CSF had the fastest increase in PMN count (mean values were >1,000/mL in all three subgroups), with a significant increase in ANC value noted in G-CSF group within 48 hours. No significant difference in effect on mortality, length of stay or later complication could be observed amongst the treated group or placebo. Treatment with G-CSF (but not GM-CSF) showed a trend toward a "prophylactic" effect on the incidence of later infections.[39]

ROLE OF G-CSF OR GM-CSF IN OTHER NEUTROPENIAS

Granulocyte colony-stimulating factor is highly effective in other immune-mediated neutropenias, like neonatal alloimmune neutropenia, neonatal autoimmune neutropenia and autoimmune neutropenia of infancy. It not only increases neutrophil production but also delays apoptosis and downregulates the antigen expression and renders the neutrophils less vulnerable to circulating antibodies, increases additional antibody mopping sites and corrects some of the functional impairment induced by antineutrophil antibody.[40,41]

Severe congenital neutropenia is a rare, heterogeneous group of disorders with different patterns of inheritance. Some like Kostmann syndrome are autosomal recessive and present in early infancy with ANC often <200/μL, a compensatory eosinophilia and monocytosis, splenomegaly and recurrent bacterial infections, like omphalitis, otitis media, pneumonitis, skin abscess and liver abscess. G-CSF is highly effective in most patients with this disease and has reduced the need for antibiotics and hospitalization and has improved the survival of these patients.[42,43] The response is seen 7–10 days after initiation of treatment. The dose to be begun is 5 μg/kg/day and after response, it can be titrated up or down to the lowest effective dose. Patients who require >8 μg/kg/day or higher doses are at higher risk of developing myelodysplastic syndrome or acute myeloid leukemia (MDS or AML) than those who are more G-CSF responsive (40% vs 11% after 10 years of therapy). Hematopoietic stem cell transplantation is the only curative treatment.[44]

In cyclic neutropenia,a disorder with a characteristically regular drop in neutrophil counts for 3–5 days after 3 weeks intervals, G-CSF use can reduce the number of days with neutropenia can be reduced by G-CSF use although the cycles may still continue. In contrast to G-CSF, these patients respond poorly to GM-CSF.[45]

Glycogen storage disease-Ib (GSD-Ib) is an autosomal-recessive disorder with intermittent neutropenia and defects in neutrophil respiratory burst chemotaxis and calcium flux. GSD-Ib also leads to hepatomegaly and metabolic crisis with hypoglycemia and lactic acidosis. The defect resides in the glucose 6-phosphatase translocase enzyme. Bone marrow biopsies of GSD-Ib patients are consistent with reduced neutrophil production. G-CSF has also been effective in treating GSD-Ib patients.

Flow chart 44.1 Algorithm to identify the use of recombinant G-CSF in case of suspected severe congenital neutropenia

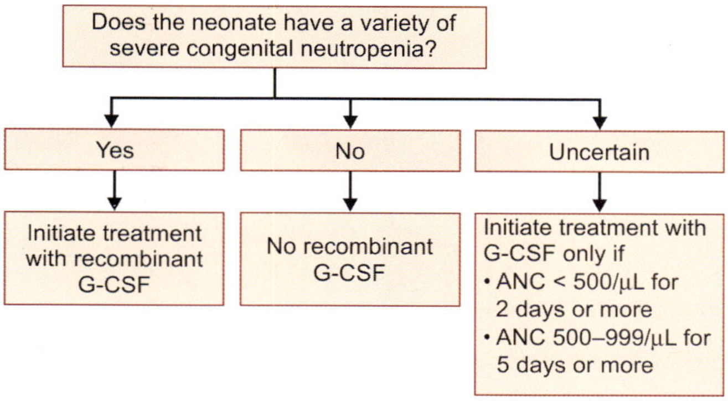

Abbreviations: ANC, absolute neutrophil count; G-CSF, granulocyte-colony-stimulating factor

Indications for G-CSF use include the following:
- Persistent neutrophil count $\leq 0.2 \times 10^9$/L;
- Life-threatening infections requiring antibiotics;
- Serious inflammatory bowel disease; or
- Severe diarrhea requiring hospitalization or disrupting normal life.[46]

Barth syndrome (BS) is characterized by mild to severe neutropenia, dilated cardiomyopathy, skeletal myopathy and 3-methylglutaconic aciduria. Barth syndrome patients have a deficiency in cardiolipin synthesis. Because of the cardiomyopathy, of these patients are unable to compensate for the decreased systemic vascular resistance that occurs during sepsis. Therefore, despite a moderately increased risk of infection, clinicians have a lower threshold for G-CSF use in this disease **(Flow chart 44.1)**.[47]

FUTURE PROPOSED USES OF G-CSF OR GM-CSF IN NEONATAL INTENSIVE CARE UNIT

Neuroprotection

Granulocyte colony-stimulating factor has been tested as a neuroprotectant in a rodent model of neonatal hypoxic-ischemic brain damage. Subcutaneous G-CSF administration beginning 1 hour after injury prevented brain atrophy, preserved reflexes and improved motor coordination and memory. In addition, animals treated with G-CSF had better somatic growth. Clinical studies are planned to test the safety and efficacy of G-CSF as a neuroprotectant for neonates with hypoxic-ischemic encephalopathy.[48]

Prevention of Feed Intolerance

Granulocyte-colony stimulating factor is found in amniotic fluid, which is swallowed by the fetus in large quantities—up to 200 mL/kg/day. The G-CSF swallowed binds to receptors on enterocytes and conveys antiapoptotic actions. A sterile, isotonic, simulated amniotic fluid containing G-CSF has been administered to neonatal intensive care unit (NICU) patients who are otherwise NPO (nil per os) with the hypothesis that such will prevent disuse atrophy of the intestinal villi that otherwise occurs during the NPO period. Safety and early efficacy studies of this approach seem promising.[49,50]

SIDE EFFECTS OF G-CSF OR GM-CSF

Common minor side effects of use of G-CSF or GM-CSF are low-grade fever and bone pain. Rarely, when high doses are administered, capillary leak and pulmonary infiltrates are reported. There is a theoretical risk of these drugs causing an increase in the inflammatory disease of neonate, such as bronchopulmonary dysplasia (BPD) and necrotizing enterocolitis (NEC). It is also associated with sickling crisis in patients with hemoglobinopathies. The long-term use in severe congenital neutropenia patients has also been associated with increased incidence of MDS and acute myeloid leukemia when used for >8–10 years. Suggested contraindications to G-CSF administration in donors include the presence of active inflammatory conditions, hypercoagulable states and in adults with known atherosclerotic vascular disease.

Serious side effects of G/GM-CSF have not been observed in neonates. There is one study that reported the long-term hematological, immunological effects and developmental outcomes at the age of 2 years and 5 years after use of G-CSF in PROGRAMS trial. The hematological profile, serum immunoglobulin and complement levels were normal and there was no difference in the fine motor and gross motor development skills.[35-37] But still mostly the late long-term side effects of these growth factors are largely unstudied.

ERYTHROPOIETIN AND ERYTHROPOIETIN STIMULATING AGENTS

The principal growth factor that regulates erythropoiesis is erythropoietin. The human erythropoietin gene is situated at chromosome 7q11-22. Erythropoietin is a glycoprotein that helps in erythropoiesis by inhibiting apoptosis of erythroid progenitors and by stimulating their proliferation and differentiation into normoblasts. It also has immunomodulatory functions.

Fetal and Neonatal Erythropoiesis

The fetus independently produces its own erythrocytes which is affected by factors produced by the fetus itself and placental factors also. Mother's erythropoietin does not effect fetal erythropoiesis as it cannot cross the placenta. The fetus produces approximately 50×10^9 RBCs per day to cope with the fetal growth. The fetal erythropoietin is lesser in quantity despite such large production and fetal erythropoiesis is much more efficient than adult erythropoiesis due to other growth factors synergizing with erythropoietin **(Fig. 44.2)**.

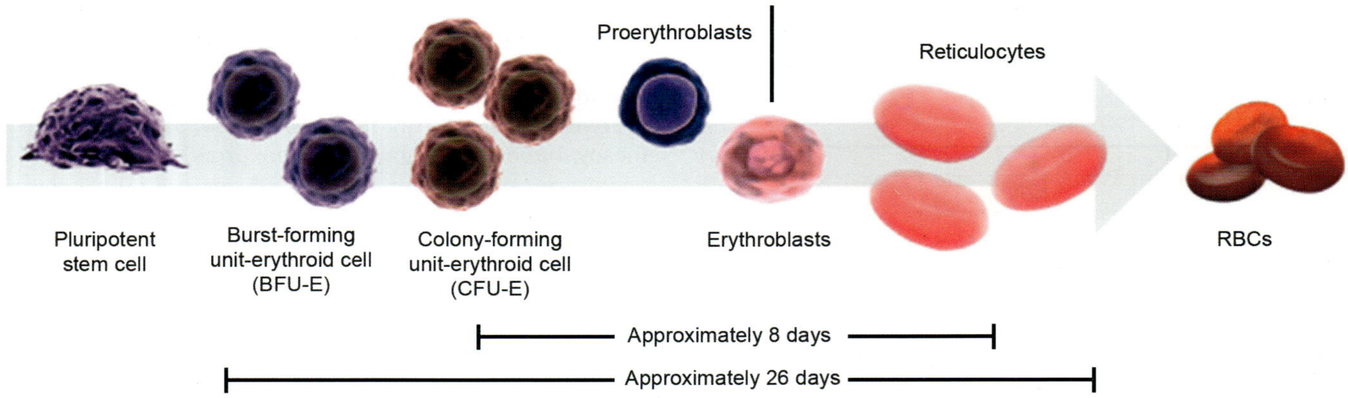

Figure 44.2 Erythropoiesis in humans

In a neonate postnatal improvement in oxygenation leads to loss of the hypoxic stimulus that increases erythropoietin production and hence the nadir is seen around 4th–6th week after birth usually. This leads to decreased erythropoiesis and the hemoglobin decreases by 8th week. The kidney then takes over production of erythropoietin and hemoglobin starts rising in 4th to 6th month.[51] By 10–12 weeks of life, they reach adult concentrations (approximately 15 mU/mL). These changes in erythropoietin concentrations are consistent with physiologic anemia seen in healthy term infants.

ANEMIA OF PREMATURITY

The anemia of prematurity is a normocytic, normochromic anemia occurring in neonates born before 32 weeks gestation. In preterm infants, the fall in erythropoietin is more profound and persists longer, leading to anemia of prematurity. In these babies, the nadir appears sooner and hemoglobin falls to a lower level. In preterm infants, circulating erythropoietin concentrations in this population are low relative to the degree of anemia. The hepatic phase of erythropoietin continues in preterms during neonatal period even postnatally. These liver cells producing erythropoietin are less sensitive to hypoxia and anemia as compared to kidney and require more prolonged hypoxia to generate adequate erythropoietin for stimulating erythropoiesis. Neonatal RBCs have a short life span and a rapid expansion of blood volume as the preterm is growing along with repeated blood sampling contributes to development of anemia of prematurity. The severity of this anemia is dependent on gestation age of the baby and the amount of phlebotomy losses inflicted. In VLBW (birth weight 1,000–1,500 g) infants, the hematocrit falls to approximately 24% at around 6 weeks of age, and to 21% in the extremely low birth weight (ELBW) (birth weight < 1,000 g) infants.[52,53] The anemia due to these reasons usually resolves by 3–6 months of life. The erythroid progenitor cells in marrow and circulation are highly sensitive to erythropoietin in vitro.

As many as 80% of VLBW infants and 95% of ELBW infants receive RBCs transfusions during their hospitalization.[54] As many as 80% of these infants require multiple RBCs transfusions. The main problem related with these blood transfusions is infection and due to multiple blood donor exposure, the preterm babies are more vulnerable to catch these infections. Hence, preventive strategies for blood transfusion are mainly focused on this clinical end point.

Use of Erythropoietin for Anemia: Evidence from *in vivo* Studies and Clinical Studies

The primary objective of recombinant human erythropoietin (rHuEPO) therapy in neonatology is to reduce the number of blood donors neonates are exposed to. The neonates have a large volume of distribution and hence there is a more rapid clearance of rHuEPO[55] and due to this reason initial studies of rHuEPO which were conducted with smaller doses did not show good benefits.

Maier et al. conducted a multicenter randomized controlled trial in six European countries including 241 VLBW premature infants with gestation <35 weeks.[56] On day 3 the infants were randomized to receive either no treatment or 250 IU/kg rHuEPO subcutaneously three times per week from day 3 to day 42 (17 doses). Oral iron supplementation (2 mg/kg/day) was given to all the neonates from day 14, and increased according to serum ferritin levels. Success of treatment was defined by no transfusion requirement and venous hematocrit above 32% during the entire study period. They showed only a modest reduction in transfusions from 1.25 per infant during the study period, in the untreated group, to 0.87 transfusions in the treated group.

The first limitation of this study was that it had excluded sick preterm neonates who require the most transfusions in the postnatal period and therefore the most likely to get benefits of an alternative therapy to RBC transfusions. The second limitation was the imbalance in the control and intervention group with 28 (23%) in the rHuEPO group and 17 (14%) in the RBC transfusion group. RBC transfusions reduces hypoxia and suppress endogenous erythropoietin production and erythropoiesis, and the need for repeated transfusion increases. In the babies who received treatment of rHuEPO in this trial, this supplementation overcame the suppressed endogenous erythropoietin production and hence the effect was exaggerated. A further exaggeration of this result could have been due to the liberal transfusion practices in that period.

To answer the question that whether erythropoietin caused a reduction in probability of bronchopulmonary dysplasia a study on 55 preterm was done by Al-Kharfy et al.[57] He found that infants who received 200 IU/kg of rHuEPO subcutaneously (sc) three times a week for 6 weeks received 2.2 less transfusion as compared to the control group (3.48 transfusions in rHuEPO group, 5.68 transfusions for infants in the control group). These results favored the hypothesis that rHuEPO was effective at reducing transfusion requirements in those infants at high-risk of having BPD. However, the authors included the subjects from 10th–14th day of life and they did not exclude babies who may have received prior transfusion thus it is likely many of the recruited infants received RBC transfusions prior to the study period, once again confounding the results.

Ohls et al. conducted a multicentric study in 2 sets of preterm babies with birth weights between 400–1250 g.[58] They enrolled 290 preterm neonates who were given rHuEPO in a dose of 400 IU/Kg given 3 times a week and its effect on decreasing the number of RBC transfusions in infants with birth weights between 400 and 1000 g (Trial I), and between 1000 and 1250 g (Trial II). Neonates were randomized between 1 and 4 days of age, and erythropoietin therapy was commenced by the 5th day and continued till the 35th postmenstrual week. They found no statistically significant decrease in the number of RBC transfusions in trial I [4.3 (rHuEPO) vs 5.2 (control) transfusions, p = 0.09], and no significant decrease in the number of VLBW infants who received any transfusions in trial II [37% (rHuEPO) vs 46% (control), p = 0.25]. One strong point of this study was that it included sick preterm infants. However, there were certain limitations of this study too. Firstly, 37% infants in the ELBW group received transfusions prior to the study period and were not excluded. Secondly, this study reported very high phlebotomy losses in sick ELBW as compared to other studies—84 mL (rHuEPO) and 87 mL (control) per infant which may have given the above nonsignificant results.[59]

Franz et al. found that RBCs transfusions to VLBW infants can be reduced to the rate reported during rHuEPO administration if restrictive transfusion guidelines are applied.[60] Most neonatal units have adopted restricted blood transfusion in most preterms in the last decade. When rHuEPO use is seen in combination with restrictive transfusion guidelines, it does not significantly reduce the use of one or more red blood cell transfusions and thus does not further reduce donor exposure to the neonate.[58] Using restrictive transfusion policies has not resulted in an increased need for respiratory support or oxygen therapy or poorer weight gain or increased length of hospital stay. Most studies show no increased incidence of important neonatal complications, such as intraventricular hemorrhage (IVH), necrotizing enterocolitis (NEC), chronic lung disease of prematurity (CLD) or sepsis in preterm neonates managed with a restrictive blood transfusion policy.[58,61] However, a recent study comparing liberal and restrictive transfusion guidelines for preterm neonates found that infants in the restrictive transfusion group were more likely to suffer IVH and periventricular leukomalacia (PVL).[62] These complications were not increased in the premature infants in need of transfusion (PINT) study of neonatal RBCs transfusion thresholds.[63]

For sick preterm infants, particularly ELBW infants, rHuEPO is unlikely to avoid RBCs transfusions in this period. Because of small blood volume and the relatively larger phlebotomy volumes that are required during hospital stay in ELBW, they often end up requiring multiple transfusions in this period. Most preterm infants who require blood transfusions will receive their first transfusion during first 2 weeks.[59] EPO takes approximately 1–2 weeks to produce effect on erythropoiesis, reflecting the time needed for proliferation, differentiation and maturation of RBCs precursors.

The administration of erythropoietin has not been accepted widely because it appears to have limited efficacy in decreasing the number of blood donors to which the infant is exposed via transfusion, whether erythropoietin is administered early (within the 1st week of life) or late (at or after 8 days of life).

Early Erythropoietin Use

Although, early administration of erythropoietin appears to reduce the number of transfusions required in preterm infants, the small reduction may be of limited clinical importance, because erythropoietin does not decrease the number of donor exposures due to the use of satellite packs. In addition, some trials suggest that early erythropoietin administration increased the risk of retinopathy of prematurity (ROP).

These findings were best illustrated in a meta-analysis of 27 trials (2,209 preterm infants) that evaluated the effect of early administration of erythropoietin (given before 8 days of age) compared with placebo or no intervention.[64] Many of these infants had received blood transfusions prior to enrollment in the trials. The following findings were noted:

- Early erythropoietin reduced the risk of receiving one or more RBC transfusions (RR 0.79, 95% CI 0.73–0.85) with number needed to treat benefit was 7, 95% CI 6–10 in 16 studies enrolling 1,661 infants.
- In 13 trials of 1,115 infants, erythropoietin slightly reduced the number of RBC transfusions (weighted mean difference of –0.27, 95% CI –0.42 to –0.12). The total volume of RBC transfused per infant was also less in erythropoietin-treated group (typical mean difference was 7 mL/kg, 7 studies, 581 infants).
- In three studies on 254 infants, erythropoietin use (EPO group) helped in reducing the number of donors to whom the infants were exposed to (mean difference –0.54, 95% CI –0.89 to –0.20)

- In 10 trials of 1,425 infants, EPO increased the risk of ROP (RR 1.18, 95% 0.99–1.40). In a subanalysis of six trials of 930 infants in which information was available, EPO appeared to increase the risk of severe ROP. With early EPO use, there was no significant increase in the risk of stage ≥3 ROP (typical RR 1.37, 95% CI 0.87–2.17; I2 = 0%; typical RD 0.03, 95% CI –0.01 to 0.06; I2 = 29%; seven studies, 801 infants). A post-hoc analysis including all studies that reported on ROP stage ≥3, regardless of the age of the infant when EPO treatment was started, showed a significantly increased typical RR of 1.48 (95% CI 1.02–2.13; p = 0.04; I2 = 0%) and typical RD of 0.03 (95% CI 0.00–0.06; p = 0.03; I2 = 50%; 10 studies, 1,303 infants) with a number needed to harm (NNH) of 33 (95% CI 17 to infinity).
- There were no differences between the EPO and placebo groups in the rates of mortality, sepsis, IVH, PVL, NEC, BPD, hypertension, length of hospital stay, or long-term neurodevelopmental outcome.

In summary, early erythropoietin is associated with only a small reduction in the number of transfusions, but no clinically significant reduction in exposure to the number of donors, and has no impact on clinical outcomes.

In a follow-up study from one of the trials included in the meta-analysis, erythropoietin and placebo-treated infants at 18–22 months corrected age with birth weights <1,000 g had similar weight and length, number of rehospitalizations, transfusions after discharge and developmental outcomes.[65]

Late Erythropoietin Use

Late administration of erythropoietin reduces the number of transfusions, but the limited benefit does not justify its use. This was illustrated in a 2014 meta-analysis that evaluated the effects of late erythropoietin administration (at or later than 8 days of age) compared with placebo or no intervention.[66] Most of these infants had received blood transfusions prior to enrollment in the trials. The following findings were noted:

- EPO reduced the risk of receiving one or more RBC transfusions (RR 0.71, 95% CI 0.64–0.79)
- EPO reduced the number of RBC transfusions (weighted mean difference of –0.22, 95% CI –0.38 to –0.06)
- There was no difference in the volume of blood transfused (mean difference –1.6 mL/kg, 95% CI –5.8–2.6)
- Erythropoietin had no effect on the rates for ROP, mortality, sepsis, IVH, PVL, NEC, BPD, hypertension, length of hospital stay, or long-term neurodevelopmental outcome. However, there was a trend toward an increased risk of ROP associated with erythropoietin administration (RR 1.27, 95% CI 0.99–1.64).

Late administration of erythropoietin reduced the mean number of transfusions by a little less than one transfusion per infant. This small benefit of erythropoietin was diminished due to the exposure of previous blood transfusions before 8 days of life, and the use of satellite packs that would mitigate against additional donor exposure in the control group. As a result, it is not recommended to routinely administer erythropoietin after 8 days because its limited benefit of limiting exposure to blood donors does not justify its cost.

Comparison Early versus Late Use

There appears to be no benefit of early erythropoietin administration compared with late administration in reducing the number of transfusions, the amount of red cells transfused, or number of donor exposures per infant. This was illustrated in a meta-analysis of two trials (262 patients), which was updated in 2012, that found no statistical benefit of early erythropoietin administration.[67,68] However, there appeared to be an increased risk of ROP associated with early administration. Early erythropoietin administration resulted in a nonsignificant reduction in the "number of transfusions per infant" compared with late erythropoietin [typical MD –0.32 (95% CI –0.92–0.29)]. There was no significant reduction in total volume of blood transfused per infant or in the number of donors to whom the infant was exposed. Early erythropoietin led to a significant increase in the risk of ROP (all stages) [two studies, 191 infants; typical RR 1.40 (95% CI 1.05–1.86); typical RD 0.16 (95% CI 0.03–0.29); NNT 6 (95% CI 3–33)]. These data support the recommendation of not administering erythropoietin in the first 8 days of life.

COMPLICATIONS

Use of erythropoietin in premature infants appears to be safe. Hypertension, rash, bone pain, seizures, or later development of anti-EPO antibodies have not been reported in premature infants. In adults, complications of erythropoietin treatment for erythropoiesis include polycythemia, rash, seizures, hypertension, shortened time to death, myocardial infarction, congestive heart failure, progression of tumors and stroke. None of these adverse effects have been reported in randomized controlled studies of erythropoietin treated neonates receiving up to 2,100 U/kg/week, nor have differences been noted in the incidence of neonatal morbidities, including IVH, ROP, NEC, CLD, and late-onset sepsis.[69]

Complications noticed in trials on neonates include the following:

- A transient neutropenia that resolves with cessation of therapy is occasionally observed. In one trial, mean ANCs after 20 days were lower in premature infants, who received erythropoietin compared with RBC transfusion (1.8×10^3 vs 3.9×10^3).[70] This side effect, however, has not been seen in many recent studies.
- Iron deficiency occurs if supplementation is inadequate.[71,72]
- As discussed above, early administration of erythropoietin has been associated with increased risk of ROP. The role of erythropoietin in the development of ROP in preterm infants is controversial. ROP occurs in two phases, the first involving loss of retinal vasculature following birth, and the second involving uncontrolled proliferation of retinal vessels. EPO induces angiogenesis and prevents vascular apoptosis which is important in preventing the first phase

of ROP, while in the second phase its angiogenic effect could increase abnormal neovascularization leading to a worsening of ROP. According to this hypothesis and with the aim to prevent ROP, rHuEPO can be given to induce angiogenesis and to inhibit apoptosis of retinal vasculature in the first phase when low IGF-1 levels prevent the angiogenic effect of vascular endothelial growth factor (VEGF), but as proliferative ROP begins rHuEPO could be avoided as hypoxia and ischemia.[73,74] A Cochrane meta-analysis of prospective studies of erythropoietin (for which ROP was not a primary outcome measure) showed an increased in rate of ROP (any grade) and of ROP stage more than or equal to three after early erythropoietin exposure.[64] This analysis could not separate out confounders such as effects of anemia or iron treatment. Also, this meta-analysis reflected a misclassification of a single-center erythropoietin study by Romagnoli and colleagues into the early erythropoietin administration group. When this study was correctly grouped with other studies of late erythropoietin use, the revised meta-analysis showed no significant difference in ROP with the use of early or late erythropoietin. Evaluation for ROP continues to be a priority in most clinical trials of erythropoietin use for preterm infants.

DOSE

If erythropoietin is given, it can be administered intravenously 3 times a week as a once daily infusion of 200 units/kg per dose or as a continuous infusion over 24 hours of 300 units/kg; or subcutaneously (400 units/kg/dose, 3 times per week).[75,76] When given intravenously, erythropoietin should be mixed in a protein-containing solution (5% albumin) and given over at least 4 hours, or continuously over 24 hours, often as an addition to total parenteral nutrition. The undiluted drug (2,000 units/mL) can be given subcutaneously in a volume of 0.2 mL/kg for infants <1,000 g. Erythropoietin preparation with higher concentrations (up to 10,000 units/mL) can be used as the infant grows. When administered intravenously over a short period of time, the increased excretion of rHuEPO results in decreased bioavailability and less effective erythropoiesis. Studies infusing rHuEPO over 24 hours, either with TPN or as a separate infusion intravenously, or as a single subcutaneous dose, showed greater bone marrow response. Thus, having peak serum levels that are sustained over a prolonged period of time results in more effective red cell production. For this reason, the preferred route of administration is by subcutaneous injection for ease of administration.

In a small clinical trial, preterm infants who received 1,200 units/kg once a week and control infants who received the standard 3 times a week dosing (400 units/kg) had similar increases in absolute reticulocyte counts and hematocrits at the end of the 4-week trial period.[77] However, further studies are needed to confirm that weekly dosing provides the same benefit as more frequent administration.

Infants treated with erythropoietin require iron supplementation. A proposed regimen is a daily elemental iron dose of 6 mg/kg for infants on full enteral feedings and 3 mg/kg for those taking at least 60 mL/kg/day.[78] The reticulocyte count, central hematocrit or hemoglobin concentration and ANC are measured before as well as 1–2 weeks after starting erythropoietin treatment. Erythropoietin is withheld if the ANC is <1,000/μL. Serum ferritin levels may be useful in evaluating those infants who are not responding to therapy to detect iron deficiency.[75] Iron can be increased to 9–12 mg/kg/day if ferritin is below 100 μg/L **(Table 44.2)**.

USE IN RHESUS SENSITIZATION

In the neonate, a postnatal hyporegenerative anemia may complicate hemolytic disease of newborn. The main reason for this is depressed erythropoiesis and low reticulocyte counts typically noticed. This spontaneously resolves by around 16 weeks of age but may require RBC transfusions.

Table 44.2 Recommendation for use of erythropoietin in neonates

Drug: Erythropoietin	*Special measure, dose and administration*
Erythropoietin use in IV route	• 200 U/kg/day added to TPN • Begin dosing when infant is receiving protein • IV administration (if not added to TPN) to run over at least 4 hours, use protein-containing solution to dilute
Erythropoietin SC route use	• 400 U/kg given 3 times a week • Begin dosing at 7–10 days of life, or when IV access is gone • For preterm infants being discharged, or for infants with late anemia due to Rh or ABO isoimmunization, a dose of 1,000 U/kg SC once a week can be used to enhance erythropoiesis
Erythropoietin length of treatment	• Continue dosing until 34–36 weeks' corrected gestational age • Erythropoietin is contraindicated in infants with thromboembolic disease, hypertension, or seizures
Iron and other nutrients	• Iron dextran, 3–5 mg/kg once a week added to TPN solution if available (1 mg/kg/day is acceptable; check ferritin after 2 weeks of dosing) • Ferrous sulfate 4–6 mg/kg/day, depending on formula (4 mg/kg/day) vs EBM (6 mg/kg/day) • Vitamin E 25 IU/day PO • Folate 50 μg/day

Abbreviations: EBM, expressed breastmilk; IV, intravenous; SC, subcutaneous; TPN, total parenteral nutrition

The possible mechanisms for this anemia in Rh sensitization are either of the three, i.e. intramedullary destruction of red blood cells precursors, bone marrow suppression from intrauterine transfusions, or erythropoietin deficiency relative to the degree of the anemia. The benefit of rHuEPO in the treatment of this hyporegenerative anemia is uncertain at present, and treatment with rHuEPO may be ineffective when anti-Rh(D) titers are high; stimulating red cell production may merely contribute to the ongoing hemolysis. Further large-scale controlled trials are needed to elucidate the potential role of rHuEPO in these patients.

USE IN JEHOVAH'S WITNESS

There are 55,00,000 Jehovah's witnesses (JWs) worldwide. Their position is based on biblical passages forbidding the eating of blood, which they interpret to preclude transfusion of blood. Legally, except in an emergency, parental consent is necessary to perform any medical procedure on a child, including the transfusion of blood based products. Although the courts can become involved to protect the child's welfare when consent is withheld, on the doctrine that the child's welfare is paramount, consideration should nevertheless be given to parental beliefs, particularly when the situation is not imminently life-threatening.

OTHER USES: NEUROPROTECTION

Erythropoietin is also produced in developing brain where it functions as both an important growth factor and neuroprotective agent for the central nervous system. Erythropoietin is produced in brain by multiple cell types, including astrocytes, oligodendrocytes, neurons and microglia. Erythropoietin production is stimulated by hypoxia; in the brain, this is mediated by the transcription factor hypoxia-inducible factor (HIF)-1.[79]

Erythropoietin is shown to have neuroprotective effects through different mechanisms such as direct neurotrophic effect, decreased susceptibility to glutamate toxicity, induction of antiapoptotic factors, decreased inflammation, decreased nitric oxide-mediated injury, direct antioxidant effects and protective effects on glia. Interestingly, the antioxidative effect of erythropoietin may be enhanced by the increased erythropoiesis utilizing the free-iron, which has accumulated following hypoxia-ischemia.[79] Erythropoietin also stimulates and interacts with other protective factors such as brain-derived neurotrophic factor (BDNF) and glial cell derived neurotrophic factor (GDNF). Erythropoietin along with VEGF promotes angiogenesis and repair **(Flow chart 44.2)**.

Many nonclinical studies have suggested that erythropoietin has a neuroprotective effect following hypoxia-ischemia and reperfusion;[80] in neonatal models systemically administered erythropoietin is neuroprotective[81] with early and high-dose treatment (5,000 U/kg) required to reduce brain injury and promote neurogenesis.[82] Multiple doses of erythropoietin would result in a more sustained neuroprotection.

The neuroprotective action of rHuEPO is usually seen at much higher doses than the one used in anemia. The CSF demonstrated neuroprotective concentrations of erythropoietin only after high-dose rHuEPO administration in nonhuman primates and sheep.[83] Whether higher doses of erythropoietin can improve outcomes without inducing complications are unknown. Concerns over the use of high doses of erythropoietin include possible thrombotic

Flow chart 44.2 Effects of erythropoietin on brain cells: short-term and long-term effects

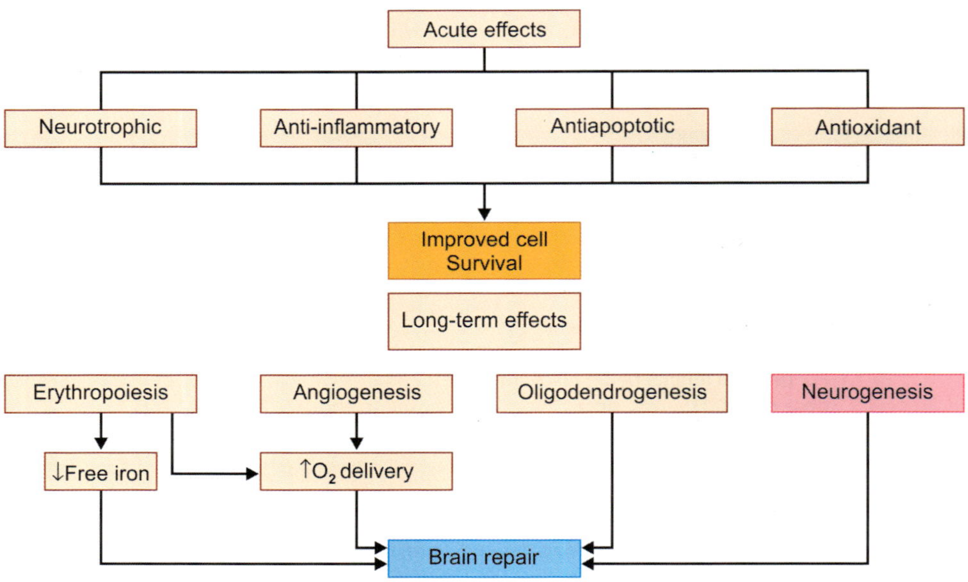

and hematological complications and real safety concerns have arisen in two recent adult studies. Brines and associates demonstrated that high-dose erythropoietin (5,000 U/kg IP) penetrates the blood-brain barrier and provides neuroprotection in adult models of brain injury.[84] The highest doses (20,000–30,000 U/kg) lose protective properties, may cause harm, and are not recommended. However, the minimum effective dose has not yet been established and may depend on whether the blood-brain barrier is intact. Thus, the mechanism of brain injury may dictate the dose of erythropoietin required for neuroprotection, as does the age of the individual.

In a study designed to test the erythropoietic effects of erythropoietin, infants weighing 1,250 g or less at birth were prospectively randomized to erythropoietin or placebo or control from day 4 of life until 35 weeks corrected gestational age. Their follow-up revealed no difference in developmental outcomes at 18–22 months.[65] Infants weighing <1,000 g with serum erythropoietin concentrations greater than 500 mU/mL had higher mental development index (MDI) scores than infants with erythropoietin concentrations <500 mU/mL when tested at 18–22 months corrected age.[85] Another retrospective review of ELBW infants compared 89 erythropoietin-treated versus 57 untreated neonates at 10–13 years of age. Erythropoietin-treated neonates had better outcomes with 55% of the erythropoietin group assessed as normal versus 39% untreated ($p < 0.05$). Intelligence quotient (IQ) scores were also higher in erythropoietin-treated patients (90.8 vs 81.3 in untreated infants; $p < 0.005$).[86]

Two-phase I or II studies evaluating the safety[87] and pharmacokinetics[88] of erythropoietin using escalating doses in preterm infants and term infants with hypoxic-ischemic encephalopathy (HIE)[89] being treated with hypothermia showed that a dose of 1,000 U/kg produced plasma concentrations similar to those found to be neuroprotective in animals and was well tolerated. Follow-up of patients treated with erythropoietin in these phase I or II trials allow for optimism that erythropoietin may be beneficial.[90] Ohls and colleagues showed that both erythropoietin and darbepoetin had neuroprotective effects (improved cognitive performance assessed by Bayley-III) when compared with placebo in preterm infants followed up at 18–22 months. There was no cerebral palsy among recipients of darbepoetin or erythropoietin, whereas five cases of cerebral palsy were identified in the placebo group (p < 0.001). The incidence of neurodevelopmental impairment in the erythropoiesis stimulating agents group (ESAs) was significantly lower compared with placebo (odds ratio, 0.18; 95% CI, 0.05–0.63).[91]

Term infants with hypoxia-ischemia were studied in a prospective case-control study of 45 infants, 15 of whom had HIE and received erythropoietin (HIE-EPO group) (2,500 IU/kg subcutaneously daily for 5 days); 15 were HIE controls, and 15 were normal term infants. Electroencephalogram (EEG) backgrounds improved (p = 0.01) and nitric oxide concentrations decreased (p <0.001) in the HIE-erythropoietin group compared with the HIE-control group. More important, infants in the HIE-erythropoietin group had fewer neurologic (p <0.05) and developmental (p <0.05) abnormalities at 6 months.[92]

A recent randomized controlled study in 167 infants reported that repeated low-dose (300 or 500 U/kg) rHuEPO was safe and resulted in improved neurological outcome in moderate-to-severe neonatal encephalopathy at 18 months of age. Recombinant erythropoietin was administered every other day for 2 weeks, starting by 48 hours after birth. Outcomes were not different between the two erythropoietin doses. Subgroup analyses indicated that erythropoietin improved long-term outcomes only for infants with moderate HIE and not those with severe HIE. No negative hematopoietic side effects were observed.[93]

A preliminary finding of a phase II study of erythropoietin neuroprotection in preterm infants has shown improved white matter integrity at term equivalent age.[94] Long-term neurodevelopmental outcomes of this study, which used three doses of 3,000 U/kg in the first 3 days of life, are pending. Other phase III studies of erythropoietin neuroprotection for preterm infants are ongoing in the United States [preterm EPO neuroprotection trial (PENUT), NCT01378273] and Europe [efficacy of erythropoietin to improve survival and neurologic outcome in HIE (Neurepo), NCT01732146]. Each of these studies is using different dosing strategies and different durations of therapy. The results from these initial trials will inform future studies as to the optimal dose and duration of therapy for individual pathologies.

Many cost benefit analyses were conducted in 1990s for use of erythropoietin as compared to RBCs transfusion with variable results. The relative benefit of erythropoietin is related to the study design (early vs late treatment, liberal vs restrictive transfusion), patient population and value assigned to different complex outcomes. One item that is perhaps most difficult to evaluate is the psychosocial burden imposed on family, patient, and caregivers by transfusion or the potential risk of transfusion-related infection, however rare transmission may be. Although most such infections can now be cured (bacterial infection) or managed as chronic diseases (human immunodeficiency virus, hepatitis C), significant social stigma and psychological burden may be associated with acquisition. The value assigned to avoiding such infection is highly subjective and, therefore, difficult to model accurately.

Necrotizing Enterocolitis

Animal studies have reported a protective effect of rHuEPO against NEC[95] and Ledbetter et al. reported a decreased incidence of NEC rates in neonates treated with rHuEPO.[96] Ohlsson and Aher included an analysis of NEC rates in their systematic review.[65] The data of 1,471 infants from 10 studies were analyzed; no difference in NEC rates was found between treated and untreated groups. In a very recent trial which included 90 preterm babies of ≤33 weeks gestational age. The cohort was randomized to receive either G-CSF, or erythropoietin or both or placebo group. This trial revealed that neonates who received enteral G-CSF and/or rHuEPO had a better feed tolerance and had a shorter duration of hospital stay. The risk of NEC was also corrected. No adverse effects were also noticed of this treatment strategy.[97]

Darbepoetin

A modified version of erythropoietin, known as darbepoetin alfa (Darbe), or novel erythropoiesis stimulating protein (NESP) was developed by Amgen in 1998. Darbepoetin has a longer serum half-life than erythropoietin in adults and preterm infants, allowing increased dosage intervals to be used. Darbepoetin alfa has been used in preterm infants using a weekly dose of 10 μg/kg. In one of the recently concluded and published trials 102 preterm infants with weight <1,250 g were randomized to receive weekly darbepoetin or erythropoietin or placebo when they were <48 hours of age and they were continued through 35 weeks of gestation. Infants in the darbepoetin and erythropoietin groups received significantly fewer transfusions ($p = 0.015$) and were exposed to fewer donors ($p = 0.044$) than the placebo group (Darbepoetin: 1.2 ± 2.4 transfusions and 0.7 ± 1.2 donors per infant; erythropoietin: 1.2 ± 1.6 transfusions and 0.8 ± 1.0 donors per infant; placebo: 2.4 ± 2.9 transfusions and 1.2 ± 1.3 donors per infant). Hematocrit and reticulocyte counts were higher in the darbepoetin and erythropoietin groups compared with placebo ($p = 0.001$, darbepoetin and erythropoietin versus placebo for both hematocrit and absolute reticulocyte count).[98] Importantly, nearly half of the infants treated with darbepoetin or erythropoietin could completely avoid transfusions. There was no significant difference in the incidence of ROP, ICH, NEC, or other complications seen frequently in the NICU. There are occasional case reports, which have proved the safety and pharmacokinetics of this drug and hence now it is mostly preferred to erythropoietin in most centers now.

CONCLUSION

Hematopoietic growth factors like G-CSF, GM-CSF, erytropoietin, drabepoietin, etc. are essential for growth and functional development of various hematopoietic stem cells. These have been tested and found to be of some use in hematological and nonhematological conditions like NEC prevention and neuroprotection. Their side effects may have potentially bad consequences and hence they need to be used judiciously in a sick neonate.

KEY POINTS

- G-CSF and GM-CSF are especially useful in severe congenital neutropenias and in neonatal sepsis in preterm babies with neutropenia they do increase the neutrophil counts earlier but do not give any advantage in reducing the mortality or improving the long-term neurological outcome. Their role in prevention of sepsis is not proven on many clinical trials and hence should not be routinely practiced.
- Erythropoietin is beneficial in increasing the hematocrit but usually not found to reduce the decrease in exposure to donors in RBCs transfusion.
- When used, rHuEPO should be administered subcutaneously 3 times a week, 250 IU/kg/dose. The use of restrictive transfusion guidelines in neonatal medicine reduces the number of transfusions given to preterm and sick neonates.
- The neuroprotective role of erythropoietin is being studied in term and preterm neonates in prospective clinical trials and may find a clinical role in neonatal medicine.

REFERENCES

1. Bradley TR, Metcalf D. The growth of mouse bone marrow in vitro. Aust J Exp Biol Med Sci. 1966;44(3):287-99.
2. Pluznik DH, Sachs L. The cloning of normal "mast cells" in tissue culture. J Cell Physiol. 1965;66(3):319-24.
3. Metcalf D. Hemopoietic regulators and leukemia development: a personal retrospective. Adv Cancer Res.1994;63:41-91.
4. Clark SC, Kamen R. The human hematopoietic colony stimulating factors. Science. 1987;236(4806):1229-37.
5. Christensen RD, Rothstein G: Pre- and postnatal development of granulocytic stem cells in the rat. Pediatr Res. 1984;18:599-602.
6. Parravicini E, van de Ven C, Anderson L, Cairo MS. Myeloid Hematopoietic growth factors and their role in prevention and/or treatment of Neonatal sepsis. Transfusion medicine reviews. 2002;1(16):11-24.
7. Christensen RD, MacFarlane JL, Taylor NL, et al. Blood and marrow neutrophils during experimental group B streptococcal infection: Quantification of the stem cell, proliferative, storage and circulating pools. Pediatr Res. 1982;16:549-53.
8. Eisenfeld L, Krause PJ, Herson V, et al. Longitudinal study of neutrophil adherence and motility. J Pediatr.1990;117:926-9.
9. Harris MC, Shalit M, Southwick FS. Diminished actin polymerization by neutrophils from newborn infants. Pediatr Res .1993;33:27-31.
10. Wolach B, Ben Dor M, Chomsky O, et al. Improved chemotactic ability of neonatal polymorphonuclear cells induced by mild membrane rigidification. J Leukocyte Biol. 1992;51:324-8.
11. Anderson DC, et al. Impaired motility of neonatal PMN leukocytes: relationship to abnormalities of cell orientation and assembly of microtubules in chemotactic gradients. J Leukoc Biology. 1984;36:1-15.
12. Dos Santos C, Davidson D. Neutrophil chemotaxis to leukotriene B4 in vitro is decreased for the human neonate. Pediatr Res. 1993;33: 242-6.
13. Lorant DE, et al. P-selectin expression by endothelial cells is decreased in neonatal rats and human premature infants. Blood. 1999;94:600-9.
14. Calhoun DA, Christensen RD. Human developmental biology of granulocyte colony stimulating-factor. Clinic Perinatol. 2000;27(3):559-76.
15. Cairo MS, Suen Y, Knoppel E, et al. Decreased G-CSF and IL-3 production and gene expression from mononuclear cells of newborn infants. Pediatric Research 1992;31:574–8.
16. Cairo MS, Plunkett JM, Mauss D, et al. Seven-day administration of recombinant human granulocyte colony-stimulating factor to newborn rats: Modulation of neonatal neutrophilia, myelopoiesis, and group B streptococcus sepsis. Blood. 1990;76:1788-94.

17. Cairo MS, Manss D, Kommareddy S, et al. Prophylactic or simultaneous administration of recombinant human granulocyte colony stimulating factor in the treatment of group B streptococcal sepsis in neonatal rats. Pediatr Res. 1990;27:612-6.
18. Frenck RW, Sarman G, Harper TE, et al. The ability of recombinant murine granulocyte-macrophage colony-stimulating factor to protect neonatal rats from septic death due to *Staphylococcus aureus*. J Infect Dis. 1990;165:109-14.
19. Cairo MS, Mauss D, Plunkett JM, et al. Modulation of neonatal myelopoiesis in newborn rats following 7-day administration of either GM-CSF or IL-3 (granulocyte-monocyte colony stimulating factor or interleukin-3). Pediatr Res. 1991;29:504-9.
20. Cairo MS, van de Ven C, Toy C, et al. Recombinant human granulocyte-macrophage colony stimulating factor primes neonatal granulocytes for enhanced oxidative metabolism and chemotaxis. Pediatr Res. 1989;26:395-9.
21. Cairo MS, van de Ven C, Toy C, et al. Lymphokines: Enhancement by granulocyte-macrophage and granulocyte colony-stimulating factors of neonatal myeloid kinetics and functional activation of polymorphonuclear leukocytes. Rev Inf Dis. 1990;12:492-7.
22. Cairo MS, van de Ven C, Toy C, et al. GM-CSF primes and modulates neonatal PMN motility: up-regulation of C3bi (Mol) expression with alteration in PMN adherence and aggregation. Am J Ped Hematol/Oncol. 1991;13:249-57.
23. Lopez AF, Nicola NA, Burgess AW, et al. Activation of granulocyte cytotoxic function by purified mouse colony-stimulating factors. J lmmunol.1983;131:2983-8.
24. Roberts RL, Szelc CM, Scates SM, Boyd MT, Soderstrom KM, Davis MW, Glaspy JA. Neutropenia in an extremely premature infant treated with recombinant human granulocyte colony-stimulating factor. Am J Dis Child. 1991;145:808-12.
25. Gillan ER, Christensen R, Suen Y, et al. A randomized, placebo-controlled trial of recombinant human granulocyte colony stimulating factor administration in newborn infants with presumed sepsis: significant induction of peripheral and bone marrow neutrophilia. Blood. 1994;84:1427-33.
26. Kocherlakota P, LaGamma EF. Preliminary report: rhG CSF may reduce the incidence of neonatal sepsis in prolonged preeclampsia-associated neutropenia. Pediatr. 1998;102: 1107-11.
27. Kuhn P, Messer J, Paupe A, Espagne S, et al. A multicentre, randomized, placebo controlled trial of prophylactic recombinant granulocyte-colony stimulating factor in preterm neonates with neutropenia. J Peds. 2009;155:324-30.
28. Miura E, Procianoy RS, Bittar C, et al. A randomized, double-masked, placebo-controlled trial of recombinant granulocyte colony-stimulating factor administration to preterm infants with the clinical diagnosis of early-onset sepsis. Pediatr. 2001;107:30-35.
29. Bernstein HM, Pollock BH, Calhoun DA, et al. Administration of recombinant granulocyte colony-stimulating factor to neonates with septicemia: A meta-analysis. Journal of Pediatrics. 2001;138:917-20.
30. Carr R, Modi N, Doré CJ. G-CSF and GM-CSF for treating or preventing neonatal infections. Cochrane Database of Systematic Reviews 2003, Issue 3. Art. No.: CD003066.
31. Borjianyazdi L , Froomandi M, Noori Shadkam M, Hashemi A, Fallah R. The Effect of Granulocyte Colony Stimulating Factor Administration on Preterm Infant with Neutropenia and Clinical Sepsis: A Randomized Clinical Trial. Iranian Journal of Pediatric Hematology Oncology. 2013;3(2):64-68.
32. Gathwala G, Walia M, Bala H, Singh S. Recombinant human granulocyte colony-stimulating factor in preterm neonates with sepsis and relative neutropenia: a randomized, single-blind, non-placebo-controlled trial. J Trop Pediatr. 2012;58(1):12-8.
33. Russell B, Emmerson AJ, Wilkinson N, Chant T, Sweet DG, Halliday HL, et al. A trial of recombinant human granulocyte colony stimulating factor for the treatment of very low birthweight infants with presumed sepsis and neutropenia. Arch Dis Child Fetal Neonatal Ed- 2001;84:F172-F176.
34. Cairo MS, Agosti JM, Ellis R. A randomized, double blind, placebo-controlled trial of prophylactic recombinant human granulocyte-macrophage colony-stimulating factor to reduce nosocomial infections in very low birth weight neonates. J Pediatr. 1999;134:64-70.
35. Carr R, Brocklehurst R, Dore CJ, Modi N. Granulocyte-macrophage colony stimulating factor administered as prophylaxis for reduction of sepsis in extremely preterm, small for gestational age neonates (the PROGRAMS trial): a single-blind, multicentre, randomised controlled trial. Lancet. 2009; 373:226-33.
36. Marlow N, et al. A randomised trial of granulocyte-macrophage colony-stimulating factor for neonatal sepsis: outcomes at 2 years. Arch Dis Child Fetal Neonatal Ed. 2013;98:F46-F53.
37. Marlow N, et al. A randomised trial of granulocyte-macrophage colony-stimulating factor for neonatal sepsis: childhood outcomes at 5 years. Arch Dis Child Fetal Neonatal Ed. 2015; 0:F1-F7.
38. Venkateswaran L, Wilimas JA, Dancy R, Wang WC, Korones S, Hayden J, et al. Granulocyte–macrophage colony-stimulating factor in the treatment of neonates with neutropenia and sepsis. Pediatr Hematol Oncol. 2000;17:469-73.
39. Ahmad A, Laborada G, Bussel J, et al. Comparison of recombinant granulocyte colony-stimulating factor, recombinant human granulocyte-macrophage colony-stimulating factor and placebo for treatment of septic preterm infants. Pediatr Infect Dis J. 2002;21:1061-5.
40. Rodwell RL, Gray PH, Taylor Km, Minchinton R. Granulocyte colony stimulating factor treatment for alloimmune neonatal neutropenia. Arch Dis Child Fetal Neonatal Ed. 1996;75(1):F57-8.
41. Kerst JM, de Haas M, van der Schoot CE, et al. Recombinant granulocyte colony-stimulating factor administration to healthy volunteers: induction of immunophenotypically and functionally altered neutrophils via an affect on myeloid progenitor cells. Blood. 1993;82(11):3265-72.
42. Zeidler C. Congenital neutropenias. Hematology. 2005;10 (Suppl 1):306-11.
43. Christensen RD, Calhoum DA. Congenital neutropenia. Clin Perinatol. 2004;31(1):29-38.
44. Rosenberg PS, Alter PB, Bolyard AA, et al. The incidence of leukemia and mortality from sepsis in patients with severe congenital neutropenia receiving long term G-CSF therapy. Blood. 2006;107(12):4628-35.
45. Schmitz S, Franke H,Wichmann HE, Diehl V. The effect of continuous G-CSF application in human cyclic neutropenia: a model analysis. Br J Hematol. 1995;90(1):41-7.
46. Calderwood S, Kilpatrick L, Douglas SD, et al. Recombinant human granulocyte colony-stimulating factor therapy for patients with neutropenia 1 and/or neutrophil dysfunction secondary to glycogen storage disease type 1b. Blood. 2001;97:376-82.
47. Rivers A, WB Slayton. Congenital cytopenias and Bone marrow Failure syndromes.Semin Perinatol. 2009;33:20-8.

48. Fathali N, Lekic T, Zhang JH, Tang J. Long-term evaluation of granulocyte-colony stimulating factor on hypoxic-ischemic brain damage in infant rats. Intensive Care Med. 2010;36:1602-8.
49. Christensen RD, Havranek T, Gerstmann DR, Calhoun DA. Enteral administration of a simulated amniotic fluid to very low birth weight neonates. J Perinatol. 2005;25:380-5.
50. Barney CK, Lambert DK, Alder SC, Scoffield SH, Schmutz N, Christensen RD. Treating feeding intolerance with an enteral solution patterned after human amniotic fluid: A randomized, controlled, masked trial. J Perinatol. 2007;27:28-31.
51. Kling PJ, Schmidt RL, Roberts RA, Widness JA. Serum erythropoietin levels during infancy: associations with erythropoiesis. J Pediatr. 1996;128:791-6.
52. Dallman PR. Anemia of prematurity. Annu Rev Med. 1981; 32:143-60.
53. Wardrop CA, Holland BM, Beale KE, Jones JG, Gray OP. Nonphysiological anemia of prematurity. Arch Dis Child. 1978;53:855-60.
54. Widness JA, Seward VJ, Kromer IJ, Burmeiser LF, Bell EF. Changing patterns of red blood cell transfusion in very low birth weight infants. J Pediatr. 1996;129:680-7.
55. Widness JA, Pedersen PV, Modi NB, Schmidt RL, Chestnut DH. Developmental changes in erythropoietin pharmacokinetics: increased clearance and distribution in fetal and neonatal sheep. Pharmacol Exp Ther. 1992;261:977-84.
56. Maier RF, Obladen M, Scigalla P, Linderkamp O, Duc G, Hieronimi G, et al. The effect of epoetin beta (recombinant human erythropoietin) on the need for transfusion in very-low-birth-weight infants. European Multicentre Erythropoietin Study Group. N Engl J Med. 1994;330:1173-8.
57. Al-Kharfy T, Smyth JA, Wadsworth L, Krystal G, Fitzgerald C, Davis J, et al. Erythropoietin therapy in neonates at risk of having bronchopulmonary dysplasia and requiring multiple transfusions. J Pediatr. 1996;129:89-96.
58. Ohls RK, Ehrenkrantz RA, Wright LL, Lemons JA, Korones SB, Stoll BJ, et al. The effects of early erythropoietin therapy on the transfusion requirements of preterm infants below 1250 grams birth weight: a multicenter, randomized controlled trial. Pediatrics. 2001;108:934-42.
59. Ohls RK, Harcum J, Schibler KR, Christensen RD. The effect of erythropoietin on the transfusion requirements of preterm infants weighing 750 grams or less: a randomized, double blind, placebo controlled study. J Pediatr. 1997;131:661-5.
60. Franz AR, Pohlandt F. Red blood cell transfusions in very and extremely low birthweight infants under restrictive transfusion guidelines: is exogenous erythropoietin necessary? Arch Dis Child Fetal Neonatal Ed. 2001;84:96-100.
61. Shannon KM, Keith III JF, Mentzer WC, Ehrenkranz RA, Brown MS, Widness JA, et al. Recombinant human erythropoietin stimulates erythropoiesis and reduces erythrocyte transfusions in very low birth weight preterm infants. Pediatrics. 1995;95:1-8.
62. Bell EF, Strauss RG, Widness JA, Mahoney LT, Mock DM, Seward VJ, et al. Randomized trial of liberal versus restrictive guidelines for red blood cell transfusion in preterm infants. Pediatrics 2005;115(6):1685-91.
63. Kirpalani H, Whyte RK, Andersen C, Asztalos EV, Heddle N, Blajchman MA, et al. The Premature Infants in Need of Transfusion (PINT) study: a randomized, controlled trial of a restrictive (low) versus liberal (high) transfusion threshold for extremely low birth weight infants. J Pediatr. 2006;149:301-7.
64. Ohlsson A, Aher SM. Early erythropoietin for preventing red blood cell transfusion in preterm and/or low birth weight infants. Cochrane Database Systematic Rev. 2014.CD004863.
65. Ohls RK, Ehrenkranz RA, Das A, Dusick AM, et al. Neurodevelopmental outcome and growth at 18 to 22 months' corrected age in extremely low birth weight infants treated with early erythropoietin and iron. Pediatrics. 2004;114(5):1287-91.
66. Aher S, Ohlsson A. Late erythropoietin for preventing red blood cell transfusion in preterm and/or low birth weight infants. Cochrane Database Syst Rev. 2014. CD004868.
67. Aher SM, Ohlsson A. Early versus late erythropoietin for preventing red blood cell transfusion in preterm and/or low birth weight infants. Cochrane Database Syst Rev. 2012;10: CD004865
68. Aher SM, Ohlsson A. Early versus late erythropoietin for preventing red blood cell transfusion in preterm and/or low birth weight infants. Cochrane Database Syst Rev. 2006; CD004865.
69. Ohls RK. The use of erythropoietin in neonates. Clin Perinatol. 2000;27(3):681-96.
70. Ohls RK, Christensen RD. Recombinant erythropoietin compared with erythrocyte transfusion in the treatment of anemia of prematurity. J Pediatr. 1991;119(5):781-88.
71. Halpérin DS. Use of recombinant erythropoietin in treatment of the anemia of prematurity. Am J Pediatr Hematol Oncol. 1991;13(3):351-63.
72. Carnielli VP, Da Riol R, Montini G. Iron supplementation enhances response to high doses of recombinant human erythropoietin in preterm infants. Arch Dis Child Fetal Neonatal Ed. 1998;79(1):F44-8.
73. Sears JE. Stimulating angiogenesis to prevent ischemic retinopathy. Ophthalmology. 2009;116:1597-8.
74. Chen J, Smith LEH. A double-edged sword: erythropoietin eyed in retinopathy of prematurity. Ophthalmology. 2009;116:221-2.
75. Calhoun DA, Christensen RD, Edstrom CS, Juul SE, Ohls RK, Schibler KR, Sola MC, Sullivan SE. Consistent approaches to procedures and practices in neonatal hematology. Clin Perinatol. 2000;27(3):733-53.
76. Costa S, Romagnoli C, Zuppa AA, Cota F, Scorrano A, Gallini F, Maggio L. How to administer erythropoietin, intravenous or subcutaneous? Acta Paediatr. 2013;102(6):579-83.
77. Ohls RK, Roohi M, Peceny HM, et al. A randomized, masked study of weekly erythropoietin dosing in preterm infants. J Pediatr. 2012;160:790.
78. American Academy of Pediatrics, Committee on Nutrition. Nutritional needs of the preterm infant. In: Kleinman RE (Ed). Pediatric nutrition handbook. 5. Chapel Hill, NC: American Academy of Pediatrics; 2004. pp. 23-54.
79. Juul S, Pet GC. Erythropoietin and neonatal neuroprotection. Clin Perinatol. 2015;42:469-81.
80. Maiese K, Li F, ZZ C. New avenues of exploration for erythropoietin. JAMA. 2005;293:90-5.
81. Kellert BA, McPherson RJ, SE J. A comparison of high-dose recombinant erythropoietin treatment regimens in brain-injured neonatal rats. Pediatr Res. 2007;61:451-5.
82. Gonzalez FF, McQuillen P, Mu D, Chang Y, Wendland M, Vexler Z, et al. Erythropoietin enhances long-term neuroprotection and neurogenesis in neonatal stroke. Dev Neurosci. 2007;29:321-30.
83. Juul SE, McPherson RJ, Farrell FX, Jolliffe L, Ness DJ, CA G. Erythropoietin concentrations in cerebrospinal fluid of nonhuman primates and fetal sheep following high-dose recombinant erythropoietin. Biol Neonate. 2004;85:138-44.
84. Brines ML, Ghezzi P, Keenan S, et al. Erythropoietin crosses the blood-brain barrier to protect against experimental brain injury. Proc Natl Acad Sci USA. 2000;97(19):10526-31.

85. Bierer R, Peceny MC, Hartenberger CH, Ohls RK. Erythropoietin concentrations and neurodevelopmental outcome in preterm infants. Pediatrics. 2006;118(3):e635-640.
86. Neubauer AP, Voss W, Wachtendorf M, Jungmann T. Erythropoietin improves neurodevelopmental outcome of extremely preterm infants. Ann Neurol. 2010;67(5):657-66.
87. Fauchere JC, Dame C, Vonthein R, et al. An approach to using recombinant erythropoietin for neuroprotection in very preterm infants. Pediatrics. 2008;122(2):375-82.
88. Juul SE, McPherson RJ, Bauer LA, et al. A phase I/II trial of high-dose erythropoietin in extremely low birth weight infants: pharmacokinetics and safety. Pediatrics. 2008;122(2):383-91.
89. Wu YW, Bauer LA, Ballard RA, et al. Erythropoietin for neuroprotection in neonatal encephalopathy: safety and pharmacokinetics. Pediatrics. 2012;130(4):683-91.
90. Rogers EE, Bonifacio SL, Glass HC, et al. Erythropoietin and hypothermia for hypoxic-ischemic encephalopathy. Pediatr Neurol. 2014;51(5):657-62.
91. Ohls RK, Kamath-Rayne BD, Christensen RD, et al. Cognitive outcomes of preterm infants randomized to Drabepoietin, erythropoietin or placebo. Pediatrics. 2014;133:1023-30.
92. Elmahdy H, El-Mashad AR, El-Bahrawy H, El-Gohary T, El-Barbary A, Aly H. Human recombinant erythropoietin in asphyxia neonatorum: Pilot trial. Pediatrics. 2010;125(5):e1135-42.
93. Zhu C, Kang W, Xu F, et al. Erythropoietin improved neurologic outcomes in newborns with hypoxic-ischemic encephalopathy. Pediatrics. 2009;124(2):e218-26.
94. Leuchter RH, Gui L, Poncet A, et al Association between early administration of high-dose e.rythropoietin in preterm infants and brain MRI abnormality at term equivalent age. JAMA. 2014;312(8):817-24.
95. Kumral A, Baskin H, Duman N, Yilmaz O, Tatli M, Ozer E, et al. Erythropoietin protects against necrotizing enterocolitis of newborn rats by the inhibiting nitric oxide formation. Biol Neonate. 2003;84:325-9.
96. Ledbetter J, Juul SE. Erythropoietin and the incidence of necrotizing enterocolitis in infants with very low birth weight. J Pediatr Surg. 2000;35:178-82.
97. El Ganzoury MM, Awad HE, El-Farrash RA, et al. Enteral granulocyte-colony stimulating factor and erythropoietin early in life improves feeding tolerance in preterm infant: a randomized controlled trial. Journal of Pediatrics. 2014;165(6):1140-5.
98. Ohls RK, Christensen RD, Kamath-Rayne BD, et al. A randomized, masked, placebo-controlled study of darbepoetin alfa in preterm infants. Pediatrics. 2013;132:e119-e127.

SECTION 8

Immunological Disorders

Section Editors

Manisha Madkaikar, Nita Radhakrishnan

CHAPTER

45

Introduction to Immunology

Amit Rawat, Biman Saikia, Jitendra K Shandilya

THE IMMUNE SYSTEM

The immune system has evolved to protect plants and microorganisms from invasion and damage by pathogenic organisms which abound in the environment. Thucydides (430 BC) is credited for perhaps the first written account of the concept of immunology. In his description of the Great Plague of Athens, he writes that only those individuals who have survived and recovered from the illness could take care of the sick, as they are unlikely to contract the illness again.

Immunity is the state of defense which protects an individual from invading microorganisms.

Immune system comprises two important components—(1) Innate immunity, mediated by phagocyte cells and molecules which recognize certain patterns of pathogens; (2) Adaptive immunity mediated by T- and B-lymphocytes.

Innate-like lymphoid cells are recently characterized group of cells. These cells lack surface expression of lineage specific molecules. Receptor subunits of cytokines (IL-25, IL7) are present on surface of these innate lymphoid cells (ILCs).

Innate immune system comprises anatomical barriers (skin, mucosa), soluble components (complement proteins, MBL, CRP, defensins, lysozymes, histitins) and cellular components (PMNs, macrophages, DC) and ILCs. Natural killer cells and cytotoxic ILCs provide protection against tumor and viruses. ILCs are further divided into distinct groups (ILC1, 2 and 3) based on transcription factors required for their development, cytokine expression and effector functions.

Innate immune response is triggered within minutes to hours on encounter with a pathogen with robust response with limited specificity and diversity and no immunological memory. Innate immune system recognizes pathogens via their specific pattern molecules (PAMPs) on binding to their cognate pattern recognition receptors (PRRs). Binding of ligand to toll-like receptor (TLR) activates downstream signaling which mediates the immune response.

Adaptive immune response comprises two key elements; humoral (antibody mediated) response to neutralize toxins and extracellular pathogen, while intracellular pathogens are eradicated by cellular arm of adaptive immune response.

Antigen-presenting cells engulf the foreign particle, digest it into small parts and present this antigenic peptide to T-lymphocytes via major histocompatibility complex (MHC) molecule (Class-I to TC cells or Class-II to TH cells). TH cells further activate B-cell to generate memory and plasma cells to secrete antibodies.

Functions of the Immune System

The major functions of the immune system are as follows:

- Protection from infections by pathogenic microorganisms
- Defense against tumors by an active immune surveillance
- Immune tolerance for self and the commensal microbiota cohabit the skin and mucosal surfaces including the gut
- Induction and maintenance of a state of immune homeostasis.

Aberrations of the Immune System

Although the immune system is an exquisitely designed system, it is not infallible and can go awry. Autoimmune diseases result from a breach in the state of immune tolerance for self. Primary immune deficiencies are experiments of nature, caused by defects in different components of the immune system. Over 300 single gene defects have been reported to be responsible for various primary immune deficiencies. Hypersensitivity diseases results from an exaggerated immune response to harmless agents in the environment.

Immune System as a Barrier to Transplantation and Gene Therapy

The immune system poses a formidable barrier to transplantation as the transplanted antigens are recognized as nonself and a robust immune response is mounted against the transplanted organ leading to rejection. Immune response also develops against viral vectors used for correction of the gene defect by gene therapy.

Organs of the Immune System

The organs of the immune system can be broadly classified into primary, secondary and tertiary lymphoid organs.

- *Primary lymphoid organs*: These are the organs in which the development and maturation of lymphoid cells take places. In humans, there are two primary lymphoid organs, namely the bone marrow and the thymus. Immune cells develop from a common progenitor in the bone marrow known as the hematopoietic stem cell. The development of B-lymphocytes is completed in the bone marrow or the bursa of Fabricius in birds. T-cell progenitors however migrate from the bone marrow to the thymus for completion of their maturation.
- *Secondary lymphoid organs*: The secondary lymphoid organs include the lymph nodes, spleen and mucosa associated tissue in the gut and other mucosal surfaces. The mature, but naive lymphocytes encounter pathogens in these secondary lymphoid organs. Lymphocytes bearing receptors with specificity for their cognate antigens borne on pathogens get activated upon recognition and develop into effectors and memory cells.
- *Tertiary lymphoid organs*: The tertiary lymphoid organs comprise of organs such as skin, liver and lung, which are sites of infectivity.

Subdivisions of the Immune System

The immune system is broadly classified into two phylogenetically distinct subgroups namely:

1. Innate immune system.
2. Adaptive immune system.

Innate Immune System

The innate immune system is an evolutionarily and phylogenetically ancient immune system, which has been conserved in different species and some elements of this system have also been observed in plants. The innate immune system responds rapidly to microbial invasion and does not require prior contact with the offending microbe for a robust and effective immune response.[1]

Adaptive Immune System

Adaptive immune system is an evolutionary more recent system, which is present only in jawed vertebrates. As the name suggests, it evolves upon the first encounter with the pathogenic microbes. It is further subdivided into two major closely co-operating arms, i.e. humoral immunity mediated by B lymphocytes and cellular arm of adaptive immunity by T lymphocytes.

It is however important to note that the innate and adaptive immune systems do not function in isolation, there is a fair degree of cross-talk between these two systems. This two-way communication is essential for an efficient immune response.

COMPONENTS OF THE INNATE IMMUNE SYSTEM

The different components of the innate system are follows:

- *Anatomical barriers*: Skin and mucosa of respiratory, urogenital and gastrointestinal tracts.
- *Chemical barriers*: Acid secreted in stomach, antimicrobial proteins and peptides in tears, sebum and gastrointestinal mucosa.
- *Soluble components:* Complement components and their fragments (C1q); *Collectins*: Mannan-binding lectin (MBL), surfactant proteins (SP-A, SP-D); *Ficolins*: L-ficolins and H-ficolins and pentraxins: C-reactive protein (CRP).
- Cellular components of the innate immune system
  - Phagocytic and antigen presenting cells
    - Neutrophils
    - Macrophages
    - Dendritic cells
  - *Innate lymphoid cells (ILCs)*
    - *Cytotoxic ILCs*: Natural killer cells
    - LTi (Lymphoid tissue inducer)
    - Noncytotoxic ILCs: ILC1, ILC2 and ILC3.

Innate lymphoid cells (ILCs) are a recently characterized group of cells of innate immune system, which comprise of the cytotoxic natural killer cells, the lymphoid tissue inducer cells and the most recently described noncytotoxic ILCs. Members of the ILC family lack the surface expression of molecules that are present on other immune cells and ascribe a particular lineage. They are therefore described as lineage negative (Lin-) cells.[2-9]

Receptor subunits of cytokines such as IL-2 (CD25) and IL-7 (CD127) are present on the surface of the ILCs. Somatically rearranged antigen receptors present on the adaptive immune cells, i.e. T and B lymphocytes are characteristically absent on ILCs.

Natural killer cells, which subserve an important function of protection against tumors and viruses, were the first described members of the ILC family. They were discovered in 1975. LTi cells were described next in 1997. The LTi cells promote formation of lymph nodes during embryogenesis.

The noncytotoxic ILCs are the newest addition to the ILC family. They have been subdivided into three distinct groups, namely group I ILCs (ILC1s), group 2 ILCs (ILC2s) and group 3 ILCs (ILC3s) based on the transcription factors required for their development, their cytokine expression pattern and their effector functions **(Fig. 45.1 and Flow chart 45.1)**. There is a striking resemblance of effector function and cytokine expression of the ILC subsets with the T-helper subsets, which will be described later in the chapter.

Soluble Components of the Innate Immune System

The soluble components of the innate immune system include several proteins present in the blood and the body

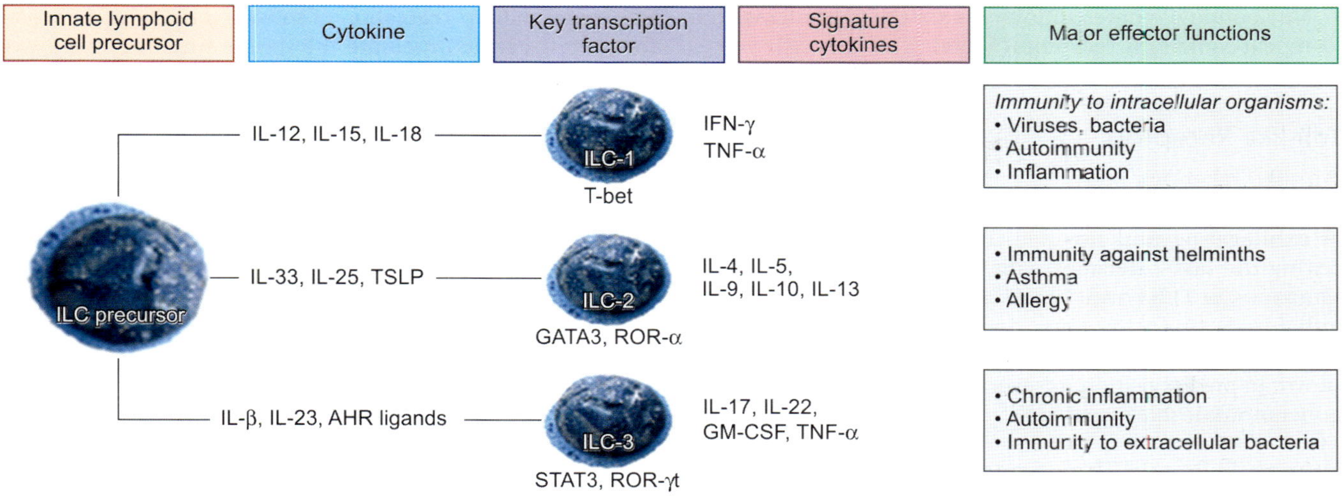

Figure 45.1 Key transcription factors, signature cytokines and effector functions of innate lymphoid cells

Abbreviations: STAT3, signal transducer and activation of transcription 3; GM-CSF, granulocyte macrophage colony stimulating factor; IFN-γ, interferon gamma; TNF-α, tumor necrosis factor-alpha; ROR-γt, retinoic acid orphan receptor-gamma *t*; TSLP, thymic stromal lymphopoietin; AHR, aryl hydrocarbon receptor

Flow chart 45.1 Development of innate lymphoid cells

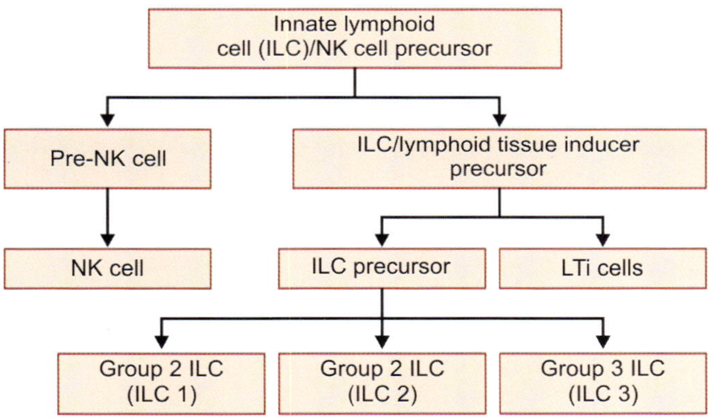

Abbreviation: NK cell, natural killer cell

secretions which protect us from microbial invasion. These include:

- Complement proteins and their breakdown products
- *Pentraxins*: C-reactive protein (short pentraxin)
- *Collectins*: Mannan binding lectin (MBL), surfactant proteins (SP-A and SP-D)
- *Ficolins*: Ficolin L and Ficolin H
- *Antimicrobial peptides*: Defensins, cathelicidins, lysozyme, histatins, dermcidin, granulysin and psoriasin.

Key Characteristics of the Innate Immune System

- Prior contact with the invading microbe is not a prerequisite for a robust and effective innate immune response.
- Triggered within minutes to hours of first encounter with an offending pathogen
- Restricted repertoire of receptors, which respond to broad classes of pathogens rather than specific epitopes
- Limited diversity and specificity in contrast to the cells of the adaptive immune system
- Stereotypic response with little or no immunologic memory
- Usually targets moieties in pathogens which are essential for their survival and not present on host cells.

Pathogen Recognition by the Innate Immune System

The cells of the innate immune system display an array of receptors on their plasma membranes and endosomes, which recognize structures, known as pathogen-associated molecular patterns (PAMPs), which are present exclusively on pathogenic microorganisms and not host cells. The receptors on innate immune cells for the PAMPs are known as pattern recognition receptors or PRRs. The PRRs are strategically located to recognize extracellular microorganisms such as extracellular bacteria and intracellular pathogens such as viruses.

In addition to recognizing pathogenic moieties, cells of the innate immune system also recognize endogenous substances released from injured and dead self-cells through the PRRs. The endogenous components recognized by the PRRs are known as death-associated molecular patterns or damage-associated molecular patterns (DAMPs).

Pattern Recognition Receptors in Human

There are predominantly four major classes of PRRs in humans. They are:

- Toll-like receptors (TLRs)
- C-type lectin receptors (CLRs)

- Nucleotide oligomerization domain (NOD)/leucine-rich repeat containing receptors (NLRs)
- Retinoic acid-inducible gene-I-like receptors (RLRs).

Toll-like Receptors

Toll-like receptors are the best characterized PRRs which were also the first PRRs to be discovered. A number of exhilarating and novel discoveries have been made during the last 2 decades with regard to these receptors. Mutations in TLR3 have been shown to predispose affected individuals to encephalitis due to *Herpes simplex* virus. Single nucleotide polymorphisms in various TLRs have seen shown to predisposition to several communicable as well as noncommunicable diseases.[10,11]

Human TLRs and Their Specific Ligands

A total of 10 TLRs, TLR 1 to 10, have been described so far in humans. TLRs bind specifically to their corresponding ligands present on microbes. Human TLRs with their cognate ligands are listed in **Table 45.1**.

Signaling through TLRs

The binding of the various TLRs with their cognate ligands triggers downstream signaling pathway culminating in transcriptional up-regulation of several genes which encode for proteins which mediate the innate immune response. The most important of these genes are the ones encoding for various cytokines. The downstream signaling pathway, which gets activated, is determined by the TLR and the adaptor protein to which it binds through its cytoplasmic domain.

The cytoplasmic domain of TLRs, which bind to the adaptor proteins, is called the Toll/Interleukin-1 (IL-1) receptor (TIR) domain. Most of the TLRs bind to the adaptor protein myeloid differentiation factor 88 (MyD88). MyD88 activates the nuclear factor-kappa B (NF-κB), which is the key transcription factor for upregulating the transcription of several genes which are important for innate immunity.

Toll/Interleukin-1 (IL-1) receptor (TIR)-domain-containing adaptor-inducing Interferon-β (TRIF) is the other adaptor protein for the TLRs. The cytoplasmic portion of TLR3 binds exclusively to TRIF, whereas TLR4 binds both to MyD88 and TRIF depending on its location on the cell surface or the endosome respectively. The binding of the TLRS to the TRIF results in the activation of interferon regulatory factors (IRFs). The IRFs exponentially increase the transcription of genes encoding for type I interferons, which are responsible for antiviral immunity.

Table 45.1 Human toll-like receptors with their ligands

Toll-like receptor (TLR)	*Ligands*	*Microbe*	*Location*	*Gene defects polymorphisms*
TLR 1	Triacyl lipopeptides	Gram-negative bacteria Mycobacteria	Plasma membrane	Susceptibility to tuberculosis
TLR 2	Peptidoglycan Zymosan Lipoproteins Phosphatidylserine GPI-linked proteins	Gram-positive bacteria Yeasts and fungi Mycobacteria Schistosomes Trypanosome	Plasma membrane	Susceptibility to tuberculosis, leprosy, Staphylococcal infection
TLR 3	Double stranded RNA (dsRNA)	Viruses	Endosome Lysosome	Herpes simplex encephalitis
TLR 4	Lipopolysaccharide Mannans F-protein	Gram-negative bacteria Fungi Respiratory syncytial virus	Plasma membrane Endosome Lysosome	Excessive TLR4 signaling in Gram-negative septicemia
TLR 5	Flagellin	Bacteria	Plasma membrane	Associated with increased risk of Legionnaires' disease
TLR 6	Zymosan Diacyl lipopeptides	Yeasts and fungi Mycobacteria	Plasma membrane	Associated with increased risk of Legionnaires' disease
TLR 7	Single stranded RNA (ssRNA)	Viruses	Endosome Lysosome	Association with hepatitis C infection
TLR 8	Single stranded RNA (ssRNA)	Viruses	Endosome Lysosome	Association with pulmonary TB and hepatitis C infection
TLR 9	CpG dinucleotide Hemozoin	Bacterial DNA Malarial pigment	Endosome Lysosome	Polymorphisms associated with SLE
TLR 10	Unknown	Influenza virus	Endosome Lysosome	Not known

NUCLEOTIDE OLIGOMERIZATION DOMAIN RECEPTORS/NUCLEOTIDE OLIGOMERIZATION DOMAIN LEUCINE-RICH REPEAT CONTAINING RECEPTORS

The NLRs or NOD receptors consists of large family of cytosolic pattern recognition receptors that are stimulated by several PAMPs, DAMPs and other harmful endogenous substances. Human NLRs are subdivided into three major categories based on the N-terminal domain. These are as follows:

- *NLRCs:* Caspase recruitment domain (CARD)
- *NLRBs:* Baculovirus inhibitory repeat (BIR) domain
- *NLRPs:* Pyrin domains (PYDs).

Nucleotide oligomerization domain 1 and NOD2 are the most well-described members of the NLRC family. They are triggered by components of peptidoglycans present on bacterial cell walls. These components are generated during the production or destruction of the bacterial cell walls. Both NOD1 and NOD2 form signaling complexes that activate NF-κB which leads to the upregulation of transcription of several proinflammatory cytokines.

Inflammasome

Some of the NLRs do not activate signaling pathways culminating in the transcriptional upregulation of genes important for an effective immune response. Instead, these NLRs form complexes with proteins that activate proteases that cleave inactive forms of interleukins, most commonly IL-1 and IL-8 into their active forms. These complexes of NLRs with proteins and proteases are collectively known as inflammasomes.[12-14]

NLRP1, NLRC4 and NLRP3 are the three NLRs that form inflammasomes. The inflammasome formed by NLRP3 is the best characterized and present rather ubiquitously on several cells such as monocytes, macrophages, dendritic cells, neutrophils, some lymphocyte subsets and epithelial cells. NLRP3 inflammasome is composed of several copies of NLRP3, the adaptor protein ASC (apoptosis-associated speck-like protein containing a caspase recruitment domain) and caspase 1 arranged in a pentameric or hexameric fashion.

Activators of NLRP3 Inflammasome

The various activators of NLRP3 inflammasome are as follows:

- *Self-derived molecules and substances*: Glucose, cholesterol and urate crystals, amyloid β protein, adenosine triphosphate (ATP)
- *Nonself environmental substances*: Asbestos, silica, alloys, alum
- *Bacterial activators*: Flagellin, peptidoglycans, pore-forming toxins
- *Virus*: Viral RNA, influenza M2 protein
- *Fungus*: Mannan, zymosan, β-glucans
- *Protozoa*: Hemozoin (malarial parasite).

Mutations in any of the several genes encoding for the constituents of the inflammasome result in a group of rare, heritable disorders known as autoinflammatory syndromes. These would be discussed in detail in a subsequent chapter.

ADAPTIVE IMMUNE SYSTEM

The adaptive immune system can be broadly classified into two major divisions also known as the "Two arms of the Immune system". These are the humoral arm which is mediated by the antibodies produced by the B lymphocytes and the cellular arm which is realized by the T lymphocytes. The humoral arm, so called is affected by antibodies present in the blood and body fluids (Greek humor meaning fluid), is designed to neutralize and eliminate extracellular microbes and the toxins produced. It is however inconsequential in the eradication of intracellular pathogens which are eliminated by cellular arm of the adaptive immunity.

Key Features of the Adaptive Immune System

The predominant features of the adaptive immune response, which distinguish it from the innate immune response, are:

- *Diversity*: Adaptive immune cells are endowed with antigen receptors that undergo somatic recombination, a process which is unique and exclusive to the immune cells of the adaptive immunity. This results in a broad and extensive repertoire of antigen receptor diversity which is lacking in the innate immune cells.
- *Specificity*: The somatically rearranged antigen receptors on the adaptive immune cells are capable of recognizing subtle differences in antigenic epitopes present on microbes.
- *Immunological memory*: The ability to mount an enhanced and heightened immune response to antigen upon re-exposure is a unique property of the adaptive immunity. This is mediated by the process of clonal selection and proliferation.

  A comparison of the key features of the innate and adaptive immune system is depicted in **Table 45.2**.

Phases of an Adaptive Immune Response

The temporal progression of the adaptive immune response is achieved by a coordinated effort of several types of immune cells including the antigen presenting cells, the T and B lymphocytes and effector cells. The antigen presenting cells include the dendritic cells and mononuclear phagocytes which phagocytose the microbes, digest the proteins into smaller peptides and present these peptides to T-cells in the context of major histocompatibility complex (MHC) molecules (MHC class I in case of CD8+ cytotoxic T-cells and MHC class II in the case of CD4+ helper T-cells). Lymphocytes include B lymphocytes, CD4+ helper T lymphocytes and CD8+ cytotoxic T lymphocytes. The effector cells included the activated T-cells and their various subsets and antibody-producing plasma cells.

Key feature	Innate immunity	Adaptive immunity
Rapidity of response	Immediate within hours	Delayed with a lag phase between exposure and response
Antigenic specificity	Broad, limited repertoire and fixed	Highly specific and evolves with time during the course of an immune response
Immunologic memory	None	Exquisite memory, rapid and heightened response to previously encountered antigens
Self/nonself recognition	Present	Present, occasional lapses resulting in autoimmunity

Table 45.2 Comparison of the key features in innate versus adaptive immunity

The adaptive immune response can thus be arbitrarily divided into three distinct phases which occur in temporal sequence. These are:

- Antigen recognition and presentation
- Lymphocyte activation and proliferation
- Effector phase.

Antigen Recognition and Presentation

The first prerequisite in the initiation of the adaptive immune response is the recognition and ingestion of microbial antigens and their presentation to lymphocytes by antigen presenting cells. Mature, naïve lymphocytes exit the thymus and enter circulation. However, the likelihood of these naïve lymphocytes encountering antigen for which they have specific receptors is very low.

This is due to the fact that the number of lymphocytes with the same antigenic receptor is very small. To overcome this challenge, dendritic cells, which are strategically located at sites of microbial entry, avidly ingest microbial antigen and ferry their antigenic cargo to the T-cells zones of the lymph node. This exponentially increases the likelihood of the lymphocytes engaging their specific antigens as the antigens are concentrated in the lymph nodes by the dendritic cells. Dendritic cells and other antigen presenting cells display antigens in the most suitable fashion to the lymphocytes.

Dendritic Cells: Remarkable Antigen Presenting Cells

Dendritic cells were first described in mid-1970 by Ralph Steinmann, a discovery for which he received the Nobel Prize in Physiology or Medicine in 2011, albeit posthumously. The dendritic cells are so called as they have long filamentous processes like the dendrites of a neuron to scan the surface of the lymphoid cells. Dendritic cells are the most efficient antigen presenting cells and indeed the most effective stimulator of naïve B lymphocytes.

Unique Properties of Dendritic Cells

- *Tactful location*: Dendritic cells are tactfully located at the sites of antigen entry such as skin and other epithelial surfaces.
- *Presence of toll-like receptors and other pattern recognition receptors*: They can easily capture invading microorganism by pattern recognition receptors that adorn their surfaces.
- Constitutive expression of self MHC molecules and costimulatory which increases after activation
- Migration to the T-cell-rich zones of the lymph node and presentation of antigens in the most suited form.

Major Histocompatibility Complex

T-lymphocytes can recognize peptides presented in the context of self MHC molecules. The antigenic peptides are displayed on the antigen/peptide binding groove of the MHC molecule. There is a great degree of allelic heterogeneity in the MHC molecules and different MHC molecules bind different antigenic peptides. The specific alleles that an individual inherits determine the T-cell immune response in that individual. It also accounts for predisposition to different diseases with underlying immune defects including autoimmune diseases.

There are two major classes of MHC molecules, MHC I and MHC II. CD4+ T helper cells recognize antigens presented in the context of MHC class II molecules whereas CD8+ cytotoxic T-cells recognize antigen present in context of MHC class I molecules. Genetic deficiencies of MHC molecules result in severe primary immunodeficiencies which are commonly known as bare lymphocyte syndromes. MHC class I deficiency results in decreased or absent CD8+ TCR-$\alpha\beta$ cells whereas MHC class II deficiency causes a deficit or absence of CD4+ TCR-$\alpha\beta$ lymphocytes.

Lymphocyte Activation

The process of lymphocyte activation begins with the engagement of the T- or the B-cell receptor with its cognate antigenic epitope. This generates the first signal for lymphocyte activation; however, the first signal by itself is not capable of completing the feat of lymphocyte activation. A second signal from costimulatory molecules is required to accomplish lymphocyte activation.

T-cell Activation

In addition to the T-cell receptor (TCR), several other molecules are involved in the activation of T lymphocytes. Some of these constitute an integral part of the TCR complex. These include CD3 and the zeta protein ζ, both of which are important for signal transduction. CD4 and CD8 coreceptors bind to the nonpolymorphic region of the MHC molecules. The adhesion molecules such as LFA-1 (Leukocyte-function associated antigen 1) and VLA-4 increase the strength of binding of T-cell to the antigen presenting cells. Finally, receptors for costimulatory molecules provide the much needed second signal for an effective immune response.

Costimulatory Molecules and Their Receptors

The expression of costimulatory molecules on antigen presenting cells is induced by microbial products during the early innate immune response. The best studied costimulatory molecules are B7-1 (CD80) and B7-2 (CD86). The receptors for these on the T-cells are CD28 and CTLA-4 (CD152). Engagement of CD28 by costimulatory molecules leads to T-cell activation whereas CTLA-4 engagement abrogates T-cell activation. Recently heterozygous germ line mutations in CTLA-4 have been identified in patients with immune dysregulation.[15]

Consequences of T-cell Activation

T-cell activation results in the following consequences:

- Production of proinflammatory cytokines
- Clonal proliferation of antigen-specific clones
- Differentiation into different effector cell depending on cytokine milieu and type of infection
- Generation of memory cells for a heightened secondary immune response.

B-cell Activation

Antigen binding to the surface B-cell receptor (BCR) of a mature naïve B-cell causes BCR cross linking resulting in signal transduction through associated Igα and Igβ. Igα and Igβ are disulfide linked to one another and noncovalently associated with the surface Ig receptor. The second signal for B-cell activation is provided by products of complement activation such as C3d which bind to complement receptor CR2 on the B-cell, which forms a part of B-cell receptor complex. This B-cell receptor complex is formed by CD19, CD81 and CR2 (CD21).

The engagement of the cognate antigen by BCR brings about proliferation, and increased expression of MHC class II, B7-1 and B7-2. These render the B-cells capable of activating T helper cells through binding to CD28. T helper cells secrete cytokines which cause clonal expansion, isotype switching, affinity maturation and differentiation into memory B-cells. B-cell activated T helper cells also express CD40 ligand (CD40L, CD154) which binds to CD40 on the B-cell and brings about B-cell maturation and isotype switching. Defects in the CD40L and CD40 results in X-linked and autosomal recessive forms of hyper IgM syndrome.

Effector Mechanisms in the B-cell-mediated Humoral Response

Effector functions of the humoral immune response are mediated by the constant region of the heavy chain; these effector functions are also determined by the specific antibody isotype. The mechanisms by which effector mechanisms of the humoral immune response are accomplished are as follows:

- Neutralization of microbes and/or their toxins
- *Opsonization and phagocytosis of microbes*: Opsonization or coating of the microbes with antibodies promotes their phagocytosis by binding of the Fc portion of the antibody to the FcR on the phagocyte.
- *Antibody-mediated cytotoxicity*: Fc receptors on natural killer (NK) cells, called Fc-γRIII, (CD16) bind to IgG antibodies attached to cells, resulting in NK cell-mediated lysis of the cell through release of perforin and granzyme from granules.
- Complement-mediated lysis of microbes.

Effector Mechanisms of T-cell Immune Response

The effector function of T lymphocytes is mediated by different subsets. The two major subdivisions of T-lymphocytes are the CD4+ helper T lymphocytes and the CD8+ cytotoxic T-lymphocytes. CD4+ helper T lymphocytes upon activation differentiate into various subsets. The cytokine milieu generated by the antigen presenting cells and activated T-cells at the site of antigen recognition determines the differentiation pathway of the T-cells. Commitment to a particular subset is driven by key transcription factors for that particular subset.

T-cell differentiation can be arbitrarily divided into three phases. These include:

- *Induction*: This phase is characterized by production of subset-specific transcription factors and cytokines.
- *Commitment*: Epigenetic changes in cytokine gene loci occur during this phase.
- *Amplification*: Development of increased numbers of effectors of the same subset and suppression of other subsets take place during the amplification phase.

The different subsets of helper T-cells, their key transcription factors, signature cytokines and effector functions are summarized in **Figure 45.1**. There is a striking resemblance of the differentiation of helper T-cell subsets with that of the three subtypes of innate lymphoid cells (ILCs).

The major well-characterized subsets of helper CD4+ are Th1, Th2 and Th17. Other subsets include Th9 and Th22. A markedly decreased population of Th17 cells is seen in different forms of mucocutaneous candidiasis and in autosomal dominant hyper IgE syndrome.[16,17] A mutation in the retinoic acid orphan receptor gamma C (RORC), the key transcription factor for Th17 and ILC3 differentiation has recently been described in patients with an unusual combination of mycobacterial infections and mucocutaneous candidiasis without any known genetic defects for the same.[18]

KEY POINTS

- Immunity is the state of protection of an individual from invading microorganisms.
- Innate immune response is triggered within minutes to hours after encountering a pathogen. Prior exposure to

an offending pathogen is not a prerequisite for an innate immune response.

- Engagement of pathogen-associated molecular patterns on the pathogen and their cognative ligands, i.e pattern recognition receptors is required for an effective innate response.
- Adaptive immune response is mediated by T and B lymphocytes which work in close concert to elicit an exquisite immune response.
- Innate and adaptive immune response function in coordination for better defense mechanism.
- A robust innate response is important to initiate and affect an effective adaptive immune response.
- Dysfunction in various components of immune system can lead to autoimmune diseases, primary immune deficiencies and hypersensitivity.

CONCLUSION

Immune system protects the host from microorganisms and tumors. Certain elements of innate system are evolutionarily conserved across species. Defects in the immune system can result in autoimmunity, primary immunodeficiency and hypersensitivity.

REFERENCES

1. Beutler B, Rietschel ET. Innate immune sensing and its roots: the story of endotoxin. Nat Rev Immunol. 2003;3(2):169-76.
2. Hazenberg MD, Spits H. Human innate lymphoid cells. Blood. 2014;124(5):700-9.
3. Hwang YY, McKenzie AN. Innate lymphoid cells in immunity and disease. Adv Exp Med Biol. 2013;785:9-26.
4. Kugelberg E. Innate lymphoid cells: breathing into allergic inflammation. Nat Rev Immunol. 2014;14(5):281.
5. Eberl G, Colonna M, Di Santo JP, McKenzie AN. Innate lymphoid cells. Innate lymphoid cells: a new paradigm in immunology. Science. 2015;348(6237):aaa6566.
6. Artis D, Spits H. The biology of innate lymphoid cells. Nature. 2015;517(7534):293-301.
7. Barlow JL, McKenzie AN. Type-2 innate lymphoid cells in human allergic disease. Curr Opin Allergy Clin Immunol. 2014;14(5):397-403.
8. Walker JA, Barlow JL, McKenzie AN. Innate lymphoid cells--how did we miss them? Nat Rev Immunol. 2013;13(2):75-87.
9. Eberl G, Di Santo JP, Vivier E. The brave new world of innate lymphoid cells. Nat Immunol. 2015;16(1):1-5.
10. Medvedev AE. Toll-like receptor polymorphisms, inflammatory and infectious diseases, allergies and cancer. J Interferon Cytokine Res. 2013;33(9):467-84.
11. Netea MG, Wijmenga C, O'Neill LA. Genetic variation in Toll-like receptors and disease susceptibility. Nat Immunol. 2012;13(6):535-42.
12. Davis BK, Wen H, Ting JP. The inflammasome NLRs in immunity, inflammation and associated diseases. Annu Rev Immunol. 2011;29:707-35.
13. Heymann MC, Rosen-Wolff A. Contribution of the inflammasomes to autoinflammatory diseases and recent mouse models as research tools. Clin Immunol. 2013;147(3):175-84.
14. Ozkurede VU, Franchi L. Immunology in clinic review series; focus on autoinflammatory diseases: role of inflammasomes in autoinflammatory syndromes. Clin Exp Immunol. 2012;167(3):382-90.
15. Kuehn HS, Ouyang W, Lo B, Deenick EK, Niemela JE, Avery DT, et al. Immune dysregulation in human subjects with heterozygous germ line mutations in CTLA4. Science. 2014;345(6204):1623-7.
16. Marodi L, Cypowyj S, Toth B, Chernyshova L, Puel A, Casanova JL. Molecular mechanisms of mucocutaneous immunity against Candida and Staphylococcus species. J Allergy Clin Immunol. 2012;130(5):1019-27.
17. Puel A, Cypowyj S, Marodi L, Abel L, Picard C, Casanova JL. Inborn errors of human IL-17 immunity underlie chronic mucocutaneous candidiasis. Curr Opin Allergy Clin Immunol. 2012;12(6):616-22.
18. Okada S, Markle JG, Deenick EK, Mele F, Averbuch D, Lagos M, et al. Immunodeficiencies. Impairment of immunity to Candida and Mycobacterium in humans with bi-allelic RORC mutations. Science. 2015;349(6248):606-13.

CHAPTER

46

Fetal and Neonatal Immunity

Biman Saikia, Parikshaa Gupta

INTRODUCTION

Humans live in intimate synergy with microbes that are abundantly distributed in the environment. In fact, it is believed that human body has 10 times more microbes than the number of cells.[1] Whereas on one hand these microbes help to synthesize and excrete vitamins, prevent colonization by pathogens, antagonize other pathogenic bacteria and stimulate the production of natural antibodies, they can also cause bacterial synergism promoting the pathogenic bacteria, compete for nutrients and cause disease.

Human embryos, like all other mammalian embryos, develop in the maternal womb, which provides a sterile environment.[2] At the maternofetal interface, placenta forms an impermeable barrier to most of the macromolecules present in the maternal circulation. Once the fetus is delivered, it enters an environment with abundance of antigens to which the neonate has never been exposed and hence has no protection against. Here comes the role of the immune system, which allows the neonate to live in symbiosis with the entire plethora of endogenous as well as exogenous antigens.

The word "immune" is derived from Latin word "immunis" meaning free from taxes. The immune system plays many important roles in the human body; one of the most important being discrimination of pathogenic from nonpathogenic organisms and protection of the body against the pathogenic ones.

The human fetus has a genetically programmed immune system to recognize and respond to a variety of antigens. However, the neonatal immune system is not experienced with the extrauterine environment and hence does not allow the neonate to elicit a very effective and specific immune responses compared to adults.[3]

FETAL IMMUNITY

The human fetus develops inside the maternal uterus but never comes in direct physical contact with the uterine walls. It is surrounded by two membranes—the chorion and the amnion and the inner space contains the amniotic fluid. Only the umbilical cord passes through these membranes to establish a connection between the fetus and the mother and the maternal and fetal circulatory systems are not continuous with each other. The entire physiological exchange between mother and fetus occurs at the interface where the umbilical cord joins the uterine walls. This interface is represented by the placenta, which ensures normal development of the two immunologically different organisms.[4]

In a fully developed placenta, the trophoblast forms finger like chorionic villi that penetrate into the endometrium. These constitute the major structural and functional units of the placenta. The fetal circulation extends from the umbilical cord and divides into the numerous capillaries inside the villi. Large intervillous spaces filled with maternal blood surround these villi. Thus, there is a continuous circulation of maternal blood around the villi, and this serves as the site for exchange of material between the mother and the fetus. The fetal circulation in the placenta contains lymphocytes along with many macrophages that are capable of phagocytosis, fixation of maternal antibodies and cytokine secretion. Maternal blood cells are not normally transferred to the fetus, although the antibodies produced by maternal B-lymphocytes do cross the placenta.[5]

The fetal immune system is generally skewed towards a suppressive direction to prevent immune reactions against maternal human leukocyte antigen (HLA) and to avoid development of a graft-versus-host disease (GvHD). There is enough evidence in the literature indicating that both fetus and placenta express HLA antigens, and half of the fetal HLA antigens are encoded by paternal genes. The fetus thus acts as a paternal allograft to the mother.[6] This degree of antigenic variability is potentially sufficient to trigger an immune response but the fetus is normally not rejected by the maternal immune system. This is because a number of complex factors lead to establishment of a maternofetal immunological balance. Several factors contribute to this:

- The syncytiotrophoblast layer expresses HLA class-I and class-II negative antigens and is positioned between maternal uterine cells and the fetus. Therefore, it acts as a partial barrier to the maternal immune system[6]
- There is production of class II-dependent antibodies, but not of class I-restricted cytotoxic T lymphocytes (CTL)[7]
- Some specific antibodies are produced, which prevent development of cell-mediated immunity (CMI) against the paternal antigens at the syncytiotrophoblast level[7]
- Many studies suggest that a successful pregnancy is associated with an altered Th1/Th2 balance, which is an important prerequisite for the maternal immune system not to reject the fetus[8,9]
- Moreover, the maternal immune response in pregnancy is biased towards humoral immunity and not toward CMI
- Several studies have shown that abundance of Th1-like interleukins (ILs) during pregnancy, without a shift to Th2 T-cells, induces immune-mediated abortions or recurrent spontaneous abortions of unexplained etiology[9,10]
- During the entire pregnancy, Th2 T lymphocytes produce IL-4, IL-5 and IL-10 at the maternofetal interface. This inhibits the action of suppressor Th1 T-cells and production of Th1-like ILs, thereby ensuring fetal survival until birth[9]
- It has also been observed that fetal T lymphocytes tend to suppress proliferative responses and further differentiation into adult lymphocytes, mainly because of Th2-like ILs produced in the fetus.[11] This prevents maternal T-cells from mounting a GvHD in the fetus[7]
- It is believed that IL-10 along with IL-2 stimulates the activity of lymphokine-activated killer (LAK) cells, which help in discriminating between self and nonself, thereby contributing to fetal protection by shutting down maternal immune responses biased toward humoral immunity[12]
- Trophoblasts do not express HLA-A or HLA-B molecules, however, when in contact with maternal cells, they express HLA-G molecules[13]
- At the end of pregnancy, there occurs a shift to humoral immunity and a gradual increase in production of Th1 ILs, like interferon-gamma (IFN-γ) and tumor necrosis factor-alpha (TNF-α)
- During the last trimester, fetus has mature B-cells, capable of producing antibodies against various antigens that are transplacentally transmitted from the mother.

It is therefore, the bias toward Th2-skewed IL response that maintains a successful pregnancy by limiting the cellular damage in the fetus.[9] Later on, during the postnatal period, multiple contacts with various antigens redirect the Th2-skewed fetal immunity toward a Th1-skewed immunity.

DEVELOPMENT OF THE IMMUNE SYSTEM

Development of the immune system in humans begins as early as 2 weeks of gestation from the hematopoietic stem cells (HSCs) **(Table 46.1)**.[14] These HSC originally develop in the yolk sac of the embryo. Thereafter, as the newly forming blood vessels start making connections with the developing embryo, the HSCs migrate into the liver and transiently into the spleen. Thus, the liver serves as the first hematopoietic organ of the embryo. Finally, these stem cells reach the bone marrow and then serve as the source of immune cells, not only during fetal life but also during adulthood.

Table 46.1 Development of the immune system[15]

Gestational age (weeks)	
2	First hematopoietic stem cells (HSCs) appear in yolk sac
4–8	Complement synthesis detected (5.5 weeks) Myelopoiesis starts (6 weeks) HSCs seen in fetal liver (7 weeks) Lymphocytes (1,000/mm^3) seen in peripheral blood (7–8 weeks) Pro-B-cells seen in liver (7–8 weeks)
8–12	Lymphocytes detected in thymus (8–9 weeks) T cell receptors (TCRs) seen in thymus (8.5–10 weeks) Pro-B-cells mature in liver and spleen; immunoglobulin A (IgA), IgD, IgM, IgG surface markers, serum IgM levels detectable (9.5–11 weeks) Lymphocytes seen in bone marrow and intestines (10–11 weeks) Hematopoietic cells in thymus and spleen (12 weeks) Mononuclear cells in spleen, antigen recognition (12 weeks) Stem cells in bone marrow (12 weeks)
12–16	Thymus becomes lymphoid (12–15 weeks) Complete differentiation of T- and B-cells (15 weeks) Langerhans cells appear in tonsils (15 weeks)
16–20	Lymphocytes migrate into lymph nodes (20 weeks) Complement levels detectable (20 weeks) Thymus and memory lymphocytes mature (20 weeks) Ability to synthesize immunoglobulins complete (20 weeks)
20–24	Lymphocytes increase in blood approximately to10,000/mm^3
33	IgG levels reach maternal levels

NEONATAL IMMUNITY

It is generally believed that neonates are more susceptible to infections because of their immature immune system. However, recent studies on experimental animals have shown that neonates are immunocompetent and thus their immune responses against various antigens do not differ much from those of adults.[16-18] Hence, the neonatal period should also be regarded as an immunologically active period. Some studies have also shown that the relative immunosuppression, exhibited by the neonates, is actually an active strategy to allow colonization of the gut mucosa by normal microbial flora in a noninflammatory manner.[19,20] Neonatal immune system, as in adults, can be classified into two types **(Table 46.2)**:

1. Innate or inborn or nonspecific immune system
2. Acquired or adaptive or specific immune system.

Innate Immune System in Neonates

Innate immune system serves as the first line of defense against invasion by foreign agents. Due to the sterile environment inside the maternal uterus, the extent of antigenic exposure of the fetus is quite limited. As a consequence, the adaptive immune system, which requires prior antigenic stimulation, is relatively underdeveloped after birth. Hence, neonates have to rely mainly on their innate immune responses for protection.[21]

Components of Innate Immune System

The components of innate immune system are similar in both neonates and adults and include:

- *Physical barriers*: Skin and mucous membranes
- Antimicrobial peptides
- Complement proteins
- Toll-like receptors
- *Immune cells*: Monocytes-macrophages, dendritic cells, mast cells, neutrophils, eosinophils, basophils and natural killer cells (NKCs)
- Cytokines.

Neonatal Skin as an Immunological Barrier

The skin serves as an anatomical as well as a functional barrier and protects the neonate from harmful extraneous stimuli, both passively by virtue of its integrity and impermeability and actively by mediating both stimulatory and modulatory immune responses. The stratum corneum plays a major role in maintaining the integrity of the skin barrier due to its lipid content and very low permeability, thereby restricting water and electrolyte loss from more hydrated, deeper layers.[22]

The skin immune system (SIS) includes mast cells, T-lymphocytes, Langerhans cells (LCs) and keratinocytes.[23] About 95% of the cell mass of human epithelium is made by the keratinocytes alone. In addition to the immune cells, the keratinocytes also participate in immune responses by releasing a wide array of proinflammatory factors in response to stimuli, like physical trauma, ultraviolet (UV) irradiation and bacterial products. These factors transmit signals in an autocrine manner to the keratinocytes themselves as well as in a paracrine manner to other cells, such as leukocytes, endothelial cells and fibroblasts. Consequently, there is activation of the innate immune system with recruitment of other inflammatory cells and upregulation of gene expression of epidermal proinflammatory cytokines.[24]

At 23–26 weeks of fetal life, the epidermis is immature. It is formed by only 2–3 cell layers and the stratum corneum is poorly developed. At birth, the epidermis undergoes accelerated maturation and around 2 weeks of age, it is almost similar to that of adults.[25] LCs start entering the fetal epidermis in first trimester, and thereafter continue to increase during the entire fetal life. HLA expression in LCs is seen very rapidly after birth.[25]

The neonatal skin is relatively fragile at birth and even a small breach in the integrity of the skin can lead to infection. Immediately after birth, a waxy coating can be seen on newborn skin, the *vernix caseosa*. It is secreted by the fetal sebaceous glands and contains a variety of antimicrobial peptides including lysozyme, alpha-defensins, ubiquitin, psoriasin and antimicrobial free fatty acids that can act synergistically to kill various microorganisms.[26] In addition, it has been observed that the skin from embryonic as well as newborn mice shows a robust expression of antimicrobial peptides, like cathelicidin and beta-defensin by epidermal cells and this exceeds that of adult skin.[27]

Mucosal Barrier: Neonatal Gastrointestinal Tract

The gastrointestinal (GI) tract during the fetal life is exposed to sterile amniotic fluid that is continuously being swallowed.

Table 46.2 Differences between innate and adaptive immunity

Innate	*Adaptive*
Nonspecific	Specific
Antigen independent	Antigen dependent
Predominant in early stage of infection	Predominant in middle and late stages of infection
Maximal response in hours	Maximal response in days
Response is limited and fixed	Response is diverse and improves over time
No immunological memory	Immunological memory is seen
Response to repeat infection is same as the initial response	Response to repeat infection is more rapid than initial response

However, after birth, rapid colonization of the neonatal gut takes place.

The human fetal enterocytes express toll-like receptor-2 (TLR-2) and TLR-4 on their basolateral surface, beginning around 18–21 weeks of gestation. Some studies have shown that fetal intestinal villous and crypt epithelial cells express TLR-4 and MD2, which are the key components of lipopolysaccharide (LPS) receptor. Thus, stimulation of fetal intestinal cells with LPS results in higher levels of nuclear factor-κβ (NF-κβ) activation and increased production of CXCL8 and CXCL2 as compared to adult intestinal epithelial cells.[28] Fortunately, this type of response is seen only in fetal life, as such robust intestinal inflammatory responses to LPS could pose a great danger after birth, when the gut is being colonized by commensal intestinal flora, including LPS-bearing gram-negative bacterial species.[29] On the other hand, exposure of neonatal intestinal cells to LPS results in the loss of responsiveness of the enterocytes to LPS, due to downregulated expression of IL-1-receptor-associated kinase 1 (IRAK1), which is important for TLR4 signaling.[28] This postnatal endotoxin (LPS) tolerance helps in normal microbial colonization in the neonates. Simultaneously, the developing paneth cells produce a variety of antimicrobial peptides and help in clearance of bacteria such as *Escherichia coli*. Recent studies have implicated a role of endotoxin and intestinal TLR4 expression in the development of neonatal necrotizing enterocolitis (NNEC), which is commonly seen in preterm infants.[30] The inability of preterm neonates to appropriately downregulate the intestinal immune responses to LPS seems to be significantly responsible for their increased susceptibility to NNEC.

There are several nonimmunological components of the mucosal barrier:[15,29]

- *Gastric acidity and enzymes of the GI tract*: Neonates have a physiological deficit of such factors in the form of:
  - Achlorhydria, thereby facilitating the microbial proliferation
  - Enzyme deficiencies leading to an impaired digestion of ingested macromolecules, thereby favoring antigen absorption
- *Gut microflora*: The neonatal gut microflora is different in composition than adults and this has been proposed to play a role in the development of allergy
- Peristaltic movements
- Intestinal secretions, such as:
  - *Saliva*: Contains lytic enzymes (lysozyme) and polymers that limits the attachment of bacteria to the epithelium
  - *Gastric secretions*: Contains hydrochloric acid and peptidases that denature various ingested antigens
  - *Pancreatic and other enteric proteolytic enzymes*: Denaturation of intraluminal antigens.
- *Mucosal surface*: Includes the microvilli of the lining epithelial cells and the overlying mucus layer. This acts as a mechanical barrier to a variety of foreign antigens. However, it is believed that in neonates, its thickness is reduced due to specific phospholipid changes in the composition of this layer and this may contribute to weakened defense.[31] Moreover, malnutrition in neonates reduces mucus secretion and bottle-feeding may reduce the intrinsic qualities of the mucus, thereby impairing the mucosal defense.[32]
- *Hepatic filtration of GI antigens*: Kupffer cells in the liver serve as the second line of mucosal defense, after secretory IgA (sIgA) and the anatomical, functional and enzymatic barriers of intestinal mucosa. Neonatal intestinal immunity is significantly modified by breastfeeding.[33]

Complement System

The synthesis of complement proteins usually begins around 6 weeks of gestation in the fetal liver. The neonates have a physiological deficiency of complement proteins, both quantitatively and qualitatively. The levels of various complement proteins, like C_1q, C_2, C_3, C_4 and C_5 are low in term neonates and even lower in preterm neonates. These generally vary from 0.41% to 0.79% of the mean adult values. This deficiency contributes towards the inability of neonates to halt the replication of certain bacteria in the blood as well as towards the impairment of neonatal adaptive immunity.[34] Moreover, the levels of mannose binding lectin, which normally activates the complement via the alternate pathway, are also low.

Toll-like Receptors

Toll-like receptors are one of the major components of mammalian innate immunity. These were first identified in *Drosophila*. Janeway et al. in 1997 identified the first human analogue of TLR and it was named as TLR4.[35]

The TLRs act as the major pattern recognition receptors (PRRs) for identification of specific pathogen associated molecular patterns (PAMPs). After recognition of a ligand, there occurs activation of the TLR, which then utilizes an adapter protein and leads to activation of downstream signaling pathways. As a consequence, there is increased transcription of NF-κβ, which leads to increased expression of a variety of cytokine genes. Eventually, many inflammatory cytokines, chemokines and colony stimulating factors are produced that play a role in immunological response against the intruding microbe. Ten different types of TLRs **(Table 46.3)** have been recognized in humans.[36]

It is believed that the expression levels of TLRs, accessory proteins and adaptor proteins on neonatal immune cells are comparable to those in adults. However, there is impaired activation of the downstream signaling pathways in response to TLR activation thereby hindering the innate immune responses against various microbes.[20] Recent studies on animal models have suggested a relation between enhanced expression of TLRs (especially TLR2 and TLR4) and development of neonatal sepsis.[37]

Chemokines and Antimicrobial Peptides

Chemokines and antimicrobial peptides are an important link between innate and adaptive immunity. Many cytokines often

Table 46.3 Toll-like receptors (TLRs)[36]

TLR	*Agonist*	*Expression*	*Adapter*
TLR 1	• Triacyl lipopeptides on gram-negative bacteria and mycoplasma	• Monocytes or macrophages • Dendritic cells (DCs) • B-lymphocytes	MyD88
TLR 2	• Bacterial lipopeptides • Lipoteichoic acid, lipoarabinomannan on gram-positive bacteria • Zymosan on fungi • tGPI-mucin from *Trypanosoma cruzi* • Hemagglutinin from measles virus	• Monocytes or macrophages • Myeloid dendritic cells (mDCs) • Mast cells	MyD88
TLR 3	• Double-stranded RNA • Polyinosinic polycytidylic acid (poly I:C)	• DC • B-lymphocytes	TRIF
TLR 4	• Lipopolysaccharide on gram-negative bacteria • F-protein on respiratory syncytial virus	• Monocytes or macrophages • mDC • Mast cells	MyD88/TRIF
TLR 5	Bacterial flagellin	• Monocytes or macrophages • DC	MyD88
TLR 6	Diacylated lipopeptides from gram-positive bacteria and mycoplasma	• Monocytes or macrophages • Mast cells • B-lymphocytes	MyD88
TLR 7	• Viral single-stranded RNA (ssRNA) • Imidazoquinoline derivates (imiquimod, R-848) • Guanine analogs (loxoribine)	• Monocytes or macrophages • Plasmacytoid dendritic cells (pDCs) • B-lymphocytes	MyD88
TLR 8	• Viral ssRNA • R-848	• Monocytes or macrophages • pDC • B-lymphocytes	MyD88
TLR 9	Unmethylated CpG-DNA motifs on bacteria and viruses	• Monocytes or macrophages • pDC • B-lymphocytes	MyD88
TLR 10	Unknown	• Monocytes or macrophages • B-lymphocytes	Unknown

also act as antimicrobial peptides and many antimicrobial peptides have chemoattractant and immunomodulatory properties. Serum levels of the chemokine CCL5 (RANTES) are lower in preterm neonates. Production of CCL3 by term neonatal mononuclear cells is impaired. However, certain chemokines, such as CXCR3, are upregulated in neonatal bacterial infection and have a use as diagnostic marker. A unique feature of neonatal immune response is the impaired production of Th1-cell associated cytokines. It has been seen that stimulus-induced production of certain cytokines such as IL-6, IL-10 and IL-23 in neonates exceeds that of adults.[38]

Neonatal Immune Cells

Neutrophils

Neonates have a quantitative deficiency of neutrophils due to diminished granulocyte and monocyte progenitors. Qualitatively, neonatal neutrophils show impairment of multiple functional aspects, including chemotaxis, rolling, adhesion, transmigration, lamellipodia formation and microbicidal mechanisms. These neutrophil defects are more pronounced with prematurity. There is impaired recruitment of neonatal neutrophils to inflammatory sites due to decreased expression of integrin and selectin and increased production of IL-6 that inhibits neutrophil migration.[39]

The decreased microbicidal action is due to reduced amounts of:

- Antimicrobial proteins and peptides (APPs), like lactoferrin (~50% of adult levels)
- Bactericidal or permeability-increasing protein (BPI) (~30% of adult levels)
- Impaired oxidase, e.g. nicotinamide adenine dinucleotide phosphate (NADPH) oxidase activity
- Impaired priming in response to LPS.

Monocyte-Macrophages and Antigen Presenting Cells

Neonatal monocytes and antigen-presenting cells (APCs) differ from those in adults, both quantitatively and qualitatively.

Major differences include:[2]

- Reduced expression of major histocompatibility complex (MHC) class II molecules
- Diminished response to antigenic stimulation, mainly LPS and also protein antigens. This is due to much higher intracellular concentration of the cyclic AMP (cAMP) that inhibits the LPS-induced production of TNF
- Diminished production of TNF compared to adults
- Impaired production of type I IFNs (that is, IFN-α and IFN-β) and deficient IFN-γ receptor signaling
- Significantly decreased phosphorylation of STAT-1 in response to IFN-γ, in spite of comparable expression of STAT-1 protein in cord blood and adult macrophages
- Impaired production of Th1-type immune responses. However, some exceptions do exist with regards to the impairment of Th1-cell responses in neonates. Agonists of TLR8, such as antiviral imidazoquinoline and single-stranded viral RNAs, can induce production of TNF and IL-12/IL-23 in neonates, similar to that of adults[40]
- Increased production of TLR-mediated IL-6, IL-10 and IL-23, compared to adults
- Increased production of IL-23 by neonatal DCs, increases expression of IL-17
- Reduced expression of the TLR adaptor molecule, MyD88 protein with normal levels of mRNA for MyD88, leading to impaired TLR-mediated responses
- Defective chemotaxis and phagocytosis due to diminished opsonin levels (complement proteins, IgS, fibronectin, etc.) as well as defective intracellular killing mechanisms
- cAMP is also known to inhibit the production of several other cytokines for which production is impaired in newborns (such as IFN-α, IFN-γ and IL-12), while enhancing the production of other cytokines, like IL-6, IL-10 and IL-23. This "cAMP hypothesis" is yet not proven, and the duration for the high cytosolic cAMP content of neonatal mononuclear cells is not known.[2]

Natural Killer Cells

Natural killer cells play a pivotal role in innate immunity. NK response is not clonally restricted due the monomorphic nature of NK receptors. NK cells mediate antibody-dependent cell-mediated cytotoxicity (ADCC) and lysis of virus-infected and tumor cells lacking MHC molecules. In healthy adults, NK cells constitute 10–15% of peripheral blood lymphocytes and mediate cytotoxic activity against virus infected and tumor cells.

Phenotypically, neonatal NK cells are different compared to adults. In neonates, the levels are only 50% of the adult values, but reach adult levels at 1–5 months of age.[41] There are no significant differences between the percentages of NK cells synthesizing IFN-γ and TNF-β in neonates and adults but those producing TNF-α were significantly lower in cord blood compared to adults. Moreover, the neonatal NK cells are functionally immature.[42]

Mast Cells

Mast cells in neonates secrete increased amounts of histamine on stimulation as compared to adults. This increased histamine, in turn, elicits increased secretion of IL-10 and decreased secretion of IL-12 from the dendritic cells, thereby further augmenting the Th2 polarization in neonates.[43] They are known to have a role in development of common neonatal rash and erythema toxicum.

ADAPTIVE IMMUNE SYSTEM

This serves as the second line of body's defense since it develops only after prior exposure to foreign antigens (and sometimes self-antigens). The effector cells of adaptive immune system are the T- and the B-lymphocytes.

T- and B-Cell Development

In the fetus, T- and B-lymphocytes develop from pluripotent HSCs in the liver. Further, differentiation occurs in the thymus for T-cells and in the bone marrow for B-cells, where they undergo an irreversible differentiation consisting of genetic rearrangements leading to TcR (T-cell receptor) and BcR (B-cell receptor) expression. By 18–20 weeks of gestation, T lymphocytes are provided with TcR. T- and B-cells start showing clonal diversity from the first trimester. However, CTL production begins in the middle of fetal life.[44] Simultaneously, a specific antibody response also develops, which is quantitatively and qualitatively different from adults. This is because fetal and neonatal B-cells have a limited ability to synthesize IgG and IgA antibodies. This is followed by a selection process, wherein the cells interact with HLA proteins expressed on the APCs in thymus. In the selection, lymphocytes with affinity for self-antigens (self-reactive clones) are removed and die by apoptosis. Thus, only lymphocytes with specificity for foreign antigens survive.

T-Cells

T-cells arise from bone marrow HSCs and undergo differentiation in thymus. In humans, thymus develops from the third branchial pouch around 6 weeks of gestation. Around 7–8 weeks of gestation, lymphoid cells with the CD7 phenotype migrate into the prethymic mesenchyme where these thymocytes undergo differentiation. Immature thymocytes are identified in the cortical zone at 8–9 weeks and in the medulla at 10 weeks, where these undergo further differentiation. By 10 weeks, thymocytes acquire CD1, CD2 and CD3. However, TCR-γδ T-cells can be identified before thymic development around 6–8 weeks of gestation in fetal liver and even in cord blood. This is followed by negative selection mediated by APCs, thereby eliminating autoreactive cells by clonal deletion or anergy.

Some immature T-cells are triple-negative cells, and express the IL-2 receptor (CD25), CD34 and CD117. Cortical cells express both CD4 and CD8 (double positive cells), which in the medullary stage divide into two subpopulations with TcR-αβ expressing either CD4 or CD8 (single positive cells). The TcR-γδ is the first receptor associated with CD3, followed by TcR-αβ expression (around 9–10 weeks of fetal life).[45] Further, thymocytes expressing TcR-γδ progressively decrease in number. At 12 weeks of gestation, antigen recognition is present. Around 14 weeks, T-cells acquire surface markers and lose CD45RA (naïve) and gain CD45RO (memory) expression. At 18–20 weeks of intrauterine life, CD4 T-cells are twice the number of CD8 T-cells. Compared to adults, fetus has reduced numbers of CD3 and a reversed CD4/CD8 ratio due to the lower numbers of CD8. Around 19 weeks of gestation, CD3+, CD4+ and CD8+ T-cells gradually increase in number; and finally reach a peak at about 6–7 months after birth.[46]

B-Cells

By 12 weeks of gestation, bone marrow becomes the major site of generation of B-cells. Around 7–8 weeks of gestation, in the liver, pro-B-cells develop from lymphoid HSCs, which are characterized by expression of CD45, TdT enzyme, IL-7, CD117 and DJ rearrangement on both pairs of chromosome 14. Around 9 weeks of gestation, the pre-B I cells appear following a VDJ rearrangement and production of μ cytoplasmic (heavy) chains, but not light chains. The cytoplasmic μ chains combine with surrogate light chains and are expressed on the surface at very low levels as pre-B-cell receptor. Pre-B-cells do not express the TdT enzyme, but immunoglobulin M (IgM) or IgD (pre-BCR), C3, CD20 and CD19 persist. λ light chains are expressed when pre-B I cells differentiate into pre-B II cells, combine with the cytoplasmic μ heavy chains and gets displayed as IgMs (surface). Although the BCR function is present right from the pro-B stage, it becomes active from the pre-B stage. Around 12–14 weeks of gestation, differentiation of immature B-cells into B-cells coexpressing IgM and IgD occurs, both with the same V region, and they acquire the Fc receptors for IgG molecules. Mature B-cells lack surface IgD but express other isotypes in sequence on their membrane. Differentiation into plasma cells is the final stage of B-cell development, when surface immunoglobulins, HLA-DR, CD19, CD20, CD21 and CD22 expression are lost[15] and CD138 is expressed at high levels.

ORGANS OF THE IMMUNE SYSTEM

The lymphoid organs can be divided into two categories—central and peripheral lymphoid organs. The central lymphoid organs are:

- *Bone marrow*: Bone marrow is the main organ of hematopoiesis throughout life; contains the HSCs which are the precursors of cells mediating both innate and adaptive immunity
- *Thymus*: The thymus is the main organ that produces T-cells.

The mature lymphocytes leave bone marrow or thymus and are distributed through lymph and blood to peripheral lymphoid organs. The peripheral organs include:

- Lymph nodes
- Spleen
- Lymphoid tissue associated with upper respiratory tract [bronchial-associated lymphoid tissue (BALT)]
- *Lymphoid tissue associated with GI tract [gut-associated lymphoid tissue (GALT)]*: Composed of the adenoids, tonsils, appendix, Peyer's patches, intraepithelial lymphocytes and lymphoid tissue contained in lamina propria
- Lymphoid tissue associated with skin [skin-associated lymphoid tissue (SALT)]
- Lymphoid tissue associated with nasopharynx [nasopharynx-associated lymphoid tissue (NALT)].

NEONATAL HUMORAL RESPONSES

At birth, neonates have a full repertoire of antigen-specific B-cells in the bone marrow and are able to produce low concentrations of IgM and even IgG and IgA. However, the B-cell responses gradually mature during the 1st years of life.

Immunoglobulin G and IgA levels are appreciable in the fetus by 17 and 30 weeks of gestation, respectively. IgE antibodies are practically absent during fetal life and are synthesized mainly after birth. A normal fetus has to rely on transplacentally transported maternal IgG antibodies, until around 33 weeks of gestation, when fetal IgG reaches maternal levels.[47]

It has been seen that supplementation of neonatal B-cells with IL-2, IL-4 and IL-6 results in the correction of the antibody deficit and production of all major immunoglobulin isotypes, thereby implying that the deficiency of these ILs may be resulting in an inconsistent antibody synthesis by neonatal B-cells.[48]

Most of the antibodies in the fetal circulation at birth are of maternal origin. Maternal IgG transfer across the placenta increases during the last 4 weeks, thus explaining higher IgG concentrations in term neonates than maternal levels and lower concentrations in preterm infants due to their short gestational age. Neonatal antibody status and susceptibility to bacterial infections are closely associated. Neonates are capable of mounting their own antibody responses to some extent. However, these responses are mainly of IgM type and this may be partly contributed by relative deficiency of CD40 on the surface of neonatal B-cells.[49]

NEONATAL CELL-MEDIATED RESPONSES

Absolute numbers of T lymphocytes in neonates are higher than in adults but these are functionally immature as compared to adults. Neonatal T-cell immaturity is evident by their reduced proliferation after CD2 and CD3 stimulation. Transiently, there are increased T-cells, reflecting an excessive activation in response to the first exposure of the immature immune system to environmental antigens. Prior to any antigenic exposure, naïve, CD45RA + CD45RO – T-cells predominate among neonatal circulating lymphocytes. This relative T-cell immunodeficiency usually persists until 4–5 years of age. Afterward, the levels of CD45RO + T-cells gradually increase until they reach adult levels around 10–15 years of age. Simultaneously, CD45RA + T-cell levels progressively decrease.[15] Earlier it was believed that being immature, neonatal T-cells are not able to mount a cytotoxic response against viruses, and hence, are unable to kill infected cells. However, recently many studies have shown that neonatal T-cells can develop a cytotoxic response under certain circumstances, in spite of the activation of CTLs being only 60% of that in adults.[49]

An important feature of neonatal CMI is the defective production of Th1 cytokines. Neonates have a biased T-cell development toward Th2 cells, influenced by immune status during pregnancy. Moreover, the meager population of neonatal Th1 cells lacks intracellular IFN-γ and produces low concentrations of IFN-γ, even after antigenic stimulation.[49] The Th1 cells play an important role in delayed-type hypersensitivity and in autoimmune diseases. The cytokines produced by Th1 cells play a role in immunity as well as in promoting the growth of other T-cell subsets. The bias in neonatal cytokine production makes the neonates particularly vulnerable to infection with a broad array of microorganisms, including intracellular pathogens requiring efficient Th1-cell responses for clearance, such as *Listeria monocytogenes* and herpes simplexvirus.[2] The mechanism of Th1 deficiency is however not completely understood. After birth, the neonatal T-cells rapidly lose their Th2 phenotype by 1 week due to diminished production of IL-4.[50] In addition, recent studies have shown that neonatal T-cells can mount efficient Th1 responses under certain conditions.[40]

PASSIVE IMMUNITY IN NEONATES

Passive humoral immunity involves direct transfer of maternal antibodies to the fetus and the neonate. There are two major routes for transfer of the maternal antibodies:
1. Transplacental transfer
2. Colostrum and breast milk.

These maternal antibodies confer a considerable degree of protection to the neonates from a variety of pathogens. However, in addition to the protective effect, maternal antibodies may hamper certain immune responses.

The protective effect is pivotal during the highly vulnerable neonatal period. Protection is provided against those viruses and bacteria that the mother has been exposed to. This is best exemplified by the enhancement of neonatal immunity subsequent to maternal immunization against pathogens that cause severe infections during the 1st months of life. For example, vaccination of pregnant women with tetanus toxoid protects the mothers against puerperal tetanus and also elicits specific IgG antibodies that are transplacentally transferred and protect the neonates against tetanus neonatorum. If the level of maternal antibodies decreases, before the neonate synthesizes sufficient amounts of his own antibodies, then the frequency of infections increases. In other words, maternal immunological experience and memory is essential for the survival of newborns during the early periods of life.

Another important aspect is the protection conferred against vertically transmitted infections. The rate of vertical transmission of human immunodeficiency virus (HIV) varies from 30–65%. It has been seen that there is presence of maternal antibodies specific for epitopes of the hypervariable loop of gp120 in the sera of both HIV-infected mothers and their uninfected children, thereby implying that such antibodies block the spread of HIV from mother to fetus.[49]

The maternal antibodies, in spite of their protective effect, can inhibit the vaccination-induced immune responses in infants. This inhibition occurs due to formation of immune complexes between antibodies and vaccine components. The antigen in these immune complexes is degraded and cleared by the reticuloendothelial system and the infant's B-cells are not able to recognize specific antigenic epitopes. However, the antigen degradation by APCs may generate peptides that can activate T-cells. Thus, maternal antibodies inhibit neonatal humoral responses without blocking T-cell-mediated responses.

Besides these properties, maternal antibodies also exert a regulatory effect on the B-cell development in the form of increased generation of pre-B-cells and subsequently mature B-cells. In addition, the number of IgM-producing plasma cells is decreased with consequent lowered levels of IgM.[49]

TRANSPLACENTAL TRANSFER

Immunoglobulin G can be transferred from mother to fetus through the placenta and in humans, IgG1, IgG3, and IgG4 fractions are more efficiently transferred than IgG2. This transfer occurs actively via the Fc receptors (FcRc), located on placental syncytiotrophoblasts, which bind to Fc fragments of maternal IgG. Each IgG molecule binds to two FcRcs. The FcRc has higher affinity for IgG at an acidic pH but low affinity at a neutral pH. Maternal IgG is taken up by the trophoblasts through pinocytosis. Pinocytotic vacuoles fuse with apical vesicles, having an acidic pH, thereby strongly binding IgG to the FcRc. The vesicles then fuse with the basal membrane of the syncytiotrophoblast and due to neutral pH of the fetal circulation, there occurs dissociation of IgG from the FcRc. This transplacental transfer of IgG becomes evident around 24 weeks of gestation and then increases exponentially. At birth, the neonatal blood level of IgG (15 g/dL) exceeds the maternal level (13 g/dL).[51,52] IgM antibodies are not transferred through the placenta due to lack of receptor for IgM on syncytiotrophoblasts.

COLOSTRUM AND BREAST MILK

After birth, IgG along with sIgA and lactoferrin are transferred to the infant through colostrum and breast milk. Breast milk has factors that not only augment the neonatal immunity against infections, but also regulates the potentially lethal immune responses. It is the richest and the most inexpensive source of immune factors for a newborn. It not only provides nourishment but also protects the vulnerable neonate during its most critical period. Breast milk provides T and B-lymphocytes, macrophages, neutrophils, immunoglobulins, IFN-γ, complement components and many other bioactive molecules to the newborn. Breast milk-fed infants have higher NK cell levels and IL-2 production compared to bottle-fed babies. This helps in strengthening neonatal defense against various bacterial and viral infections. In addition, breast milk stimulates active secretion of IgA and sIgA, thereby promoting the maturation of the neonatal immune system, unlike bottle-fed neonates.[15]

Colostrum and breast milk, both mostly contain sIgA with IgM and IgG in small amounts. sIgA is the major antibody of breast milk.[31] The maternal antibodies transferred through milk protect the neonate against the gut pathogens such as *Escherichia coli, Vibrio cholerae, Shigella, Campylobacter*, and some parasites such as *Giardia*. Simultaneously, IgA and sIgA antibodies inhibit the penetration of harmful luminal antigens. The ingested IgG from colostrum and breast milk on the other hand is transported into the circulation, across the intestinal wall by binding to FcRns that are expressed at high levels in neonatal intestinal epithelial cells. The IgM antibodies transferred via milk have a very short half-life of 1–2 days. This might explain the high incidence of otitis, meningitis, and pulmonary infections in human neonates caused by bacteria such as *Streptococcus pneumoniae, Neisseria meningitidis* and *Haemophilus influenzae.*[49]

Breast-milk also contains:[15]

- ω-6 long-chain polyunsaturated fatty acids (LCPUFAs) that protect the infants against atopy and respiratory diseases by favoring Th2/Th1 switching and potentiation of the Th1 response
- Spermine and spermidine that prevent the development of food allergy
- *Nucleotides and nucleic acids*: Nucleotides, influence several aspects of neonatal immunity, are essential for normal development and maturation of the GI tract and in energy metabolism. The nucleic acids present in breast milk help in inhibiting the Th2-mediated responses, thereby, directing the original fetal immune responses toward the Th1 phenotype
- TLR signaling regulator (sTLR2), which helps in regulating cellular responses to bacterial antigens. This helps in preventing the development of excessive local inflammation of the neonatal gut following bacterial colonization.
- Antimicrobial peptides are also secreted in the breast milk such as defensins and cathelicidin. Cathelicidin has effective antimicrobial activity against both gram-positive and negative bacteria.

To conclude, the immune defense provided by colostrum and breast milk is fundamental for the neonate whose GI maturation and antibody secretion are still inefficient **(Table 46.4)**.

DELETERIOUS EFFECTS OF MATERNAL ANTIBODIES

Occasionally, transfer of pathogenic autoantibodies from the mother to the fetus or the newborn can occur and may lead to fetal or neonatal diseases of varying severity. Natural passive transfer of maternal pathogenic autoantibodies to a fetus from a mother having an autoimmune disease can lead to various autoimmune diseases such as transient myasthenia

Table 46.4 Immunology of breast milk[15]

Components	*Properties*
sIgA	Does not activate complement, suppresses PMN chemotaxis, blocks adhesion of microbial pathogens, prevents infections, limits the allergenic penetration
IgM	Activates complement, forms antibodies against bacteria and virus, retains opsonic activity after traversing the intestinal canal
IgG	Activates complement, has heat-stable opsonic activity, blocks toxins and virus
IgD	Forms antibodies against bacteria
α-2-glycoprotein	Inhibits the lymphocytes, lymphocyte blastogenesis, ADCC and immunoglobulin production
Antioxidants: Ascorbic acid, cysteine, β-carotene, α-tocopherol	Contrast superoxide production
Arylsulfatase	Degrades leukotrienes
Catalase	Degrades H_2O_2
Glycoproteins, glycolipids Fibronectins	Antiviral activity, offer protection against bacterial colonization Membrane protein, mediates cell interactions and adhesion Plasma protein with opsonic functions
Protease inhibitors	Reduce inflammation Degrades the enzymes active in the inflammatory reactions
Lysozyme	Inhibits PMN chemotaxis and free radical formation, antibacterial activity
Macrophages	Have sIgA, produce lysozyme and PGE2, which reduces intestinal permeability
Polyamines	Spermine and spermidine

Contd...

Contd...

Components	*Properties*
Prostaglandins	Inhibit degranulation of neutrophils, activation of lymphocytes, are cytoprotective, promote intestinal and cellular integrity, release brush-border enzymes
Cytokines IFN-γ IL-1 IL-6 IL-10 M-CSF, GM-CSF TNF-α TGF-β	Increases chemotaxis and opsonization, enhances Th1 and antagonizes Th2 cells Activates T-lymphocytes Enhances IgA production and favors oral tolerance Carries out anti-inflammatory activity in the infant gut, has effects opposed to those of IFN-g on Th1 and Th2 cells Induces macrophage differentiation Enhances isotype switching to IgA + B-cells and favors oral tolerance Induces proliferation of epithelial cells from G-CSF activates macrophage motility and SC production

Abbreviations: G-CSF, granulocyte colony-stimulating factor; GM-CSF, granulocyte-macrophage colony-stimulating factor; SC, subcutaneous; TGF, transforming growth factor; IFN, interferon; IL, interleukin; ADCC, antibody-dependent cellular cytotoxicity; PMN, polymorphonuclear neutrophils

gravis, neonatal Graves' disease [maternal antithyroid-stimulating hormone receptor (TSHR) autoantibodies], neonatal lupus and complete heart block (maternal anti-Ro and anti-La antibodies) and neonatal pemphigus (maternal anti-desmoglein antibodies).[49]

Besides these, some other neonatal autoimmune diseases can also occur by transfer of alloantibodies from normal mothers against the paternal antigens. These include alloautoimmune diseases, like hemolytic diseases of fetuses and newborns resulting from transplacentally transferred maternal antibodies directed against the paternal blood group antigens. These alloantibodies cause immune-mediated destruction of fetal red blood cells.

CONCLUSION

Many studies in the recent years have challenged the long held belief that neonates have an immature immune system. In fact, it has now become obvious that basically the neonatal immune responses are highly regulated and tailored to match the distinct requirements of the neonatal environment.

Major differences exhibited by the neonatal immune system as compared to the adults include:

- Weak mucosal immunity
- Deficiency of complement components
- Diminished TLR signaling mechanisms
- Deficient activation in response to stimulation by LPS and protein antigens
- Deficient rolling, adhesion and chemotaxis of neutrophils and monocytes
- Decreased opsonins
- Defective phagocytosis by neutrophils and macrophages
- Defective intracellular killing mechanisms
- Reduced number and activity of NK cells
- Decreased levels of G-CSF, GM-CSF, IL-3, IL-5, IL-6, IL-12, INF-γ and TNF-α
- Deficient Th1 immune response with Th2 skewing
- Deficient T-cell IL secretion
- Reduced cytotoxic activity of CTLs
- Deficient B-cell immunoglobulin production
- Deficient CD154/CD40 expression on B-cells.

REFERENCES

1. Berg RD. The indigenous gastrointestinal microflora. Trends Microbiol. 1996;4(11):430-5.
2. Levy O. Innate immunity of the newborn: basic mechanisms and clinical correlates. Nat Rev Immunol. 2007;7(5):379-90.
3. Wilson CB, Lewis DB, Penix LA. The physiologic immunodeficiency of immaturity. In: Stiehm ER (Ed). Immunologic Disorders in Infants and Children, 4th edition. Philadelphia, PA, USA: WB Saunders; 1996. pp. 253-95.
4. Weetman AP. The immunology of pregnancy. Thyroid. 1999;9(7):643-6.
5. Ben-Hur H, Gurevich E, Tchanyshev R, Berman V, Gurevich E, Zusman I. The secretory immune system as a part of the placental barrier in the second trimester of pregnancy in humans. In Vivo. 2001;15(5):429-35.
6. Daya S, Clark DA. Immunoregulation at the maternofetal interface. Immunol Allergy Clin North Am. 1990;10:49-64.
7. Wood GW. Is restricted antigen presentation the explanation for fetal allograft survival? Immunol Today. 1994;15(1):15-8.
8. Reinhard G, Noll A, Schlebusch H, Mallmann P, Ruecker AV. Shifts in the TH1/TH2 balance during human pregnancy correlate with apoptotic changes. Biochem Biophys Res Commun. 1998;245(3):933-8.
9. Wegmann TG, Lin H, Guilbert L, Mosmann TR. Bidirectional cytokine interactions in the maternal-fetal relationship: is successful pregnancy a TH2 phenomenon? Immunol Today. 1993;14(7):353-6.
10. Hill JA, Polgar K, Anderson DJ. T-helper 1-type immunity to trophoblast in women with recurrent spontaneous abortion. JAMA. 1995;273(24):1933-6.
11. Quie PG. Antimicrobial defenses in the neonate. Semin Perinatol. 1990;14(4 Suppl 1):2-9.
12. Warner JA, Jones CA, Jones AC, Warner JO. Prenatal origins of allergic disease. J Allergy Clin Immunol. 2000;105(2 Pt 2):S493-8.
13. Pazmany L, Mandelboim O, Valés-Gómez M, Davis DM, Reyburn HT, Strominger JL. Protection from natural killer cell-mediated lysis by HLA-G expression on target cells. Science. 1996;274(5288):792-5.

14. Gutman GA. Immunology core notes. University of Califiornia. [online] Available from http://jeeves.mmg.uci.edu/immunology/CoreNotes/CoreNotes.htm. [Accessed October, 2016].
15. Cantani A. Pediatric Allergy, Asthma and Immunology. Berlin: Springer Berlin Heidelberg; 2008.
16. Forsthuber T, Yip HC, Lehmann PV. Induction of TH1 and TH2 immunity in neonatal mice. Science. 1996;271(5256):1728-30.
17. Ridge JP, Fuchs EJ, Matzinger P. Neonatal tolerance revisited: turning on newborn T cells with dendritic cells. Science. 1996;271(5256):1723-6.
18. Sarzotti M, Robbins DS, Hoffman PM. Induction of a protective CTL response in newborn mice by a murine retrovirus. Science. 1996;271(5256):1726-8.
19. Elahi S, Ertelt JM, Kinder JM, Jiang TT, Zhang X, Xin L, et al. Immunosuppressive CD71+ erythroid cells compromise neonatal host defence against infection. Nature. 2013;504(7478):158-62.
20. Kollmann TR, Crabtree J, Rein-Weston A, Blimkie D, Thommai F, Wang XY, et al. Neonatal innate TLR-mediated responses are distinct from those of adults. J Immunol. 2009;183(11):7150-60.
21. Kenzel S, Henneke P. The innate immune system and its relevance to neonatal sepsis. Curr Opin Infect Dis. 2006;19(3):264-70.
22. Holbrook KA, Pincus S, Parker F, Holloway Jr GA, Kraning KB, Yancey K. Structure, function, and immunology of the skin. Middleton E Jr, Reed CE, Ellis EF, Adkinson NF Jr, Yunginger JW, Busse WW (Eds). Allergy: Principles and Practice, 4th edition. St Louis, USA: CV Mosby; 1993. pp. 390-427.
23. Bos JD, Kapsenberg ML. The skin immune system: progress in cutaneous biology. Immunol Today. 1993;14(2):75-8.
24. Luger TA, Schwarz T. The role of cytokines and neuroendocrine hormones in cutaneous immunity and inflammation. Allergy. 1995;50(4):292-302.
25. Rutter N. The immature skin. Eur J Pediatr. 1996;155 Suppl 2:S18-20.
26. Tollin M, Bergsson G, Kai-Larsen Y, Lengqvist J, Sjövall J, Griffiths W, et al. Vernix caseosa as a multi-component defence system based on polypeptides, lipids and their interactions. Cell Mol Life Sci. 2005;62(19-20):2390-9.
27. Dorschner RA, Lin KH, Murakami M, Gallo RL. Neonatal skin in mice and humans expresses increased levels of antimicrobial peptides: innate immunity during development of the adaptive response. Pediatr Res. 2003;53(4):566-72.
28. Lotz M, Gütle D, Walther S, Ménard S, Bogdan C, Hornef MW. Postnatal acquisition of endotoxin tolerance in intestinal epithelial cells. J Exp Med. 2006;203(4):973-84.
29. Fanaro S, Chierici R, Guerrini P, Vigi V. Intestinal microflora in early infancy: composition and development. Acta Paediatr Suppl. 2003;91(441):48-55.
30. Jilling T, Simon D, Lu J, Meng FJ, Li D, Schy R, et al. The roles of bacteria and TLR4 in rat and murine models of necrotizing enterocolitis. J Immunol. 2006;177(5):3273-82.
31. Walker WA. The role of immunologic immaturity in neonatal food allergy. In: Chandra RK (Ed). Food Allergy. Philadelphia, PA, USA: St John's: Nutrition Research Education Foundation; 1987. pp. 45-66.
32. Turck D, Feste AS, Lifschitz CH. Age and diet affect the composition of porcine colonic mucins. Pediatr Res. 1993;33(6):564-7.
33. Newburg DS, Walker WA. Protection of the neonate by the innate immune system of developing gut and of human milk. Pediatr Res. 2007;61(1):2-8.
34. Drossou V, Kanakoudi P, Diamanti E, Tzimouli V, Konstantinidis T, Germenis A, et al. Concentrations of main serum opsonins in early infancy. Arch Dis Child Fetal Neonatal Ed. 1996;72(3):F172-5.
35. Medzhitov R, Preston-Hurlburt P, Janeway CA Jr. A human homologue of the Dorosophila Toll protein signals activation of adaptive immunity. Nature. 1997;388(6640):394-7.
36. Belderbos ME. Neonatal innate immunity. A translational perspective [dissertation on internet]. [online] Available from *http://www.researchgate.net/profile/Louis_Bont/publication/51818432_Breastfeeding_modulates_neonatal_innate_immune_responses_a_prospective_birth_cohort_study/links/00b7d52bec905437ca000000.pdf.* [Accessed October, 2016].
37. Martin CR, Walker WA. Intestinal immune defences and the inflammatory response in necrotizing enterocolitis. Semin Fetal Neonatal Med. 2006;11(5):369-77.
38. Angelone DF, Wessels MR, Coughlin M, Suter EE, Valentini P, Kalish LA, et al. Innate immunity of the human newborn is polarized toward a high ratio of IL-6/TNF-alpha production in vitro and in vivo. Pediatr Res. 2006;60(2):205-9.
39. Schultz C, Rott C, Temming P, Schlenke P, Möller JC, Bucsky P. Enhanced interleukin-6 and interleukin-8 synthesis in term and preterm infants. Pediatr Res. 2002;51(3):317-22.
40. Levy O, Suter EE, Miller RL, Wessels MR. Unique efficacy of Toll-like receptor 8 agonists in activating human neonatal antigen-presenting cells. Blood. 2006;108(4):1284-90.
41. Yabuhara A, Kawai H, Komiyama A. Development of natural killer cytotoxicity during childhood: marked increases in number of natural killer cells with adequate cytotoxic abilities during infancy to early childhood. Pediatr Res. 1990;28(4):316-22.
42. Krampera M, Tavecchia L, Benedetti F, Nadali G, Pizzolo G. Intracellular cytokine profile of cord blood T-, and NK-cells and monocytes. Haematologica. 2000;85(7):675-9.
43. Mazzoni A, Young HA, Spitzer JH, Visintin A, Segal DM. Histamine regulates cytokine production in maturing dendritic cells, resulting in altered T cell polarization. J Clin Invest. 2001;108(12):1865-73.
44. Marshall-Clarke S, Reen D, Tasker L, Hassan J. Neonatal immunity: how well has it grown up? Immunol Today. 2000;21(1):35-41.
45. Haas W, Tonegawa S. Development and selection of γδ-T cells. Curr Opin Immunol. 1992;4(2):147-55.
46. Rognum TO, Thrane PS, Stoltenberg L, Vege A, Brandtzaeg P. Development of intestinal mucosal immunity in fetal life and the first postnatal months. Pediatr Res. 1992;32(2):145-9.
47. Landor M. Maternal-fetal transfer of immunoglobulins. Ann Allergy Asthma Immunol. 1995;74(4):279-83.
48. Splawski JB, Jalinek DF, Lipsky PE. Delineation of the functional capacity of human neonatal lymphocytes. J Clin Invest. 1991;87(2):545-53.
49. Constantin B. Neonatal Immunity. Totowa, New Jersey, USA: Humana Press; 2009.
50. Adkins B, Ghanei A, Hamilton K. Develpmental regulation of IL-4, IL-2, and INF-γ production by murine peripheral T lymphocytes. J Immunol. 1993;151(12):6617-26.
51. Kohler PF, Farr RS. Elevation of cord over maternal IgG immunoglobulin: evidence for an active placental IgG transport. Nature. 1966;210(5040):1070-1.
52. Auestad N, Montalto MB, Hall RT, Fitzgerald KM, Wheeler RE, Connor WE, et al. Visual acuity, erythrocyte fatty acid composition, and growth in term infants fed formulas with long chain polyunsaturated fatty acids for one year. Ross Pediatric Lipid Study. Pediatr Res. 1997;41(1):1-10.

CHAPTER 47

Infections in Neonatal Period: Primary Immunodeficiency Perspective

Vinod Gunasekaran, Nita Radhakrishnan

INTRODUCTION

Infections lead the list of causes for neonatal morbidity and mortality. Apart from neonatal factors, maternal and environmental factors are also contributory for the incidence of neonatal sepsis. The manifestations of neonatal sepsis are myriad and subtle. The progression may be rapid and delay in initiation of treatment leads to disastrous outcome. Hence, practicing pediatricians and neonatologists should be trained to identify early symptoms of neonatal infections, perform a judicious laboratory evaluation and initiate early and effective treatment. Nonetheless, preventive measures including hygiene techniques, exclusive breastfeeding, etc. should be given due importance. This chapter briefly discusses the current evidence in the diagnosis and management of neonatal infections, with a special consideration to the clues for primary immunodeficiency (PID) during the neonatal period.

NEONATAL SEPSIS

Neonatal sepsis is the presence of systemic features of infection occurring in neonates (0–28 days of life) with isolation of bacteria from at least one sterile site. It includes septicemia, pneumonia, arthritis, urinary tract infections and osteomyelitis.[1] The term probable sepsis is used where the clinical and laboratory features are consistent with an underlying bacterial infection without a positive culture. Fungal and viral infections can also occur in neonates that must be differentiated from bacterial infections.[2] Sepsis, if untreated, can rapidly progress to cause organ dysfunction, shock and multiorgan failure. It is broadly classified into two: early onset neonatal sepsis (EONS) and late onset sepsis (LOS).

EPIDEMIOLOGY

The data from National Neonatal Perinatal Database (2002–03) reports the incidence of neonatal sepsis in our country to be 30 per 1,000 live births. *Klebsiella pneumoniae* followed by *Staphylococcus aureus* and *Pseudomonas* were the most common organisms isolated.[1] The other common bacteria isolated include *Escherichia coli*, coagulase-negative *Staphylococcus*, streptococcal species, *Listeria monocytogenes*, enterococci, *Enterobacter* species, *Haemophilus influenzae*, *Acinetobacter* species, etc.[2] Fungal infections (especially *Candida* species) are rare but should be thought of especially in premature babies. Sepsis accounted for 19% of all neonatal deaths.

EARLY ONSET NEONATAL SEPSIS

Early onset neonatal sepsis (EONS) is defined as the onset of bacteremia in a neonate within first 72 hours of life.[2] A cut-off period of 7 days is used by some practitioners in term neonates. Infections occurring during this period are mainly attributable to maternal factors and the perinatal conditions. Various studies have found the following factors to be associated with an increased risk for EONS:[1,2]

- Low-birth-weight (<1,500 g) or prematurity.
- Perinatal asphyxia (APGAR score ≤ 6 at 5 minutes).
- Intrapartum per vaginal examinations (single unclean or > 3 sterile).
- Foul smelling liquor.
- Prolonged labor (>24 hours).
- Prolonged rupture of membranes (>24 hours).
- Clinical chorioamnionitis in mother (characterized by maternal fever, tachycardia, uterine tenderness, leukocytosis and foul smelling liquor).
- Any evidence of bacterial infection in mother less than 2 weeks prior to delivery.
- Male sex.

Babies meeting the criteria to be at high-risk for EONS should be started on empirical antibiotics after sending sepsis screen.

LATE ONSET SEPSIS

Late onset sepsis is defined as the onset of sepsis after 72 hours and up to 90 days of life. The causative factors can be broadly classified as nosocomial (hospital-acquired) and community-acquired. Factors leading to prolonged hospitalization including prematurity, low-birth-weight, perinatal asphyxia, requirement for intensive care unit admission, mechanical ventilation, parenteral therapy, invasive procedures, etc. predispose to nosocomial LOS. Factors leading to community-acquired LOS include poor socioeconomic status, poor living conditions, bottle feeding, poor hygiene, etc.

CLINICAL FEATURES

As discussed previously, the features of infections in the newborn are myriad, subtle and nonspecific, which may be missed unless one has a high index of suspicion. Common presentations include hypothermia (commoner than fever especially in premature babies), lethargy, poor feeding, feed intolerance, diarrhea, jaundice, rashes, weak cry, high-pitched cry, excessive irritability, fast breathing, apnea, seizures, etc. Examination findings may be normal or may reveal hypothermia, unexplained tachycardia or bradycardia, respiratory distress, hypotonia, poor perfusion, hypotension, neck retraction, abdominal distension, dyspnea, skin pustules, etc.

INVESTIGATIONS

Any neonate with suspected sepsis is an emergency and has to be evaluated immediately. Sepsis screen is done for such babies, which include a combination of inflammatory markers including total leukocyte count (abnormal if < 5,000/μL), absolute neutrophil count (low as per reference charts), ratio of immature to total neutrophils in blood (ITR > 0.27 in term and > 0.2 in preterm babies is abnormal), micro erythrocyte sedimentation rate (ESR) (>10 mm in 1st hour), C-reactive protein (CRP) (quantitative > 10 mg/L or qualitative).[1] Different cut-off values and reference charts are available for these parameters. Generally, if any two of these parameters are abnormal, sepsis screen is considered to be positive. If clinical suspicion is high, a negative sepsis screen should not preclude a physician from starting antibiotics. A repeat screen has to be performed after 12–24 hours in negative cases.[1] Two consecutively negative sepsis screen results done 12 hours apart certainly rule out sepsis. The other inflammatory markers tried for this purpose include procalcitonin, interleukin-6, interleukin-8, gamma interferon, etc.[2]

Blood culture is the gold standard investigation to diagnose bacteremia in neonates.[1] Proper aseptic techniques have to be followed during collection to avoid contamination and adequate volume of blood (minimum 1 mL blood in a pediatric blood culture bottle) has to be inoculated to yield best results. BACTEC and BACT/ALERT culture systems help in early identification of organism in 12–24 hours with high sensitivity. The antibiotic sensitivity report guides in optimizing antibiotic policy once available.

Lumbar puncture is indicated in all cases of suspected neonatal sepsis. It is not indicated in suspected EOS if antibiotics are started only on the basis of high-risk features. The prevalence of meningitis in suspected sepsis is around 5% and in case of proven sepsis is around 13–17%. Other investigations including chest X-ray, urine culture, evaluation for viral and fungal etiologies, etc. are done if clinically indicated.

MANAGEMENT

Initial stabilization of temperature, respiration, oxygen saturation, circulation and glycemic status has to be performed in all cases. The indication for starting antibiotics must be made clear. The choice of empirical antibiotics must be customized to the culture and sensitivity patterns of the treating unit and the source and focus of infection. Positive culture or changing clinical course should guide modifications in antibiotics. The duration of antibiotics is guided by organism isolated and the focus of infection.

PREVENTION OF LATE ONSET SEPSIS

Preventive strategies including hand hygiene, use of skin antiseptics (2% chlorhexidine), removal of unnecessary catheters, avoiding unnecessary handling and sampling of babies, etc. have significantly decreased the incidence of LOS among admitted babies.[3] Early initiation of trophic feeding in a sick or a low-birth-weight baby helps in establishing the normal commensal flora of gut, maintains mucosal integrity and improves feed tolerance, thereby avoiding the need for parenteral nutrition in these babies. This prevents the incidence of sepsis significantly. Gut of a normal term baby is immediately colonized by commensals from maternal vaginal tract (anaerobes, *E. coli*, etc.), which are largely replaced by *Bifidobacterium* and *Lactobacillus* once breastfeeding is initiated. It may be delayed or disturbed in case of prematurity, antibiotic use, formula feeding and prolonged hospital stay. Normal probiotic flora is essential for maintaining integrity of gut mucosa and preventing translocation of pathogenic microbes. Administration of probiotics, however, has not found to decrease the incidence of sepsis in studies.[3] Breast milk along with abundant nutrients has secretory antibodies, lactoferrin, immune cells and probiotics, all of which improves gut immunity. Lactoferrin chelates iron in the local environment, thereby depriving iron required for bacterial growth. It also has immunomodulatory effects, decreases production of reactive oxygen species and maintains gut integrity.[3]

NEONATAL IMMUNE SYSTEM AND PREDISPOSITION TO INFECTIONS

The adaptive immune system of neonates is immature. Hence, neonates depend on the innate immune system and passively derived adaptive immunity from mother (immunoglobulin transfer) for fighting infections.[4] Outer layer of skin (stratum corneum) is the first line of defense. Vernix caseosa gives an additional line of defense. Neutrophils in neonates are also found to have a diminished recruitment capacity and oxidative burst response.[4] Pattern recognition receptors (PRRs) are present on the membrane of phagocytes, which recognize the pathogen-associated molecular patterns (PAMPs) present on the surface of the pathogenic microbes. Activation of PRRs by PAMPS leads to further activation on signaling cascades and cytokine production. Toll-like receptors (TLRs) are the extensively studied PRRs. Defects in PRRs lead to susceptibility for specific type of organisms.[4] Preterm babies are immunologically more vulnerable to infections due to decreased passive transfer of maternal immunoglobulins, diminished barrier effect of skin and mucous membranes and increased requirement of invasive procedures. Defects in certain steps of innate and acquired immunity predispose neonates to uncommon infections that may be severe.

Approach to Diagnosis of Primary Immunodeficiency in the Newborn Period

T-cell defects and phagocytic defects typically present in the newborn period as maternal antibodies offer protection in those with antibody deficiencies. Severe PIDs that present in the neonatal period include severe combined immunodeficiency (SCID), Omenn syndrome, leukocyte adhesion defect 1, IL-1 receptor affected kinase-4 deficiency (IRAK-4), DiGeorge syndrome, severe congenital neutropenia, etc. Antibody defects typically present later in life where as phagocytic defects such as chronic granulomatous disease (CGD) can present at any age. The approach for detecting PIDs in newborn period is similar to those at other ages and pattern of infections and sites involved should be given consideration. Unlike in other age groups, early detection of PIDs such as SCID is vital as they are usually life-threatening and may not give a window of opportunity later. Also, evaluation of the family history including consanguinity, early childhood mortality in other family members gives us clues regarding the inheritance and possible etiologies.

Delayed separation of umbilical cord beyond 6–8 weeks suggests leukocyte adhesion deficiency-1 (LAD-1) and IRAK-4 deficiencies. Infection with minimal features of inflammation such as pus formation, omphalitis and perianal ulcers again suggest LAD-1 deficiency as neutrophils are not mobilized to the site of infection. Erythroderma in newborn period can suggest Omenn syndrome, whereas neonatal-onset eczema or atopic dermatitis should suggest Wiskott-Aldrich syndrome (WAS) or hyper-immunoglobulin (IgE) syndrome. Hypocalcemia, facial dysmorphism and congenital cardiac defects should suggest evaluation for DiGeorge syndrome. Early onset refractory diarrhea with failure to thrive merits evaluation for immunodysregulation, polyendocrinopathy, enteropathy, X-linked (IPEX) syndrome in addition to other causes intestinal malabsorption. Reticular dysgenesis is subtype of SCID that presents in the newborn period with severe cytopenias.

Careful evaluation of complete blood count with differential gives invaluable clues to the diagnosis of primary immune deficiencies. Absolute lymphopenia is a hallmark of SCID and age appropriate values should be taken into consideration, as lymphocytosis is the norm in this age group. Low neutrophil count again warrants evaluation for congenital neutropenias. Persistent neutrophilic leukocytosis despite the absence of infections merits evaluation for LAD. Neonatal-onset thrombocytopenia especially if associated with skin changes and colitis needs to be evaluated for WAS.

UNCOMMON INFECTIONS IN NEONATE AND ROLE OF PRIMARY IMMUNODEFICIENCY

Fungal Infections in Neonate

The common risk factors for fungal infections in newborn include colonization of mother's vagina with Candida, prematurity, low-birth-weight, neonatal intensive care unit (NICU) admission, use of broad-spectrum antibiotics and multiple invasive procedures. Congenital candidiasis usually involves skin with maculopapular rashes, abscesses and desquamation followed by invasion of fungus. Occurrence of severe congenital candidiasis in a term baby should alert physician to suspect underlying immunodeficiency.[2] Human immunodeficiency virus (HIV), the most common acquired immunodeficiency, has to be ruled out before evaluating any child for PID. *Candida albicans* and *Candida parapsilosis* are normal commensals of digestive tract and skin respectively in healthy individuals. However, persistent or recurrent Candidal infections of skin, nails, hairs and mucosal surfaces of intestinal tract (chronic mucocutaneous candidiasis CMC) can be seen in HIV infection or with inherited T-cell deficiency (SCID and idiopathic CD4 + lymphopenia).[5] Other inherited conditions including DOCK8, STAT3 (seen in hyper-IgE syndrome), TCR-α, CARD9 or CD25 deficiencies also have T cell abnormalities and present with CMC.[5] Invasive candidiasis can be associated with certain PIDs, like LAD type 1 (CD18 deficiency) and CGD. Infants with CGD can also present with invasive aspergillosis, as phagocytes defective in reactive oxygen species are unable to kill *Aspergillus*. *Cryptococcal* infections involving central nervous system (CNS), commonly seen in HIV-infected individuals, can also be seen in association with certain PIDs including idiopathic CD4 lymphopenia, X-linked CD40L deficiency (hyper-IgM syndrome) and gamma interferon deficiency.[5] *Pneumocystis jirovecii* is an extracellular air borne fungus seen ubiquitously. It causes fulminant interstitial pneumonia in HIV-infected individuals as well as in those with inherited CD4 + T cell defects (SCID, idiopathic CD4 + lymphopenia, WAS, Hyper-IgM syndrome, etc.).

Viral Infections in Neonate

The presence of rash, seizures, encephalitis, transaminitis or myocardial dysfunction should alert the possibility of viral etiologies in a sick neonate.[2]

Herpes Simplex Virus

Herpes simplex virus (HSV) infections spread vertically from mother usually in the peripartum period (85%) and also during *in utero* or postnatal period. HSV in neonates manifests in three distinct forms: skin, eye and mouth (SEM) disease (in 45% cases), meningoencephalitis (30%) or disseminated (25%).[2] Intrauterine infection with HSV may present with sequelae during birth including skin scarring, hyperpigmentation, microcephaly with intracerebral calcifications and chorioretinitis. Diagnostic accuracy has improved with the use of polymerase chain reaction (PCR) techniques, magnetic resonance imaging of brain (showing focal temporal or multifocal hyperintensities) and electroencephalogram showing focal epileptiform discharges, burst suppression or diffuse slowing.[2] Treatment with intravenous acyclovir for 21 days (in CNS and disseminated disease) and for 14 days (in SEM disease) improves outcome successfully.

Cytomegalovirus

Congenital infections with cytomegalovirus (CMV) present with sequelae including microcephaly, sensorineural hearing loss and mental retardation. Perinatally acquired infections from mother may present with organomegaly, low platelet counts, cholestasis, retinitis, pneumonia or sepsis-like presentation.[6] They may be life-threatening and lead to long-term sequelae. Postnatal acquisition of CMV through transfusions and breast milk is known to occur especially in preterm babies. Children with defective function of T cells, natural killer (NK) cells, polymorphisms in TLRs-3, TLRs-4 are at an increased risk of developing serious infections with CMV.[6]

Respiratory Syncytial Virus

Respiratory syncytial virus (RSV) causes bronchiolitis and pneumonia in early infancy. The severity of RSV infection is increased in babies with prematurity, heart diseases, chronic lung disease and an underlying immunodeficiency. A younger infant evokes a poor immune response and hence the illness may be severe. Babies with T-cell defects are unable to clear the virus and the infection may be lethal.[7] RSV infection has also been identified in children with PID undergoing stem cell transplantation, where it was treated with Ribavirin and specific immunoglobulin. Palivizumab is a monoclonal antibody approved for prophylaxis against RSV.

Enteroviruses and *Parechoviruses* are the other common viruses isolated in newborns.[2] These present with gastrointestinal illness or meningoencephalitis.

Bacille Calmette-Guérin Infection in Neonate

Bacille Calmette-Guérin (BCG) vaccine is a live attenuated strain of *Mycobacterium bovis* used against tuberculosis. In all normal babies, a red indurated tender nodule develops at the injection around 2 weeks after the administration, which may ulcerate. Formation of superficial scar may take time period of 2–5 months. Ipsilateral axillary lymphadenopathy with suppuration may occur in some babies, which resolve spontaneously. Dissemination of BCG with fatal outcome may occur in 30% of children with SCID receiving BCG vaccine.[8] SCID is characterized by inadequate T-lymphocyte production with a varying combination of defects in B and NK cell production. As these babies are asymptomatic at birth and BCG is given for all children at birth or at the first contact, early identification of these vulnerable babies prior to BCG administration becomes difficult in the absence of a screening program. Presence of a family history suggestive of SCID or severe complications with BCG vaccine should raise the clinical suspicion.[8] Persistent lymphopenia in a neonate (<2,500/µL) should also raise the possibility of underlying SCID. A case series of nine children presenting with BCG infections reported an underlying diagnosis of SCID in two children (both of them presented with cutaneous nodules at BCG site and died of disseminated BCG before 1 year of age), undiagnosed cellular immunodeficiency in four children (presenting with regional lymphadenitis resistant to treatment), three children with CGD (Two X-linked boys and one autosomal recessive girl presenting with regional lymphadenitis).[9] Hence, a suspicion of and underlying T-cell defect or a phagocytic defect should arise in any neonate with unusual reaction to BCG.

Pneumocystis jirovecii

Pneumocystis pneumonia (PCP) implies immunodeficiency at any age. PCP is commonly observed in patients with severe T-cell lymphopenia such as those observed in SCID. It merits rapid evaluation as these babies often do not survive this infection and a diagnosis is vital for genetic counseling.

CONCLUSION

Bacterial infections remain the most common cause for neonatal infections in our country. Recognition of early signs and symptoms of neonatal sepsis is of paramount importance to decrease morbidity and mortality. An updated protocol to neonatal sepsis in each center is helpful. PIDs should be suspected in neonates in case of unusual infections or infections with unusual severity.

KEY POINTS

- Neonates depend on innate immune system and passive transfer of adaptive immunity to ward off infections.
- T-cell deficiencies and phagocytic disorders present with infections in neonatal period and early infancy.
- Detailed physical examination and evaluation of complete blood count provide vital clues to identifying severe immunodeficiencies
- Recognition of early signs and symptoms of neonatal sepsis is of paramount importance to decrease morbidity and mortality.

8 SECTION Immunological Disorders

REFERENCES

1. Sankar MJ, Agarwal R, Deorari AK, Paul VK. Sepsis in the newborn. Indian J Pediatr. 2008;75(3):261-6.
2. Simonsen KA, Anderson-Berry AL, Delair SF, Davies HD. Early-onset neonatal sepsis. Clin Microbiol Rev. 2014;27(1):21-47.
3. Dong Y, Speer CP. Late-onset neonatal sepsis: recent developments. Arch Dis Child Fetal Neonatal Ed. 2015;100(3):F257-63.
4. Marchant EA, Boyce GK, Sadarangani M, Lavoie PM. Neonatal sepsis due to coagulase-negative staphylococci. Clin Dev Immunol. 2013;2013:586076.
5. Lanternier F, Cypowyj S, Picard C, Bustamante J, Lortholary O, Casanova JL, et al. Primary immunodeficiencies underlying fungal infections. Curr Opin Pediatr. 2013;25(6):736-47.
6. Schleiss MR. Cytomegalovirus in the neonate: immune correlates of infection and protection. Clin Dev Immunol. 2013;2013:501801.
7. Lanari M, Vandini S, Capretti MG, Lazzarotto T, Faldella G. Respiratory syncytial virus infections in infants affected by primary immunodeficiency. J Immunol Res. 2014;2014:850831.
8. Roxo-Junior P, Silva J, Andrea M, Oliveira L, Ramalho F, Bezerra T, et al. A family history of serious complications due to BCG vaccination is a tool for the early diagnosis of severe primary immunodeficiency. Ital J Pediatr. 2013;39:54.
9. Gonzalez B, Moreno S, Burdach R, Valenzuela MT, Henriquez A, Ramos MI, et al. Clinical presentation of Bacillus Calmette-Guérin infections in patients with immunodeficiency syndromes. Pediatr Infect Dis J. 1989;8(4):201-6.

CHAPTER

48

Approach to Newborns with Immunodeficiency

Manisha Madkaikar, Mukesh Desai, Jahnavi Aluri

INTRODUCTION

A newborn's immune system is naïve and lacks an exposure to antigens. The adaptive immune responses are poor at birth. Gradually, with antigenic exposure, the immunologic competence of the neonate progresses for the next 3–6 months of life. During this period, the neonate mainly depends upon components of the innate or antigen-independent immune system including phagocytes, natural killer (NK) cells, antigen-presenting cells (APCs), humoral mediators of inflammation, and complement and maternally transferred immunoglobulins to fight the infections.[1-3] Hence, infections in newborns are not uncommon. However, when these infections are recurrent or when the severity is disproportionate to the virulence of the organisms, one must suspect an underlying immunodeficiency. Primary immunodeficiency disorders (PIDs) are a heterogeneous group of inherited disorders of immune system. They affect the development and/or functioning of immune system leading to increased susceptibility to infections and also autoimmunity and malignancies.[4] The clinical manifestations including the age at presentation depend largely on the underlying immune defect. The common and overlapping clinical manifestations and rarity and complexity of PIDs poses a diagnostic challenge to the treating pediatricians and results in significant delay in diagnosis.

There are some PIDs that are clinically severe and present very early in the neonatal period. It is extremely important to suspect these PIDs as the early diagnosis and initiation of specific therapy significantly reduces the mortality and morbidity in these patients. The organisms causing the infection and associated clinical manifestations provide very important clue to underlying immune defects. This chapter will give a brief background of PIDs, common neonatal presentations of PIDs and approach to diagnosis of these disorders.

PRIMARY IMMUNODEFICIENCY DISORDERS

There are more than 200 different forms of primary immune deficiency diseases. The prevalence of these diseases varies. In the United States, it is estimated to be one in 1,200 persons.[5] Though, the overall incidence of PID in India is not known, it is expected to be on the higher side due to high rate of consanguinity in some of the Indian communities.[6] The International Union of Immunological Societies (IUIS) expert committee on primary immunodeficiency classifies PID into nine different categories.[4]

1. Combined T-cell and B-cell immunodeficiencies
2. Predominantly antibody deficiencies
3. Other well-defined immunodeficiency syndromes
4. Diseases of immune dysregulation
5. Congenital defects of phagocyte number and function
6. Defects in innate immunity
7. Autoinflammatory disorders
8. Complement deficiencies
9. Phenocopies of PID.

Majority of these PIDs are not clinically apparent at birth. It is the recurrent infections and observation of clinical alarm signs associated with PID that direct the need for considering immunodeficiency in a child.[7]

Apart from recurrent infections affecting different organs, PIDs can also present with organ-specific inflammation or autoimmunity and increased cancer risk, especially hematopoietic malignancies. This genetic and clinical diversity of PIDs often makes the early diagnosis difficult.

Clinical Clues to Primary Immunodeficiency Disorders in Newborn

Recurrent infections are the most common presenting manifestation of PIDs. Evaluation for immunodeficiency should be specifically considered in a clinical scenario of severe infections affecting multiple sites, infections by unusual organisms (for example, *Pneumocystis jirovecii, Burkholderia cepacia*) and systemic bacterial infection like sepsis. Importantly, if any newborn develops vaccine-associated paralytic poliomyelitis (VAPP) and BCGosis due to routine administration of live vaccines like oral poliovirus vaccine (OPV) and Bacillus Calmette-Guérin (BCG) given at birth in India, he/she should be evaluated for PID. As infections give very important clue to underlying defect, every effort must be made to identify the causative organism in patients with unusual infections rather than treating empirically with broad-spectrum antibiotics. Especially children presenting in early infancy with persistent or recurrent bronchiolitis or interstitial pneumonia with no obvious infective cause must be evaluated with bronchoalveolar lavage or lung biopsy to isolate the organism like parainfluenza virus, cytomegalovirus or *Pneumocystis jirovecii*, which strongly suggests underlying immunodeficiency especially severe combined immunodeficiency (SCID), CD40 ligand deficiency or other combined immunodeficiency.[8] Chronic infection-related diarrhea with failure to thrive (FTT) is often seen with SCID whereas noninfective persistent diarrhea in boys with recurrent respiratory tract infections and eczema is suggestive of immunodysregulation, polyendocrinopathy, enteropathy or X-linked (IPEX) syndrome.[9] Hepatic abscess and other deep-seated infections especially small bone osteomyelitis due to *Staphylococcus aureus* are typically seen in patients with chronic granulomatous disease (CGD).[10] Disseminated BCGosis is common in patients with SCID or severe forms of Mendelian susceptibility to mycobacterial diseases (MSMDs)[11] whereas localized BCG adenitis is common in patients with CGD **(Fig. 48.1)**. Patients with MSMD are susceptible to infections from the ubiquitous, environmental nontuberculous strains of mycobacteria, such as *Mycobacterium avium*. Staphylococcal lung infections leading to pneumatocele formation associated with eczema is typically seen in patients with hyper-immunoglobulin E (IgE) syndrome.[12] Severe gram-negative sepsis is common in patients with phagocytic defect especially severe congenital neutropenia (SCN), CGD and leukocyte adhesion deficiency (LAD).[13] Persistent mucosal candidiasis and oropharyngeal thrush are seen in patients with SCID or chronic mucocutaneous candiadiasis (CMC).[14]

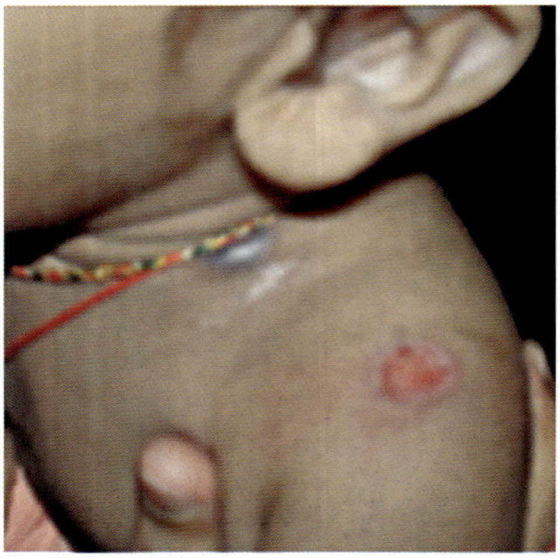

Figure 48.1 BCGosis in a patients with Mendelian susceptibility to mycobacterial diseases (MSMDs)

Other organ-specific manifestations also give clue to underlying specific immunodeficiencies. Eczema, which resembles "cradle cap" or severe diaper rash with petechiae is seen in Wiskott-Aldrich syndrome (WAS).[15] Mucocutaneous albinism is seen in Chediak-Higashi syndrome (CHS) or Griscelli syndrome **(Figs 48.2A to C)**.[8] Neurodevelopmental delays are observed in some forms of SCID, like adenosine deaminase (ADA) deficiency, purine nucleoside phosphorylase (PNP) deficiency and DiGeorge syndrome.[16] Absent thymus with cardiac anomalies is seen in DiGeorge syndrome.[8] Neurological manifestations like, seizures, irritability and other focal neurological defects are common in patients with familial hemophagocytic lymphohistiocytosis (FHL).[17] Skeletal abnormalities, like cupping at the end of the ribs on X-ray chest are seen in ADA deficiency. Rib cage abnormalities and metaphyseal dysostosis are seen in Shwachman-Diamond syndrome,[8] hyperextensibility and increased fractures in hyper-IgE syndrome.[12]

Careful evaluation of family history is important while evaluating patient for PID. History of previous sibling death in early childhood due to infection should raise a strong suspicion of underlying PID. PIDs have different modes of inheritance including autosomal recessive (AR), autosomal dominant (AD) and X-liked. There are selected few X-linked diseases and hence a clear X-linked family history with affected male siblings or maternal uncle narrow your search to selected few X-linked diseases. Consanguinity in parents with both males and females being affected suggests an autosomal recessive inheritance.

Primary Immunodeficiency Disorders Presenting during Neonatal Period

Combined T-cell and B-cell Immunodeficiencies

Cell-mediated immunity plays an important role in the immune response and due to the lack of maternally acquired cellular immunity, the clinical manifestations associated with these disorders become apparent in the neonatal period.[18] These include:

- SCID referred to as a case of pediatric emergency. The critical component affected in SCID is the T-cell compartment with an effect on the B and/or NK cells number/function. Signs and symptoms typically observed are to FTT, infections by opportunistic organisms, fungal infections and chronic diarrhea.[19]
  - Omenn syndrome (OS) refers to a rare SCID phenotype that presents in the neonatal period with erythroderma, massive lymphadenopathy and hepatosplenomegaly. It is caused by hypomorphic or partial loss of function mutations in the classical SCID genes.

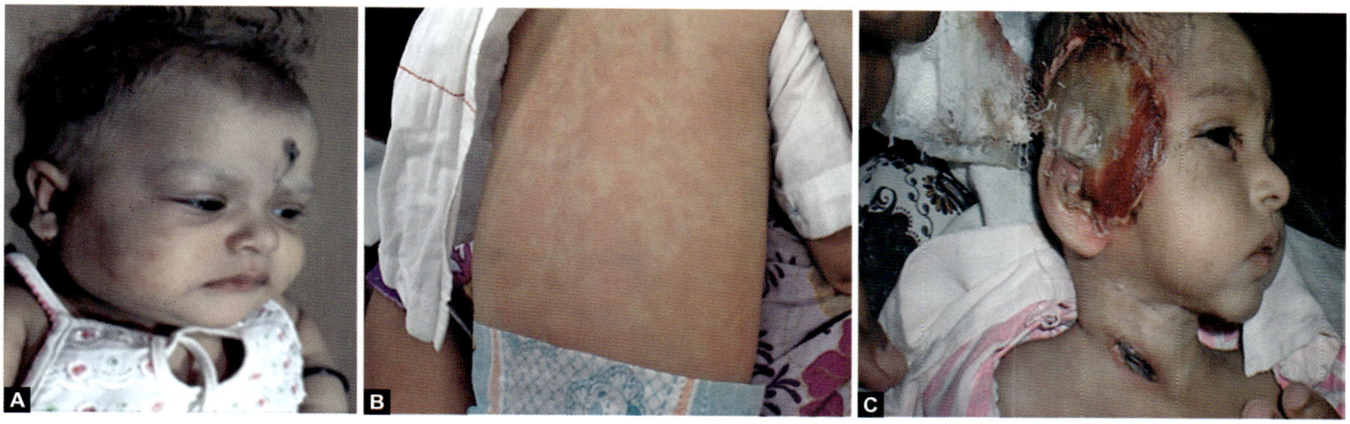

Figures 48.2A to C (A) Griscelli syndrome patient with hypopigmented skin and hair; (B) A child with periodic rash associated with fever and (C) A child with severe brain abscess

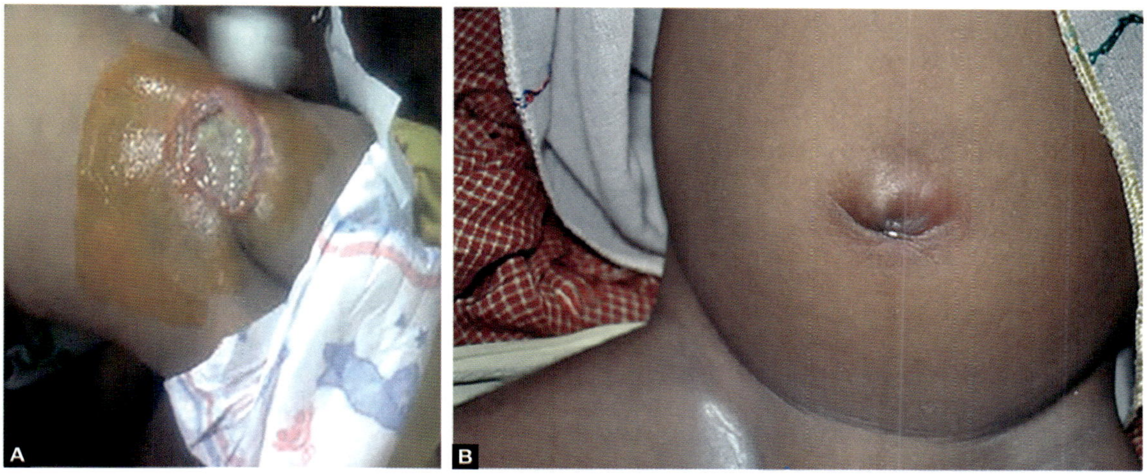

Figures 48.3A and B (A) Child with a large bone deep ulceration; (B) Picture depicting omphalitis, infection of the umbilical stump. Bone marrow (BM) aspiration site; child had persistent neutrophilic leukocytosis and otitis media

Histological findings resemble graft-versus-host disease because of a few expanded clones of aberrant autoreactive autologous T lymphocytes.[20]

- DiGeorge syndrome is associated with thymic and parathyroid hypoplasia or aplasia leading to T-cell immunodeficiency and hypoparathyroidism. This leads to severe hypocalcemia with tetany and seizures that are seen within a few days after birth. T-cell lymphopenia presents the newborn at risk of viral and fungal infections.[21]

Phagocytic Defects

- LAD is associated with a failure of innate host defense mechanism against bacteria, fungi, and other microorganisms due to defective tethering and adhesion of myeloid leukocytes (neutrophils and monocytes) to sites of microbial invasion.[21] LAD presents in the neonatal period with severe infections, delayed separation of the umbilical stump and persistent leukocytosis **(Figs 48.3A and B)**.
- *CGD*: This is the most common phagocytic disorder with a defect in phagocytic cell microbicidal function.[21] CGD is suspected because of a clinical presentation of severe, often recalcitrant infections with catalase-positive bacteria or fungi during the neonatal period.
- *SCN*: This is associated with a high degree of neutropenia, which usually manifests in the neonatal or early infancy period and presents with life-threatening sepsis and cutaneous pyogenic infections such as skin pustules, cellulitis and cutaneous abscess. Delayed umbilical cord blood separation is also a common observation.[22]

Other Well-defined Immunodeficiency Syndromes

- *WAS*: Wiskott-Aldrich syndrome (WAS) patients are susceptible to infections and problems with abnormal bleeding due to the presence of small dysfunctional

platelets. This leads to unique health challenges that are not typically seen in other immunodeficiency disorders.[15] Neonatal presentation of WAS includes bloody stools and prolonged nosebleeds and eczema of the skin.
- *MSMD*: This is characterized by increased susceptibility to infections by weakly pathogenic *Mycobacterium* species[11] and can be especially identified in India in early infancy due to the routine administration of BCG at birth.

Diseases of Immune Dysregulation

Familial hemophagocytic lymphohistiocytosis: Neonatal presentation of hemophagocytic lymphohistiocytosis (HLH) is often confused with sepsis and presents with severe anemia and respiratory problems at birth.[23] During the neonatal period, episodes of fever are misinterpreted as systemic infection; hence, repeated microbiological examinations (bacterial cultures and serologic tests) become important to rule out bacterial infections. Herpes simplex virus and enterovirus are common triggers of severe HLH in the neonatal period.

Diagnosis of Specific Primary Immunodeficiency Disorder

Although immunodeficiency can be suspected by careful reviewing the clinical presentation and by physical examination, specific diagnosis requires the use of certain laboratory tests. The pattern of infection and other symptoms help design a stepwise laboratory approach. Recognizing the underlying cause of immunodeficiency assists in better management of the patient. Furthermore, a molecular confirmation of the underlying disorder also helps in genetic counseling and offering prenatal diagnosis.

Laboratory Evaluation

One of the common causes of immunodeficiency in neonates is the maternally acquired HIV infection. Without antiretroviral intervention for mother and child, about one-third of mothers transmit the virus to the child.[24] Laboratory investigations for immunodeficiency disorders therefore, should first begin by ruling out HIV in case the infants presents with diarrhea, FTT and unusual opportunistic infections as HIV infection clinically resembles a T-cell immunodeficiency disorder. HIV DNA polymerase chain reaction testing or HIV RNA assay testing in newborns is recommended during the first 14–21 days of life, at 1 month of age, and again at 4–6 months of age to identify those who have perinatal-acquired HIV infection.[25] Also, the mother's HIV status can be determined to rule out the possibility of HIV in the newborn.

Once the secondary causes of lymphopenia (HIV, malnutrition) are ruled out, the recommended laboratory tests are complete blood counts (CBCs) with differential, serum immunoglobulin profile and complement levels.

Abnormal CBC findings may point out to a specific disease such as lymphopenia in SCID, WAS, AT, DiGeorge.[26] The finding of low absolute lymphocyte count (ALC) in a newborn with recurrent or persistent infection should prompt further investigation and is highly suggestive of SCID. Importantly, a low ALC also needs to be confirmed by repeat CBC testing as low ALC can also be due to an immunosuppressive state resulting from overwhelming sepsis. Neutrophilia is an observation associated with leukocyte adhesion defect (LAD). In case of suspicion of SCN, it is necessary to periodically repeat the absolute neutrophil count (ANC) to establish a diagnosis. Neutropenia is also observed in hyper-IgM syndrome and autoimmune-mediated neutropenia. A CBC finding of eosinophilia is associated with OS and an observation of eosinophilia with thrombocytopenia is suggestive of WAS. The serum immunoglobulin profile in the neonates is misleading as it can look very similar to those of normal infants because of the presence of passive maternal antibody, hence, antibody deficiency diseases are missed during the neonatal period and infancy.

Organisms isolated from the patients may point out a specific immune defect such as encapsulated bacteria in antibody, T-cell and complement deficiencies, opportunistic organisms observed in T-cell deficiencies, recurrent *Staphylococcus* infections in CGD, LAD and hyper-IgE syndrome and recurrent catalase-positive organism infections in CGD.[26]

ADVANCED TESTS FOR SPECIFIC DISORDERS

Investigations for Cellular Immunity

Cell-mediated immunity is governed by T and B cells, and can be assessed by measurement of T and T cell surface markers including T helper and T cytotoxic cells by flow cytometry. The results of the initial tests usually give an important clue to the underlying immune defect. Patients with low T and B-cell counts are likely to have combined immunodeficiency (CID) disorders. Based on T, B, NK populations and the associated clinical and laboratory evaluation, patients can be categorized as SCID, DiGeorge or WAS. This also requires flow cytometric assays for specific protein expression, like the WASP expression to rule out WAS, CD132, CD127, pSTAT5 to rule out T-B + SCID and assessment of lymphocyte function. An observation of low total T-cell numbers with elevated (above three) ratios of CD4 to CD8 T-cells supports diagnosis of DiGeorge anomaly. Low or normal T and low B cell numbers with oligoclonal expansion of T cells are a classic flow cytometric characteristic associated with OS.

Biochemical tests like ADA levels (for ADA SCID), uric acid level (for PNP SCID) and calcium levels (for hypocalcemic tetany to rule out DiGeorge syndrome) also provide clues in understanding the type of T-cell deficiency.

Newborn Screening for Severe Combined Immunodeficiency

The first group of PIDs targeted for newborn screening (NBS) was SCID. As SCID encompasses a genetically heterogeneous group of inherited disorders resulting from defects in T-cell development, measurement of T-cell receptor excision circles helps in early diagnosis of SCID. Recently, a similar method for analysis of B cell κ-deleting recombination excision circles (KRECs) was developed, allowing identification of patients with B cell lymphopenia for the detection of patients with X-linked agammaglobulinemia (XLA).[27] For detailed information on this topic refer the chapter on "Neonatal Screening and Prenatal Diagnosis of PID".

Evaluation of Phagocytic Defects

Patients suspected with CGD can be diagnosed by nitroblue tetrazolium (NBT) test and dihydrorhodamine (DHR) test. These tests can also detect carrier mothers in X-linked CGD.[28] Final confirmation of underlying defect can be done by studying the intracellular expression of gp91 for X-CGD and p22, p67 or p47 for autosomal recessive CGD followed by molecular analysis of the affected gene.[28] Patients with LAD-I can be easily diagnosed by flow cytometric analysis of CD18, CD11a, CD11b and CD11c expression on peripheral blood leukocytes.[28]

Evaluation for Mendelian Susceptibility to Mycobacterial Disease

Patients without any apparent cause for recurrent TB need further investigation for IL-12–23 or interferon-gamma (IFN-γ) loop defects. Mutations in one of the following genes IL-12, the IL-12 receptor β1 chain, or either of the two protein subunits, R1 and R2, of the receptor for IFN-γ[29] is responsible for a genetic predisposition to MSMD.

Evaluation of Familial Hemophagocytic Lymphohistiocytosis

Diagnosis of HLH in neonatal period is complicated as it may mimic a number of other diseases such as congenital infection, sepsis or inherited metabolic disorders. The diagnosis of HLH is based on clinical and laboratory criteria, which involve complete hemogram, bone marrow aspiration studies, liver function tests, estimation of S bilirubin, S ferritin, S triglyceride, S fibrinogen and sCD25 levels.[28] In the presence of cytopenias and hyperferritinemia, further evaluation using NK cell cytotoxicity assay, perforin expression studies, granule release by NK cells and SAP and XIAP expression on lymphocytes and MUNC 13-4 and SYNTAXIN-11 by western blot help significantly in diagnosis of genetic HLH.[23]

PREVENTION

There is no way to prevent a congenital immunodeficiency disorder. However, families with an affected child can benefit from genetic counseling and prenatal diagnostic facilities that help to find out if the future child will be carrying the defect.[30]

CONCLUSION

As immaturity of the neonatal immune system already puts a neonate at risk to many infections, it is important to specifically differentiate the clinical signs of infection arising due to immaturity from those which are related to PIDs. Further, as PIDs are rare, they are often unrecognized or attributed to other common etiologies. Knowledge of clinical presentation of these disorders, correct interpretation of initial laboratory tests aids in suspecting a PID and guides choosing the appropriate test for specific diagnosis. As early and judicious use of prophylactic antibiotics and replacement, immunoglobulin can prevent significant end organ damage, diagnosing PID in the early infancy helps reduce the morbidity associated with the disease and improve the overall quality of life. Importantly, children with SCID succumb to infection or malignancy unless the condition is corrected with bone-marrow transplantation before the age of 2 years. The best prognosis is for those infants transplanted before 6 months of age,[31] hence a number of countries in the west have implemented the NBS program, which helps identify babies with combined immunodeficiency disorders at birth. Notably, a simple CBC in correlation with the clinical manifestation can also direct our attention to an underlying immunodeficiency, highlighting the importance of a routine CBC for newborns.

REFERENCES

1. Maródi L. Neonatal innate immunity to infectious agents. Infect Immun. 2006;74(4):1999-2006.
2. PrabhuDas M, Adkins B, Gans H, King C, Levy O, Ramilo O, et al. Challenges in infant immunity: implications for responses to infection and vaccines. Nat Immunol. 2011;12(3):189-94.
3. Ygberg S, Nilsson A. The developing immune system—from foetus to toddler. Acta Paediatr. 2012;101(2):120-7.
4. Picard C, Al-Herz W, Bousfiha A, Casanova JL, Chatila T, Conley ME, et al. Primary Immunodeficiency Diseases: an Update on the Classification from the International Union of Immunological Societies Expert Committee for Primary Immunodeficiency 2015. J Clin Immunol. 2015;35(8):696-726.
5. Boyle JM, Buckley RH. Population prevalence of diagnosed primary immunodeficiency diseases in the United States. J Clin Immunol. 2007;27(5):497-502.
6. Madkaikar M, Mishra A, Desai M, Gupta M, Mhatre S, Ghosh K. Comprehensive report of primary immunodeficiency disorders from a tertiary care center in India. J Clin Immunol. 2013;33(3):507-12.
7. Primary Immunodeficiency Association (PIA). Publications: 10 warning signs of a primary immunodeficiency. [online] Available from *www.pia.org.uk/publications/10_signs_of_pia/10_signs_01.htm*. [Accessed October, 2016].
8. Slatter MA, Gennery AR. Clinical immunology review series: an approach to the patient with recurrent infections in childhood. Clin Exp Immunol. 2008;152(3):389-96.
9. Torgerson TR, Ochs HD. Immune dysregulation, polyendocrinopathy, enteropathy, X-linked: forkhead box protein 3 mutations and lack of regulatory T cells. J Allergy Clin Immunol. 2007;120(4):744-50.
10. Goldblatt D, Thrasher AJ. Chronic granulomatous disease. Clin Exp Immunol. 2000;122(1):1-9.
11. Al-Muhsen S, Casanova JL. The genetic heterogeneity of Mendelian susceptibility to mycobacterial diseases. J Allergy Clin Immunol. 2008;122(6):1043-51.

12. Freeman AF, Holland SM. The Hyper-IgE syndromes. Immunol Allergy Clin North Am. 2008;28(2):277-91.
13. Andrews T, Sullivan KE. Infections in patients with inherited defects in phagocytic function. Clin Microbiol Rev. 2003;16(4):597-621.
14. Barrett DJ, Sleasman JW. Immunodeficiency disorders in infants and children. In: Kass EH, Platt R (Eds). Current Therapy in Infectious Disease. Philadelphia, PA, USA: BC Decker; 1990. pp. 51-68.
15. Buckley RH. Primary cellular immunodeficiencies. J Allergy Clin Immunol. 2002;109(5):747-57.
16. Cole TS, Cant AJ. Clinical experience in T cell deficient patients. Allergy Asthma Clin Immunol. 2010;6(1):9.
17. Kim MM, Yum MS, Choi HW, Ko TS, Im HJ, Seo JJ, et al. Central nervous system (CNS) involvement is a critical prognostic factor for hemophagocytic lymphohistiocytosis. Korean J Hematol. 2012;47(4):273-80.
18. Paul ME, Shearer WT. Approach to the evaluation of the immunodeficient patient. In: Rich RR, Fleisher TA (Eds). Clinical Immunology, Principles and Practice, 2nd edition. St. Louis, USA: CV Mosby; 2001. pp. 33.1-33.11.
19. Janeway CA Jr, Travers P, Walport M, Shlomchik MJ. Immunobiology: The Immune System in Health and Disease, 5th edition. New York: Garland Science; 2001.
20. Santagata S, Villa A, Sobacchi C, Cortes P, Vezzoni P. The genetic and biochemical basis of Omenn syndrome. Immunol Rev. 2000;178:64-74.
21. Behrman RE, Kliegman RM, Nelson WE. Nelson Essentials of Pediatrics, 7th edition. Philadelphia, PA, USA: WB Saunders Co; 2002.
22. Maheshwari A. Neutropenia in the newborn. Curr Opin Hematol. 2014;21(1):43-9.
23. Whaley BF. Familial hemophagocytic lymphohistiocytosis in the neonate. Adv Neonatal Care. 2011;11(2):101-7.
24. Cooper ER, Charurat M, Mofenson L, Hanson IC, Pitt J, Diaz C, et al. Combination antiretroviral strategies for the treatment of pregnant HIV-1-infected women and prevention of perinatal HIV-1 transmission. J Acquir Immune Defic Syndr. 2002;29(5):484-94.
25. Burgard M, Blanche S, Jasseron C, Descamps P, Allemon MC, Ciraru-Vigneron N, et al. Performance of HIV-1 DNA or HIV-1 RNA tests for early diagnosis of perinatal HIV-1 infection during anti-retroviral prophylaxis. J Pediatr. 2012;160(1):60-6.
26. Case based Pediatrics for medical students and resident. Second edition, copyright 2013, 2014, 2015, Loren Yamamoto. [online] Available from *https://www.hawaii.edu/medicine/pediatrics/pedtext/pedtext.html*. [Accessed October, 2016].
27. Somech R, Lev A, Simon AJ, Korn D, Garty BZ, Amariglio N, et al. Newborn screening for severe T and B cell immunodeficiency in Israel: a pilot study. Isr Med Assoc J. 2013;15(8):404-9.
28. Madkaikar M, Mishra A, Ghosh K. Diagnostic approach to primary immunodeficiency disorders. Indian Pediatr. 2013;50(6):579-86.
29. Ramirez-Alejo N, Santos-Argumedo L. Innate defects of the IL-12/IFN-γ axis in susceptibility to infections by mycobacteria and salmonella. J Interferon Cytokine Res. 2014;34(5):307-17.
30. Mishra A, Gupta M, Dalvi A, Ghosh K, Madkaikar M. Rapid flow cytometric prenatal diagnosis of primary immunodeficiency (PID) disorders. J Clin Immunol. 2014;34(3):316-22.
31. Brown L, Xu-Bayford J, Allwood Z, Slatter M, Cant A, Davies EG, et al. Neonatal diagnosis of severe combined immunodeficiency leads to significantly improved survival outcome: the case for newborn screening. Blood. 2011;117(11):3243-6.

CHAPTER 49

Neutrophil Functions and Disorders of Neutrophils in Newborns

Sagar Bhattad, Surjit Singh

INTRODUCTION

Neutropenia is an important problem noted in neonates. It could be benign and self-limiting on one hand and harbinger of a serious underlying illness on the other. Neutropenia is noted in 6–58% of neonates.[1] This wide variation is due to difference in cut-offs used to define neutropenia in various studies. It is more common among preterm neonates compared to term neonates. Neonates are predisposed to serious infections in severe neutropenia. This review aims to highlight important causes of neutropenia and disorders of neutrophil dysfunction in children, particularly neonates. An approach to these disorders has been presented that may guide clinicians managing these diseases.

NORMAL DEVELOPMENT AND FUNCTION OF NEUTROPHILS

Neutrophils are phagocytes that form an important component of innate immune defense. They are produced in the bone marrow from pluripotent stem cells. Under the influence of growth factors like granulocyte-monocyte colony-stimulating factor (GM-CSF) and granulocyte colony-stimulating factor (G-CSF), myeloblasts differentiate through various stages and form mature neutrophils. Myeloblasts are the first cells committed to form neutrophils. They differentiate to form promyelocyte and myelocyte, all of which have ability to divide actively. Further differentiation results in development of metamyelocytes, band forms and mature neutrophils. Several factors influence release of neutrophils from the marrow pool to the circulating pool. During infections and stress and in presence of glucocorticoids and catecholamines, there is accelerated release of neutrophils resulting in neutrophilia. Neutrophils have a half-life of about 7–10 hours in circulation.[2] Antiapoptotic factors prolong their survival.

Neutrophils migrate to the sites of infection and inflammation from the blood stream, which involves several important but complex steps. Defect in any of these steps results in several distinct disorders. Rolling of neutrophils along the vessel wall is selectin mediated, while adhesion to endothelial cells is via integrins. CD11/18 integrin plays an important role in the same.[3] Neutrophils undergo transmigration through intercellular junctions and reach the sites of infection. This process is driven by chemical gradients (chemotaxis). Bacterial peptides, complement C5a, monocyte chemotactic factor, interleukin-8 and leukotrienes act as chemoattractants which induce movement of neutrophils to the site of inflammation.[4,5] Neutrophils carry a variety of cell surface receptors that recognize pathogens which are then engulfed by the process called phagocytosis. Opsonization of the pathogens is an important step that aids phagocytosis. Mannan-binding lectin, immunoglobulins and complement fragment C3b act as opsonic proteins.[6]

Studies suggest that phagocytic ability in neonatal life is dependent on the size of the infecting particle. Neutrophils in adults and neonates demonstrate similar capabilities in phagocytosing bacteria such as *Staphylococcus aureus* and *Escherichia coli*; however, capacity to phagocytose *Candida* is diminished in neonates.[7] This is most probably linked to deficit of neonatal neutrophils to engulf larger particles.[8] This deficiency gets resolved by 2 weeks of life, as chemotactic response gets matured.[9]

In the neutrophils, respiratory burst results in production of reactive oxygen species like hydrogen peroxide and superoxide ions.[10] These play a pivotal role in killing the intracellular pathogens.

Normal Neutrophil Counts in Term and Preterm Neonates

Neutropenia is diagnosed on the basis of reduced neutrophil concentration in the blood.

Following formula can be used to enumerate blood neutrophil count:

Absolute neutrophil count (ANC) = White blood cells/μL × % neutrophils noted in the differential count.

The total neutrophils include metamyelocytes, band neutrophils and segmented neutrophils. Normal ranges expected for healthy babies for blood neutrophil counts have been defined by several investigators. There exists a wide variation in the definition of neutropenia. It has been reported variously as 1,100/µL, 1,500/µL and 1,800/µL by different workers.[11-13] The ranges of neutrophil counts provided by Manroe et al.[13] are widely used for term and near-term infants, while that provided by Mouzinho et al.[11] are appropriate for usage in very low birth weight (VLBW) infants. Both systems demonstrate that blood neutrophil concentrations in the neonate sharply increase during the first 12 hours of life and gradually decline toward a steady 2.0–6.0 × 10^9/L range between 2 days and 3 days.[14] However, these systems do not account for variations in altitude, gender, and maternal status that could each affect neonatal blood neutrophil concentrations.[15]

An ANC below 500/µL predisposes to serious infections, while with an ANC above 1,000/µL, the risk is minimal.[16,17] While this has been stated in some studies, this relationship is not consistent. Transient neutropenia does not pose problems, but severe and persistent neutropenia increases the morbidity and mortality several fold.

DISORDERS IN NEUTROPHILS

Disorders in neutrophils may be quantitative or qualitative:

- Disorders affecting neutrophil number
- Disorders affecting neutrophil function.

Disorders of Neutrophil Number

Production of neutrophils is markedly enhanced in the bone marrow in presence of bacterial infection.[18,19] As a response to stress, there is increased release of neutrophils from the marrow to circulation. As 99% of neutrophils are stored in marrow during steady state, a large number can be released into periphery whenever required.[20] Subsequently, marrow progenitors proliferate and result in increased production of neutrophils. In the process, both mature and immature neutrophils are released into circulation. This results in increased immature to mature ratio (I/T) in times of stress or infection. As a result, more immature forms of neutrophils (band forms, metamyelocytes) are seen in periphery; and this is known as left shift. The response to infection in neonates is significantly different. This is partly because of immaturity of immune response and partly due to poor marrow reserve. Unlike older children and adults where neutrophil counts often rise in presence of infection, neonates with fulminant sepsis present with neutropenia. Maternal hypertension, twin-twin transfusion, alloimmunization and hemolytic disease are the other common causes of neonatal neutropenia.

Neutropenia due to Maternal Hypertension

About 50% of neonates whose mothers had pregnancy-induced hypertension develop neutropenia. This is usually mild and transient; however, on occasions it may drop below 500/µL. It is due to an inhibitory factor produced in placenta and transferred by the cord blood. As marrow is suppressed, there is no left shift in this form of neutropenia. It usually resolves by 72 hours. If it persists beyond day 5, further work up to look for alternate causes is warranted **(Box 49.1)**.[21-23]

Box 49.1 Causes of neutropenia

- *Decreased synthesis*
  - Pregnancy-induced hypertension
  - Hemolytic disease of newborn or Rh-hemolytic disease
  - Donors of twin-twin transfusions
  - Syndromes associated with bone marrow failure:
    - Kostmann syndrome
    - Shwachman-Diamond syndrome
    - Cartilage-hair hypoplasia
    - Reticular dysgenesis
    - Cyclic neutropenia
  - Inherited errors of metabolism
    - Organic acidemias
    - Storage diseases like glycogen storage disease type 1b
  - Viral infections
    - Cytomegalovirus infection
    - Rubella infection
- *Increased destruction*
  - Septicemia (bacterial of fungal)
  - Necrotizing enterocolitis (NEC)
  - Antibody induced neutropenia
    - Alloimmune neutropenia
    - Neonatal autoimmune neutropenia
    - Autoimmune neutropenia of infancy

Neutropenia in Twin-Twin Transfusion Syndrome

Neutropenia occurs in donor twin in twin-to-twin transfusion syndrome. It is secondary to marrow suppression and thus there is no left shift. It is self-limiting and resolves in 72 hours.[24]

Neutropenia in Rh Hemolytic Disease

Severe Rh hemolytic disease of newborn may be associated with neutropenia. As a result of hemolysis in the periphery, there is increased erythropoiesis in the marrow. The erythroid lineage expands rapidly leading to decreased production of neutrophils and platelets.[25] This, however, is a self-limiting condition that recovers rapidly, usually by 72 hours.

Syndromes-associated with Bone Marrow Failure

Kostmann Syndrome: This is the most severe form of congenital neutropenia with ANC below 500/µL, usually below 200/µL. Children with Kostmann syndrome present with life-threatening infections in early infancy. They have neutropenia that is severe and persistent. Bone marrow examination reveals maturation arrest at the promyelocyte to myelocyte stage. Initially, it was described as an autosomal recessive disorder,[26] but later autosomal dominant (AD) form of inheritance has also been noted.[27] Sporadic forms are also described. Genetic studies have revealed mutations in G-CSF receptor that result in defective downstream signaling.[28] Children usually present in early childhood with infections like omphalitis, lymphadenitis, pneumonia, septicemia, meningitis and peritonitis. Gram-positive pathogens like *Staphylococcus aureus* and gram-negative organisms like *Pseudomonas* and *Escherichia coli* cause infections in the majority. In the absence of definitive therapy, it is universally fatal in the first decade of life. With the usage of G-CSF injections, outlook has changed and life expectancy has increased significantly. Although G-CSF treatment results in resolution of neutropenia and cutaneous abscesses, but gingivitis and periodontal disease fail to respond. The periodontal disease in these children is said to be associated with the deficiency of antimicrobial peptide LL-37.[29] In children who continue to have life-threatening infections, stem cell transplant must be carried out.[29]

Reticular Dysgenesis: This is a form of severe combined immunodeficiency (SCID) that presents in early infancy with fulminant infections. It is a rare condition characterized by the presence of lymphopenia, agranulocytosis and thymic hypoplasia. Severe neutropenia and lymphopenia are noted on routine hemogram; however, platelet count and hemoglobin are within normal limits. Flow cytometric evaluation of lymphocyte subsets shows marked reduction in all the types of lymphocytes. The bone marrow examination reveals marked hypoplasia. It is universally fatal in absence of stem cell transplant.[30,31]

Shwachman-Diamond Syndrome: Shwachman-Diamond syndrome is a rare autosomal recessive disorder. Pancreatic insufficiency and neutropenia are the hallmarks of this disorder. Majority of children present in infancy with diarrhea due to fat malabsorption and failure to thrive. Less commonly children may become symptomatic from neonatal life onward. They are predisposed to bacterial and fungal infections secondary to neutropenia. Metaphyseal chondrodysplasia associated with dwarfism has been noted in a few. As the disease progresses, other blood cell lineages become affected resulting in pancytopenia. G-CSF is initially helpful but once marrow failure sets in, stem cell transplant is required.[32]

Cyclic Neutropenia: Cyclic neutropenia is a disorder characterized by cyclic fluctuations or oscillations of blood neutrophil counts. It is better known as "cyclic hematopoiesis" because cyclic fluctuations or oscillations are noted in all the formed elements of blood. Typically, a 21-day periodicity is noted, wherein the neutrophil count reaches a nadir. It may remain low for 3–10 days in each cycle. The duration of cycle may vary from 15 days to 35 days; however, it is fixed in a given individual. Children usually present in first decade of life with recurrent episodes of fever, mucositis and infections. Diagnosis is often missed until a note is made of neutrophil counts on repeated occasions. For diagnosis, neutrophil counts need to be monitored weekly twice for at least 6 weeks. Autosomal dominant pattern of inheritance is noted with mutations in ELANE gene.[33,34] Human recombinant G-CSF is the treatment of choice. Majority do well on therapy; however, neutropenic episodes may be associated with serious infections. Mortality as high as 10% has been previously reported.[35]

Antibody-mediated Neutropenia

These include immune neutropenia noted in neonates and the autoimmune neutropenia of infancy.

Immune-mediated Neonatal Neutropenia: Neonatal neutropenia can be caused by antineutrophil antibodies produced in the mother and transferred to the fetus across placenta. Antineutrophil antibodies may be seen in autoimmune disorders like lupus, rheumatoid arthritis, etc. Pregnant women suffering from such disorders can transfer these antibodies and their babies manifest with neutropenia in early neonatal life. There is another mechanism by which antineutrophil antibodies can be produced in mother in a subset of pregnancies. Mother's immune system recognizes paternal antigens present on fetal neutrophils and this results in production of antineutrophil antibodies. Transplacental transfer of these results in neutropenia in the neonate and this is called alloimmune neonatal neutropenia (ANN).[36] These antibodies have been demonstrated in up to 20% of pregnant women in a survey. However, alloimmune neutropenia has been documented in about 0.2–2% of newborns.[37] The antigenic targets for these antibodies are HNA-1, HNA-2 and HNA-3 antigen groups; and CN1, LEA, SH, and NC1.[38-43] Delayed separation of umbilical cord, omphalitis, pneumonia and cutaneous infections may be noted in the first 2 weeks of life in these neonates. In majority of the cases, this is a self-limiting disorder with neutropenia resolving in about 2 months (2 weeks–6 months).[42,44] A small proportion of neonates develop fulminant sepsis and a mortality of up to 5% has been reported.[45]

Autoimmune Neutropenia of Infancy: This is the most common cause of chronic neutropenia in infancy and childhood. It is due to presence of antineutrophil antibodies. These cause peripheral destruction of mature neutrophils; however, in some cases suppression of marrow elements has been documented. Spontaneous disappearance of these antibodies is known to occur and thus this condition may resolve with time in many.[46] Bux et al.[47] have reported 240 cases of autoimmune neutropenia of infancy. Mean age at diagnosis in their series was 8 months. Mild infections affecting skin, ear and those involving upper respiratory tract were noted in majority. However, severe infections like meningitis, sepsis and pneumonia were documented in 12%. On an average, neutropenia lasted 7–24 months in majority and then spontaneously resolved. Antineutrophil antibodies are also seen in ANN; however, these resolve within 6 months of life. Autoimmune neutropenia can be differentiated from severe congenital neutropenia as ANI presents later in life with less severe infections. Demonstration of antigranulocyte antibodies would be definitive.

Drug-induced Neutropenia: Sick neonates in intensive care units are exposed to several drugs, many of which are known to produce neutropenia. Beta-lactam antibiotics, thiazides, ranitidine[48-50] are commonly implicated drugs. Neutropenia is a well-known side effect of ganciclovir caused by marrow suppression.[51] Multiple mechanisms have been proposed to explain drug-induced neutropenia. Drugs may suppress marrow progenitors or stromal cells or result in production of antineutrophil antibodies or combination of mechanisms may be operating in a given patient.[52] Neutropenia usually resolves once the offending drug is withdrawn.

Approach to Diagnosis in a Child Presenting with Neutropenia

As the list of conditions that may cause neutropenia in a neonate or an infant is overwhelming, a systematic approach is required in order to arrive at an appropriate diagnosis in reasonable time. Good history and focused clinical examination may shortlist the possibilities. A sensible laboratory work up may then follow.

Maternal history of hypertension in an intrauterine growth restricted baby, twins with weight discrepancies and history suggestive of chorioamnionitis in mother are diagnostic in themselves. Clinical condition of the baby like necrotizing enterocolitis, blood culture proven sepsis may lead to neutropenia. Presence of neutropenia or autoimmune disorder in mother indicates transplacental transfer of antineutrophil antibodies.

Examination findings of skeletal dysplasia like absent thumb and radial abnormalities point to syndromic causes with inherited marrow failure. Presence of organomegaly and retinitis indicates intrauterine infections. Organomegaly may also be seen storage disorders like glycogen storage disease 1b.

On evaluation, one must note whether child has isolated neutropenia or involvement of multiple cell lineages. Immature to mature (I/T) neutrophil ratio helps in classifying neutropenia. Low I/T ratio along with neutropenia suggests decreased production, while high ratio indicates peripheral destruction with good marrow response.

Bone marrow biopsy is warranted in cases where neutropenia is persistent and no obvious cause is ascertained. Various stages in development of neutrophils need to be assessed. A reduced pool of proliferative neutrophils (like myeloblasts, promyelocytes, etc.) indicates marrow suppression. An arrest in maturation during promyelocyte/myelocyte development is noted in Kostmann syndrome. Increased proliferative pool suggests peripheral destruction. Although marrow examination provides important clues to the etiology, it does not help in confirming a particular diagnosis. Mutation studies may help in diagnosing conditions like Kostmann syndrome, cyclic neutropenia and others.

Role of Granulocyte-colony Stimulating Factor (G-CSF)

Neonates, who are sick and neutropenic, mandate usage of antimicrobials targeting common pathogens based on local sensitivity. Recombinant G-CSF stimulates myeloid proliferation, decreases apoptosis of neutrophils and causes increased release of neutrophils from the marrow, thus leading to increased neutrophils in the circulation. This effect is usually seen in 48 hours. Role of G-CSF in neonatal sepsis is controversial. Some studies report significant rise in blood neutrophil concentration with G-CSF.[53] Several studies report usage of G-CSF in neonatal sepsis.[54-57] A meta-analysis has showed survival benefit; however, no statistical significance was noted on exclusion of nonrandomized studies.[58]

Granulocyte-colony stimulating factor has a definite role in the management of Kostmann syndrome and cyclic neutropenia. The usual dosage is 5–10 μg/kg/day given subcutaneously. The target is to keep ANC above 1,000/μL.

In ANI and ANN, intravenous immunoglobulin has been used with variable success. Studies report improvement in neutrophil counts in about 50% of cases.[59,60]

Disorders of Neutrophil Functions

Children presenting with recurrent infections may have defective neutrophil function despite having normal neutrophil counts. Defect may be seen at any of the several steps involved in normal functioning (described earlier). Neutrophils may fail to extravasate to the sites of infections. Neutrophils may not reach sites of infection due to defective chemotaxis. There may be defect in intracellular killing of phagocytosed pathogens **(Box 49.2)**. Some of these conditions are elaborated further.

Defect in Intracellular Killing

Chronic Granulomatous Disease: This is the most common symptomatic defect involving intracellular killing of pathogens. Generation of reactive oxygen species like superoxide ions is dependent on NADPH oxidase system in neutrophils. A mutation in genes coding this protein complex results in chronic granulomatous disease (CGD). X-linked

Box 49.2 Disorders with neutrophil dysfunction

Defect in intracellular killing
- Chronic granulomatous disease
- Myeloperoxidase deficiency
- Glutathione synthetase deficiency
- Severe G6PD deficiency

Diseases with defect in neutrophil chemotaxis
- Leukocyte adhesion defect
- Wiskott-Aldrich syndrome
- Juvenile periodontitis

Diseases involving defect in degranulation
- Chediak-Higashi syndrome
- Specific granule deficiency

form is the most commonly reported worldwide. While the X-linked form is caused by mutations in *CYBB* gene, the autosomal recessive variants are caused by mutations in *CYBA, NCF1, NCF2 and NCF4*. Children present with recurrent pneumonia, suppurative lymphadenitis, recurrent otitis media and colitis. They are predisposed to catalase-positive bacterial infections. Aspergillus species and candida are other important pathogens. Marked neutrophilic leukocytosis, thrombocytosis and hypergammaglobulinemia suggest exaggerated inflammatory response secondary to persistent infection.

Nitroblue tetrazolium dye reduction test (NBT) and flow cytometry based dihydrorhodamine dye oxidation (DHR) tests help in laboratory confirmation. Gp91phox, p47phox, p22phox, p67phox and p40phox are the components of NADPH oxidase and their expression can be studied by flow cytometry. With the increasing usage of flow cytometry, not only the diagnosis of CGD has become easier, the exact subtype may be pointed out in a short span of time.

Infections in CGD need to be treated with prolonged courses of antimicrobials. In the long run, majority do well on antibacterial and antifungal prophylaxis, while the severe forms require stem cell transplant.

Myeloperoxidase Deficiency: This is the most common phagocytic defect noted in around 1:2,000 people.[61] As majority of affected individuals are asymptomatic or have mild infections, it is not diagnosed often. Granulocytes with myeloperoxidase (MPO) deficiency have defective generation of hypochlorite ion, but have normal superoxide ion production and hence intracellular killing of phagocytosed microbes is only minimally affected.

Leukocyte Adhesion Defect: Children with leukocyte adhesion defect (LAD) present in neonatal life with omphalitis, delayed cord fall and septicemia. They have recurrent infections and cutaneous ulcers that heal to form scars. There is no pus formation at the site of lesions which is a characteristic finding in these disorders. Marked neutrophilic leukocytosis, often more than 50×10^9/L is a hallmark finding. The basic defect lies in adhesion of neutrophils to the endothelium. As they fail to extravasate, the sites of infections have no neutrophilic infiltrate, thus the lack of pus formation. There are three different forms, all being inherited in autosomal recessive fashion. Type 1 is the most common due to CD18 deficiency. The severity of infections and complications is related to the severity of CD18 deficiency; cases with less than 1% expression are clinically severe, whereas those with 2.5–10% expressions are moderate to mild. In LAD type 1, establishing an early diagnosis is possible with the demonstration of reduced or absent CD18 expression on flow cytometry. Children with severe form of LAD 1 require stem cell transplant, without which this form is almost always fatal.

Diseases Involving Defect in Degranulation

Chediak-Higashi Syndrome: This is a rare autosomal recessive disorder with defect in granule morphogenesis. It is caused by mutation in *LYST* gene which is present on the long arm of chromosome 1.[62] As a result, there is defective targeting of proteins to the membranes. Neutrophils, melanosomes and Schwann cells contain giant and defective granules. As all cells containing granules are affected, Chediak-Higashi syndrome (CHS) is a multisystemic disease. Children are born with partial albinism and later develop recurrent infections. Some of them develop peripheral neuropathy. Large cytoplasmic granules are noted in the neutrophils and lymphocytes in the peripheral smear. Specialized tests that demonstrate neutrophil functions reveal abnormal chemotaxis and defect in intracellular killing.

When children with albinism present with bleeding, recurrent infections and/or neurological abnormalities, conditions like CHS, Griscelli syndrome and Hermansky-Pudlak syndrome should be thought of. Stem cell transplant is the therapy of choice in severe forms of CHS.[63]

Approach to Child/Neonate with Dysfunction of Neutrophil

Children who present with recurrent pyogenic infections or fungal infections should be evaluated for defect in phagocytic function. A detailed family history must be taken in all cases as it may provide clue to the pattern of inheritance.

Routine hemogram provides clues to many disorders. Marked neutrophilic leukocytosis may suggest LAD. Neutropenia with neutrophil dysfunction is noted in CHS. Giant granules in neutrophils on the peripheral smear points toward CHS.

Simple laboratory tests like NBT test can diagnose serious diseases like CGD. This can be further confirmed on flow cytometry by DHR test.

Enzyme assays for G6PD and glutathione synthetase must be carried out in appropriate setting. NBT can be abnormal in severe deficiency of G6PD or glutathione synthetase. If children present with features that suggest CGD; however, tests have excluded CGD beyond doubt, one must think of deficiencies involving G6PD or glutathione synthetase and workup accordingly.

CD11/CD18 expression can be studied on flow cytometry. Reduced expression of these, make the diagnosis of LAD certain.

CONCLUSION

Neutropenia is a common problem noted in neonates. It can be benign and self-limited. When severe and persistent, detailed evaluation is warranted. Severe neutropenia has been associated with increased morbidity and mortality. A variety of conditions may present with neutropenia. A good history and examination followed by investigations that are apt for the given setting help in arriving at the correct diagnosis. Classifying neutropenia based on I/T ratio is useful. G-CSF has important role in management of several conditions like Kostmann syndrome and cyclic neutropenia.

A variety of disorders with defect in phagocytic function may be seen with normal or elevated counts. Chronic granulomatous disease, LAD and CHS are the important ones. With the usage of flow cytometry, many of these complex disorders can now be reliably and quickly diagnosed.

REFERENCES

1. Al-Mulla ZS, Christensen RD. Neutropenia in the neonate. Clin Perinatol. 1995;22(3):711-39.
2. von Vietinghoff S, Ley K. Homeostatic regulation of blood neutrophil counts. J Immunol. 2008;181:5183-8.
3. Hughes BJ, Hollers JC, Crockett-Torabi E, Smith CW. Recruitment of CD11b/CD18 to the neutrophil surface and adherence-dependent cell locomotion. J Clin Invest. 1992;90(5):1687-96.
4. Middleton J, Neil S, Wintle J, et al. Transcytosis and surface presentation of IL-8 by venular endothelial cells. Cell. 1997;91:385-95.
5. Baggiolini M, Dewald B, Moser B. Human chemokines: an update. Annu Rev Immunol. 1997;15:675-705.
6. Hart SP, Smith JR, Dransfield I. Phagocytosis of opsonized apoptotic cells: roles for 'old-fashioned' receptors for antibody and complement. Clin Exp Immunol. 2004;135(2):181-5.
7. Falconer AE, Carr R, Edwards SW. Impaired neutrophil phagocytosis in preterm neonates: lack of correlation with expression of immunoglobulin or complement receptors. Biol Neonate. 1995;68(4):264-9.
8. Carr R. Neutrophil production and function in newborn infants. Br J Haematol. 2000;110(1):18-28.
9. Al-Hadithy H, Addison IE, Goldstone AH, Cawley JC, Shaw JC. Defective neutrophil function in low-birth-weight, premature infants. J Clin Pathol. 1981;34:366-70.
10. Dahlgren C, Karlsson A. Respiratory burst in human neutrophils. J Immunol Methods. 1999;232(1-2):3-14.
11. Mouzinho A, Rosenfeld CR, Sanchez PJ, Risser R. Revised reference ranges for circulating neutrophils in very-low-birth weight neonates. Pediatrics. 1994;94:76-82.
12. Xanthou M. Leucocyte blood picture in healthy full-term and premature babies during neonatal period. Arch Dis Child. 1970;45:242-9.
13. Manroe BL, Weinberg AG, Rosenfeld CR, Browne R. The neonatal blood count in health and disease. I. Reference values for neutrophilic cells. J Pediatr. 1979;95:89-98.
14. Christensen RD, Calhoun DA, Rimsza LM. A practical approach to evaluating and treating neutropenia in the neonatal intensive care unit. Clin Perinatol. 2000;27:577-601.
15. Schmutz N, Henry E, Jopling J, Christensen RD. Expected ranges for blood neutrophil concentrations of neonates: the Manroe and Mouzinho charts revisited. J Perinatol. 2008;28:275-81.
16. Engle WD, Rosenfeld CR. Neutropenia in high-risk neonates. J Pediatr. 1984;105:982-6.
17. Gray PH, Rodwell RL. Neonatal neutropenia associated with maternal hypertension poses a risk for nosocomial infection. Eur J Pediatr. 1999;158:71-3.
18. Demetri GD, Griffin JD. Granulocyte colony-stimulating factor and its receptor. Blood. 1991;78:2791-808.
19. Marodi L, Goda K, Palicz A, Szabo G. Cytokine receptor signalling in neonatal macrophages: defective STAT-1 phosphorylation in response to stimulation with IFN-gamma. Clin Exp Immunol. 2001;126:456-60.
20. Semerad CL, Liu F, Gregory AD, Stumpf K, Link DC. G-CSF is an essential regulator of neutrophil trafficking from the bone marrow to the blood. Immunity. 2002;17:413-23.
21. Koenig JM, Christensen RD. Incidence, neutrophil kinetics, and natural history of neonatal neutropenia associated with maternal hypertension. N Engl J Med. 1989;321:557-62.
22. Fraser SH, Tudehope DI. Neonatal neutropenia and thrombocytopenia following maternal hypertension. J Paediatr Child Health. 1996;32:31-4.
23. Sharma G, Nesin M, Feuerstein M, Bussel JB. Maternal and neonatal characteristics associated with neonatal neutropenia in hypertensive pregnancies. Am J Perinatol. 2009;26(9):683-9.
24. Koenig JM, Hunter DD, Christensen RD. Neutropenia in donor (anemic) twins involved in the twin-twin transfusion syndrome. J Perinatol. 1991;11(4):355-8.
25. Koenig JM, Christensen RD. Neutropenia and thrombocytopenia in infants with Rh hemolytic disease. J Pediatr. 1989;114:625-31.
26. Kostman R. Infantile genetic agranulocytosis. A review with presentation of ten new cases. Acta Paediatr Scand. 1975;64:362-8.
27. Briars GL, Parry HF, Ansari BM. Dominantly inherited severe congenital neutropenia. J Infect. 1996;33:123-6.
28. Dong F, Dale DC, Bonilla MA, Freedman M, Fasth A, Neijens HJ, et al. Mutations in the granulocyte colony-stimulating factor receptor gene in patients with severe congenital neutropenia. Leukemia. 1997;11:120-5.
29. Zeidler C, Welte K. Kostmann syndrome and severe congenital neutropenia. Semin Hematol. 2002;39:82-8.
30. Ohashi Y. [Reticular dysgenesis]. Ryoikibetsu Shokogun Shirizu. 2000;(32):35-7.
31. Cham B, Bonilla MA, Winkelstein J. Neutropenia associated with primary immunodeficiency syndromes. Semin Hematol. 2002;39(2):107-12.
32. Burroughs L, Woolfrey A, Shimamura A. Shwachman-Diamond syndrome: a review of the clinical presentation, molecular pathogenesis, diagnosis, and treatment. Hematol Oncol Clin North Am. 2009;23(2):233-48.
33. Horwitz M, Benson KF, Person RE, Aprikyan AG, Dale DC. Mutations in ELA2, encoding neutrophil elastase, define a 21-day biological clock in cyclic haematopoiesis. Nat Genet. 1999;23(4):433-6.
34. Bellanné-Chantelot C, Clauin S, Leblanc T, Cassinat B, Rodrigues-Lima F, Beaufils S, et al. Mutations in the ELA2 gene correlate with more severe expression of neutropenia: a study of 81 patients from the French Neutropenia Register. Blood. 2004;103:4119-25.
35. Bar-Joseph G, Halberthal M, Sweed Y, Bialik V, Shoshani O, Etzioni A. Clostridium septicum infection in children with cyclic neutropenia. J Pediatr. 1997;131:317-9.
36. Curtis BR, Reno C, Aster RH. Neonatal alloimmune neutropenia attributed to maternal immunoglobulin G antibodies against the neutrophil alloantigen HNA-1c (SH): a report of five cases. Transfusion. 2005;45(8):1308-13.
37. Maheshwari A, Christensen RD, Calhoun DA. Immune neutropenia in the neonate. Adv Pediatr. 2002;49:317-39.
38. Lalezari P. Alloimmune neonatal neutropenia and neutrophil-specific antigens. Vox Sang. 1984;46:415-7.
39. Lalezari P, Murphy GB, Allen FH Jr. NB1, a new neutrophil-specific antigen involved in the pathogenesis of neonatal neutropenia. J Clin Invest. 1971;50:1108-15.
40. Lalezari P. Neutrophil antigens: immunology and clinical implications. Prog Clin Biol Res. 1977;13:209-25.
41. Bux J, Jung KD, Kauth T, Mueller-Eckhardt C. Serological and clinical aspects of granulocyte antibodies leading to alloimmune neonatal neutropenia. Transfus Med. 1992;2:143-9.
42. Gilmore MM, Stroncek DF, Korones DN. Treatment of alloimmune neonatal neutropenia with granulocyte colony-stimulating factor. J Pediatr. 1994;125:948-51.
43. Maheshwari A, Christensen RD, Calhoun DA. Resistance to recombinant human granulocyte colony-stimulating factor

in neonatal alloimmune neutropenia-associated with anti-human neutrophil antigen-2a (NB1) antibodies. Pediatrics. 2002;109:e64.

44. Latini G, Del Vecchio A, Rosati E, Borzini P, Chirico G, Rondini G. Different responses to granulocyte colony-stimulating factor treatment in siblings with alloimmune neonatal neutropenia. Acta Paediatr. 1999;88:1407-9.
45. Minchinton RM, McGrath KM. Alloimmune neonatal neutropenia—a neglected diagnosis? Med J Aust. 1987;147(3):139-41.
46. Boxer LA, Greenberg MS, Boxer GJ, Stossel TP. Auto-immune neutropenia. N Engl J Med. 1975;293:748-53.
47. Bux J, Behrens G, Jaeger G, Welte K. Diagnosis and clinical course of autoimmune neutropenia in infancy: analysis of 240 cases. Blood. 1998;91:181-6.
48. Taniuchi S, Masuda M, Yamamoto A, Hasui M, Tsuji S, Takahashi H, et al. Two cases of autoimmune neutropenia possibly induced by beta-lactam antibiotics in infants. J Pediatr Hematol Oncol. 2000;22:533-8.
49. Schotland MG, Grumbach MM. Neutropenia in an infant secondary to hydrochlorothiazide therapy: with a review of hematologic reactions to "thiazide" drugs. Pediatrics. 1963;31:754-7.
50. Shields LI, Files JA, Doll DC, Greenberg BR. Ranitidine and agranulocytosis. Ann Intern Med. 1986;104:128.
51. Kimberlin DW, Lin CY, Sanchez PJ, Demmler GJ, Dankner W, Shelton M, et al. Effect of ganciclovir therapy on hearing in symptomatic congenital cytomegalovirus disease involving the central nervous system: a randomized, controlled trial. J Pediatr. 2003;143:16-25.
52. Guest I, Uetrecht J. Drugs toxic to the bone marrow that target the stromal cells. Immunopharmacology. 2000;46:103-12.
53. Gillan ER, Christensen RD, Suen Y, Ellis R, van de Ven C, Cairo MS. A randomized, placebo-controlled trial of recombinant human granulocyte colony-stimulating factor administration in newborn infants with presumed sepsis: significant induction of peripheral and bone marrow neutrophilia. Blood. 1994;84:1427-33.
54. Schibler KR, Osborne KA, Leung LY, Le TV, Baker SI, Thompson DD. A randomized, placebo-controlled trial of granulocyte colony-stimulating factor administration to newborn infants with neutropenia and clinical signs of early-onset sepsis. Pediatrics. 1998;102:6-13.
55. Bedford Russell AR, Emmerson AJ, Wilkinson N, Chant T, Sweet DG, Halliday HL, et al. A trial of recombinant human granulocyte colony stimulating factor for the treatment of very low birthweight infants with presumed sepsis and neutropenia. Arch Dis Child Fetal Neonatal Ed. 2001;84:F172-6.
56. Miura E, Procianoy RS, Bittar C, Miura CS, Miura MS, Mello C, et al. A randomized, double-masked, placebo-controlled trial of recombinant granulocyte colony-stimulating factor administration to preterm infants with the clinical diagnosis of early-onset sepsis. Pediatrics. 2001;107:30-5.
57. Barak Y, Leibovitz E, Mogilner B, Juster-Reicher A, Amitay M, Ballin A, et al. The in vivo effect of recombinant human granulocyte-colony stimulating factor in neutropenic neonates with sepsis. Eur J Pediatr. 1997;156:643-6.
58. Bernstein HM, Pollock BH, Calhoun DA, Christensen RD. Administration of recombinant granulocyte colony-stimulating factor to neonates with septicemia: a meta-analysis. J Pediatr. 2001;138:917-20.
59. Huizinga TW, Kuijpers RW, Kleijer M, Schulpen TW, Cuypers HT, Roos D, et al. Maternal genomic neutrophil FcRIII deficiency leading to neonatal isoimmune neutropenia. Blood. 1990;76:1927-32.
60. Yoshida N, Shikata T, Sudo S, Matsumura A, Tsujii H, Doi Y, et al. Alloimmune neonatal neutropenia in monozygous twins. High-dose intravenous gammaglobulin therapy. Acta Paediatr Scand. 1991;80:62-5.
61. Parry MF, Root RK, Metcalf JA, Delaney KK, Kaplow LS, Richar WJ. Myeloperoxidase deficiency: prevalence and clinical significance. Ann Intern Med. 1981;95:293-301.
62. Barrat FJ, Auloge L, Pastural E, Lagelouse RD, Vilmer E, Cant AJ, et al. Genetic and physical mapping of the Chediak-Higashi syndrome on chromosome 1q42–43. Am J Hum Genet. 1996;59:625-32.
63. Haddad E, Le Deist F, Blanche S, Benkerrou M, Rohrlich P, Vilmer E, et al. Treatment of Chediak-Higashi syndrome by allogenic bone marrow transplantation: report of 10 cases. Blood. 1995;85:3328-33.

CHAPTER

50

Combined T- and B-Cell Defects

Mamta Vijay Manglani, Omkar Nagesh Khandkar, Savita Khadse

INTRODUCTION

Lymphocytes are divided into three types—(1) T-cells (thymus cells), (2) B-cells (bone marrow or bursa derived cells) and (3) natural killer (NK) cells. The T-cells, which are further divided into T helper cells and T cytotoxic cells, are involved in cell-mediated immunity, whereas B-cells in humoral immunity (antibody-mediated). They both function together and identify nonself-antigens (invaders): B-cells through antibody production and T-cells by producing cytokines directing the immune response as well as toxic granules that kill the pathogen infected cells. NK cells protect the host from tumors and viruses.

Combined T- and B-cell immunodeficiencies are a group of disorders resulting from genetic defects in both cellular and humoral immunity. It could be a quantitative or a qualitative defect, i.e. defect in production or maturity of T-cells, coupled with deficient antibody production or, defective antibody production even in the presence of mature B-cells as T-cell help is absent. NK cell function may or may not be affected. These defects lead to extreme susceptibility to serious infections with bacterial, fungal and viral pathogens and can cause significant morbidity and mortality. The most common prototype of combined T- and B-cell disorders is severe combined immunodeficiency (SCID).

EPIDEMIOLOGY

The prevalence of primary immunodeficiency (PID) disorders as reported in literature is 1 in 10,000 live births, though in a population survey by Boyle et al. in USA, it was found to be 1 in 1,200 persons in population.[1,2] The estimated incidence of SCID is 1 per 50,000–100,000 live births in the developed world.[3] In view of the significantly high prevalence of SCID, neonatal screening for SCID has been nationally recommended in USA in the uniform screening panel and has been made mandatory in many states of America.[1] There is paucity of literature depicting the incidence or prevalence of either PID or SCID in India.

ETIOLOGY AND PATHOPHYSIOLOGY

The common ancestor for lymphoid cells is the common lymphoid progenitor, which differentiates into intermediate progenitors. These further continue to develop in the bone marrow through an antigen-independent process called primary lymphopoiesis **(Fig. 50.1)**. Secondary B and T-cell lymphopoiesis, which occurs in germinal centers of peripheral lymphoid organs and thymus respectively, is an antigen-dependent process.

There are a number of genes coding for various important proteins required for the process of lymphopoiesis **(Table 50.1, Figs 50.2 and 50.3)**: T-cell *lineage development and defective genes*). Defects or mutations in any of these genes hampering the proliferation, maturation and/or function of T-cells and consequently B-cells with variable affection of NK cells cause various types of combined T- and B-cell immunodeficiency syndromes as depicted in **Table 50.1**.

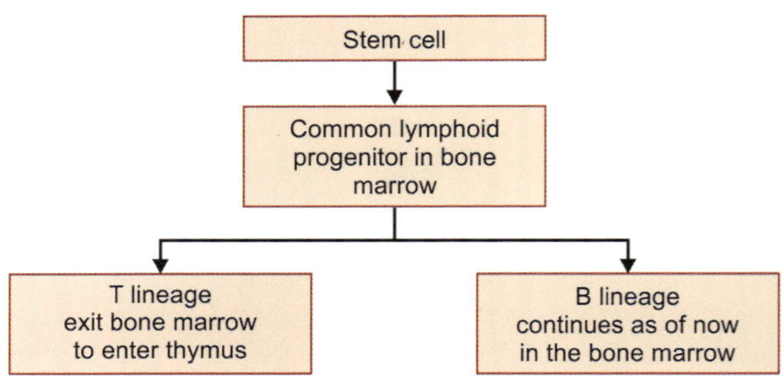

Figure 50.1 Primary lymphopoiesis in the bone marrow

Table 50.1 Characteristics of various combined T- and B-cells immunodeficiencies

Serial No.	*Diseases*	*Types*	*Gene responsible*	*Locus*	*Inheritance*	*Features*
1.	T-/B+ SCID	X-linked (γc deficiency)	*IL-2 RG*	Xq12-13.11	XLR	NK–
		JAK3 deficiency	*JAK3*	19p13.11	AR	NK–
		IL-7 R α deficiency	*IL-7 R*	5p13.2	AR	NK+
		CD45 deficiency	*LCA*	1q31.3-q32.1	AR	NK+/–
		CD3 chain deficiency (γ, δ, ε, ξ)	*CD3 (G, D, E and Z)*		AR	
2.	T-/B–SCID	*RAG1* deficiency	*RAG1*		AR	NK+
		RAG2 deficiency	*RAG2*		AR	
		Artemis deficiency	*DCLRE1C*		AR	
		ADA deficiency	*ADA*		AR	NK–
		Reticular dysgenesis	*AK2*		AR	NK–, granulocytopenia, thrombocytopenia
3.	Omenn syndrome		*RAG1/2, Artemis and IL-7R*		AR	NK+, erythroderma, eosinophilia, lympho-proliferation
4.	DNA ligase IV deficiency		*LIG-4*		AR	Microcephaly; radiation sensitivity
	Cernunnos deficiency		*NHEJ1*		AR	Microcephaly; radiation sensitivity, growth retardation
5.	Immunoglobulin class switch recombination deficiencies	CD40 ligand deficiency and CD40 deficiency	*TNFS5B and TNFRSF5*		XLRAR	Decreased IgG, IgA and normal or increased IgM
6.	PNP deficiency		*PNP*	14q11.2	AR	Neurological impairment, autoimmunity
7.	CD8 deficiency	CD8 α chain defect	*CD8A*	2p11.2	AR	Absent CD8 T-cells
		ZAP 70 deficiency	*ZAP-70*	2q11.2	AR	

Contd...

Contd...

Serial No.	Diseases	Types	Gene responsible	Locus	Inheritance	Features
8.	MHC class II deficiency	CIITA deficiency	*CIITA*	16p13.13	AR	Decreased CD4 T-cells
		RFX5 deficiency	*RFX5*	1q21.3	AR	
		RFXAP deficiency	*RFXAP*	13q13.3	AR	
		RFXANK deficiency	*RFXANK*	19p13.11	AR	
	MHC class I deficiency	TAP1 deficiency	*TAP1*	6p21.32	AR	Decreased number of CD8 T-cells
		TAP2 deficiency	*TAP2*	6p21.32	AR	
		Tapasin deficiency	*TAPBP*	6p21.32	AR	
9.	CD4 deficiency	p56lck deficiency	*LCK*	1p35.2	AR	Decreased number of CD4+ T-cells
10.	CD25 deficiency		*IL2RA*	10p15.1	AR	Autoimmunity
11.	Winged helix nude deficiency		*WHN/FOXN1*	17q11.2	AR	Normal number of B-cells
12.	STAT5b deficiency		*STAT5b*	17q21.2	Not known	Dwarfism not responding to growth hormone, dysmorphic features
13.	Coronin 1A deficiency		*CORO1A*	16p11.2	AR	EBV-induced lymphoproliferation
14.	CRAC		*ORAI1*	12q24.31	AR	Hypergammaglobulinemia, myopathy
Other Immunodeficiency Syndromes						
1.	DNA repair defects	Bloom syndrome	*RECQL3*	15q26.1	AR	Chromosomal instability, growth deficiency, sun sensitivity, predisposition to malignancy
		Ataxia Telangiectasia	*ATM*	11q22.3	AR	Cerebellar ataxia, telangiectasis, increased predisposition to malignancy
		Nijmegen breakage syndrome	*NBN*	8q21.3	AR	Microcephaly, growth retardation, increased predisposition to malignancy
2	Wiskott-Aldrich syndrome (WAS)		*WAS*	Xp11.23	XLR	Microthrombocytopenia, immune defects and eczema
3.	Immune osseous dysplasia	Cartilage hair hypoplasia	*RMRP*	9p13.3	AR	Short limbed dwarfism

Abbreviations: ADA, adenosine deaminase; JAK, Janus-associated kinase; SCID, severe combined immunodeficiency; NK, natural killer; NHEJ, nonhomologous end joining; RAG, recombination-activating genes; TNF, tumor necrosis factor; XLR, X-linked recessive; ZAP, zeta chain-associated protein

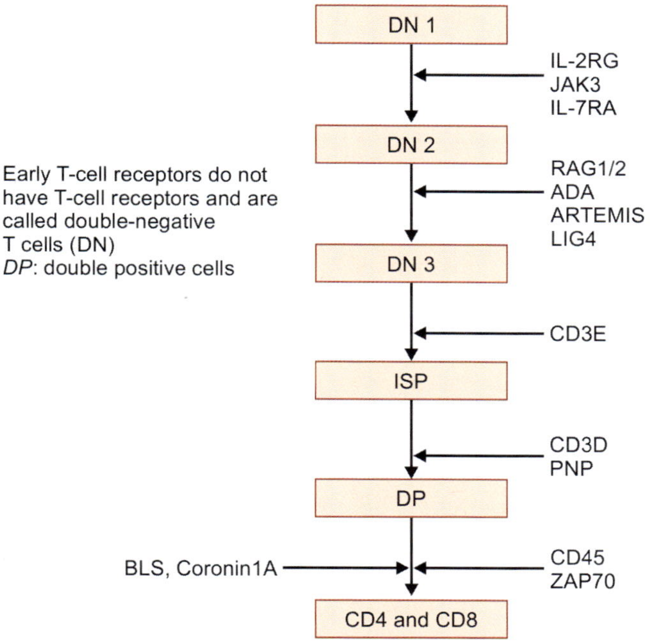

Figure 50.2 T-cell lineage development and defective genes
Abbreviations: ADA, adenosine deaminase; IL, interleukin; JAK, Janus-associated kinase; ZAP, zeta chain-associated protein; PNP, purine nucleoside phosphorylase; BLS, bare lymphocyte syndrome; RAG, recombination activating gene

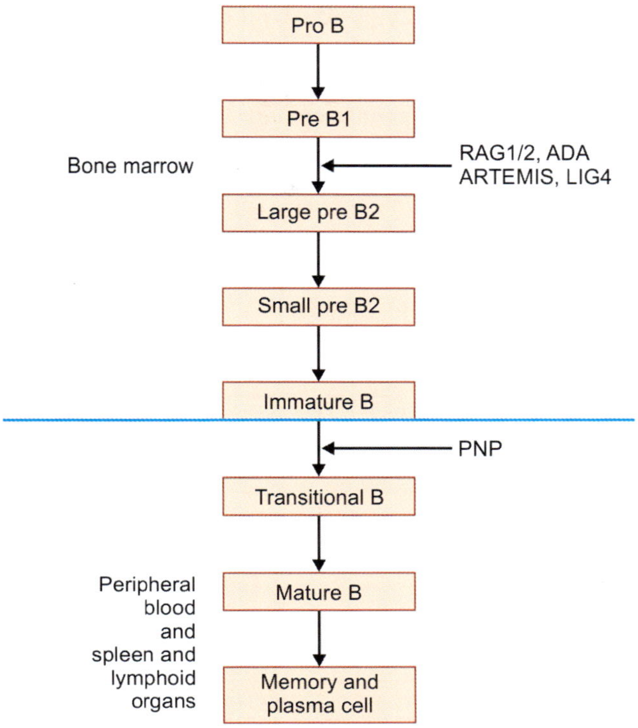

Figure 50.3 B-cell lineage development and defective genes
Abbreviations: ADA, adenosine deaminase; PNP, purine nucleoside phosphorylase; RAG, recombination activating gene

TYPES OF COMBINED T- AND B-CELLS DISORDERS (CLASSIFICATION)

T–B+ Severe Combined Immunodeficiency (T-cells Predominantly Absent)

X-linked (γc-Chain Deficiency) Severe Combined Immunodeficiency (T–B+ NK–)

X-linked SCID is the most common genetic condition (1 in 150,000–200,000 live births) responsible for SCID, accounting for 50% of patients.[2] It is caused by a mutation of the *IL2RG* gene leading to γc chain deficiency of the interleukin-2 receptor (IL-2). The γ chain is called the common γ chain as it is shared by the receptors for IL-2, IL-4, IL-7, IL-9, IL-15 and IL-21 (T–B+ NK–). This can explain the complex phenotype of XL SCID as several IL receptors affecting multiple cytokine pathways are affected, leading to severe T-cell maturation defects. There is a suggestion that this may not be the exclusive defect and the IL-7 alpha gene too may be involved.[2]

X-linked SCID is characterized by decreased number of peripheral T-cells and abnormal T-cell proliferation, normal B-cell development and autoimmune features.

Janus-associated Kinase 3 Deficiency (T–B+ NK–)

Janus-associated kinase 3 (JAK3) is a tyrosine kinase that belongs to the Janus family. JAK3 functions in signal transduction and interacts with members of the STAT (signal transduction and activators of transcription) family. JAK 3 deficiency is caused by a mutation in a gene on chromosome 19 that encodes the enzyme JAK3. When T, B and NK lymphocyte counts are done, infants with this type look very similar to those with X-linked SCID, i.e. they are T–B+ NK–. JAK3 deficiency accounts for less than 10% of cases of SCID.

Deficiency of the Alpha Chain of the IL-7 Receptor (T–B+ NK+)

It is the third most common amongst the SCIDs, accounting for 11% of all SCIDs. Interaction between IL-7 and γc-containing IL-7 receptor complex is necessary during lymphoid development. This plays a pivotal role during early T lineage development. IL-7-Rα plays a role in lymphoid development as a part of the IL-7 receptor complex. Deficiency of IL-7-Rα results from mutations in a gene on chromosome 5.[4] These infants have normal B-cells (may even be elevated) and NK cells, but T-cells are absent.

CD45 Deficiency (T–B+ NK+/–)

CD45 is also known as common leukocyte antigen and functions as a regulator of certain kinases involved in B and T-cell antigen receptor signaling. Deficiency of CD45 leads to arrest in maturation from immature CD4+ CD8+ to mature CD4+ CD8 + stage[5], causing significant reduction in peripheral circulating T-cells.

Deficiencies of CD3/T-cell Receptor Complex (γ, δ, ε or ζ Chains) (T–B+ NK+)

T-cell receptor (TCR) has an extracellular component, transmembrane segment and an intracellular segment. The antigen specificity of the TCR is dependent on a heterodimer composed of either $\alpha\beta$- or $\gamma\delta$-chain. This is linked with CD3γ, δ, ε or ζ chains. Mutations in any one of the genes coding for the CD3 chains, i.e. the transmembrane proteins causes an abnormality in the TCR signaling. This signaling via CD3 dimers is necessary for T-cell lineage commitment, development and maturation of naïve T-cells. Thus, a mutation in the development of these CD3 chains leads to moderate-to-severe immunodeficiency.[6]

T–B– Severe Combined Immunodeficiency

Recombination Activating Genes (RAG1/RAG2) Deficiency (T–B– NK+)

Both T-cell receptors as well as the immunoglobulins or B-cell receptors require the recombination of genetic elements for achieving diversity in the variable region. These receptors are required during the T-cell development at the stage of transforming from CD4– CD8– double negative T-cells to CD4+ CD8+ immunocompetent T-cells, as well as from pro-B to mature B-cells. The genes responsible for the recombination of these genetic elements to confer appropriate configuration to the receptor for specific antigen detection are *RAG1* and *RAG2*. The lack of these recombination-activating genes, therefore, blocks the T-cells at the double negative stage and prevents the B-cells from being released from the bone marrow into circulation, resulting in T– B– NK+ SCID. Along with Artemis deficiency, this accounts for 20–30% of all SCID patients. Attenuated forms of *RAG1* and *RAG2* deficiency have also been identified leading to milder phenotypes.[7,8]

Omenn syndrome is one of the variants with missense mutations in the *RAG1* and *RAG2* genes, leading to partial abrogation of the V(D)J recombination. This partial activity of the recombination activating genes allows some T-cell clones to survive; however, these being oligoclonal patients develop immune deficiency. But, the severity may be variable with some being as severe as the *RAG* genes mutations. The molecular basis is not necessarily linked with *RAG* genes, but could be due to Artemis or *IL7Rα genes.*[9,10]

Artemis Deficiency (T–B– NK+)

It results from mutation in Artemis protein resulting in defective V(D)J recombination. It is one of the several genes including ligase IV and Cernunnos/XLF (XRCC4 like factor), which is important for maintaining genomic stability during the process of recombination of genetic elements. As these genes are also involved in the DNA double strand break repair, it also leads to sensitivity to radiation. Aberrant expression of Artemis gene leads to T–B– SCID. The "hypomorphic" mutations (last exon causing truncation of the Artemis protein) of Artemis gene has also led to a milder phenotype with B- and T-cell lymphopenia along with lesser radiosensitivity and propensity to B-cell lymphomas.[2]

Adenosine Deaminase Deficiency (T–B– NK–)

Adenosine deaminase (ADA) is an enzyme necessary for breaking down toxic products of purine scavenging pathway. Mutations in the *ADA* gene lead to accumulation of deoxyadenosine in the cells causing apoptosis of lymphocytes, resulting in SCID **(Flow chart 50.1)**. It is the second most common cause of SCID, accounting for 15% of patients.[2] Severity is related to 29 known genotypes associated with the disorder, thus presenting variably in infancy, childhood and adolescence or even later.[11]

Reticular Dysgenesis (T–B– NK–)

Reticular dysgenesis (RD) is the most severe form of SCID. As late as 2009, it has been shown that mutation in adenylate kinase 2 is responsible for RD.[12,13] Adenylate kinase 2 is expressed in the mitochondrial intermembrane space, involved in regulating the adenine nucleotides. There is a hypothesis that it may impose oxidative stress on precursor cells in the marrow leading to defective maturation of immune cells from stem cells. It is characterized by markedly decreased T, B and NK cells, granulocytopenia and thrombocytopenia.[14]

Ligase IV Deficiency (T–B– NK+)

It is associated with impaired DNA damage response mechanisms. Ligase IV syndrome results from mutations in the DNA Ligase IV gene encoding an enzyme that plays a pivotal role in repairing double strand DNA breaks and V(D)J recombination.[15,16] Carriers heterozygous for those mutations usually develop moderate defects in V(D)J recombination, mild immune abnormalities and malignancies.

Flow chart 50.1 Effect of adenosine deaminase (ADA) deficiency on lymphocytes

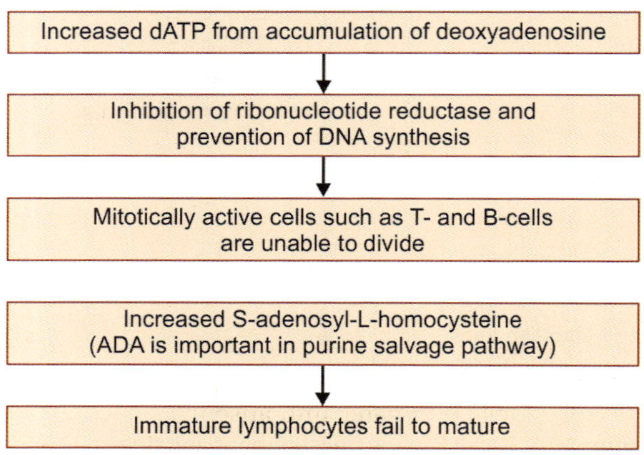

Abbreviations: dATP, deoxyadenosine triphosphate; ADA, adenosine deaminase

Cernunnos Deficiency (T–B– NK+)

Besides the Artemis, Ligase IV, DNA-PKcs deficiencies/ mutations, leading to defective DNA repair mechanisms affecting the nonhomologous end joining (NHEJ) pathways. Cernunnos is another factor responsible for the same, affecting the signal fidelity in V(D)J recombination process.

Immunoglobulin Class Switch Recombination Deficiencies (CD40-CD40 Ligand Deficiency)

CD40-CD40 ligand interaction is important to the T-cell dependent B-cell proliferation and differentiation. This in return, leads to germinal center formation with secondary antibody repertoire production. Mutations in either CD40 or CD40L result in lack of immunoglobulin class switch leading to hyper-immunoglobulin M (IgM) type III syndrome. Various mutations implicated in these disorders are missense mutations, insertions, deletions, splice site mutations and nonsense mutations.[17-19]

Purine Nucleoside Phosphorylase Deficiency (T–B+ NK+/–)

It is an autosomal recessive metabolic disorder resulting from mutation of purine nucleoside phosphorylase (PNP) gene located on chromosome 14q13.1. PNP is an enzyme from purine salvage pathway required for purine degradation. PNP deficiency leads to accumulation of PNP lymphotoxic substrates responsible for immunodeficiency. T-cell number and function are the most affected. B-cell number, immunoglobulin levels and antibody production are normal in these patients. The number of NK cells varies.[20]

CD8 Deficiency (CD8 α-chain Defect, ξ-chain-associated Protein-70 Deficiency)

The differentiation and activation of T-cells require TCR-dependent signal transduction through phosphorylation of various substrates within the cell. This happens via CD3 dimers, which evoke downstream signaling effecting the recruitment by ξ chain of ξ chain-associated protein-70 (ZAP-70), which in turn is phosphorylated and activated by tyrosine kinase p56lck. Consequently, ZAP-70 phosphorylates the other substrates within the cell differentiating it into an immune competent cell. Deficiency of ZAP-70 thus leads to severe forms of immune deficiency. CD8α polypeptides are mandatory molecules for expression of CD8β polypeptides, without which the CD8 coreceptor cannot function in recognizing the major histocompatibility complex (MHC) class I peptide. Both these defects, i.e. ZAP-70 deficiency and CD8α deficiency culminates into absence or deficiency of peripheral CD8+ T-cells; peripheral CD4+ T-cells are abundant in both these conditions, however, they are refractory to T-cell receptor-mediated activation in ZAP-70 deficiency, while they function normally in CD8α deficiency.[21]

Bare Lymphocyte Syndrome (MHC Class I and II Deficiency, Milder Variety)

Bare lymphocyte syndrome (BLS) is caused by mutations in genes for MHC class I and II. There are two types:

1. BLS 1, also called human leukocyte antigen (HLA) class I deficiency, is rare and is associated with mutations of TAP2 (encodes the protein antigen peptide transporter 2), TAP1 (transporter associated with antigen processing 1 is a protein that in humans is encoded by the *TAP1* gene), or TAPBP (TAP-associated glycoprotein also known as tapasin or TAPBP is a protein that is encoded by the *TAPBP* gene).
2. BLS 2 is the result of mutations in genes that code for proteins (transcription factors) that normally regulate the expression (gene transcription) of the *MHC II* genes.[22,23]

Mutation in any one of the four genes can lead to BLS II. The four genes responsible for the deficiency are as follows:

1. Class II transactivator (*CIITA*)
2. Regulatory factor of the X box 5 (*RFX5*)
3. RFX-associated protein (*RFXAP*)
4. RFX ankyrin repeats (*RFXANK*; also known as *RFXB*).

CD4 Deficiency

It is also called as idiopathic CD4 lymphocytopenia and is characterized by less than 1 × 10^3/mL in children above 23 months of age or less than 20% of the total T-cell count on two occasions, absence of acquired causes of low CD4 counts [human immunodeficiency virus-1 (HIV-1), HIV-2, human T-cell lymphotropic virus (HTLV)], absence of other immunodeficiency disorder or therapy known to be associated with reduced CD4 T-cell count.[24]

Various mechanisms that have been proposed include abnormal cytokine related reduced T-cell generation in bone marrow, defective T-cell maturation in thymus, spontaneous apoptosis of T lymphocytes due to overexpression of FAS-FAS ligand. Another possibility that has been depicted is low expression of p56lck consequently affecting T-cell proliferation and activation through ZAP70.

CD25 Deficiency

IL-2 receptor is composed of three chains, α, β and γ.[25] Mutation in the gene *IL-2Rα* results in deficiency of IL-2 receptor alpha chain required for optimal proliferative responses to IL-2 after stimulation of T-cell receptor. CD25 is also expressed on T regulatory cells.[26,27] The studies on two patients with CD25 deficiency indicate critical role played by CD25 in central as well as peripheral tolerance.[28,29]

Winged-Helix-Nude Deficiency

Winged-Helix-Nude deficiency results from mutation in the gene called *WHN/FOXN1* localized on chromosome 17. This gene is mainly expressed in thymus and skin and plays an important role in differentiation of thymic and skin epithelial cells. Therefore, deficiency of this gene leads to athymia and alopecia affecting scalp, eyebrows and eyelashes.[30-32]

Signal Transducers and Activators of Transcription 5b (STAT5b) Deficiency

Signal transducers and activators of transcription are latent transcription factors responsible for transcription of several genes.[33] STAT5b plays an important role in cellular differentiation in response to pulsatile pattern of growth hormone.[34,35] Deficiency of STAT5b leads to defective or absent cellular differentiation and proliferation and, consequently growth retardation in a child born with normal birth length.[36] Many cytokines use STAT5 for their intracellular signaling cascade in lymphocytes. Additionally, STAT5a and STAT5b cause decreased NK cell numbers in mice; STAT5b deficiency also causes loss of function of NK cells.[37]

Coronin 1A Deficiency

Coronins are actin-binding proteins, which are involved in cytokinesis, cell motility and in immune homeostasis and calcium-calcineurin signaling. Deficiency of coronin 1A leads to absence of T lymphocytes culminating in severe immunodeficiency, whereas hypomorphic mutations result in defective naïve T-cells with defective expansion of oligoclonal memory T-cells, leading to increased susceptibility to Epstein-Barr virus (EBV) associated B-cell lymphoproliferation.[38]

Calcium++ Release-activated Calcium Channels Deficiency

Calcium plays an important role as second messenger in immune and nonimmune cells. Calcium release-activated calcium channels deficiency (CRAC) is associated with absence of intracytoplasmic calcium increase in response to immunoreceptor engagement. Homozygous missense mutations in *ORAI1* gene are responsible for this deficiency.

OTHER IMMUNODEFICIENCY DISORDERS

DNA Repair Defects

Bloom Syndrome

Bloom syndrome is a type of chromosomal breakage syndrome characterized by chromosomal instability, sun sensitivity, growth deficiency (prenatal as well as postnatal), telangiectatic, hypo- and hyperpigmented skin and increased predisposition to malignancy. It is an autosomal recessive condition caused by mutation in the gene named *RECQL3* on long arm of chromosome 15.

Ataxia Telangiectasia

Ataxia telangiectasia is a type of chromosomal breakage disorder characterized by cerebellar ataxia, telangiectasis, immune defects, increased ionizing radiation sensitivity and increased predisposition to malignancy. It is an autosomal recessive disorder caused by mutation in *ATM* gene on long arm of chromosome 11. Defects in immune mechanism and hypoplastic thymus have been observed in these patients. There is decrease or absence of serum IgG2 and IgA. Serum IgE and IgM may be decreased.[39] Carbonari et al. found that the number of circulating immature T-cells is much more in these patients when compared to number of mature T-cells accounting for the defective immune function of these patients.[40]

Nijmegen Breakage Syndrome

Nijmegen breakage syndrome is an autosomal recessive condition caused by mutation in *NBN* gene on long arm of chromosome 8. Patients present with growth retardation, microcephaly and there is increased predisposition to malignancy. Individuals with this condition demonstrate structural aberrations with multiple rearrangements, preferentially involving chromosomes 7 and 14, in a proportion of metaphase. Patients exhibit severe humoral and cellular immune defects.

Wiskott-Aldrich Syndrome

It is a rare X-linked recessive disease caused by mutation of the gene located on Xp11.22-23 coding for Wiskott-Aldrich syndrome (WAS) protein (WASp). This protein functions as a bridge between signaling and movement of the actin filaments in the cytoskeleton. Actin cytoskeleton is responsible for growth, endocytosis, exocytosis and cytokinesis. Absence of WAS protein leads to defective T-cell function due to abnormal cytoskeletal reorganization further culminating into impaired migration, adhesion and interaction with other cells due to abnormal synapse formation. WAS is characterized by triad of microthrombocytopenia, eczema and immune deficiency. But the classic presentation may not always be present. With increased longevity, there has been increased incidence of autoimmunity and hematological malignancies in patients with WAS.

Immuno-osseous Dysplasia

Cartilage Hair Hypoplasia

Cartilage hair hypoplasia is an autosomal recessive disorder resulting from mutation in *RMRP* gene located on short arm of chromosome number 9. It is characterized by short-limbed dwarfism, variable immunodeficiency and predisposition to malignancy in some cases. Immunodeficiency is in the form of mild-to-moderate form of lymphopenia, decreased delayed type of hypersensitivity reaction and impaired responses to phytohemagglutinins. Profound impairment of T-cell function is attributed to intrinsic defect in cell proliferation. This may lead to severe infections early in life.

Others

Hermansky-Pudlak syndrome type 2, hyper-IgE syndrome, etc. are some of the rarer syndromes with combined immunodeficiencies.

CLINICAL PRESENTATION

The clinical manifestations in different forms of SCID are quite similar barring few characteristic features based on the cell type affected.

Typically, symptoms begin early in life by 3–6 months of age. However, some may present in the neonatal period with skin rashes due to graft-versus-host disease (GvHD) owing to maternal T-cell engraftment. Infants present with recurrent infections with unexpected severe and prolonged course coupled with unusual complications. The most common manifestations include chronic/recurrent diarrhea, oral thrush and respiratory infections. Opportunistic infections such as *Pneumocystis jirovecii* (PCP), *Cryptosporidium*, mycobacteria, cytomegalovirus (CMV), EBV as well as fungal infections are known.

Besides, failure to thrive or inability to gain weight may also be present. Dermatologic manifestations (Eczematous rash, recurrent warts, molluscum contagiosum, seborrheic dermatitis, etc.), nonresponsiveness to antibiotics and recurrent symptoms should alarm the physician for diagnosis of immunodeficiency. Absence of lymph nodes, tonsils, thymic shadows in chest X-ray corroborate the diagnosis of SCID. History of consanguinity further favors the diagnosis as most of the SCIDs have autosomal recessive inheritance. Inadvertently administered live vaccines can be hazardous in babies with SCID. In our country, bacillus Calmette-Guérin (BCG) is given at birth, thereby posing these infants to grave risk of BCGosis. Live polio vaccines can lead to bulbar poliomyelitis in these infants.

Graft-versus-host disease may occur due to maternal alloreactive T-cells or transfusion of nonirradiated blood products, later being often fatal.

There are some combined B- and T-cell disorders with peculiar clinical features. These include the following:

Adenosine Deaminase Deficiency

All the manifestations of SCID in variable proportions based on the mutation as well as neonatal hepatitis, delayed development, deafness, seizures and characteristically cupping at the end of ribs on chest radiograph.[41,42] Besides, it can manifest with hypotonia and movement disorders too.[2]

Reticular Dysgenesis

Sensorineural deafness is a well-known feature of this condition and may not be apparent in the neonatal period unless specifically tested for. Additionally, there is pancytopenia, especially leukopenia and thrombocytopenia due to defect in the hematopoietic stem cell in the bone marrow.

Omenn Syndrome

Though manifestations overlap with SCID disorders, lymphadenopathy and hepatosplenomegaly are characteristically seen in infants with Omenn syndrome. Additionally these infants suffer from hair loss and recurrent staphylococcal skin infections accompanied by sepsis.

DNA Ligase IV Deficiency

It is characterized by clinical features such as microcephaly, growth retardation, developmental delay, skin anomalies, radiosensitivity, dysmorphic facies and propensity to malignancies especially lymphoreticular ones.

Cernunnos Deficiency

Patients with this condition manifest with microcephaly and developmental defects especially bone and urogenital malformations.

Purine Nucleoside Phosphorylase Deficiency

Besides typical features of SCID, PNP deficient patients present typically during 1st year of life with a triad of neurologic abnormalities, autoimmune manifestations and recurrent infections. Neurologic manifestations include features suggestive of cerebral palsy, hypotonia, ataxia, tremors, developmental delay, hyperactivity and mental retardation. Autoimmune manifestations include autoimmune hemolytic anemia, autoimmune neutropenia, autoimmune thrombocytopenia, systemic lupus erythematosus (SLE) and serositis.

CD40-CD40 Ligand Deficiency

Most of the children with this disorder present between 3 months and 2 years of life. Manifestations are similar to any other SCID with neutropenia being most typical hematological abnormality in this disorder.

Major Histocompatibility Complex Class I Deficiency

Symptoms occur at around 4–7 years of age. Chronic infections of respiratory tract and granulomatous lesions of skin are unique manifestations of this condition.

CD 4 Deficiency

Besides the manifestations of typical SCID, children with this disorder often manifest with autoimmune phenomena such as Behçet disease, Sjögren syndrome, psoriasis, vasculitis and thrombotic thrombocytopenic purpura. Secondary malignancies especially lymphomas and Kaposi's sarcoma are also reported.

Calcium Release-activated Calcium Channels Deficiency

They manifest early in life by 3 months of age with serious opportunistic infections. Among the seven reported cases, myopathy was seen in four and in one patient hypohidrotic ectodermal dysplasia has been noted.

Winged-Helix-Nude Deficiency

The characteristic features include alopecia, nail dystrophy and bilateral epicanthal folds. Other manifestations are those similar to Omenn syndrome.

CD25 Deficiency

They manifest by 6 months of age with recurrent infections as well as autoimmune phenomena.

STAT 5b Deficiency

They manifest with a short stature without a deficiency of growth hormone and low insulin, like growth factor levels. They are susceptible to infections due to immunodeficiency.

DIAGNOSIS

History of recurrent infections in the index case should prompt a suspicion of immune deficiency state; similar history of infections, autoimmune diseases and/or malignancies in other family members can additionally give a clue. Inquiry of any infant deaths without a known diagnosis as well as history of consanguinity is equally important. SCID being an inherited disorder (AR/XLR), a good family history with pedigree is crucial for diagnosis.

Early diagnosis, preferably by neonatal screening, is imperative as outcomes with hematopoietic stem cell transplantation (HSCT) (irrespective of graft source) are significantly better (reaching up to 90% survival), if done before onset of infections.[47]

Laboratory Parameters

A complete blood count forms the backbone of diagnosing SCID. Reduced absolute lymphocyte count (<1,000/μL) is common, though not a necessary finding. Persistence of maternal T-cells may interfere with lymphocyte count and this can be resolved by performing chimerism assays (in males by XX/XY hybridization of CD3+ cells and in girls by molecular biological methods). HIV DNA PCR would help in excluding acquired immunodeficiency and should be performed before confirming diagnosis of SCID based on lymphocyte count. Eosinophilia may be present.

Complete evaluation of humoral and cellular immunity needs to be done in a suspected case of T- and B-cell deficiency. This includes determination of immunoglobulin levels, specific antibody titers, lymphocyte subset assay and evaluation of T-cell function.

Diagnosis of SCID should be made on the basis of the following:

T-cell Evaluation

Quantitative analysis: A T-cell count less than 20% of the total lymphocytes and absolute lymphocyte count less than 3,000/μL response to mitogens below 10% of control and presence of maternal T-cells.

T-cell function: This can be done using mitogen assays for lymphocyte proliferation or response to antigens through either vaccines or infections. Impaired T-cell maturation can be confirmed further by estimating T-cell receptor excision circles (TRECs) in the patient. TREC are DNA circles, which are generated during the V(D)J recombination by endjoining of the removed genomic DNA segments. These can be measured by PCR.

B-cell Evaluation

Serum immunoglobulin levels along with IgG subclass help to confirm B-cell deficiency. However, these levels may not be useful or may be normal in the early months of life due to maternal antibodies. If the levels are normal and B-cell defect is suspected, antibody responses to vaccine antigens should be looked at. In a child suspected to have immunodeficiency, antitetanus or antidiphtheria antibodies (IgG1), antipneumococcal antibodies (IgG2) and antirespiratory virus antibodies (IgG3) titers will be lower than expected despite immunization. A fourfold rise in antitetanus and twofold rise for antipneumococcal titers 3–4 weeks after vaccination is a normal response. Immunoglobulin deficiency can also be corroborated by an absent response to A and B blood group antigens (isohemagglutinins).

Age-specific values should be used when interpreting immunoglobulin assays. Normal age-specific values of lymphocyte subsets and immunoglobulins and specific subclass are cited in literature for Western countries, but till date, there is no published Indian data for the same.[43,44] In immunodeficiency disorders involving IgG, generally, the levels will be below 200 mg%. Other immunoglobulins may be variably affected. In a subclass deficiency, the decrease of the specific subclass would be greater than two standard deviations below the normal mean for age.

Molecular Diagnosis

Defining the genetic defect and achieving a molecular diagnosis is of paramount importance in a SCID. It not only helps confirm the diagnosis in the index case, but also assists in prenatal diagnosis for the unborn sibling of the patient. For most SCIDs, the genetic defect has been elucidated. This has been described in the chapter under each of the conditions.

TREATMENT

If one suspects SCID in a neonate or infant, prompt diagnosis and treatment of acute infections are mandatory. Prevention of recurrence of infections is a priority. The infant should be referred to a specialized center as suspicion of SCID is a "pediatric-immunological-emergency" and the work-up for confirmatory diagnosis should be initiated at the earliest. Once the blood is drawn for immunoglobulin assays, intravenous substitution of immunoglobulin should be begun along with prophylaxis for other infections, as indicated, especially *Pneumocystis jirovecii pneumonia* (PCP). Preparation for curative treatment should also be started at the earliest, thereby improving the chances of long-term survival in them. Definitive treatment includes HSCT, enzyme replacement and gene therapy. If HSCT is the treatment of choice, HLA typing of the infant, siblings and parents should be sent immediately. While awaiting the final diagnosis and planning for the curative treatment, all the general measures for infection control should be strictly adhered to.

General Treatment

Prevention of Infections

It is crucial to prevent any infection in the infant with SCID. This can be achieved to an extent by isolating them, especially from other young children, as far as possible, to avoid possibility of any viral or bacterial infections. Thus, settings such as day care, play schools or groups, family get-togethers need to be avoided. Amongst infections that spread most frequently and easily among infants and children, varicella is of grave concern. Hence, all children in close contact should receive varicella vaccine. In case, a close contact such as a sibling or neighbor contracts varicella, the patient should receive varicella zoster immunoglobulin (VZIG) or immunoglobulin replacement therapy immediately. If the infant develops varicella before or despite giving the immunoglobulin, intravenous acyclovir is the treatment option.

Immunization

No live vaccines, like *rotavirus*, chickenpox, mumps, measles, oral polio or BCG should be given to the child with SCID. Additionally, children who are household contacts (such as siblings) should receive the killed polio vaccine and not the live oral vaccine.

Personal Hygiene

As a general measure to control or prevent infections, all the caretakers and the patient should follow all measures of personal hygiene including frequent hand-washing.

Prevention and Management of Opportunistic Infections

Trimethoprim-sulfamethoxazole given as a part of PCP prophylaxis is mandatory. If infection is suspected, antifungal and antiviral treatment, or prophylaxis should also be initiated. CMV and adenovirus infections can be fatal and hence, a high index of suspicion as well as prompt treatment is indicated. If respiratory syncytial virus (RSV) infection is suspected, palivizumab may be administered. TB prophylaxis may be required in those at risk due to contact. In case of suspected BCGosis, one needs to give a four drug antituberculous regimen.

Blood Products

Infants and children with SCID should always get irradiated (CMV-negative, leukocyte-depleted) blood products. This precaution is necessary in order to prevent fatal GvHD from T-cells in blood products as well as to prevent infection with CMV, which also could be fatal.

Specific Treatment Other than Hematopoietic Stem Cell Transplantation

Intravenous Immunoglobulin Replacement Therapy

This should be given to SCID infants who are more than 3 months of age and/or who have already had infections. The overall consensus among clinical immunologists is that a monthly dose of 400–600 mg/kg of intravenous immunoglobulin (IVIG) or a dose that maintains through serum IgG levels greater than 500 mg/dL is desirable.[45] Although immunoglobulin therapy will not restore the function of the deficient T-cells, it does replace the missing antibodies resulting from the B-cell defect and is, therefore, of some benefit.

Adenosine Deaminase Enzyme Replacement Therapy

For patients with SCID due to *ADA* deficiency, replacement therapy with a modified form of the enzyme [from a cow, called pegademase bovine (PEG)-*ADA*] has been used with some success. The immune reconstitution effected by PEG-*ADA* is not a permanent cure and requires two subcutaneous injections weekly for the rest of the child's life. PEG-*ADA* treatment is not recommended if the patient has an HLA-matched sibling available as a donor for a marrow transplant.

Hematopoietic Stem Cell Transplant

The goal of HSCT in infants with SCID is to correct the immune dysfunction at the level of stem cell. The ideal donor for a SCID infant is a perfectly HLA-type matched normal brother or sister. In absence of a fully matched sibling donor, haploidentical (half-matched) related donors such as a mother or a father would be the next best choice. Pretransplant chemotherapy is usually not necessary or a reduced intensity conditioning may be sufficient, especially in NK-patients.

It is interesting to note that the survival rates for HSCTs have been reported to be highest regardless of donor type among infants who received transplants at 3.5 months of age or younger (94%) and among older infants without prior infection (90%) as compared to those with prior infection that had resolved (82%) and they were worst in cases where an ongoing infection or sepsis was present during the HSCT (50%).[46]

In utero marrow stem cell transplantation has been tried with limited success and has no special advantage over the transplant carried out immediately after birth; and in fact, it poses a risk of GVHD to both mother and child, hence is not preferred.[47]

Gene Therapy

The future of SCID lies in success of gene therapy. This would transform the management of SCIDs drastically. Although, there has been some success achieved in both X-linked and *ADA*-deficient SCID, it has not yet reached a level to become the standard of care.

PROGNOSIS

Severe combined immunodeficiency syndrome is generally considered to be the most serious of the primary immune deficiencies. Without a successful bone marrow transplant or gene therapy, the patient is likely to succumb to a severe or fatal infection, sooner or later in infancy or early childhood for severe types and in later childhood for less severe types of combined immune deficiencies.

NEONATAL SCREENING

Though SCID manifests generally by 3–6 months of age, and a neonate is generally asymptomatic and healthy, except for a few with syndromic manifestations and GVHD due to maternal T-cells, it is in reality a prenatal T lymphocyte disorder. Hence, it is possible to diagnose it in neonates and the importance to diagnose it early, even before symptoms and signs appear, is evident from the results of HSCT; an early diagnosis confers an advantage of being transplanted well before the first infection in the infant, leading to excellent outcomes with an overall survival of more than 90%. Mandatory neonatal screening, therefore, is a very crucial step in bringing down the otherwise inevitable mortality in these disorders.

T-cell receptor excision circles, which are by products of T-cell maturation and can be measured by PCR on DNA extracted from dried blood spots, are either absent or very low in numbers in neonates with SCID. Wisconsin state in the USA was the first to start the mandatory neonatal screening for SCID by TREC in 2008. Since 2010, the Department of Health and Human Services has recommended universal screening of all neonates for SCID.

CONCLUSION

- Combined T- and B-cell deficiency is predominantly T-cell deficiency with B-cell dysfunction, though some may have low or absent B-cells
- There are numerous genetic defects with complete or "hypomorphic" forms, hypomorphic also known as "leaky forms", are less severe
- It is a prenatal T lymphocyte disorder, though clinical manifestations are generally seen by 3–6 months of age. Neonates may present with GVHD due to maternal T-cell engraftment and can be fatal
- A good family history with pedigree chart can give an important clue in diagnosing combined immunodeficiencies
- Neonatal screening by evaluating TRECs can diagnose SCID, thereby lending an opportunity to perform HSCT before even the first infection occurs with a great survival advantage
- If not diagnosed early, these infants will present with recurrent infections, especially due to intracellular organisms. Diagnosis of SCID can then be suspected on the basis of lymphopenia
- Live vaccines are an absolute contraindication in these infants
- All blood products should be irradiated as well as leukodepleted and CMV-negative
- HSCT is the curative treatment for most forms of SCID.

REFERENCES

1. Boyle JM, Buckley RH. Population prevalence of diagnosed primary immunodeficiency diseases in the United States. J Clin Immunol. 2007;27(5):497-502.
2. Le Deist F, Moshous D, Howe SJ. Combined T and B cell immunodeficiencies. In: Rezaei N, Aghamohammadi A, Notarangelo LD (Eds). Primary Immunodeficiency Diseases: Definition, Diagnosis and Management. Berlin, Germany: Springer Science and Business Media; 2008. pp. 39-95.
3. Puck JM; SCID Newborn Screening Working Group. Population-based newborn screening for severe combined immunodeficiency: steps toward implementation. J Allergy Clin Immunol. 2007;120(4):760-8.
4. Giliani S, Mori L, Basile G, Le Deist F, Rodriguez-Perez C, Forino C, et al. Interleukin-7 receptor α (IL-7R α) deficiency: cellular and molecular bases. Analysis of clinical, immunological, and molecular features in 16 novel patients. Immunol Rev. 2005;203:110-26.
5. Kishihara K, Penninger J, Wallace VA, Kündig TM, Kawai K, Wakeham A, et al. Normal B lymphocyte development but impaired T cell maturation in CD45-exon6 protein tyrosine phosphatase-deficient mice. Cell. 1993;74(1):143-56.
6. Alarcon B, Regueiro JR, Arnaiz-Villena A, Terhorst C. Familial defect in the surface expression of the T- cell receptor-CD3 complex. N Engl J Med. 1988;319(18):1203-8.
7. Geha RS, Notarangelo LD, Casanova JL, Chapel H, Conley ME, Fischer A, et al. Primary immunodeficiency diseases: an update from the international Union of Immunological Societies Primary Immunodeficiency Diseases Classification Committee. J Allergy Clin Immunol. 2007;120(4):776-94.
8. Notarangelo L, Casanova JL, Conley ME, Chapel H, Fischer A, Puck J, et al. Primary immunodeficiency diseases: an update from the International Union of Immunological Societies Primary Immunodeficiency Diseases Classification Committee Meeting in Budapest, 2005. J Allergy Clin Immunol. 2006;117(4):883-96.
9. Gennery AR, Hodges E, Williams AP, Harris S, Villa A, Angus B, et al. Omenn's syndrome occurring in patients without mutations in recombination activating genes. Clin Immunol. 2005;116(3):246-56.
10. Ege M, Ma Y, Manfras B, Kalwak K, Lu H, Lieber MR, et al. Omenn syndrome due to ARTEMIS mutations. Blood. 2005;105(11):4179-86.
11. Arredondo-Vega FX, Santisteban I, Daniels S, Toutain S, Hershfield MS. Adenosine deaminase deficiency: genotype-phenotype correlations based on expressed activity of 29 mutant alleles. Am J Hum Genet. 1998;63(4):1049-59.
12. Lagresle-Peyrou C, Six EM, Picard C, Rieux-Laucat F, Michel V, Ditadi A, et al. Human adenylate kinase 2 deficiency causes a profound hematopoietic defect associated with sensorineural deafness. Nat Genet. 2009;41(1):106-11.

13. Pannicke U, Hönig M, Hess I, Friesen C, Holzmann K, Rump EM, et al. Reticular dysgenesis (aleukocytosis) is caused by mutations in the gene encoding mitochondrial adenylate kinase 2. Nat Genet. 2009;41(1):101-5.
14. Cham B, Bonilla MA, Winkelstein J. Neutropenia associated with primary immunodeficiency syndromes. Semin Hematol. 2002;39(2):107-12.
15. Chistiakov DA, Voronova NV, Chistiakov AP. Ligase IV syndrome. Eur J Med Genet. 2009;52(6):373-8.
16. O'Driscoll M, Cerosaletti KM, Girard PM, Dai Y, Stumm M, Kysela B, et al. DNA ligase IV mutations identified in patients exhibiting developmental delay and immunodeficiency. Mol Cell. 2001;8(6):1175-85.
17. Lee WI, Torgerson TR, Schumacher MJ, Yel L, Zhu Q, Ochs HD. Molecular analysis of a large cohort of patients with the hyper immunoglobulin M (IgM) syndrome. Blood. 2005;105(5):1881-90.
18. Notarangelo LD, Peitsch MC, Abrahamsen TG, Bachelot C, Bordigoni P, Cant AJ, et al. CD40lbase: a database of *CD40L* gene mutations causing X-linked hyper-IgM syndrome. Immunol Today. 1996;17(11):511-6.
19. Seyama K, Nonoyama S, Gangsaas I, Hollenbaugh D, Pabst HF, Aruffo A, et al. Mutations of the CD40 ligand gene and its effect on CD40 ligand expression in patients with X-linked hyper IgM syndrome. Blood. 1998;92(7):2421-34.
20. Cohen A, Doyle D, Martin DW Jr, Ammann AJ. Abnormal purine metabolism and purine overproduction in a patient deficient in purine nucleoside phosphorylase. N Engl J Med. 1976;295(26):1449-54.
21. Elder ME, Lin D, Clever J, Chan AC, Hope TJ, Weiss A, et al. Human severe combined immunodeficiency due to a defect in ZAP-70, a T cell tyrosine kinase. Science. 1994;264(5165):1596-9.
22. Reith W, Mach B. The bare lymphocyte syndrome and the regulation of MHC expression. Annu Rev Immunol. 2001;19:331-73.
23. De Sandro A, Nagarajan UM, Boss JM. The bare lymphocyte syndrome: molecular clues to the transcriptional regulation of major histocompatibility complex class II genes. Am J Hum Genet. 1999;65(2):279-86.
24. Walker UA, Warnatz K. Idiopathic CD4 lymphocytopenia. Curr Opin Rheumatol. 2006;18(4):389-95.
25. Minami Y, Kono T, Miyazaki T, Taniguchi T. The IL-2 receptor complex: its structure, function, and target genes. Annu Rev Immunol. 1993;11:245-68.
26. Fontenot JD, Gavin MA, Rudensky AY. Foxp3 programs the development and function of CD4+CD25+ regulatory T cells. Nat Immunol. 2003;4(4):330-6.
27. Khattri R, Cox T, Yasayko SA, Ramsdell F. An essential role for Scurfin in CD4+CD25+ T regulatory cells. Nat Immunol. 2003;4(4):337-42.
28. Sharfe N, Dadi HK, Shahar M, Roifman CM. Human immune disorder arising from mutation of the alpha chain of the interleukin-2 receptor. Proc Natl Acad Sci U S A. 1997;94(7):3168-71.
29. Caudy AA, Reddy ST, Chatila T, Atkinson JP, Verbsky JW. CD25 deficiency causes an immune dysregulation, polyendocrinopathy, enteropathy, X-linked-like-syndrome, and defective IL-10 expression from CD4 lymphocytes. J Allergy Clin Immunol. 2007;119(2):482-7.
30. Nehls M, Pfeifer D, Schorpp M, Hedrich H, Boehm T. New member of the winged-helix protein family disrupted in mouse and rat nude mutations. Nature. 1994;372(6501):103-7.
31. Su DM, Navarre S, Oh WJ, Condie BG, Manley NR. A domain of Foxn1 required for crosstalk-dependent thymic epithelial cell differentiation. Nat Immunol. 2003;4(11):1128-35.
32. Frank J, Pignata C, Panteleyev AA, Prowse DM, Baden H, Weiner L, et al. Exposing the human nude phenotype. Nature. 1999;398(6727):473-4.
33. Akira S. Functional roles of STAT family proteins: lessons from knockout mice. Stem Cells. 1999;17(3):138-46.
34. Gebert CA, Park SH, Waxman DJ. Regulation of signal transducer and activator of transcription (STAT) 5b activation by the temporal pattern of growth hormone stimulation. Mol Endocrinol. 1997;11(4):400-14.
35. Udy GB, Towers RP, Snell RG, Wilkins RJ, Park SH, Ram PA, et al. Requirement of STAT5b for sexual dimorphism of body growth rates and liver gene expression. Proc Natl Acad Sci USA. 1997;94(14):7239-44.
36. Vidarsdottir S, Walenkamp MJ, Pereira AM, Karperien M, van Doorn J, van Duyvenvoorde HA, et al. Clinical and biochemical characteristics of a male patient with a novel homozygous STAT5b mutation. J Clin Endocrinol Metab. 2006;91(9):3482-5.
37. Moriggl R, Topham DJ, Teglund S, Sexl V, McKay C, Wang D, et al. Stat5 is required for IL-2-induced cell cycle progression of peripheral T cells. Immunity. 1999;10(2):249-59.
38. Moshous D, de Villartay JP. The expanding spectrum of human coronin 1A deficiency. Curr Allergy Asthma Rep. 2014;14(12):481.
39. Gatti RA, Boder E, Vinters HV, Sparkes RS, Norman A, Lange K. Ataxia-telangiectasia: an interdisciplinary approach to pathogenesis. Medicine (Baltimore). 1991;70(2):99-117.
40. Carbonari M, Cherchi M, Paganelli R, Giannini G, Galli E, Gaetano C, et al. Relative increase of T cells expressing the gamma/delta rather than the alpha/beta receptor in ataxia-telangectasia. N Engl J Med. 1990;322(2):73-6.
41. Cossu F. Genetics of SCID. Ital J Pediatr. 2010;36:76.
42. Madkaikar M, Mishra A, Ghosh K. Diagnostic approach to primary immunodeficiency disorders. Indian Pediatr. 2013;50(6):579-86.
43. Shearer WT, Rosenblatt HM, Gelman RS, Oyomopito R, Plaeger S, Stiehm ER, et al. Lymphocyte subsets in healthy children from birth through 18 years of age: the Pediatric AIDS Clinical Trials Group P1009 study. J Allergy Clin Immunol. 2003;112(5):973-80.
44. Aksu G, Genel F, Koturoğlu G, Kurugöl Z, Kütükçüler N. Serum immunoglobulin (IgG, IgM, IgA) and IgG subclass concentrations in healthy children: a study using nephelometric technique. Turk J Pediatr. 2006;48(1):19-24.
45. Garcia-Lloret M, McGhee S, Chatila TA. Immunoglobulin replacement therapy in children. Immunol Allergy Clin North Am. 2008;28(4):833-49.
46. Pai SY, Logan BR, Griffith LM, Buckley RH, Parrott RE, Dvorak CC, et al. Transplantation outcomes for severe combined immunodeficiency, 2000-2009. N Engl J Med. 2014;371(5):434-46.
47. Buckley RH. Transplantation of hematopoietic stem cells in human severe combined immunodeficiency: long term outcomes. Immunol Res. 2011;49(1-3):25-43.

CHAPTER

51

Primary Antibody Deficiencies

Deepti Suri, Vignesh P

INTRODUCTION

Primary antibody deficiencies (PADs) are the most common types of primary immunodeficiency diseases (PIDs). They constitute approximately half of all PIDs and include a wide spectrum of diseases ranging from patients with agammaglobulinemia or severe reduction in all the immunoglobulin (Ig) classes with totally absent B-cells to patients with milder disease and selective antibody deficiency with normal serum immunoglobulins.[1] Most of these patients have a similar clinical profile characterized by recurrent sinopulmonary and gastrointestinal bacterial infections, predisposition to chronic inflammation and autoimmunity. Hypogammaglobulinemia is the major hallmark of these disorders. Unlike patients with combined immunodeficiency, T-cell functions are preserved in patients with PADs.

B-cells development and differentiation terminally lead to production of plasma cells, which produce functional antibodies, the essential component of humoral immunity. Factors that hinder the development or maturation of B-cells lead to PADs.[1] Recent advances in the understanding of the genetic basis of early maturation and terminal development of B-lymphocytes and identification of the genes involved in many PADs have led to a significant increase in our understanding of the pathogenesis of this group of disorders. Identification of the genes involved in many PADs allows a definitive diagnosis of some of the PAD.

However, while evaluating a child for hypogammaglobulinemia, it must be remembered that hypogammaglobulinemia can also be acquired. It can occur secondarily to loss of protein via the kidneys, intestinal tract, lymphatic system or skin. Some common secondary causes are nephrotic syndrome, protein losing enteropathies, severe dermatitis, peritoneal dialysis, burns and intestinal lymphangiectasia.[2] Immunosuppressive drugs corticosteroids, anticonvulsants such as phenytoin, carbamazepine and some toxins may also lead to antibody deficiencies.[3] Patients with primary hypogammaglobulinemias are usually free of infection until the latter part of the first year of life. They become symptomatic as passively acquired IgG from the mother decreases to below protective level. They manifest in late infancy with recurrent respiratory and gastrointestinal tract infections. Signature manifestations are otitis media, chronic recurrent sinusitis and pneumonia.[4] Infections are usually caused by pyogenic bacteria like *Haemophilus influenzae, Moraxella catarrhalis, Streptococcus pneumoniae, Staphylococcus aureus* and *Pseudomonas aeruginosae.* Chronic diarrhea related to giardiasis is also common.[5] However, unlike patients with combined deficiencies who have increased risk with opportunist viral and fungal infections, patients with antibody deficiencies do not have problems with these organisms except patients with X-linked agammaglobulinemia (XLA), who are susceptible to *Enteroviruses* and may develop chronic enteroviral encephalomyelitis.

As a result of repeated clinically overt as well as subclinical pulmonary infections, there occurs a progressive deterioration in pulmonary function. Bronchiectasis or bronchiolitis obliterans is one of the devastating terminal complications in these patients.[6]

Immunoglobulin replacement therapy is the cornerstone in the management of humoral immunodeficiency disorders. This is to be coupled with appropriate and timely use of antibiotics to treat infections and judicious use of prophylactic antibiotic therapy.[7] Early diagnosis and adequate therapy are the keys to survival and a better quality of life. Delays in diagnosis and/or inadequate management may lead to permanent organ damage or death due to overwhelming infection.

Commonly described PADs are XLA (X-linked agammaglobulinemia), common variable immunodeficiency (CVID), transient newborn hypogammaglobulinemia, IgG subclass deficiency, selective immunoglobulin deficiency **(Table 51.1)**. Differential diagnosis between subgroups of PAD is important as they have variable clinical course and different prognosis and treatment. Clinical overviews of

Table 51.1 Classification and characteristics of primary antibody deficient disorders				
Disease	*Subtypes*	*Genetic defects*	*Immunological phenotype*	*Clinical phenotype*
Agammaglobulinemia and absent B-cells	X-linked agammaglobulinemia	BTK	Decreased levels of all immunoglobulin types; markedly decreased or absent B-cells; normal numbers of pro-B-cells	Onset of infections > 6–9 months *H. influenzae*, *S. pneumoniae*, *P. aeruginosa*. Recurrent otitis media. pneumonia, sinusitis, diarrhea. Mycoplasma arthritis, enteroviral encephalitis, giardiasis
	Autosomal recessive agammaglobulinemia	*IGHM, IGLL1, CD79A, CD79B, BLNK*		
Hypogammaglobulinemia with normal or low numbers of B-cells	Common variable immunodeficiency	Unknown	Decreased serum levels of IgG and IgA; normal or low numbers of B-cells	Onset of infections usually > 2 years-*H. influenzae*, *S. pneumoniae*, *P. aeruginosa*. Recurrent otitis media, pneumonia, sinusitis, diarrhea. Autoimmunity features, granuloma formation predisposition to malignancy
	ICOS deficiency	*ICOS*		
	TACI deficiency	*TACI*		
	CD19 deficiency	*CD19*		
Immunoglobulin class switch recombination deficiencies	*AID* deficiency	*AID*	Decreased serum levels of IgG and IgA; increased or normal numbers of IgM; normal or increased number of B-cells	Lymphoid hyperplasia, increased predisposition to bacterial infections, autoimmune and inflammatory disorders
	UNG deficiency	*UNG*		
Selective IgA deficiency	—	Unknown	Decreased or absent levels of IgA	Usually asymptomatic. Sinopulmonary and gastrointestinal infections may occur. Increased predisposition to allergies and celiac disease. Fatal anaphylaxis to blood products or IVIg containing IgA
Immunoglobulin subclass deficiency	Isolated IgG subclass deficiency	Unknown	Decreased serum levels of one or more IgG subclasses	Usually asymptomatic. Respiratory and gastrointestinal infections may occur
	IgA with IgG subclass deficiency	Unknown	Decreased serum levels of one or more IgG subclass and decreased IgA levels in serum	Same as selective IgA deficiency
Transient hypogammaglobulinemia of infancy	—	Unknown	Decreased serum levels of IgG and IgA; normal numbers of B-cells	Manifests from 6 months to 15 months usually with recurrent sinopulmonary infections. Normal functional antibodies
Specific antibody deficiency with normal immunoglobulin levels	—	Unknown	Normal serum immunoglobulins; normal numbers of B-cells; inability to produce antibodies to specific antigens	Recurrent sinopulmonary infections, diarrhea

Abbreviations: IgA, immunoglobulin A; IVIg, intravenous immunoglobulin; ICOS, inducible constimulator; TACI, transmembrane activator and calcium-modulator and cyclophilin ligand interactor; UNG, uracil-DNA glycosylase

these conditions are presented in this chapter and readers are referred to further literature for detailed molecular and immunological aberrations of these disorders. The diagnostic flow chart is presented **(Flow chart 51.1)**.

X-LINKED AGAMMAGLOBULINEMIA

X-linked agammaglobulinemia, previously called as Bruton's agammaglobulinemia, is a prototype for PID and is the first primary immunodeficiency disease for which a genetic cause was established. It was described by Colonel Bruton in 1952 while the molecular defect was identified in early 1993 by two different groups.[8] It is caused by mutations in the Bruton tyrosine kinase (*BTK*) gene, located on the long arm of the X chromosome. BTK is a member of the Tec family of nonreceptor tyrosine kinases, which are signal transduction molecules. *BTK* is critical in maturation of pre-B-cells to mature B-cells. Its major role is in promoting pre-B-cell expansion at the pre-B1 to pre-B2 stage. As a result of mutation in *BTK* gene, there is failure of B-cell development

Flow chart 51.1 The approach to antibody deficiencies

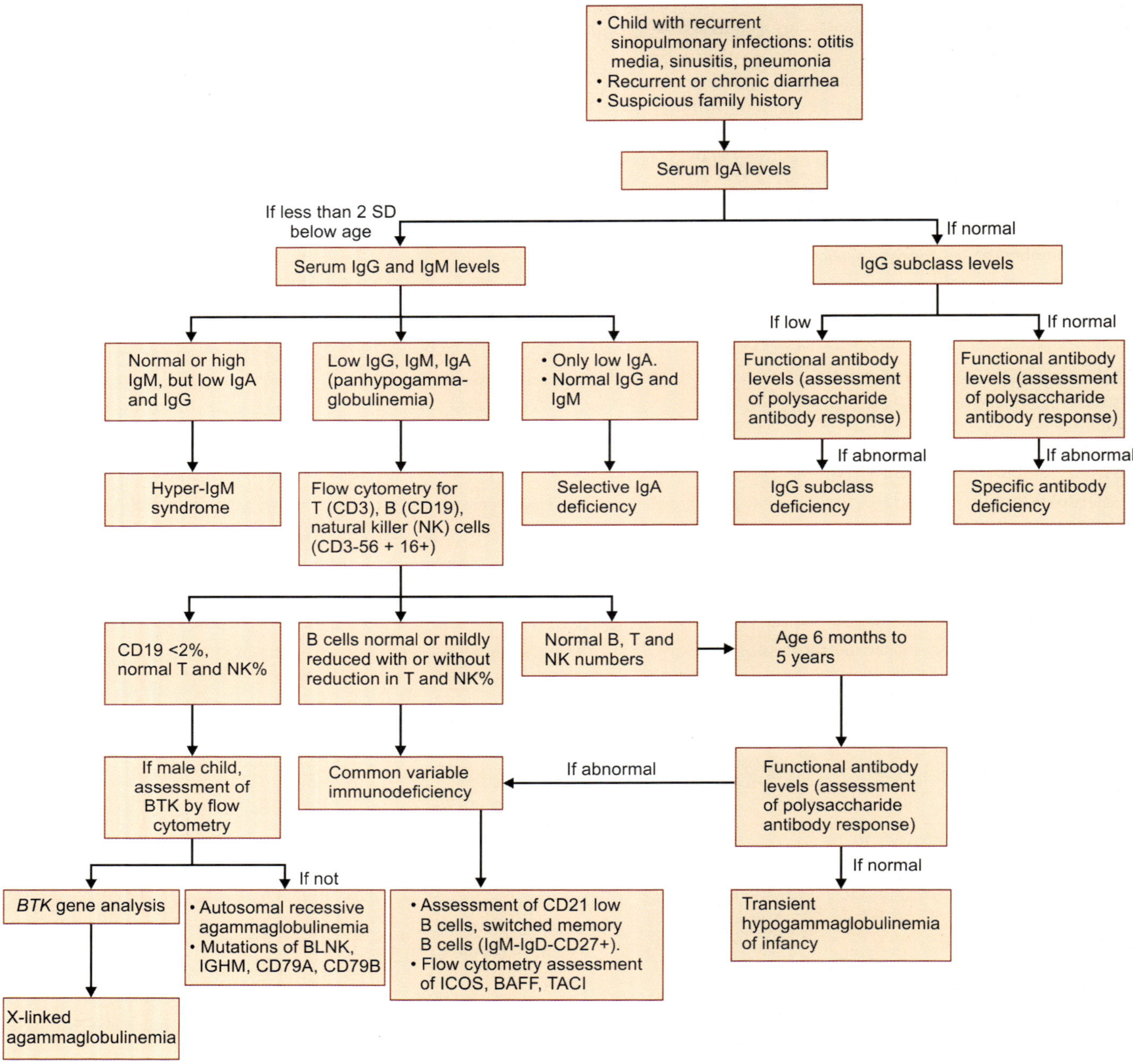

and affected patients have significantly reduced levels (<1%) of B-lymphocytes in their peripheral blood circulation. They fail to generate plasma cells and consequently have markedly low levels of all classes of immunoglobulins with virtually no humoral responses.[9] It also results in reduced size of lymph nodes and tonsils, which are highly populated by B-cells.

Bruton tyrosine kinase is located on the X-chromosome and both *de novo* as well as familial mutations can occur. Approximately, 40% of patients with XLA are born into a family with a previously affected family member and mothers are healthy carriers. Only one case of a female with agammaglobulinemia due to BTK mutation has been reported so far, due to skewed X-chromosome inactivation.

CLINICAL MANIFESTATIONS

Children with XLA become symptomatic by 6–12 months of age, once the passively transferred protective maternal

IgG fade. Most patients present with recurrent infection and more than 50% children have had serious infections by 2 years of life.[10] There are rare reports of individual patients with well-documented XLA who did not have sufficient clinical symptoms to be diagnosed with agammaglobulinemia until well into adult life. Though some children may be identified early due to a positive family history but unfortunately even in countries with high index of suspicion for PIDs, two-thirds of patients with a positive family history are not diagnosed at or soon after birth, but rather are diagnosed after the children have presented with clinical symptoms.

Recurrent bacterial upper and lower respiratory tract infections are the most common manifestation of XLA. Typically, XLA patients suffer from recurrent otitis media, sinusitis, bronchitis, pneumonia and gastrointestinal infections; however, the frequency of these manifestations is variable. The infections are usually caused by encapsulated pyogenic bacteria, namely *Streptococcus pneumoniae*, *Haemophilus influenzae* type B, *Streptococcus pyogenes* and *Pseudomonas* species.[4] Septicemia, pyogenic meningitis, osteomyelitis and septic arthritis are well described. Mycoplasma infections cause respiratory, urogenital as well as joint infections. It is worth noting that mycoplasma arthritis in patients with XLA may pose a clinical dilemma for treating physicians. The serology-based tests are typically negative, and hence all attempts should be made to culture these organisms.[11] Recurrent conjunctivitis also occurs in around 5–8% patients.

Infections of the gastrointestinal tract are frequent in XLA patients. *Giardia lamblia* is frequently isolated from stool samples from these patients, and sometimes its eradication may become difficult, resulting in chronic diarrhea and malabsorption. *Campylobacter jejuni* is also an unusual pathogen implicated in causing gastrointestinal manifestations.[5]

Patients with XLA are able to handle most of the childhood viral infections well due to intact T-cell function. However, they are susceptible to certain *Enteroviruses* namely; *Echovirus*, poliovirus and Coxsackievirus. Fatal vaccine-associated poliovirus infection has been described in children with XLA who had receive oral polio vaccine (Sabin).[12]

Enteroviral infection can take the form of chronic meningoencephalitis. The earliest signs of enteroviral meningoencephalitis may be a change in behavior and/or developmental regression, which then progresses to full blown neurologic impairment and coma over a period of months to years. Enteroviral infection of muscle and skin may occasionally masquerade as dermatomyositis like syndrome presenting with erythematous rash and peripheral edema. They may even cause chronic hepatitis manifesting with fever, rash and elevated hepatic enzymes.[13]

Neutropenia has been reported in 10–25% of XLA, although the clear involvement of BTK in neutrophil development has not been elucidated yet.

On physical evaluation, there are evidences of growth failure. Signs of recurrent and chronic sinopulmonary infections postnasal discharge, tympanic membrane perforation; digital clubbing and bronchiectasis may be seen. Absent or atrophied tonsils and lymph nodes is often the most important clinical clue in clinching the diagnosis **(Fig. 51.1)**.[14]

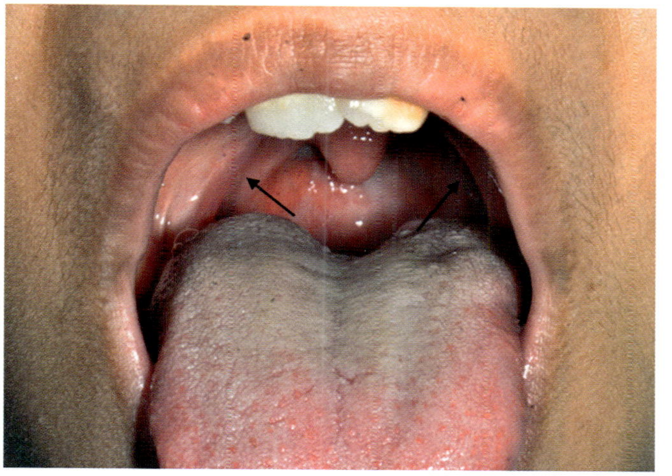

Figure 51.1 Oral cavity of a boy with X-linked agammaglobulinemia showing absent tonsils in the tonsillar fossa

LABORATORY DIAGNOSIS

The hallmark of patients with XLA is a marked reduction in all classes and subclasses of serum immunoglobulins and almost complete absence of peripheral B-cells defined as less than 2% CD19 and CD20 expression **(Figs 51.2A and B)**. Serum levels of antibodies to ubiquitous antigens (e.g. isohemagglutinins and *E. coli*) or to immunizations (e.g. polio, tetanus, diphtheria) are markedly reduced or undetectable. T-cell number and function are normal.[15]

Bruton tyrosine kinase expression can also be ascertained by flow cytometry **(Figs 51.3A and B)**.

This is a simple and robust test which aids in diagnosis. Once the clinical and laboratory findings sustain the diagnosis, molecular analysis of the *BTK* gene should be performed. Once the mutation is defined, carrier diagnosis and prenatal diagnosis can be performed where necessary. If *BTK* mutation analysis results are noncontributory, sequencing analysis of the other known uncommon genes causing antibody deficiencies can be undertaken like μ heavy chain, Igα, Igβ, λ5 and BLNK.

A definitive diagnosis is made when a male patient has hypogammaglobulinemia or agammaglobulinemia, CD19+ B-cells (<2%), and either a male family member of maternal lineage who is documented to also have agammaglobulinemia and less than 2% CD19+ B-cells or a confirmed [by deoxyribonucleic acid (DNA), messenger ribonucleic acid (mRNA), or protein analysis] defect in the *BTK* gene or BTK expression.[16]

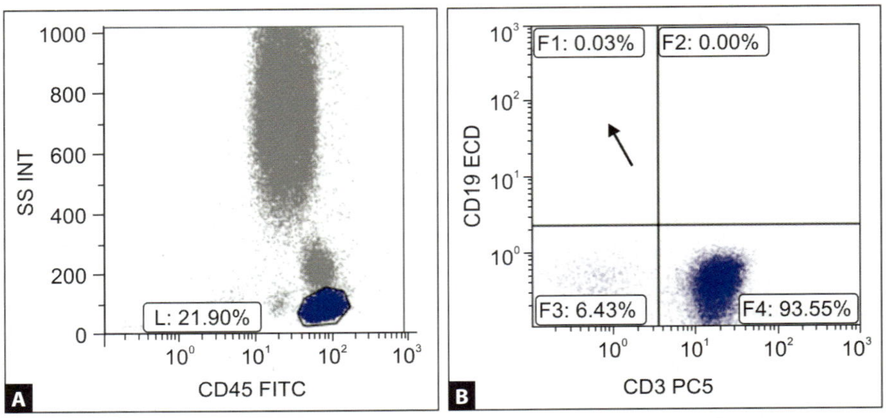

Percentage of CD3+ (T-lymphocytes) = 93.72 (N:55–78%)

Percentage of CD19+ (B-lymphocytes) = 0.03% (N:10–32%)

Figures 51.2A and B Flow cytometry results showing very low B-cell (CD 19) population; (B) Among the gated lymphocytes (blue region in A), suggestive of X-linked agammaglobulinemia

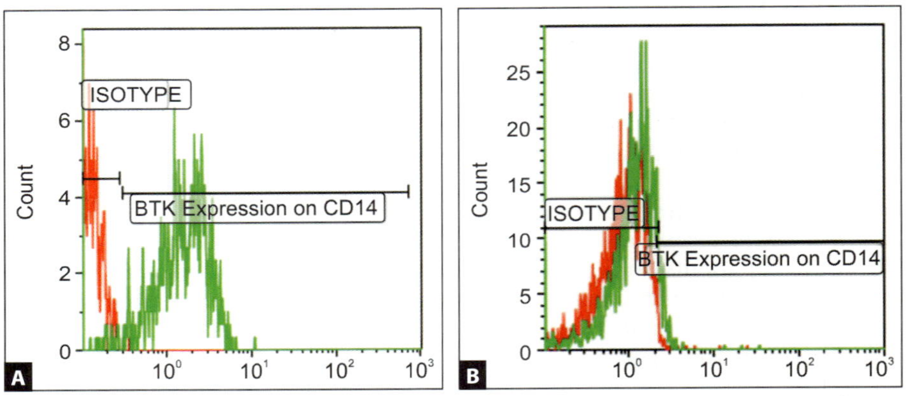

Figures 51.3A and B (A) Flow cytometry-based Bruton tyrosine kinase (BTK) protein expression in the monocytes of a normal control; (B) A case of X-linked agammaglobulinemia, where absent staining for BTK was noted in the case

A probable or possible diagnosis based upon clinical history, quantitative serum immunoglobulin levels, and response to vaccines is made if these criteria are not met, but other causes of agammaglobulinemia/hypogammaglobulinemia are ruled out. Plasma cells are generally absent in the lymphoid tissue, bone marrow and the lamina propria of the rectal mucosa.

Tests are being developed for screening of newborn babies for XLA. Studies report immunoglobulin kappa-deleting recombination excision circles (KRECs assay) to be a useful screening tool for early B-cell maturation defects. It is similar to T-cell receptor excision circles (TRECs) used to screen for T-cell defects. Dried blood spots are placed on newborn screening cards and polymerase chain reaction are performed to detect KRECs. KRECs are formed in the process of B-cell maturation during allelic exclusion and are not produced in patients with B-cell maturation defects, such as XLA.[17]

TREATMENT AND PROGNOSIS

Replacement of immunoglobulin is the cornerstone of treatment for XLA. The rationale is to provide missing antibodies, not to raise the serum IgG or IgG subclass level. The development of safe and effective immunoglobulin preparations is a major advance in the treatment of these patients. Although expensive and very difficult to sustain, especially in setting of developing countries, like ours, regular infusions of intravenous immunoglobulin can significantly alter the outcome and quality of life in these children. Most common forms of replacement therapy are either intravenous or subcutaneous immunoglobulin (IVIg or SCIg). SCIg is still not available in India. A standard initial dose of IVIg for the treatment of antibody deficient patients is 400 mg/kg (with a range of 300–500 mg/kg) every 3–4 weeks. Standard starting doses for SCIg are in the range of 100–150 mg/kg per week.

The 21 or 28 days dosing interval for intravenous infusions is based upon the half-life of IgG in the circulation, which is normally 21–22 days, although variability among individuals exists. Therapeutic levels are reached within an hour of infusion of IVIg, and consistent trough levels are usually achieved after 3–6 months of therapy. With each infusion cycle, the peak serum level is typically 2–3 times the trough level.

Dosing of both IVIg and SCIg should be adjusted based upon the patient's clinical condition. The trough serum IgG level should be monitored, but there is no single target trough level that correlates to protection from infection in all patients. Some guidelines mention that trough serum IgG levels to be maintained at least 400 mg/dL. However, some patients appear to derive clinical benefit from IVIg only at levels considerably above 700 mg/dL, especially if bronchiectasis has already set in.[18]

Patients with XLA require aggressive antibiotic therapy for any documented and/or suspected infection. In some instances, prolonged antibiotic therapy may be indicated as a treatment for ongoing pulmonary infections or chronic sinusitis. Cotrimoxazole at a dose of 5 mg/kg of trimethoprim single dose daily is usually used as a prophylactic therapy. Finally, immunizations with live viral vaccines are generally held to be contraindicated. There are no data on the safety or efficacy of other vaccines in patients with XLA. Personal hygiene and precautions, such as hand washing and avoidance of respiratory droplets must be advised. Finally, patients should avoid ingestion of untreated drinking water, if possible.

Most patients with XLA born in the last few decades and treated optimally can be expected to survive into adult life because of the improvements in initial diagnosis, immunoglobulin replacement therapy and treatment of infections. For patients who survive into adulthood, the quality of life is generally good. Adults with XLA miss more days of school or work, and they are hospitalized more frequently than males in the general population. However, most lead productive and fulfilling lives despite these limitations.[19]

AUTOSOMAL RECESSIVE HYPOGAMMAGLOBULINEMIA

There are at least six forms of genetically determined agammaglobulinemia that are caused by autosomal recessive (AR) mutations in genes contributing to the maturation and function of B-cells. These are μ heavy chain, Igα, Igβ, λ5, BLNK, CD79A and CD79B. Autosomal recessive agammaglobulinemia (ARA) should be suspected when the patient's family history is consistent with an AR pattern of inheritance, or when the patient with agammaglobulinemia is female, or when a mutation in *BTK* cannot be identified in a male with agammaglobulinemia.[20] The clinical and laboratory features of these disorders resemble those of XLA and the treatment is essentially similar.

COMMON VARIABLE IMMUNODEFICIENCY

Common variable immunodeficiency is a primary immunodeficiency disorder characterized by impaired B-cell differentiation with defective immunoglobulin production. It is the most prevalent form of severe antibody deficiency affecting both children and adults. "Variable" refers to the heterogeneous clinical manifestations of this disorder, which includes recurrent infections, chronic lung disease, autoimmune disorders, gastrointestinal disease and a heightened susceptibility to lymphoma. CVID is defined by markedly reduced serum concentrations of immunoglobulin G (IgG) in combination with low levels of IgA and/or IgM, poor or absent response to immunizations and an absence of any other defined immunodeficiency state.[16] Age of onset is also variable. Most patients are diagnosed between the ages of 20 years and 40 years. A diagnosis of CVID before age 6 years is difficult because of immunologic immaturity and the persistence of transient hypogammaglobulinemia of infancy (THI) in some children.

CLINICAL MANIFESTATIONS

Up to 73% of CVID patients (all ages) develop chronic structural pulmonary complications, including bronchiectasis and bronchial wall thickening. Other common infections include giardiasis and mycoplasma infections. Food allergy, eczema, urticaria, rhinitis, and asthma can be found in 38–83% of patients with CVID. Autoimmunity is seen in 20–25% of patients with CVID when all ages are considered together.[21] Autoimmune cytopenias are common presenting manifestations in children than adults. Autoimmune neutropenia, immune thrombocytopenia (ITP), hemolytic anemia, or combinations of these disorders (Evans syndrome) are seen. Insulin-dependent diabetes, psoriasis, systemic lupus erythematosus, rheumatoid arthritis, and juvenile idiopathic arthritis are also associated with CVID, although these are less common. Children with these diseases may be cared for in hematology, rheumatology, or endocrine clinics for a period of time before the underlying diagnosis is appreciated.[21]

Patients with CVID may develop noncaseating granulomas in the lymphoid or solid organs, including the lungs, lymph nodes, spleen, liver, intestine, brain, eyes or skin. It is estimated that 8–20% of CVID patients have some form of granulomatous disease, although the prevalence is probably underappreciated since most tissues are not biopsied. A sarcoid-like disorder with granulomatous infiltration of the liver, lungs and lymph nodes, and variable elevations in angiotensin converting enzyme (ACE) levels is recognized in CVID patients. Nodular regenerative hyperplasia of liver and idiopathic noncirrhotic portal hypertension are well described in patients with CVID.[22] In adults with CVID, the lifetime risk of malignancy has been estimated to be between 1.4% and 7%, and the most frequently diagnosed disorder is a B-cell lymphoma.[23]

defect in the production of specific functional antibodies especially to the polysaccharide antigens. The diagnosis is usually considered in adults and children above 2 years age, as younger children are normally less responsive to polysaccharide antigens. The condition may be a result of specific molecular defect or it may just represent a delayed maturation of the immune system.[34] The clinical manifestations include recurrent sinopulmonary infections due to *Streptococcus pneumoniae, Haemophilus influenzae, Moraxella catarrhalis*, or *Staphylococcus aureus.* Infections beyond the normal frequency should prompt evaluation of antibody-mediated immunity. Many patients also have atopic diseases. Polysaccharide vaccine response is assessed by measuring the protective antibody titers, as described previously in the section on CVID. Management includes prompt treatment of sinopulmonary infections. All patients with specific antibody deficiency must be vaccinated with the 13-valent conjugate pneumococcal vaccine. In patients in whom infections continue to occur despite vaccination with conjugate vaccine, management of atopic conditions and aggressive use of antibiotics during infections, administration of prophylactic antibiotics is suggested. In few patients in whom infections continue to occur despite all of the above measures, administration of immunoglobulin replacement therapy is suggested. For those patients requiring immunoglobulin replacement, interruption of therapy after 1–2 years of treatment is suggested in order to reassess the response to polysaccharide vaccine, as the condition may spontaneously improve. The prognosis in children is favorable because the condition often resolves spontaneously over time.[35]

CONCLUSION

Primary antibody deficiencies are the most common type of primary immunodeficiencies. They present with recurrent sinopulmonary and gastrointestinal bacterial infections. Autoimmune manifestations are common in CVID. Lack of functional antibodies with or without hypogammaglobulinemia is diagnostic. Replacement immunoglobulin therapy is the treatment of choice.

KEY MESSAGE

Primary antibody deficiencies are not uncommon. Clinical suspicion in patients with recurrent infections and simple laboratory tests can result in early diagnosis.

REFERENCES

1. Notarangelo L, Casanova JL, Fischer A, Puck J, Rosen F, Seger R, et al. Primary immunodeficiency diseases: an update. J Allergy Clin Immunol. 2004;114(3):677-87.
2. Ballow M. Primary immunodeficiency disorders: antibody deficiency. J Allergy Clin Immunol. 2002;109(4):581-91.
3. Wood P, Stanworth S, Burton J, Jones A, Peckham DG, Green T, et al. Recognition, clinical diagnosis and management of patients with primary antibody deficiencies: a systematic review. Clin Exp Immunol. 2007;149(3):410-23.
4. Kainulainen L, Vuorinen T, Rantakokko-Jalava K, Osterback R, Ruuskanen O. Recurrent and persistent respiratory tract viral infections in patients with primary hypogammaglobulinemia. J Allergy Clin Immunol. 2010;126(1):120-6.
5. Agarwal S, Mayer L. Pathogenesis and treatment of gastrointestinal disease in antibody deficiency syndromes. J Allergy Clin Immunol. 2009;124(4):658-64.
6. Tarzi MD, Grigoriadou S, Carr SB, Kuitert LM, Longhurst HJ. Clinical immunology review series: An approach to the management of pulmonary disease in primary antibody deficiency. Clin Exp Immunol. 2009;155(2):147-55.
7. Quartier P, Debré M, De Blic J, de Sauverzac R, Sayegh N, Jabado N, et al. Early and prolonged intravenous immunoglobulin replacement therapy in childhood agammaglobulinemia: a retrospective survey of 31 patients. J Pediatr. 1999;134(5):589-96.
8. Ochs HD, Smith CI. X-linked agammaglobulinemia: A clinical and molecular analysis. Medicine (Baltimore). 1996;75(6):287-99.
9. Vetrie D, Vorechovský I, Sideras P, Holland J, Davies A, Flinter F, et al. The gene involved in X-linked agammaglobulinaemia is a member of the src family of protein-tyrosine kinases. Nature. 1993;361(6409):226-33.
10. Conley ME, Rohrer J, Minegishi Y. X-linked agammaglobulinemia. Clin Rev Allergy Immunol. 2000;19(2):183-204.
11. Plebani A, Soresina A, Rondelli R, Amato GM, Azzari C, Cardinale F, et al. Clinical, immunological, and molecular analysis in a large cohort of patients with X-linked agammaglobulinemia: an Italian multicenter study. Clin Immunol. 2002;104(3):221-30.
12. Sarpong S, Skolnick HS, Ochs HD, Futatani T, Winkelstein JA. Survival of wild polio by a patient with XLA. Ann Allergy Asthma Immunol. 2002;88(1):59-60.
13. Halliday E, Winkelstein J, Webster AD. Enteroviral infections in primary immunodeficiency (PID): a survey of morbidity and mortality. J Infect. 2003;46(1):1-8.
14. Conley ME, Howard V. Clinical findings leading to the diagnosis of X-linked agammaglobulinemia. J Pediatr. 2002;141(4):566-71.
15. Ochs HD, Stiehm ER, Winkelstein JA. Antibody deficiencies. In: Stiehm ER, Ochs HD, Winkelstein JA (Eds). Immmunologic Disorders in Infants and Children, 5th edition. Philadelphia, PA, USA: Elsevier WB Sanders; 2004. p. 356.
16. European Society for Immunodeficiencies (ESID). 2015. [online] Available from *http://esid.org/Working-Parties/Registry/Diagnosis-criteria*. [Accessed November 2016].
17. Borte S, von Döbeln U, Fasth A, Wang N, Janzi M, Winiarski J, et al. Neonatal screening for severe primary immunodeficiency diseases using high-throughput triplex real-time PCR. Blood. 2012;119(11):2552-5.
18. Liese JG, Wintergerst U, Tympner KD, Belohradsky BH. High- vs low-dose immunoglobulin therapy in the long-term treatment of X-linked agammaglobulinemia. Am J Dis Child. 1992;146(3):335-9.
19. Howard V, Greene JM, Pahwa S, Winkelstein JA, Boyle JM, Kocak M, et al. The health status and quality of life of adults with X-linked agammaglobulinemia. Clin Immunol. 2006;118(2-3):201-8.
20. Conley ME, Rohrer J, Rapalus L, Boylin EC, Minegishi Y. Defects in early B-cell development: comparing the consequences of abnormalities in pre-BCR signaling in the human and the mouse. Immunol Rev. 2000;178:75-90.
21. Ogershok PR, Hogan MB, Welch JE, Corder WT, Wilson NW. Spectrum of illness in pediatric common variable immunodeficiency. Ann Allergy Asthma Immunol. 2006;97(5):653-6.

22. Cunningham-Rundles C, Bodian C. Common variable immunodeficiency: clinical and immunological features of 248 patients. Clin Immunol. 1999;92(1):34-48.
23. Kersey JH, Shapiro RS, Filipovich AH. Relationship of immunodeficiency to lymphoid malignancy. Pediatr Infect Dis J. 1988;7(5 Suppl):S10-2.
24. Bousfiha AA, Jeddane L, Ailal F, Al Herz W, Conley ME, Cunningham-Rundles C, et al. A phenotypic approach for IUIS PID classification and diagnosis: guidelines for clinicians at the bedside. J Clin Immunol. 2013;33(6):1078-87.
25. van de Ven AA, van de Corput L, van Tilburg CM, Tesselaar K, van Gent R, Sanders EA, et al. Lymphocyte characteristics in children with common variable immunodeficiency. Clin Immunol. 2010;135(1):63-71.
26. Piątosa B, Pac M, Siewiera K, Pietrucha B, Klaudel-Dreszler M, Heropolitańska-Pliszka E, et al. Common variable immune deficiency in children-clinical characteristics varies depending on defect in peripheral B cell maturation. J Clin Immunol. 2013;33(4):731-41.
27. Wang J, Cunningham-Rundles C. Treatment and outcome of autoimmune hematologic disease in common variable immunodeficiency (CVID). J Autoimmun. 2005;25(1):57-62.
28. Yel L. Selective IgA deficiency. J Clin Immunol. 2010;30(1):10-6.
29. Eijkhout HW, van den Broek PJ, van der Meer JW. Substitution therapy in immunodeficient patient with anti-IgA antibodies or severe adverse reactions to previous immunoglobulin therapy. Neth J Med. 2003;61(6):213-7.
30. Wilson CB, Lewis DB, Penix LA. The physiologic immunodeficiency of immaturity. In: Stiehm ER (Ed). Immunologic Disorders in Infants and Children. Philadelphia, PA, USA: WB Saunders; 1996. p. 253.
31. Doğu F, Ikincioğullari A, Babacan E. Transient hypogammaglobulinemia of infancy and early childhood: outcome of 30 cases. Turk J Pediatr. 2004;46(2):120-4.
32. Umetsu DT, Ambrosino DM, Quinti I, Siber GR, Geha RS. Recurrent sinopulmonary infection and impaired antibody response to bacterial capsular polysaccharide antigen in children with selective IgG-subclass deficiency. N Engl J Med. 1985;313(20):1247-51.
33. Moss RB, Carmack MA, Esrig S. Deficiency of IgG4 in children: association of isolated IgG4 deficiency with recurrent respiratory tract infection. J Pediatr. 1992;120(1):16-21.
34. Sanders LA, Rijkers GT, Kuis W, Tenbergen-Meekes AJ, de Graeff-Meeder BR, Hiemstra I, et al. Defective antipneumococcal polysaccharide antibody response in children with recurrent respiratory tract infections. J Allergy Clin Immunol. 1993;91(1 Pt 1):110-9.
35. Ortigas AP, Leiva LE, Moore C, Bradford N, Sorensen RU. Natural history of specific antibody deficiency after IgG replacement therapy. Ann Allergy Asthma Immunol. 1999;82:71.

CHAPTER 52

Combined Immunodeficiencies with Associated or Syndromic Features

Biman Saikia, Parvati Joshi

INTRODUCTION

Described as "Well-defined syndromes with immunodeficiency" in the 2011 International Union of Immunological Societies (IUIS) classification, this group of primary immunodeficiency disorders (PIDs) has been rechristened "combined immunodeficiencies with associated or syndromic features" in the latest 2013 IUIS classification to reflect the immunological similarity between the disorders included in "combined immunodeficiencies" without syndromic features **(Box 52.1)**.[1]

The word "syndrome" derives from the Greek σύνδρομον, meaning "concurrence". Thus, the group of diseases included under this classification have features of combined immunodeficiency (CID) that occurs in concurrence with other features, which are apparently nonimmunological and seemingly involve unrelated organ/biologic systems. Among all these diseases, the congenital thrombocytopenias, ataxia-telangiectasia (AT), hyperimmunoglobulin E (IgE) syndromes, and immunodeficiency associated with thymic defects are more likely to be clinically encountered, and hence are dealt with comparative detail.

CONGENITAL THROMBOCYTOPENIAS

Wiskott-Aldrich Syndrome

The Wiskott-Aldrich syndrome (WAS) is a rare X-linked immunodeficiency disorder characterized by a clinical triad of eczema, thrombocytopenia (with small platelets), and recurrent infections along with an associated increased risk of autoimmunity and malignancies. First described by Wiskott in 1937, the X-linked nature of the syndrome was identified by Aldrich in 1954. Another less severe X-linked disorder mainly characterized by thrombocytopenia (with small platelets) and a bleeding tendency known as X-linked thrombocytopenia (XLT) described for the first time by Wooley in 1956, was identified as a variant of WAS by Canales in 1967. The pathophysiology of both WAS and XLT remained uncertain for a long time till Derry et al. cloned the WASP gene in 1994. Identification of the molecular defect has now broadened the clinical spectrum of WAS to include chronic or intermittent XLT (now considered a relatively mild form of WAS with less severe eczema if present and normal immunological functions) and X-linked neutropenia caused by a mutation in the GTPase binding domain of the WAS gene causing arrest of myelopoiesis.[2] The latter in the IUIS classification is however classified under "congenital defects of phagocyte number, function or both".

Structural and Functional Aspects of Wiskott-Aldrich Syndrome Protein

Wiskott-Aldrich syndrome and XLT are allelic diseases caused by mutations of the Wiskott-Aldrich syndrome protein (WASP) gene located on the short arm of chromosome Xp11.2-11.3, which codes for the *WASP* protein of 502 amino acids, and expressed exclusively in the cells of the hematopoietic system. It is a member of a growing family of proteins involved in cytoskeletal rearrangement, namely actin nucleation and polymerization in response to cell activation stimuli.

At a cellular level, WASP plays a role in the formation of immunological synapses. In addition, WASP regulates the production of cell protrusions (podosomes, filopods and lamellipods), which play a key role in chemotaxis, chemokinesis and cell transport and therefore have major effects on the hematopoietic system. T-cells in WAS have stubby protrusions, impaired CD3 mediated proliferative responses, delayed and less sustained calcium flow following cell activation and defects in immunological synapse formation. As a result, natural killer (NK) cells display reduced cytotoxicity and major migration defects are observed in macrophages and dendritic cells.

Molecular Genetics of Wiskott-Aldrich Syndrome and X-linked Thrombocytopenia

Wiskott-Aldrich syndrome protein gene mutations can impair all or part of the protein's expression and function.

Box 52.1 Classification of the combined immunodeficiencies with associated or syndromic features according to International Union of Immunological Societies (IUIS) 2013 classification[1]

- Congenital thrombocytopenias
  - Wiskott-Aldrich syndrome
  - WIP deficiency
- DNA repair defects
  - Ataxia-telangiectasia
  - Ataxia-telangiectasia like disease
  - Nijmegen breakage syndrome
  - Bloom syndrome
  - Immunodeficiency with centromeric instability and facial anomalies (ICF 1) due to DNMT3B defects
  - Immunodeficiency with centromeric instability and facial anomalies (ICF 2) due to ZBTB24 defects
  - PMS2 deficiency
  - RNF16B deficiency
  - MCM4 deficiency
- Thymic defects with additional congenital anomalies
  - DiGeorge anomaly
  - CHARGE syndrome
- Immune-osseous dysplasia
  - Cartilage hair hypoplasia
  - Schimke syndrome
- Hyper-IgE syndromes (HIES)
  - AD-HIES (Job's syndrome)
  - Tyk2 deficiency
  - DOCK8 deficiency
- Dyskeratosis congenital (DKC)
  - XL-DKC
  - AR-DKC due to NHP2 deficiency
  - AR-DKC due to NOP10 deficiency
  - AR-DKC due to RTEL1 deficiency
  - AD-DKC due to TERC deficiency
  - AD-DKC due to TERT deficiency
  - AD-DKC due to TINF2 deficiency
- Defects of vitamin B_{12} and folate metabolism
  - TCN2 deficiency
  - SLC46A1 deficiency
  - MTHFD1 deficiency
- Comèl-Netherton syndrome
- Winged-helix deficiency
- ORAI-I deficiency
- STIM1 deficiency
- STA5b deficiency
- Hepatic veno-occlusive disease with immunodeficiency
- IKAROS deficiency
- FILS syndrome
- Immunodeficiency with multiple intestinal atresias

Abbreviations: AD, autosomal dominant; AR, autosomal recessive; XLI, X-linked inheritance

There is growing evidence that the severity of impaired protein expression is directly correlated to the severity of the clinical phenotype. In particular, missense mutations in exons 1 and 2 (which usually diminish but do not suppress protein expression) are associated with a mild phenotype, i.e. XLT. Splicing mutations to donor and acceptor splice sites, especially outside the conserved positions (–2, –1, +1, +2), may also lead to low levels of protein expression resulting in mild or moderate clinical phenotypes. Conversely, nonsense mutations or mutations impairing the reading frame of the RNA messenger, abolish or radically reduce protein expression and tend to be associated with a severe clinical phenotype.

Epidemiology and Clinical Phenotype

The incidence of WAS is estimated to be anywhere between 1 million and 10 million. Recent reports, however, suggest that this may be an underestimation as the phenotype of the disorder is much broader than recognized. The classical triad of eczema, thrombocytopenia (with microthrombocytes) and immune deficiency is found in less than one-third of all patients. Approximately, 5% present with infections, whereas about in 20% of cases, the only clinical manifestation can be bleeding. Microthrombocytes though pathognomonic, however, may not be a universal feature[3] and mutation proven cases of WAS without microthrombocytes have been documented. A series of WAS patients with two novel mutations have been reported from India.

Bleeding: Severe bleeding is common and occurs earlier in patients who have a defect in protein expression compared to patients with XLT where protein expression is spared.[4] The average incidence of bleeding before diagnosis is more than 80% and manifest as petechiae and ecchymoses in most cases.[5] Around 30% patients present with severe bleeding episodes,[5] like hematemesis and melena may manifest as bloody diarrhea in newborns and infants. Intracranial bleeding is uncommon but constitutes a major risk. The severity of bleeding is closely linked to the severity of thrombocytopenia and can be the cause of death in 4–20% of patients.

Infections: Wiskott-Aldrich syndrome results in susceptibility to a wide variety of bacterial, viral as well as fungal infectious pathogens but despite this, infectious complications as a sole first manifestation of WAS is uncommon and occurs in less than 5% of cases.[5] Patients are susceptible to encapsulated bacteria because of the impaired capability of patients to produce IgG2 antibodies, the major immunoglobulin subclass produced against polysaccharide antigens. Upper airway infections are common, but invasive infections viz meningitis and sepsis are also common and caused mainly by encapsulated bacteria. Herpes simplex 1 and 2 may cause recurrent severe and/or disseminated infections (6% of cases). *Molluscum contagiosum* and *verrucas* are common and often difficult to treat. In addition, candida or other fungal infections are encountered. Opportunistic infections such as *Pneumocystis carinii* have also been reported and tend to arise during the disease following diagnosis and seldom in the early months of life. Otitis media (64% of cases) and pneumonia (25% of cases) are frequent.[5]

Eczema: Eczema affects 80% of WAS patients, is more common in the first 2 years of life and tends to subside over time. Incidence of eczema in XLT patients is variable, but its occurrence is usually mild and lasts for shorter periods of time. Eczema is often observed, but not always associated with raised total IgE serum levels.

Autoimmunity: Autoimmunity is one of the most common and most significant complications of WAS and manifests in the form of autoimmune hemolytic anemia, cutaneous vasculitis (including the Schönlein-Henoch syndrome), nephropathies and arthritis, which together account for more than 80% of autoimmune manifestations. Recent emphasis has also been put on chronic inflammatory bowel disease and postsplenectomy idiopathic thrombocytopenia purpura among the autoimmune events arising in WAS.

Malignancy: Reported incidence of malignancy in WAS varies from 10% to 13% with an average age at diagnosis of 9.5 years.[5] Malignancies comprise of leukemias, myelodysplasia and lymphomas in 90% of cases, highlighting the role of the WASP protein in regulating the differentiation and function of blood elements.

Laboratory Parameters

The only consistent laboratory abnormality encountered in the WAS/XLT is thrombocytopenia with microthrombocytes. Thrombocytopenia tends to be chronic and the platelets count is usually below 70,000/μL. Rare cases present periodically low platelet counts interspersed with normal counts (X-linked intermittent thrombocytopenia). Platelet volume is typically reduced and is usually less than 5 fL (normal: 7–10 fL).

In addition, significant lymphopenia (<1,000/μL) is found in 22% of WAS patients, whereas eosinophilia (>500 eosinophils/μL) is seen in 31% of cases.[6] Anemia is common and is caused by microbleeds or autoimmune events. Average erythrocyte size is also reduced similar to what occurs in platelets.

Serum IgM levels may be reduced with elevated IgA and IgE. A significant number of WAS subjects, however, show normal or even raised IgM values, the latter being a risk factor for the development of autoimmunity. Patients have low isohemagglutinin levels and are unable to produce antibodies against polysaccharide antigens, like pneumococcal vaccine, which may account for the increased incidence of invasive infections by encapsulated bacteria. The immunological changes are however inconstant—13% of WAS patient (and most XLT subjects) having normal isohemagglutinin levels, while up to 31% of patients produce antipolysaccharide antibodies.

Wiskott-Aldrich syndrome protein expression can be easily assessed using flow cytometry[7] where lymphocytes from WAS patients show WASP^{dim} instead of WASP^{bright} populations. In addition, carrier detection by using monocytes, which is a better indicator of WASP^{dim} population detection, has also been aptly demonstrated.[8] If the flow cytometry analysis of WASP expression is normal, further testing should be dictated by the clinical suspicion of the diagnosis. For those cases in which the diagnosis is still under consideration, sequencing of the WAS gene is required.

Clinical Classification of Wiskott-Aldrich Syndrome X-linked Thrombocytopenia

A WAS disease severity scoring system[4] facilitates the clinical categorization of patients. A score of 1 or 2 defines patients with XLT, a score of 3 to 4 identifies patients with classic WAS, and a score of 5 is reserved for patients with either XLT or WAS who develop autoimmunity and/or malignancies.[4]

WASP Interacting Protein Deficiency

In T-lymphocytes, WASP is almost totally complexed with the WASP-interacting protein (WIP), which functions to stabilize WASP and prevent its degradation. It has been observed in WIP deficient mice that the WASP protein levels are severely compromised but WASP mRNA levels are normal. Langi G et al.[9] in 2012 reported an 11 days old female patient who presented with features of WAS but had reduced WASP protein, normal WASP mRNA levels and had no mutations in the WASP gene, features highly suggestive of WASP instability. WIP protein expression was also undetectable and a homozygous c.1301C more than G stop codon mutation was found in the *WIPF1 gene*, which encodes WIP.[9] Autosomal recessive (AR) WIP deficiency hence should be suspected, especially in female patients who present with typical features of WAS, or in boys with typical features of WAS but without a demonstrable mutation and normal WASP mRNA levels. Both WASP and WIP expression can be investigated by flow cytometric assays.[10]

DNA Repair Defects

Ataxia-telangiectasia is an AR disease characterized by progressive cerebellar ataxia, dysarthria, oculomotor dyspraxia, oculocutaneous telangiectasia and immune deficiency with associated chromosomal instability and increased sensitivity to ionizing radiation (IR), leading to increased susceptibility to malignancies, especially lymphomas and leukemais. Mutations in the ATM (AT mutated) gene located on chromosome 11 are responsible for majority of the cases of AT. The *ATM* gene codes for the ATM protein, which is a member of the phosphatidylinositol 3-kinase family, and is involved in numerous pathways including cell cycle checkpoint control and DNA double-stand break repair.

Patients present commonly in early childhood. Classical forms of AT are associated with truncating mutations of the *ATM* gene, resulting in undetectable functional ATM kinase. A milder form of the disease with less severe neurological features and progression and milder immune deficiency is observed in patients where some residual kinase activity is preserved.

Immune deficiency in AT patients is highly variable, seen in up to 71% of patients with evidence of CID, consisting of cellular/thymic defects in conjunction with humoral defects. Early postmortem studies on thymus morphology in AT revealed the presence of an embryonic thymus. In a more recent study, immune deficiency in AT has been suggested to be a result of premature ageing of the immune system.

The immune defects associated with AT include low total immunoglobulin levels (IgG/IgA or IgM), low IgG2, defective polysaccharide antibody responses and lymphopenia. Patients with AT often suffer from frequent respiratory tract infections, which may lead to pulmonary insufficiency. Serum levels of alpha fetoprotein (AFP) are typically raised. About 10% of children with AT present with decreased levels of IgG and A, and a normal or increased IgM due to defect in immunoglobulin isotype switching.[11] This might lead to a misdiagnosis of hyper-IgM syndrome until patients develop characteristic ocular telangiectasia and gait abnormalities.[11] Lymphopenia affects CD4+ cells, although T-cell function is preserved and B-cell numbers are commonly reduced. In a study by Azarsiz E et al.[12] low IgG was found in 45%, low IgA in 65% and elevated IgM in 60% of patients. CD3+CD4+ T-lymphocyte frequency was low in 45% patients. Thymic output, evaluated by measuring T-cell receptor (TCR) excision circle-positive T cells, is low; the peripheral T-cell population is characterized by a bias toward terminally differentiated effector cells reflected by a low ratio of naïve to memory T-cells.

Ataxia Telangiectasia-like Disorder

The AT-like disorder is an extremely rare disorder with clinical features similar to those in patients having AT with progressive cerebellar ataxia that is of later onset and slower progression than of AT. There is absence of telangiectasia and AFP is not raised. The gene defect lies in *hMRE11,* which encodes for a protein that associates in the hMre11/hRad50/Nbs1 protein complex.[13] Patients have features overlapping with both AT and Nijmegen breakage syndrome (NBS). Immunoglobulin levels seem normal, although deficiency in specific function antibodies has been reported, particularly to pneumococcal polysaccharide antigen.

Nijmegen Breakage Syndrome

Nijmegen breakage syndrome is a rare AR disease, which presents at birth with microcephaly. Other important clinical features include "bird-like" facies, short stature, mild growth delay, premature ovarian insufficiency and predisposition to recurrent infections of various organs and a very high risk to develop hematological malignancies at an early age. These manifestations develop with age. Patients however do not exhibit neurological abnormalities, telangiectasia, or increased alpha-fetoprotein levels observed in AT patients.[14] CID of both the cellular and humoral response is an essential feature of the disease. Chromosomal instability with characteristic rearrangements in peripheral T lymphocytes in the form of inversions and translocations involving chromosomes 7 and 14, and cellular sensitivity to IR *in vitro* are all characteristic for the disease and have diagnostic relevance. Identifying mutations in both alleles of the NBN gene (formerly NBS1) complete the diagnosis of NBS.

Bloom Syndrome

Bloom syndrome (BS) first described in 1954, is a rare AR disorder caused by mutations in the *BLM* gene at 15q26.1,[15] which encodes a RecQ helicase that plays a pivotal role in DNA repair and recombination. Gene cluster instability and sister chromatid exchange (SCE; homologous recombination associated with crossover) is increased during mitotic recombination in patients with BS. The disorder is characterized by growth deficiency, which leads to short stature, sun sensitive erythema of face resembling lupus, infertility and increased risk of cancer. There is evidence of immunodeficiency in form of hypogammaglobulinemia (IgM, IgG, IgA), which predominantly lead to recurrent sinopulmonary infections. Patients with BS have a predisposition to the early development of cancer due to genetic instability. A male dominance despite being an AR disorder (male ~53% and female ~47%, according to data from the Bloom syndrome registry of 2009) suggests the presence of a gene other than *BLM*, probably on the X chromosome.[16]

Immunodeficiency with Centromeric Instability and Facial Anomalies due to DNMT3B and ZBTB24 Defects

Immunodeficiency with centromeric instability and facial anomalies (ICF) syndrome is a rare AR disorder that is characterized by immunodeficiency, intellectual deficit, and mild facial dysmorphism with rearrangement in juxtracentromeric chromosome 1, 9 and 16. Facial dysmorphisms may include a round face, flat nasal bridge, hypertelorism, epicanthus, upturned nose, macroglossia, micrognathia and low-set ears. ICF 1 (60% of the cases) and 2 (40%) are caused by biallelic mutations in the DNA methyltransferase 3B gene (DNMT3B) and in the zinc-finger-and BTB-domain containing 24 gene *ZBTB24* respectively.[17] Recently mutations in the cell division cycle associated 7 (CDCA7) and the helicase, lymphoid-specific (*HELLS*) genes have been demonstrated in 10 unexplained ICF cases.[18] Most patients with ICF syndrome die of infection at a young age, usually in the first or second decade of life. Development of a combined immune defect throughout the disease course as well as putative autoimmune phenomena such as granulomatous hepatitis and nephritis has also been observed.[19]

The pattern of immunodeficiency in ICF is variable with agammaglobulinemia to hypogammaglobulinemia with normal to mildly decreased B cells. An increased proportion of circulating immature B cells and a lack of memory cells with B cells being more prone to undergo apoptosis upon in vitro activation have been reported. Interestingly, activation, differentiation and immunoglobulin class-switch recombination appear normal. T-cell levels may be normal or mildly reduced with normal proliferative responses. However, opportunistic infections with Pneumocystis and Candida albicans occur in several ICF patients irrespective of the group pointing to a functional T-cell defect. The humoral immunodeficiency is generally more pronounced in ICF1 patients, B- and T-cell compartments are both involved in ICF1 and ICF2. ICF2 patients have a significantly higher incidence of intellectual disability, congenital malformations can be observed in some ICF1 and ICF2 cases.[20]

PMS2 Deficiency

PMS2 deficiency is another rare AR disorder caused by mutation in *PMS2* resulting in defect in class switch recombination due to impaired mismatch repair. The syndrome is characterized by recurrent infections, café-au-lait spots, lymphoma, colorectal carcinoma and brain tumor. There is deficiency of switched and nonswitched B cells. IgG and IgA levels are low while IgM level is often elevated or normal.[21]

RNF16B Deficiency

Recently, RIDDLE (radiosensitivity, immunodeficiency, dysmorphic features and learning difficulties) syndrome, a novel human immunodeficiency disorder associated with defective double-strand break (DSB) repair, has been described. This is caused by mutations in *RNF168*. There is hypogammaglobulinemia in form of low level of IgA and IgG.[22]

MCM4 Deficiency

MCM4, which encodes a component of the MCM2-7 helicase complex, is required for DNA replication. A splice-site mutation in the patients causes genomic instability and is characterized by hypocortisolemia. Affected children show signs of growth failure, increased chromosomal breakage and selective NK cell deficiency. T and B cell levels are usually normal.[23,24]

Thymic Defects with Additional Congenital Anomalies

DiGeorge syndrome (DGS) first reported by Dr Angelo M DiGeorge in 1965 classically comprises T-cell deficiency (due to thymic hypoplasia resulting from a failure in development of the pharyngeal arch), hypoparathyroidism, cardiac malformations and facial abnormalities. Subsequently, it was recognized that deletion of the long arm of chromosome 22 at position q.11 was associated with DGS.[25] This deletion presents with a variety of phenotypes, including DGS and Velocardiofacial syndrome. CATCH22 (cardiac abnormality/abnormal facies, T-cell deficit due to thymic hypoplasia, cleft palate, hypocalcemia due to hypoparathyroidism resulting from 22q11 deletion) was proposed as a collective acronym for these differing presentations of a common genetic etiology. 22q11 deletion syndrome (22q11DS) is an umbrella term that describes all these various clinical phenotypes. The 3 Mb chromosomal region contains more than 35 genes, of which *TBX1* is the most important and most well characterized and implicated gene for 22q11DS.

DiGeorge syndrome may be associated with a complete range of T-cell deficiency from normal T-cell numbers and function to complete DGS (cDGS) with a T-negative severe combined immunodeficiency (T^-B^+SCID)-like picture. The term partial DGS (pDGS) is used to designate patients with incomplete and less severe forms of T-cell immunodeficiency. The proportion of affected individuals falling into the cDGS category is less and majority of individuals would be classified as pDGS. In the typical form of cDGS, the T-cell numbers are less than 50/mm^3 and mitogen responses are absent. B cells are usually present in normal numbers and NK cells are normal or high.[26]

Despite the low-for-age T-cell counts in most patients during infancy, the counts usually improve during the 1st year of life. Antibody deficiencies (hypogammaglobulinemia) have also been described in a minority of patients, most commonly IgA deficiency. An increased frequency of infections, mainly respiratory tract infections are observed, but the frequency commonly diminishes with increasing age. An increased prevalence of autoimmune conditions has been reported in both children and adults with 22q11DS.

CHARGE syndrome (coloboma, heart defects, atresia choanae, retarded growth and development, genital hypoplasia and ear abnormalities) is characterized by multiple malformations and is diagnosed using distinct consensus criteria. Although *SEMA3E* was the first gene to be implicated, mutations in the gene encoding chromodomain helicase DNA-binding protein 7 (CHD7) is the major cause of CHARGE syndrome.[27] Clinical features of CHARGE syndrome considerably overlap those of 22q11.2 deletion syndrome. The severity of immunodeficiencies in patients with CHARGE syndrome ranges from mild-to-severe T-lymphocyte deficiency and isolated humoral immunodeficiency, which is similar to that in patients with 22q11.2 deletion syndrome. Most patients with CHARGE syndrome have decreased number and poorly functional T-lymphocytes.[26]

Immune-osseous Dysplasia

The osteochondrodysplasias are a heterogeneous group of inherited disorders of skeletal growth causing disproportionate short stature.

Cartilage Hair Hypoplasia

Cartilage hair hypoplasia (CHH) is a rare metaphyseal chondrodysplasia characterized by short stature and short limbs caused by mutations in the *RMRP* gene located on chromosome 9p13.3. The disorder has several characteristic orthopedic manifestations, including joint laxity, limited elbow extension, ankle varus and genu varum. Immunodeficiency is of concern in most cases[28] associated with a broad spectrum of mild-to-moderate, cell-mediated immune dysfunction, occasionally manifesting as SCID, neutropenia, lymphopenia, disordered erythrogenesis and a predisposition to lymphoma. Recurrent infections are commonly seen in 60% of patients. Individuals can have marked impairment of T-lymphocyte function due to an intrinsic defect in cell proliferation. Morbidity and mortality to varicella is clearly increased in CHH, but there is no apparent increase in susceptibility to severe or fatal infections with other viruses. Morbidity and mortality are directly related to immune dysfunction. The presence of infections, particularly in the first 2 years of life in children, is increased in frequency and hematologic malignancy, most commonly non-Hodgkin lymphoma is increased in adults together with an excess risk of basal cell carcinoma.[29] Anemia is also common and significantly correlates with the severity of immunodeficiency and growth failure.

Schimke immuno-osseous dysplasia (SIOD) is an AR multisystem osteochondrodysplasia, characterized by dysmorphism, prominent spondyloepiphyseal dysplasia, T-cell immunodeficiency and nephrotic syndrome.[30] Approximately 80% of patients with SIOD have lymphopenia, which is predominantly due to a deficiency of CD4+ T cells, whereas B-cell counts and immunoglobulin levels are usually normal. Half of these patients develop recurrent opportunistic infections.[31] Biallelic mutations in SWI/SNF-related, matrix-associated, actin-dependent regulator of chromatin, subfamily a-like 1 (SMARCAL1) are the only identified cause of SIOD, but approximately half of patients do not have detectable mutations in SMARCAL1.[32]

HYPERIMMUNOGLOBULIN E SYNDROMES

The hyper-IgE syndrome (HIES) is an exceedingly rare, complex immunoregulatory disorder characterized clinically by raised serum IgE, recurrent bacterial infections and chronic eczematoid dermatitis usually manifesting itself early in life. It is clinically a triad of high serum levels of IgE (>2,000 IU/mL), recurring staphylococcal skin abscesses, and pneumonia with *pneumatocele* formation. Coarse facies, mild eosinophilia, lymphomas, cryptococcal meningitis, neutrophil chemotactic dysfunction, and mucocutaneous or systemic fungal disease are other variable features. Both autosomal dominant (AD) and AR forms of the disease have been identified with skeletal manifestations being a feature of the former and not seen in the latter whereas viral infections and neurologic manifestations are a feature of the AR-HIES. Patients with AD-HIES have characteristic features based on which the National Institute of Health (NIH) scoring has been devised.

History

Davis, Schaller and Wedgwood first coined the term Job's syndrome in 1966. The syndrome was further defined and clarified by Buckley et al. in 1972, who noted infectious problems in two boys with severe dermatitis characteristic facies and elevated IgE levels leading to the term Buckley's syndrome.

Clinical Features

The clinical features of HIES encompass the immune system, connective tissue, skeletal, and dental development with variations in the severity of the symptoms. The most common clinical features are eczema, recurrent skin abscesses, pneumonia with *pneumatocele* formation, mucocutaneous candidiasis, elevated serum IgE and eosinophilia. Pneumonias and skin abscesses are mainly caused by *Staphylococcus aureus*, *Streptococcus pneumoniae*, or *Haemophilus influenzae*. The *pneumatocele* that typically follows the resolution of cured bacterial pneumonias is frequently superinfected by *Pseudomonas aeruginosa* and *Aspergillus fumigatus*. The most common opportunistic infection in HIES is mucocutaneous candidiasis. Mucocutaneous fungal disease can be seen in up to 43–85% of HIES including 64% of patients with oral candidiasis during the neonatal period.[33-35] Mycobacterial infections, though reported, are not a common feature observed in HIES.[36-39]

Patients with AD and sporadic forms of the disease have facial abnormalities including *ocular hypertelorism, a prominent, protruding, triangular mandible, prominent forehead, deep set eyes, broad nasal bridge and a somewhat bulbous nose with increased interalar distance*. The facial skin appears coarse and exhibits prominent pores. The affected members look different from the other family members. Recurrent pathological fractures occur in about half of the patients and affect mainly the long bones, pelvic bones and ribs rather than the spine. Scoliosis is seen in about two-thirds of patients, but the reasons for this are complex. Craniosynostosis has been reported in HIES but is much less common than the other skeletal features.

Anomalies in dentinogenesis are consistent features of HIES. *Reduced resorption of primary tooth roots* is thought to lead to prolonged retention of primary teeth, which in turn prevents the appropriate eruption of permanent teeth, or *retention of both sets of teeth is common*. About 72% of the patients with the HIES who were older than 8 years reported *retained primary teeth, noneruption of permanent teeth, or double row of teeth* where permanent teeth erupted adjacent to primary teeth.

Ophthalmologic pathologies such as extensive xanthelasma, giant chalazia, undefined tumors of the eyelid, strabismus and several malignancies, especially lymphomas, have been observed in HIES patients. Recent reports include anaplastic large cell lymphoma, peripheral T-cell lymphoma and a pulmonary adenocarcinoma.

Genetics

Although first described in Caucasians with red hair, HIES occurs in all ethnic groups and almost equally in both genders. Most pedigrees of HIES families are consistent with an AD inheritance. The pathogenesis of HIES remained unknown till 2007 when mutations in *STAT3* (signal transducer and activator of transcription 3) were documented in patients with AD and sporadic forms of HIES by two investigating groups simultaneously.[40,41] Before this in 2006, a mutation in *TYK2* was demonstrated in a single patient of AR form of the disease from Japan.[42] STAT3-related HIES with novel mutations have also been reported from India.[43] Tyk2 functions upstream of STAT3, and hence involvement of these two molecules in the same cellular pathway further consolidated its pathogenesis.

STAT 3 in Hyper-IgE Syndrome

The janus kinase (JAK): Signal transducer and activator of transcription (STAT) signaling pathway has emerged over the past decade as a major relay between cell-surface receptors and cytokine responses. *STAT3* mutation is the predominant cause of sporadic and familial HIES, although other genomic loci may also be involved. Remarkably, only heterozygous missense mutations (predicted to affect the DNA-binding or SH2 domain) were detected, suggesting either haploinsufficiency or dominant negative mechanisms. The DNA binding domain of STAT3 is located between exon 10 and exon 16 and the SH2 domain is located between exon 20 and exon 21A. Consistent with a dominant negative mode of action, mutations within segments encoding the DNA-binding domain resulted in a protein with an impaired ability to target promoter DNA sequences and induce the expression of relevant genes. Mutations affecting the SH2 domain led to similar reductions in target-gene expression, although a dominant negative mechanism for these mutations is more difficult to envisage.

Tyrosine Kinase 2 Deficiency in Hyper-IgE Syndrome

Tyrosine kinase 2 (TYK2) is a nonreceptor tyrosine kinase that belongs to the JAK family. JAKs are critical for cytokine signaling. Mutation of *JAK3* is known to cause primary immunodeficiency. A homozygous mutation in the *TYK2* is associated with a variant form of AR-HIES. This genetic cause of HIES was identified in 2006 in a single patient, which is a null recessive mutation in *TYK2*. A homozygous four base-pair deletion in the coding region of the *TYK 2* gene in a HIES patient has been identified.[42]

DOCK8 Deficiency and Hyper-IgE Syndrome

A form of AR-HIES with the usual triad of HIES but complicated by recurrent cutaneous viral infections and resultant cancers with involvement of the central nervous system and without connective tissue and bone abnormalities has been described and now been associated with dedicator of cytogenesis 8 protein (DOCK8) mutations discovered in 2009.[44] The cutaneous viral infections are extensive, difficult to control and often occur concurrently. The most common viruses are herpes simplex virus (HSV), human papillomavirus (HPV), molluscum contagiosum and varicella-zoster virus (VZV). Chronic orolabial or ulcerative anogenital HSV infections as well as herpes simplex keratitis and eczema herpeticum are typically observed. Patients often have disfiguring flat and verrucous warts from HPV infection. Some observers indicate clinical overlaps of DOCK8 deficiency with CID and it has been shown lately that many of the patients that were initially thought to be DOCK8-associated AR-HIES are actually cases of CID. The DOCK8-associated phenotype, however, clinically very distinct unlikely to be confused with usual form of HIES.

Immunopathology of Hyper-IgE Syndrome

Hyper-IgE syndrome patients with mutated *STAT3* have been shown to have impaired development of Th17 cells and interleukin-17 (IL-17) production and this defect in the STAT3-IL-17 axis is the major pathogenic mechanism of the defective immunity against extracellular bacterial pathogens. The most recent model proposes that TGF-β and IL-6 initially drive the expression of IL-21 in a STAT3-dependent manner. STAT3 is involved in the signal transduction of many cytokines, including but not limited to IL-6, IL-10, IL-21, IL-22, and IL-23, and plays an integral role in wound healing, angiogenesis, cancer and immunity. It is an essential mediator of the immunosuppressive action of IL-10, and the loss of responsiveness of this IL may underlie much of the proinflammatory nature of the hyper-IgE syndrome.

Impaired CD19+CD27+ memory B-cell responses and decreased CD8+ cytotoxic T-cell numbers have also been documented.

Laboratory Findings in Hyper-IgE Syndrome

Serum IgE and absolute eosinophil count: Serum IgE levels from 10,000 to as high as more than 100,000 IU/mL are characteristic of HIES, but the levels are not static. Most HIES patients have eosinophilia at least 2 SDs above the normal (usually more than 700 cells/mL). However, there is no correlation between eosinophilia and IgE levels or eosinophilia and infectious complications of HIES. Total white blood cell counts are typically in the normal range when no infection is present, and they often fail to elevate even in the setting of acute infection. The eosinophilia is more severe in AR-HIES patients than in AD-HIES patients with values up to 17,500/mL (normal <700).

TH-17 cell numbers and IL-17 assessment: TH-17 cell numbers assessment requires peripheral blood mononuclear cells (PBMCs) to be stimulated for 6 hours with 10 ng/mL phorbol-12-myristate 13- acetate (PMA) and 1 μg/mL ionomycin in the presence of 10 μg/mL Golgi blocker. After cell surface staining with anti-CD4, cells are fixed, permeabilized and stained with anti-IL-17A and anti-IFN-γ, the latter as a control for cellular activation and intracellular staining. The threshold value of normal TH-17 cell numbers expressed as a percentage of CD4+ IL-17+ T cells as determined in healthy adult control subjects is set as greater than 0.6% with a range of 0.6–2.84 (mean 1.58 ± 0.72 and median 1.63) in the Indian population.[43]

Assessment of IL-17 by enzyme-linked immunosorbent assay (ELISA) can be done on the stimulation culture supernatants. Serum IL-17 is usually inadequate for assessment. Reduced memory B-cell numbers (CD19+CD27+) is another consistent finding of HIES. Reduced CD8+ cytotoxic T-cell has also been reported.

Phopho-STAT3: STAT3 phosphorylation assessed on flow cytometry using antityrosine 705 phosphorylated STAT3 (pY705-STAT3) mAb has been shown to be reduced in SH2 domain mutations whereas with mutations in the DNA binding domain, STAT3 phosphorylation is often normal. Mutations in the transactivation domain, which primarily affect the phosphorylation site, are likely to affect phosphorylation of STAT3 to a greater extent.[43]

Mutation studies: Patients with AD and sporadic forms of HIES have characteristic features based on which the NIH scoring has been devised.[45] Patients with higher NIH score, typically more than 40 are more likely to harbor a mutation in *STAT3* and hence can be subjected to mutation analysis. In AR forms of HIES, mutations in *TYK2* and *DOCK8* are advocated.

Dyskeratosis Congenita

Dyskeratosis congenita (DC) is a rare hereditary disorder characterized by bone marrow failure, cancer predisposition (11-fold increase compared to general population), ectodermal dysplasia (oral leukoplakia, abnormal skin pigmentation and nail dystrophy) and other additional somatic abnormalities.[46] Bone marrow failure ensues in around 85% of cases and is responsible for 80% of the observed mortality.

Defects in seven unique genes, all involved in telomere maintenance, have been associated with DC: *DKC1* (X-linked); *NOP10*, *TCAB1*, and *NHP2* (AR); and *TERT*, *TERC* and *TINF2* (AD). Mutations in these genes, however, account for only 50% of all patients with the clinical phenotype of DC.[46] DC patients carrying mutations in these genes possess critically short telomeres and an abnormal DNA damage response, causing selective exhaustion of cells in tissues with rapid turnover such as the bone marrow. Approximately 30% of the leukoplakic areas progress to develop squamous cell carcinoma in 10–30 years.[46]

DKC1 mutation is responsible for X-linked DC. The majority of patients with *DKC1* mutations have a classic DC phenotype, but a subgroup of *DKC1* mutations is associated with the Hoyeraal-Hreidarsson syndrome. This phenotype is characterized by growth retardation of prenatal onset, microcephaly, cerebellar hypoplasia, aplastic anemia and immunodeficiency. There is progressive decrease in T- and B-cells with variable deficiency of serum immunoglobulin.[47]

DEFECTS OF VITAMIN B_{12} AND FOLATE METABOLISM

Folate and vitamin B_{12} metabolism are essential for de novo purine synthesis, and several defects in these pathways have been associated with immunodeficiency.

In transcobalamin II deficiency, neutropenia is thought to be the primary cause of recurrent bacterial infections, although infection with opportunistic agents such as pneumocystis jirovecii pneumonia has also been described.[48]

A SCID-like phenotype is associated with functional methionine synthase deficiency, with lymphopenia and severe bacterial and viral infections.[49]

Hereditary folate malabsorption resulting from deficiency in the proton coupled folate transporter (PCFT) has similarly been linked with a SCID phenotype with severe opportunistic infections and was shown to be responsive to folate replacement therapy.[50]

Deficiency of methyl tetrahydrofolate dehydrogenase 1 (MTHFD1) represents a new form of SCID resulting from a defect in folate metabolism. Like PCFT, a beneficial response was seen with replacement of the depleted vitamins.[51]

Although uncommon, these defects collectively illustrate the range of metabolic causes of immunodeficiency and the importance of early treatment to minimize neurologic injury and/or opportunistic infections.

Comèl-Netherton Syndrome

Rare AR disorder belonging to the group of inherited ichthyoses is characterized by congenital ichthyosiform dermatitis with defective cornification, atopic diathesis with high serum IgE levels and trichorrhexis invaginata. Genetic mutation causing Netherton syndrome is located within the *SPINK5* gene on chromosome 5q32. Hyperimmunoglobulinemia E, high levels of complements (C3/C4) and a reduced number of NK cells make the patients susceptible for recurrent infections and allergic reactions, like angioedema, hay fever and food allergies.[52]

Winged-Helix Deficiency (Nude)

Autosomal recessive disorder caused by defect in *FOXN1* gene. Mutations in *FOXN1* lead to athymia together with total alopecia. A significant reduction in number of circulating T-cells with impaired T-cell maturation is found.[53]

Calcium-release Activated Calcium Channel Defect: ORAI1 and STIM1 Deficiency

Mutations in genes encoding the calcium-release activated calcium (CRAC) channel abolish calcium influx in cells of the immune system and cause severe congenital immunodeficiency. ORAI1 functions as the pore forming subunit of the CRAC channel where ORAI1-CRAC channels are activated by the endoplasmic reticulum (ER) protein stromal interaction molecule (STIM) 1. The latter senses the ER Ca^{2+} concentration and, upon release of Ca^{2+} from ER stores, multimerizes and binds to ORAI1.

A missense mutation in ORAI1 (R91W) abolishes ORAI1 and CRAC channel function and causes SCID characterized by a severe defect in T-cell activation.[54] Lack of STIM1 expression in human patients due to a nonsense mutation in STIM1 severely impairs store operated Ca^{2+} entry (SOCE) and causes immunodeficiency and autoimmunity associated with myopathy and abnormal enamel dentition.[55]

The severity of infections, their time of onset in the 1st year of life and the spectrum of pathogens in CRAC-deficient patients are similar to those with SCID. In contrast to SCID patients, T- and B-cell development is normal in CRAC-deficient patients and their immunodeficiency is due to the severely impaired function of T-cells.

STAT5b deficiency is an AR disorder caused due to mutations in STAT5b signal transducer, and transcription factor involved in IL-2 and IL-15 signaling, key factors for T and NK cells. Patients have growth hormone insensitive dwarfism, dysmorphic features, eczema, lymphocytic interstitial pneumonia and autoimmunity. T cells are modestly decreased but B cells and immunoglobulins are normal.[56]

Hepatic veno-occlusive disease with immunodeficiency (VODI) is AR and caused by mutations in *SP110*.[57] Affected patients have hepatic veno-occlusive disease, *Pneumocystis jirovecii* pneumonia along with increased susceptibility to candida and cytomegalovirus (CMV). Thrombocytopenia and hepatosplenomegaly are associated features. Patients have decreased memory T-cell and memory B-cell populations along with decreased IgG, IgA and IgM, with reduced germinal center reaction and absent plasma cells.

IKAROS Deficiency

Rare AD syndrome caused by mutation in *IKAROS* gene and characterized by profound B lymphopenia, near absent NK cells, and normal T-cell number. Associated hematological findings are anemia, neutropenia and thrombocytopenia.[58] The Ikaros family of transcription factors is critical for normal T-cell development while limiting malignant transformation.

FILS syndrome (facial dysmorphism, immunodeficiency, livedo and short stature) is caused by mutation in the POLE1 (polymerase ε 1), resulting in its haploinsufficiency. Patients have frequent upper and lower respiratory tract infections and meningitis. T cells are often reduced with reduced proliferative responses along with a more severe B-cell defect in the form of low memory B cells, low serum IgM and IgG, and lack of antibody production to polysaccharide antigens.[59]

CONCLUSION

Our understanding regarding molecular basis of diseases classified under "Combined Immunodeficiencies with Associated or Syndromic Features" has been increasing, offering tremendous insight into pathogenesis of these disorders. Specific diagnosis can now be made in most patients with appropriate work-up, which will led to early initiation of therapy and appropriate genetic counseling. Therefore high index of suspicion for PID in patients presenting with recurrent or unusual infections and referral to clinical immunologist is important.

KEY POINTS

- Combined immunodeficiencies (CID) with associated or syndromic features are a group of disorder characterized by presence of features of CID and other features which are apparently non-immunological.
- Congenital thrombocytopenias, ataxia-telangiectasia (AT), immunodeficiency associated with thymic defects are more common among this group of disorder.
- Congenital thrmbocytopenias are characterized by small platelets, eczema, recurrent infection and increased risk of autoimmune and malignant diseases.
- Ataxia-telangiectasia is characterized by progressive cerebellar ataxia, dysarthria, oculocutaneous telangiectasia, immune deficiency and chromosomal instability.
- Thymic defects with additional congenital anomalies includes DiGeorge syndrome and Velocardiofacial syndrome is associated with deletion of the long arm of chromosome 22 at position q.11.
- Specific diagnosis is possible for most of these disorders, hence high index of suspicion and referral to clinical immunologist should be sought in patients having recurrent or severe infections.

REFERENCES

1. Al-Herz W, Bousfiha A, Casanova JL, Chatila T, Conley ME, Cunningham-Rundles C, et al. Primary immunodeficiency diseases: an update on the classification from the international union of immunological societies expert committee for primary immunodeficiency. Front Immunol. 2014;5:162.
2. Thrasher AJ. New insights into the biology of Wiskott-Aldrich syndrome (WAS). Hematology Am Soc Hematol Educ Program. 2009;132-8.
3. Skoric D, Dimitrijevic A, Cuturilo G, Ivanovski P. Wiskott-Aldrich syndrome with macrothrombocytopenia. Indian Pediatr. 2014;51(12):1015-6.
4. Imai K, Nonoyama S, Ochs H. WASP (Wiskott-Aldrich syndrome protein) gene mutations and phenotype. Curr Opin Allergy Clin Immunol. 2003;3(6):427-36.
5. Sullivan KE, Mullen CA, Blaese RM, Winkelstein JA. A multi-institutional survey of the Wiskott-Aldrich syndrome. J Pediatr. 1994;125(6 Pt 1):876-85.
6. Suri D, Singh S, Rawat A, Gupta A, Kamae C, Honma K, et al. Clinical profile and genetic basis of Wiskott-Aldrich syndrome at Chandigarh, North India. Asian Pac J Allergy Immunol. 2012;30(1):71-8.
7. Kawai S, Minegishi M, Ohashi Y, Sasahara Y, Kumaki S, Konno T, et al. Flow cytometric determination of intracytoplasmic Wiskott-Aldrich syndrome protein in peripheral blood lymphocyte subpopulations. J Immunol Methods. 2002;260(1-2):195-205.
8. Yamada M, Ariga T, Kawamura N, Yamaguchi K, Ohtsu M, Nelson DL, et al. Determination of carrier status for the Wiskott-Aldrich syndrome by flow cytometric analysis of Wiskott-Aldrich syndrome protein expression in peripheral blood mononuclear cells. J Immunol. 2000;165(2):1119-22.
9. Lanzi G, Moratto D, Vairo D, Masneri S, Delmonte O, Paganini T, et al. A novel primary human immunodeficiency due to deficiency in the WASP-interacting protein WIP. J Exp Med. 2012;209(1):29-34.
10. Sasahara Y. The WASP-WIP complex in the molecular pathogenesis of Wiskott-Aldrich syndrome. Pediatr Int. 2016;58(1):4-7.
11. Rawat A, Imai K, Suri D, Gupta A, Bhisikar S, Saikia B, et al. Ataxia Telangiectasia Masquerading as Hyper IgM Syndrome. Indian J Pediatr. 2016;83(3):270-1.
12. Azarsiz E, Karaca NE, Gunaydin NC, Gulez N, Ozturk C, Aksu G, et al. Do elevated serum IgM levels have to be included in probable diagnosis criteria of patients with ataxia-telangiectasia? Int J Immunopathol Pharmacol. 2014;27(3):421-7.

13. Stewart GS, Maser RS, Stankovic T, Bressan DA, Kaplan MI, Jaspers NG, et al. The DNA double-strand break repair gene hmre11 is mutated in individuals with an ataxia-telangiectasia-like disorder. Cell. 1999;99(6);577-87.
14. Carney JP, Maser RS, Olivares H, Davis EM, Le Beau M, Yates JR 3rd, et al. The hMre11/hRad50 Protein Complex and Nijmegen breakage syndrome: linkage of double-strand break repair to the cellular dna damage response. Cell. 1998;93(3):477-86.
15. Amor-Guéret M, Dubois-d'Enghien C, Laugé A, Onclercq-Delic R, Barakat A, Chadli E, et al. Three new BLM gene mutations associated with Bloom syndrome. Genet Test. 2008;12(2):257-61.
16. Aslan D. The X chromosome: does it have a role in Bloom syndrome, a genomic instability disorder? Turk J Pediatr. 2014;56(3):327-9.
17. Wijmenga C, Hansen RS, Gimelli G, Bjorck EJ, Davies EG, Valentine D, et al. Genetic variation in ICF syndrome: evidence for genetic heterogeneity. Hum Mutat. 2000;16(6):509-17.
18. Thijssen PE, Ito Y, Grillo G, Wang J, Velasco G, Nitta H, et al. Mutations in CDCA7 and HELLS cause immunodeficiency-centromeric instability-facial anomalies syndrome. Nat Commun. 2015;6:7870.
19. von Bernuth H, Ravindran E, Du H, Fröhler S, Strehl K, Krämer N, et al. Combined immunodeficiency develops with age in immunodeficiency-centromeric instability-facial anomalies syndrome 2 (ICF2). Orphanet J Rare Dis. 2014;9:116.
20. Weemaes CM, van Tol MJ, Wang J, van Ostaijen-ten Dam MM, van Eggermond MC, Thijssen PE, et al. Heterogeneous clinical presentation in ICF syndrome: correlation with underlying gene defects. Eur J Hum Genet. 2013;21(11):1219-25.
21. Peron S, Metin A, Gardes P, Alyanakian MA, Sheridan E, Kratz CP, et al. Human PMS2 deficiency is associated with impaired immunoglobulin class switch recombination. J Exp Med. 2008;205(11):2465-72.
22. Stewart GS, Panier S, Townsend K, Al-Hakim AK, Kolas NK, Miller ES, et al. The RIDDLE syndrome protein mediates a ubiquitin-dependent signaling cascade at sites of DNA damage. Cell. 2009;136(3):420-34.
23. Hughes CR, Guasti L, Meimaridou E, Chuang CH, Schimenti JC, King PJ, et al. MCM4 mutation causes adrenal failure, short stature, and natural killer cell deficiency in humans. J Clin Invest. 2012;122(3):814-20.
24. Gineau L, Cognet C, Kara N, Lach FP, Dunne J, Veturi U, et al. Partial MCM4 deficiency in patients with growth retardation, adrenal insufficiency, and natural killer cell deficiency. J Clin Invest. 2012;122(3):821-32.
25. de la Chapelle A, Herva R, Koivisto M, Aula P. A deletion in chromosome 22 can cause DiGeorge syndrome. Hum Genet. 1981;57(3):253-6.
26. Davies EG. Immunodeficiency in DiGeorge Syndrome and Options for Treating Cases with Complete Athymia. Front Immunol. 2013;4:322.
27. Jongmans MC, Admiraal RJ, van der Donk KP, Vissers LE, Baas AF, Kapusta L, et al. CHARGE syndrome: the phenotypic spectrum of mutations in the CHD7 gene. J Med Genet. 2006;43(4):306-14.
28. Riley P Jr, Weiner DS, Leighley B, Jonah D, Morton DH, Strauss KA, et al. Cartilage hair hypoplasia: characteristics and orthopaedic manifestations. J Child Orthop. 2015;9(2):145-52.
29. Mäkitie O, Pukkala E, Teppo L, Kaitila I. Increased incidence of cancer in patients with cartilage-hair hypoplasia. J Pediatr. 1999;134(3):315-8.
30. Spranger J, Hinkel GK, Stoss H, Thoenes W, Wargowski D, Zepp F. Schimke immuno-osseous dysplasia: a newly recognized multisystem disease. J Pediatr. 1991;119(1 Pt 1):64-72.
31. Clewing JM, Antalfy BC, Lucke T, Najafian B, Marwedel KM, Hori A, et al. Schimke immuno-osseous dysplasia: a clinicopathological correlation. J Med Genet. 2007;44(2): 122-30.
32. Hunter KB, Lücke T, Spranger J, Smithson SF, Alpay H, André JL, et al. Schimke immunoosseous dysplasia: defining skeletal features. Eur J Pediatr. 2010;169(7):801-11.
33. Woellner C, Gertz EM, Schäffer A, Lagos M, Perro M, Glocker EO, et al. Mutations in STAT3 and diagnostic guidelines for hyper-IgE syndrome. J Allergy and Clin Immunol. 2010;125(2):424-32.
34. Schimke LF, Sawalle-Belohradsky J, Roesler J, Wollenberg A, Rack A, Borte M, et al. Diagnostic approach to the hyper-IgE syndromes: immunologic and clinical key findings to differentiate hyper-IgE syndromes from atopic dermatitis. J Allergy and Clin Immunol. 2010;126(3):611-7.
35. Chandesris M, Melki I, Natividad A, Puel A, Fieschi C, Yun L, et al. Autosomal dominant STAT3 deficiency and hyper IgE syndrome: molecular, cellular, and clinical features from a French National Survey. Medicine (Baltimore). 2012;91(4):1-19.
36. Lee WI, Huang JL, Yeh KW, Jaing TH, Lin TY, Huang YC, et al. Immune defects in active mycobacterial diseases in patients with primary immunodeficiency diseases (PIDs). J Formos Med Assoc. 2011;110(12):750-8.
37. Metin A, Uysal G, Güven A, Unlu A, Oztürk MH. Tuberculous brain abscess in a patient with hyper IgE syndrome. Pediatr Int. 2004;46(1):97-100.
38. Pasic S. Local bacillus Calmette-Guérin infection in hyperimmunoglobulin-E syndrome. Acta Paediatr. 2002;91(11):1271-2.
39. Pasic S, Lilic D, Pejnovic N, Vojvodic D, Simic R, Abinun M. Disseminated Bacillus Calmette-Guérin infection in a girl with hyperimmunoglobulin E syndrome. Acta Paediatr. 1998;87(6):702-4.
40. Holland SM, DeLeo FR, Elloumi HZ, Hsu AP, Uzel G, Brodsky N, et al. STAT3 mutations in the hyper-IgE syndrome. N Engl J Med. 2007;357(16):1608-19.
41. Minegishi Y, Saito M, Tsuchiya S, Tsuge I, Takada H, Hara T, et al. Dominant-negative mutations in the DNA-binding domain of STAT3 cause hyper-IgE syndrome. Nature. 2007;448(7157):1058-62.
42. Minegishi Y, Saito M, Morio T, Watanabe K, Agematsu K, Tsuchiya S, et al. Human tyrosine kinase 2 deficiency reveals its requisite roles in multiple cytokine signals involved in innate and acquired immunity. Immunity. 2006;25(5):745-55.
43. Saikia B, Suri D, Goel S, Rawat A, Minz RW, Gupta A, et al. Hyper-IgE syndrome with a novel STAT3 mutation-a single center study from India. Asian Pac J Allergy Immunol. 2014;32(4):321-7.
44. Engelhardt KR, McGhee S, Winkler S, Sassi A, Woellner C, Lopez-Herrera G, et al. Large deletions and point mutations involving the dedicator of cytokinesis 8 (DOCK8) in the autosomal-recessive form of hyper-IgE syndrome. J Allergy Clin Immunol. 2009;124(6):1289-302.
45. Grimbacher B, Schäffer AA, Holland SM, Davis J, Gallin JI, Malech HL, et al. Genetic linkage of hyper-IgE syndrome to chromosome 4. Am J Hum Genet. 1999;65(3):735-44.
46. Dokal I. Dyskeratosis congenita. Hematology Am Soc Hematol Educ Program. 2011;2011:480-6.
47. Cossu F, Vulliamy TJ, Marrone A, Badiali M, Cao A, Dokal I. A novel DKC1 mutation, severe combined immunodeficiency

(T+B-NK-SCID) and bone marrow transplantation in an infant with Hoyeraal-Hreidarsson syndrome. Br J Haematol. 2002;119(3):765-8.
48. Kaikov Y, Wadsworth LD, Hall CA, Rogers PC. Transcobalamin II deficiency: case report and review of the literature. Eur J Pediatr. 1991;150(12):841-3.
49. Zittoun J, Fischer A, Marquet J, Perignon JL, Lagrue A, Griscelli C. Megaloblastic anemia and immune abnormalities in a patient with methionine synthase deficiency. Acta Paediatr Scand. 1987;76(6):991-8.
50. Borzutzky A, Crompton B, Bergmann AK, Giliani S, Baxi S, Martin M, et al. Reversible severe combined immunodeficiency phenotype secondary to a mutation of the proton-coupled folate transporter. Clin Immunol. 2009;133(3):287-94.
51. Keller MD, Ganesh J, Heltzer M, Paessler M, Bergqvist AG, Baluarte HJ, et al. Severe combined immunodeficiency resulting from mutations in MTHFD1. Pediatrics. 2013;131(2):e629-34.
52. Smith DL, Smith JG, Wong SW, deShazo RD. Netherton's syndrome: a syndrome of elevated IgE and characteristic skin and hair findings. J Allergy Clin Immunol. 1995;95(1 Pt 1):116-23.
53. Zook EC, Krishack PA, Zhang S, Zeleznik-Le NJ, Firulli AB, Witte PL, et al. Overexpression of Foxn1 attenuates age-associated thymic involution and prevents the expansion of peripheral CD4 memory T cells. Blood. 2011;118(22):5723-31.
54. McCarl CA, Picard C, Khalil S, Kawasaki T, Rother J, Papolos A, et al. ORAI1 deficiency and lack of store-operated Ca2+ entry cause immunodeficiency, myopathy, and ectodermal dysplasia. J Allergy Clin Immunol. 2009;124(6):1311-8.
55. Picard C, McCarl CA, Papolos A, Khalil S, Luthy K, Hivroz C, et al. STIM1 mutation associated with a syndrome of immunodeficiency and autoimmunity. N Engl J Med. 2009;360(19):1971-80.
56. Varco-Merth B, Feigerlová E, Shinde U, Rosenfeld RG, Hwa V, Rotwein P, et al. Severe growth deficiency is associated with STAT5b mutations that disrupt protein folding and activity. Mol Endocrinol. 2013;27(1):150-61.
57. Roscioli T, Ziegler JB, Buckley M, Wong M. Hepatic veno-occlusive disease with immunodeficiency. In: Pagon RA, Adam MP, Ardinger HH, Wallace SE, Amemiya A, Bean LJH (Eds). GeneReviews®. Seattle (WA): University of Washington, Seattle; 1993-2015.
58. Goldman FD, Gurel Z, Al-Zubeidi D, Fried AJ, Icardi M, Song C, et al. Congenital pancytopenia and absence of B lymphocytes in a neonate with a mutation in the Ikaros gene. Pediatr Blood Cancer. 2012;58(4):591-7.
59. Pachlopnik Schmid J, Lemoine R, Nehme N, Cormier-Daire V, Revy P, Debeurme F. Polymerase ε1 mutation in a human syndrome with facial dysmorphism, immunodeficiency, livedo, and short stature ("FILS syndrome"). J Exp Med. 2012;209(13):2323-30.

CHAPTER

53

Immune Dysregulation Syndromes

Anupa Mishra, Nitin K Shah

INTRODUCTION

Dissection of the immune system down to its basic mechanisms of tolerance has been enabled by the recent clinical and molecular definition of primary immunodeficiency disorders (PIDD), which considers the primary defect to be in the immune-regulatory compartment of the immune system, coupled with the realization that autoimmunity and immune dysregulation form an important part in the spectrum of pathophysiology and clinical manifestations in patients having PIDD. Consequently, this has opened hundreds of avenues for scientists and clinicians working in the field of immunology to study the pathways and target the right molecules to correct for immune dysregulations. **Table 53.1** presents the latest classification of the various

Table 53.1 Classification of immune dysregulation syndromes [International Union of Immunologic Societies (IUIS) 2014]

	Disease		*Inheritance*	*Defect*
1.	Familial HLH syndromes			
1.1	Without hypopigmentation	FHL1	AR	
		FHL2	AR	Mutations in *PRF1*; perforin, perforin deficiency
		FHL3	AR	Mutations in *UNC13D a*; MUNC13-4 deficiency; required to prime vesicles for fusion
		FHL4	AR	Mutations in *STX11*, SYNTAXIN 11 deficiency; required for secretory vesicle fusion with the cell membrane
		FHL5	AR	Mutations in *STXBP2*, MUNC 18-2 deficiency; required for secretory vesicle fusion with the cell membrane
1.2	With hypopigmentation	Chédiak-Higashi syndrome	AR	Mutations in *LYST* impaired lysosomal trafficking
		Griscelli type 2	AR	Mutations in *RAB27A* encoding a GTPase that promotes docking of secretory vesicles to the cell membrane
		Hermansky-Pudlak type 2	AR	Mutations in *AP3B1* gene, encoding for the b subunit of the AP-3 complex
2.	Lymphoproliferative disorders			
	XLP1		XL	Mutations in *SH2D1A* encoding an adaptor protein regulating intracellular signaling
	XLP2		XL	Mutations in *XIAP/BIRC4* encoding an inhibitor of apoptosis
	ITK deficiency		AR	Mutations in *ITK* encoding IL-2 inducible T-cell kinase required for TCR-mediated activation
	CD27 deficiency		AR	Mutations in *CD27*, encoding TNF-R member superfamily required for generation and long-term maintenance of T-cell immunity

Contd...

Contd...

	Disease		*Inheritance*	*Defect*
3.	Genetic defects of regulatory T-cells			
	IPEX (immune dysregulation, polyendocrinopathy, enteropathy X-linked)		XL	Mutations in *FOXP3*, encoding a T-cell transcription factor
	CD25 deficiency		AR	Mutations in *IL-2RA*, encoding IL-2Ra chain
	STAT 5b deficiency		AR	Mutations in *STAT5B*, signal transducer, and transcription factor, essential for normal signaling from IL-2 and 15, key growth factors for T and NK cells
4.	Autoimmunity with lymphoproliferation			
	APECED (autoimmune polyendocrinopathy with candidiasis and ectodermal dystrophy)		AR	Mutations in *AIRE*, encoding a transcription regulator needed to establish thymic self-tolerance
	ITCH deficiency		AR	Mutations in *ITCH*, an E3 ubiquitin ligase catalyzes the transfer of ubiquity into a signaling protein in the cell including phospholipase Cg1 (PLCg1)
5.	Autoimmune lymphoproliferative syndrome			
	ALPS FAS		AR/AD	Germinal mutations in *TNFRSF6*, encoding CD95/Fas cell surface apoptosis receptor
	ALPS FASLG		AR	Mutations in *TNFSF6*, Fas ligand for CD95 apoptosis
	ALPS caspase-10		AD	Mutations in *CASP10*, intracellular apoptosis pathway
	ALPS caspase-8		AR	Mutations in *CASP8*, intracellular apoptosis, and activation pathways
	FADD deficiency		AR	Mutations in *FADD* encoding an adaptor molecule interacting with FAS, and promoting apoptosis
	CARD 11, Gain of function (GOF) mutations		AD	GOF mutations in *CARD11*, encoding a protein required for antigen receptor–induced NF-κB activation in B- and T-lymphocytes
	PRKC delta deficiency		AR	Mutations in *PRKCD*, encoding a member of the protein kinase C family critical for regulation of cell survival, proliferation, and apoptosis
6.	Immune dysregulation with colitis			
	IL 10 deficiency		AR	Mutations in *IL-10*, encoding IL-10
	IL10 R alpha deficiency		AR	Mutations in *IL-10RA*, encoding IL-10R1
	IL10 R beta deficiency		AR	Mutations in *IL-10RB*, encoding IL-10R2
7.	Type 1, interferonopathies			
	TREX 1 deficiency, Aicardi–Goutières syndrome 1 (AGS 1)		AR/AD	Mutations in *TREX1*, encoding nuclease involved in clearing cellular nucleic debris
	AGS 2		AR	Mutations in *RNASEH2B*, encoding nuclease subunit involved in clearing cellular nucleic debris
	AGS 3		AR	Mutations in *RNASEH2C*, encoding nuclease subunit involved in clearing cellular nucleic debris
	AGS 4		AR	Mutations in *RNASEH2A*, encoding nuclease subunit involved in clearing cellular nucleic debris
	AGS 5		AR	Mutations in *SAMHD1*, encoding negative regulator of the immunostimulatory DNA response

Contd...

Contd...

Disease		Inheritance	Defect
AGS 6		AR	Mutations in *ADAR1*, encoding an RNA-specific adenosine deaminase
SPENCD (Spondyloenchondromatosis dysplasia with immune dysregulation)		AR	Mutations in *ACP5*, encoding tartrate-resistant acid phosphatase (TRAP)

Abbreviations: HLH, hemophagocytic lymphohistiocytosis; FHL, familial hemophagocytic lymphohistiocytosis; AR, autosomal recessive; XLP, X-linked lymphoproliferative; ITK, interleukin-2-inducible T-cell kinase; XL, X-linked; NK cell, natural killer cell; AD, autosomal dominant; ALPS, autoimmune lymphoproliferative syndrome

immune dysregulation syndromes [International Union of Immunologic Societies (IUIS) 2014].[1] This chapter will give a brief overview of hemophagocytic lymphohistiocytosis (HLH) and autoimmune lymphoproliferative syndrome (ALPS), two of the most common entities amongst this gamut of unusual diseases.

HEMOPHAGOCYTIC LYMPHOHISTIOCYTOSIS

INTRODUCTION

Hemophagocytic lymphohistiocytosis (HLH) is a potentially fatal hyperinflammatory disorder with an incidence of approximately 1.2 cases per million populations. It occurs as a result of immune dysregulation and pathological immune activation that manifest into a syndrome characterized by a clinical presentation of extreme inflammation and cytopenias, eventually resulting in multiorgan failure and death if left untreated. HLH can be primary or familial (familial hemophagocytic lymphohistiocytosis—FHL) and secondary, often associated with infections, autoimmune diseases, malignancies, genetic immunodeficiencies, and some inborn errors of metabolism, such as lysinuric protein intolerance. Contrary to the initial belief that it affects only infants and children, it is now known that it can manifest even in the 7th decade of life. Research on the genetics and pathophysiology of HLH over the last decade has greatly improved our understanding of this condition. In addition, with increasing awareness of the condition and availability of better treatment options, including hematopoietic stem cell transplantation (HSCT), the outlook toward HLH has changed from a universally fatal disorder to a treatable condition with good long-term survival.

HISTORY

Before James Farquhar and Albert E Claireaux from the University of Edinburgh published an article in May 1952 describing the fatal condition in a pair of siblings, with the major findings being a marked increase in histiocytes in the bone marrow at the expense of blood-forming cells, there had been only few case reports of similar cases in adults (Robb-Smith, 1938) and infants (Reese and Levy, 1951). They coined the term "Familial Hemophagocytic Reticulosis," which is now known as HLH. Henter et al. in 1991 and Osugi in 1997 first described the role of activated lymphocytes, macrophages, and large amounts of proinflammatory cytokines in the pathophysiology of HLH. The first genetic insight into the etiology of HLH was obtained in 1999 with the discovery of perforin mutations in some affected patients.

EPIDEMIOLOGY[2,3]

Hemophagocytic lymphohistiocytosis more occurs in children born out of consanguineous marriages, thereby suggesting autosomal recessive pattern of inheritance. There is a tendency toward similar age of onset in patients from the same family. Approximately 70–80% of the patients present FHL in the first year of life with the incidence peaking at 1–6 months of age. Rare cases of *in utero* development of the disease and manifestation at birth have also been reported. However, contrary to common belief, FHL may present in later stages of life as well, with reported presentations in and after teenage. Many adults with FHL2 were believed to have missense mutations in the perforin gene, leading to partial protein expression and hence the delay in presentation. As reported in various studies, incidence varies depending on the ethnic groups being studied and also on the awareness, high index of suspicion, and improved ability to diagnose the condition by the investigators. The incidence is reportedly 0.12 per 100,000 in Sweden and 0.342 per 100,000 in Japan, whereas in Turkey, it is as high as 7.5 per 100,000 hospitalized patients, owing to a high frequency of consanguinity. A marginal male predominance is noted.

PATHOPHYSIOLOGY[4-25]

The basic pathophysiology of HLH is a hyperinflammatory uncontrolled response triggered by various stimuli. Although the mechanisms of genetic HLH have been clarified to quite an extent, those of the acquired counterpart require further research. Some triggers for secondary HLH are shown in **Table 53.2**.

Table 53.2 Conditions associated with secondary hemophagocytic lymphohistiocytosis

S No		
1.	Viral infections	HSV, EBV, CMV, HIV, Parvovirus, H1N1, Postvaccination
2.	Other infections	Bacteria; Protozoa like malaria and *Leishmania*; *Mycoplasma*; Fungi like *Candida, Aspergillus*; Mycobacteria
3.	Malignancies	Leukemias, Hodgkin's and Non-Hodgkin's lymphoma, solid tumors like germ cell tumors
4.	Rheumatological disorders [Macrophage activation syndrome (MAS)]	Systemic onset JRA, SLE, Scleroderma, Sjögren, mixed connective tissue disorder, Kawasaki disease
5.	Immune deficiency syndromes	SCID, CVID, CGD, Stem cell transplant
6.	Others	Unknown triggers

Abbreviations: HSV, herpes simplex virus; EBV, Epstein-Barr virus; CMV, cytomegalovirus; HIV, human immunodeficiency virus; JRA, juvenile rheumatoid arthritis; SLE, systemic lupus erythematosus; SCID, severe combined immunodeficiencies; CVID, common variable immunodeficiency; CGD, chronic granulomatous disease

Triggers of hemophagocytic lymphohistiocytosis: There can be a variety of triggers, including infections, autoimmune diseases, malignancies and inborn errors of metabolism.

Infectious triggers[4-6,8,24] are found in both familial and acquired HLH, and hence, the isolation of an infectious agent does not help to differentiate between the two. Viruses, particularly herpes viridae, form the largest group of triggering infectious agents. Other viruses, protozoa, bacteria, fungi, and mycobacteria have also been implicated in the pathogenesis of HLH. Cytomegalovirus (CMV) and herpes simplex virus (HSV) have been particularly found to trigger neonatal and infantile HLH, while Epstein-Barr virus (EBV) is the most common virus that causes full-blown acquired HLH postinfancy. Polymerase chain reaction (PCR) is recommended for the diagnosis as it may be missed initially during serological examination. It has been found to be useful to screen for EBV, CMV, Parvo B19, HSV, human herpes viruses-6 (HHV6) and Varicella-zoster virus (VZV) infections.

Interestingly intracellular pathogens appear to have an increased propensity to cause HLH. Visceral leishmaniasis is often a trigger that is missed because of the misconception that this protozoa does not cause infections in the temperate regions; in addition, one may rarely find microscopic evidence of the amastigote on examination of the bone marrow smear and even serology may be negative in the initial stages. Only a PCR assay of the bone marrow can confirm the absence of this infection. *Salmonella* and mycobacteria must be screened for in places endemic for these infections, such as India. Frequently, the infection trigger may be difficult to identify without extensive examination.

Nonantigen-specific triggers leading to activation of the cells involved in innate immune response via pattern recognition receptors can also trigger HLH. Among these are the toll-like receptors (TLRs) that respond to components of various bacteria, fungi, mycoplasma, and even viruses. Bacterial sepsis leading to a systemic inflammatory response syndrome can mimic HLH as it is characterized by both hemophagocytosis and decreased NK cell function, among other clinical features of hyperinflammation.

Autoimmune and Autoinflammatory Diseases[17,18]

By convention, HLH with autoinflammatory and autoimmune syndromes, such as systemic onset JIA, systemic lupus erythematosus (SLE), inflammatory bowel disease, and Kawasaki disease, has been termed as macrophage activation syndrome (MAS). It will be discussed in detail in a separate section.

Malignancy[7,9]

Hemophagocytic lymphohistiocytosis may precede, follow, or occur concurrently with a malignancy. Overall, the proportion of HLH with malignancy is higher in adults. T-cell lymphomas and leukemia and particularly anaplastic large-cell lymphoma (ALCL) have been the most commonly implicated tumors in childhood although scattered reports of precursor B-cell tumors are also there. However, one needs to remember that any chemotherapy is associated with infections and a thorough search for the same must be made. HLH occurring in such a setting should be regarded as infection associated rather than malignancy associated. Nevertheless, malignancy must be ruled out in any patient presenting with HLH beyond the toddler age without an associated perforin or degranulation defect, SAP [signaling lymphocyte activating (SLAM) associated protein] and X-linked inhibitor of apoptosis (XIAP), autoinflammatory condition and/or infectious trigger to account for the condition. It would be worthwhile to rule out SH2D1A mutation in males with lymphomas since X-linked lymphoproliferative (XLP) is associated both with HLH and lymphomas. Biallelic STXBP2, PRF1 and STX11 mutations also predispose to malignancies.

Inborn Errors of Metabolism[19-21]

Isolated case reports of HLH in various inborn errors of metabolism are found in literature; however, the association has most consistently been found with lysinuric protein intolerance. These patients have been intermittently found to satisfy the HLH criteria. Patients with Gaucher disease may present with hepatosplenomegaly, hemorrhages, cytopenia, hyperferritinemia, marginally increased transaminases and LDH. Marrow examination easily differentiates lipid-laden Gaucher cells from activated monocytes and macrophages in HLH. There is a substantial overlap in the signs and symptoms of Wolman disease and HLH.

Mechanism of Immune Dysregulation[22-25]

Defective Cytotoxic T-cell and Natural Killer Cell Functions

The pathogenesis of HLH remains controversial. Although research over the last two decades has helped elucidate the underlying defects that impaired normal functioning of T and natural killer (NK) cells despite normal effector cell numbers, the exact mechanisms linking cytotoxicity and clinical manifestations are still not understood.

Natural killer cells and cytotoxic T-cells play a major role in containing invading organisms, predominantly viruses, by secreting soluble factors such as interferon-gamma (IFN-γ), which enhances immunity, interferes with viral replication, and is also a potent macrophage activator. In an immunocompetent host, these cells kill their targets via nonsecretory pathways, which involve the Fas ligand, and more importantly through direct cytolytic pathways, which involve formation of an immunological synapse through a contact between the target cell and the effector cell. Once the NK and T-cells are activated, the cytotoxic granules or secretory lysosomes containing perforin and granzyme traffic toward the synapse along the microtubules, dock and fuse with the plasma membrane, and release their contents into the synapse. This mediates apoptotic death of the target cells, and the immune response is downregulated.

All known defects in HLH seem to involve this process as shown in **Figure 53.1**. PRF1 mutations lead to loss of cytolytic activity. RAB 27 alpha, UNC13D and LYST mutations lead to impaired docking, granule priming and granule secretion at the synapse, respectively. In XLP, impaired lymphocyte activation impairs granule-mediated cytotoxicity while Syntaxin 11 mutations may theoretically impair cytolytic pathways involving the interaction of dendritic and killer cells.

Studies in mice having one of the above defects have shown that when the cytotoxic functions are impaired, there is a disproportionate expansion of the CD8 T-cells with excessive cytokine production and macrophage activation. These excessive proinflammatory cytokines then give rise to the clinical picture of HLH as seen in humans. Although it has been postulated that the increased macrophages and histiocytes then infiltrate various organs and simultaneously damage them, whether this infiltration represents the cause or the effect of the disease remains to be elucidated.

Gene expression studies on peripheral blood mononuclear cells in patients with active HLH have revealed a downregulation of genes involved in innate and adaptive immune systems, including TLRs and B and T-cells, indicating that during active HLH, the patient is actually in an immunodeficient state and hence more vulnerable infections. This can lead to a vicious cycle of continued immune stimulation and disease activity.

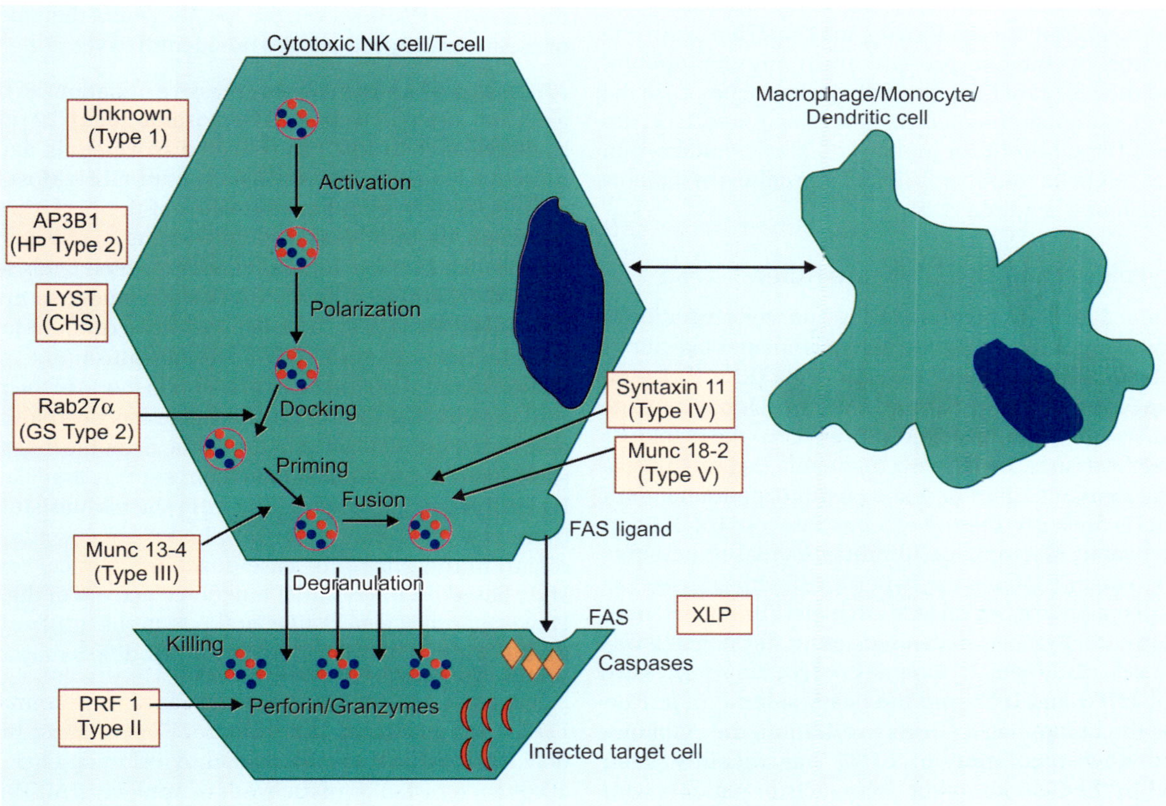

Figure 53.1 Pathways involved in primary hemophagocytic lymphohistiocytosis (HLH)

Failure of Downregulation of the Immune Response

Once the trigger is successfully eliminated in a normal host, the immune response against it is contained and contracted and hence an immune homeostasis is maintained. In experimental animals, perforin- and Fas-mediated killing of antigen-presenting cells (APCs), such as dendritic cells, by cytotoxic T lymphocytes (CTLs) and perforin-mediated killing of activated CD4 cells by NK cells are known to control the immune response. Similarly, NK cells cause lysis of dendritic cells in humans as well. Failure to kill the APCs, similar to its occurrence in HLH because of impaired perforin-mediated cytolysis that occurs in HLH, not only impedes the reduction in the viral load but also leads to continuous stimulation of the immune system. Another mechanism includes "Fratricide," wherein CTLs having acquired fragments and antigenic particles from the target cells become susceptible to destruction by other CTLs. The CD4 T regulatory cells not being able to contain the largely expanding CD8 T-cell population may also explain the failure of timely downregulation of the immune system in HLH.

Acquired Hemophagocytic Lymphohistiocytosis

In patients without the known genetic mutation for familial HLH, a temporary phase of immune-compromise may predispose them to the condition by their inability to cope with any infection. Direct activation of TLRs by intracellular organisms that persists in the histiocytes may explain a few cases of HLH that occur following *Leishmania, Mycobacterium* and *Salmonella* infections. Viruses may interfere with the CTL function by specific proteins in immunocompetent hosts, and the resultant high levels of cytokines may have the same effect, although the mechanisms of acquired HLH are yet unclear. Hypomorphic or mono- or biallelic mutations in FHL genes might be responsible for a large cohort of patients with unexplained acquired HLH.

Hypercytokinemia: The Ultimate Killer

During the active phase, there is a high serum concentration of many proinflammatory cytokines and chemokines like tumor necrosis factor-alpha (TNFα), IL6, IL8, IL10, IL12, IL18, and macrophage inflammatory protein MIP1α. Organ damage and necrosis can be caused by direct effect of the cytokines infiltrating the tissues. This hypercytokinemia explains most of the clinical signs and symptoms and laboratory parameters of HLH. Fever is caused by the endogenous pyrogens IL1, IL6 and TNFα. Activated macrophages produce increased amounts of ferritin, which explains the hyperferritinemia, as well as plasminogen activator, which leads to hyperfibrinolysis, both of which eventually cause decreased serum fibrinogen levels and increased D-dimers. Cytopenias reflect the suppressive activity of TNFα and IFNγ and the heavy subunit of ferritin as well as the hemophagocytosis. In addition, the cytokine-mediated downregulation of CD47 has recently been described in the hematopoietic stem cells of patients with HLH. CD47 prevents phagocytosis by interaction with the signal regulatory protein α (SIRPA), and its downregulation in stem cells could explain the evolution to bone marrow aplasia in patients with poorly controlled disease. The hyperlipidemia is due to suppression of the lipoprotein lipase and stimulation of triglyceride synthesis by TNFα and IFNγ. Increased number of activated lymphocytes account for the increased levels of sIL2Rα. Increased levels of Fas L as well as TNF alpha can both induce liver cell apoptosis.

GENETICS OF HEMOPHAGOCYTIC LYMPHOHISTIOCYTOSIS[26-41]

With an autosomal recessive inheritance, HLH is found to occur more commonly in children born out of consanguineous marriages. Thus far, five loci have been identified whose mutations can cause five different subtypes of HLH. The frequency of genetic abnormalities may vary with ethnicity and nationality. A variety of other genetic syndromes are associated with HLH, including Chédiak-Higashi syndrome, Griscelli syndrome (GS) type 2 and Hermansky-Pudlak type 2. Here, HLH may not be always present but can more often than not be the first manifestation of the disease. All the genes identified till date encode proteins that are essential for the granule-dependent cytotoxic functions of NK cells and T-cells. How it leads to HLH is explained in further details under the heading pathophysiology.

FHL1: Genetic mutations of the locus identified on chromosome 9 (9q21) is considered responsible for 10% of the cases of FHL; however, the specific genes, their mutations, or their specific products are not identified yet.

FHL2: More than 70 different recessive mutations in the *PRF1* gene encoding perforin on chromosome 10q21-22 (identified by Ohadi et al. in 1999) have been discovered till date. These mutations account for 30–35% cases of HLH. Most of these defects lead to quantitative defects of the perforin protein; however, certain missense mutations cause qualitative defects like inability to bind calcium, which leads to loss of cytolytic function of perforin. Certain missense mutations lead to partial loss of function and often result in late onset disease. One such example is polymorphism of C272T (Ala 91Val). It leads to partial loss of function (50%) of the perforin. Although homozygosity for this allele has been found to be associated with leukemia/lymphoma, a double heterozygous state (with a null perforin allele present) is associated with HLH. Thus, one may conclude from the various studies that there is a definitive genotype-phenotype correlation with regard to the time of disease onset and clinical severity in HLH based on the residual functional activity of the protein. However, other factors like viral infections, other alleles, or modifier genes, as well as epigenetic modifiers may affect the expression levels.

FHL3: Mutation in the *UNC13D* causing Munc13-4.3 deficiency, which was discovered by Feldman et al. in 2003, accounts for 30–35% of the cases of familial HLH. The overall age of presentation of patients with this mutation is later than the FHL2. However, two disruptive mutations are found to manifest at an earlier age when compared to two missense mutations of the same gene. In addition, there is increased incidence of central nervous system (CNS) involvement when compared to FHL2. Munc13 is essential for fusion of the cytolytic granule with other structures of the plasma membrane and a mutation in the same results in defective degranulation. The priming of the cytolytic granules docked at the plasma membrane requires the Munc13-4.3 to regulate the interactions between the v-SNARE (soluble N-ethyl maleimide sensitive factor attachment protein receptors) and t-SNARE and eventually cause the fusion of the granule. It has a similar role as a priming factor for the synaptic vesicle at the neurological synapse, which probably explains the more frequent occurrence of CNS involvement in patients with this genotype.

FHL4: The *STX11* gene, which encodes the Syntaxin11, a member of the t-SNARE protein family, involved in the membrane fusion events and produced by CTLs, NK cells and myeloid cells in large amounts, has been found to be mutated in patients with FHL4. The distribution is more worldwide. It generally has a late onset. Deleterious mutations reported are generally null mutations. The selective pairing of t-SNARE, v-SNARE synaptosome-associated proteins (SNAP) from opposing membranes results in the formation of very stable bundles of four helices. Syntaxin 11 by regulating these bundle and the resultant membrane fusions during intracellular trafficking forms a key element in the process and its deficiency leads to disruption of the same. However, it is to be noted that defects were found in the cytolytic functions of NK cells but not in those of the syntaxin11-deficient CTLs.

FHL5: Defined by the deficiency of syntaxin-binding protein or Munc-18-2 protein due to mutations in the encoding gene; STXBP2 is the latest to be identified as a culprit causing FHL5. Here, again a genotype-phenotype correlation has been found with early onset and severe manifestations in those with missense mutations and onset at more than 1 year of age with less severe course in those harboring homozygous splice site mutations or compound heterozygous splice site mutations. The STXBP2 belongs to the SM family of fusion accessory proteins, and it probably has a role in stabilizing the expression of syntaxin-11 protein. A decrease in the levels of syntaxin-11 in STXBP2-deficient lymphoblast reinforces the theory.

Primary Immune Deficiency Syndromes with Hemophagocytic Lymphohistiocytosis

X-linked Lymphoproliferative Syndromes[36-38]

Duncans disease or X-linked lymphoproliferative syndrome is a rare immunodeficiency syndrome with an estimated incidence of 1/1,000,000 live births. This condition is characterized by extreme vulnerability to EBV infection which can consequently trigger HLH, malignant lymphoproliferation, and/or humoral immunodeficiency and is believed to be caused by two mutations identified till date.

Table 53.3 X-linked lymphoproliferative 1 (XLP1)and XLP2 presentations

XLP1	*XLP2*
More severe HLH with frequent neurological involvement and fatal outcome	Recurrent splenomegaly with cytopenias. Full blown HLH even in absence of EBV more likely in XLP2
Hypogammaglobulinemia (65%) and predisposition to lymphoma	Hypogammaglobulinemia (30%) and associated with hemorrhagic colitis

Abbreviations: HLH, hemophagocytic lymphohistiocytosis; EBV, Epstein-Barr virus

X-linked lymphoproliferative type 1 is caused by hemizygous mutations in SH2D1A which encodes for a protein SAP which is important for signal transduction in a variety of immune cells and for activation of NK cells and CTLs. This mutation results in dysregulated signaling pathways and impaired cell-cell interactions at multiple levels. Humoral immunodeficiency can be explained by decreased IL10 production and inducible costimulatory molecule (ICOS) expression on CD4 T-cells, which results in impaired T-cell help and impaired development of memory B-cells and long-lived plasma cells. Besides, the polarization of cytotoxic mediators to the immunological synapse is defective as is the NK/T-cell development. Recently, another gene encoding the XIAP/(BIRC4) on the same chromosome Xq2, separated only by 0.4 Mb from the SH2D1A encoding region, has been found to be mutated in patients with XLP type 2 disease. XIAP plays a role in the antiapoptotic control as well as in the numerous signal transduction pathways, although the pathophysiology of HLH in XLP2 is not fully understood. XLP1 and XLP2 presentations are shown in **Table 53.3**.

Hemophagocytic Lymphohistiocytosis Associated with Pigmentary Dilution[39-41]

Secretory lysosomes, which are cellular organelles involved in intracellular protein trafficking and exocytosis, are not only present in NK cells and CTLs but also in many other cell types, such as melanosomes, neuronal cells, platelets, mast cells and granulocytes. Some of the proteins required for cytolysis by NK cells and CTLs are also involved in trafficking of pigmentary granules by melanocytes, and therefore, an association is found between albinism and immune dysregulation with a high risk of developing HLH. Three such distinct syndromes have been identified namely GS type 2, Chédiak-Higashi syndrome and Hermansky-Pudlak syndrome type 2.

Chédiak-Higashi syndrome: This autosomal recessive condition is caused by a mutation in the *LYST* gene mapped to 1q43, which encodes a ubiquitous cytosolic protein which is involved in regulation of protein to and from lysosomes. It is marked by neutropenia with characteristic giant intracytoplasmic lysosomal structures in all granulated cells like neutrophils, monocytes, eosinophils and large granular lymphocytes and melanocytes. It is characterized by hypopigmentation, impaired NK and T-cell cytoxicity, and the onset of HLH, typically occurring at a later age of about 2–10 years, bleeding tendencies, neurological symptoms and frequent pyogenic infections **(Figs 53.2 to 53.5)**. Approximately 85% of patients with Chédiak-Higashi syndrome (CHS) develop HLH.

Griscelli syndrome type 2: This autosomal recessive condition is characterized by pigmentary dilution with silvery grey sheen of hair **(Fig. 53.6)**. Three subtypes have been described: GS type 1 is characterized by mutations in myosine VA (MYO5a) and is associated with severe neurological abnormalities. GS type 3 has mutations in the melanophilin gene (MLPH) and has isolated hypopigmentation. The GS type 2 is associated with HLH. This type is caused by a mutation in the RAB27A, the protein encoded by this gene is a small membrane bound GTPase which interacts with Munc13-4 and is involved in cytotoxic granule exocytosis. The Munc13/Rab27a complex is required for docking of the secretory granules with the plasma membrane in the hematopoietic cells and thereby for cytolytic functions.

Hermansky-Pudlak type 2: It is characterized by oculo-cutaneous albinism, bleeding, and neutropenia, with an increased susceptibility to infections. Besides, a very fair complexion and greyish hair, which are distinctive functional abnormalities, can be seen in these patients, along with ceroid storage disease in the lungs and kidneys and a high incidence of granulomatous colitis. This can be accounted for by mutations in the *AP3B1* gene encoding adapter protein 3-subunit beta 1which is a part of the AP-3 complex involved in lysosome biogenesis as well as formation of melanosomes and platelet dense granules.

CLINICAL PRESENTATION OF HEMOPHAGOCYTIC LYMPHOHISTIOCYTOSIS[42-46]

The above-mentioned pathophysiology accounts for the clinical picture of HLH, which includes prolonged fever, splenohepatomegaly, lymphadenopathy, bleeding, cutaneous manifestations, CNS affections, jaundice, and deranged laboratory parameters in the form of bicytopenias or pancytopenias, coagulopathy, hyperlipidemias, hypo-fibrinogenemia, hyperferritinemia, transaminitis, hyper-bilirubinemia, hypoalbuminemia, hyponatremia, and hemophagocytosis on examination of various tissues, such as those of bone marrow, liver and lymph node.

Fever: It is generally prolonged, unexplained, and more often presented to the hematologist as a fever of unknown origin (FUO). Differentiating it from other causes of FUO in children including malignancy can be challenging because of the simultaneous presence of hepatosplenomegaly and pancytopenia.

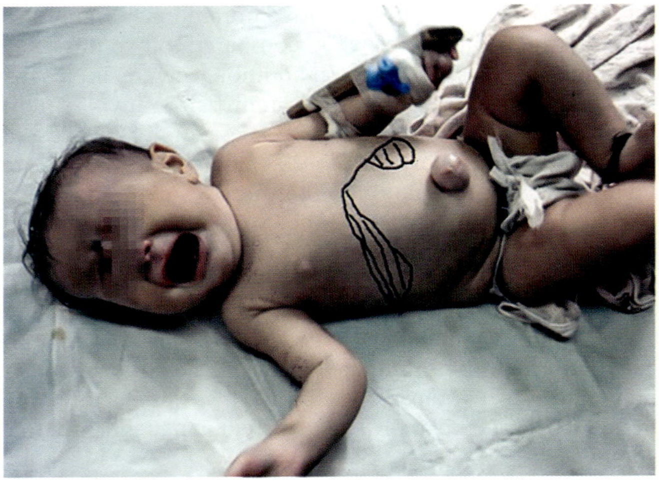

Figure 53.2 Chédiak-Higashi syndrome (Note partial albinism with HS megaly) (*Courtesy:* Dr Nitin K Shah)

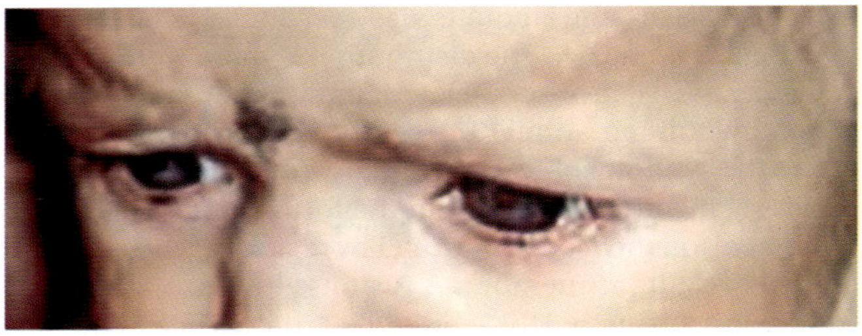

Figure 53.3 Chédiak-Higashi syndrome (Note heterochromia) (*Courtesy:* Dr Nitin K Shah)

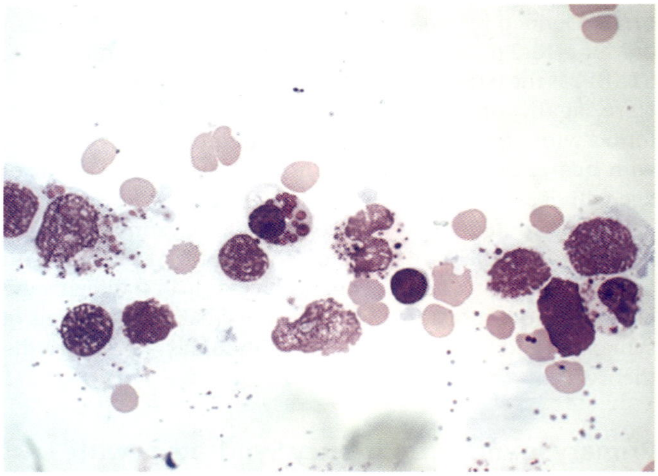

Figure 53.4 Microphotograph of peripheral smear in a case of Chédiak-Higashi syndrome (Note clumped granules) (*Courtesy:* Dr Nitin K Shah)

Hepatopathy and coagulopathy: Most patients will show some evidence of affected liver at presentation. Neonates with HLH may present with hydrops fetalis and liver failure. In fact, it would be wise to consider HLH in the differential diagnosis of all cases presenting with acute liver failure in infants,

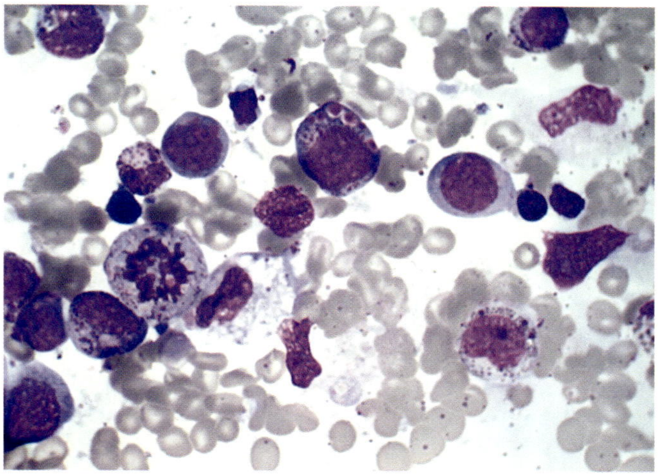

Figure 53.5 Microphotograph of bone marrow in a case of Chédiak-Higashi syndrome (Note clumped granules) (*Courtesy:* Dr Nitin K Shah)

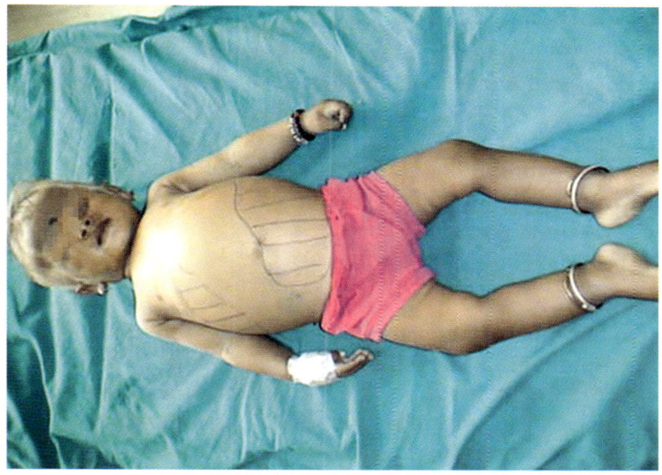

Figure 53.6 Griscelli syndrome (Note ash-colored hair with HS megaly) (*Courtesy:* Dr MR Lokeshwar and Dr Nitin K Shah)

particularly if lymphocytic infiltrates are noted on biopsy. As high as 25% of patients with veno-occlusive disease have been reported after HSCT.

Cutaneous manifestations: The cutaneous manifestations in HLH, as reported in the literature, are highly pleomorphic with incidence ranging from 6% to 65% in various studies. Generalized maculopapular rashes, generalized erythroderma, edema, panniculitis, morbilliform erythema, petechiae, and purpura are the many forms in which HLH may manifest in the skin. Occasionally, a Kawasaki disease-like presentation may also be encountered. Rashes may correlate with lymphocyte infiltration on skin biopsy, where hemophagocytes may also be found.

Pulmonary involvement: Respiratory dysfunction-mandating ventilator care has been reported in HLH with radiographic findings of alveolar and interstitial opacities; 88% of these patients could not be salvaged.

CNS manifestation: Neurological manifestations, another prominent feature of this disease, are associated with histiocytic infiltration of the CNS and are representative of advanced FHL. These are present in almost 30–40% of the patients, with younger ones manifesting with irritability, bulging fontanalle, neck stiffness, hypo or hypertonia, seizures, cranial nerve palsies, ataxia, psychomotor retardation, hemiplegia/tetraplegia, blindness, decreased level of consciousness, and other signs of raised intracranial pressure that may eventually develop. Retinal hemorrhages, swelling of the optic nerve, and infiltration of the choroid plexus have been reported in infants with HLH along with peripheral neuropathy and weakness due to myelin destruction by macrophages. Analysis of the cerebrospinal fluid suggests pleocytosis, elevated protein and/or hemophagocytosis. Elevated proteins or cell count of more than 5 cells/μL defines CNS involvement. Virtually all areas of the brain can be affected. On MRI of cerebral atrophy, diffuse white matter abnormalities, diffuse leptomeningeal enhancement, global edema, and multiple focal lesions are the typical findings. Notably, clinical, radiological, and cerebrospinal fluid (CSF) findings may not always be coherent. Also one must keep therapy-related changes in mind once the treatment has been initiated.

Reticuloendothelial system: Lymphadenopathy and splenomegaly are often present. The degree of infiltration of tissues is highly variable. Bone marrow examination is informative in many cases.

Laboratory Findings and Other Investigations[47-57]

Hematological findings: Anemia and thrombocytopenia occur in 80% of the patients. Reticulocytes are moderately raised despite severe anemia. Neutrophils are generally the last cell line to drop below the cut-off levels and can be considered as a red flag of the disease severity.

Bone marrow examination ***(Figs 53.7A and B)****:* It is mandatory not only to look for hemophagocytes but also to rule out a malignancy as a trigger of HLH. Although the disease is termed as "Hemophagocytic lymphohistiocytosis", hemophagocytes are neither a sensitive nor a specific marker of the condition because the phenomenon of hemophagocytosis is also associated with other events, such as blood transfusions, infections, autoimmune diseases, myeloproliferative disorders, bone marrow failure, or hemolysis; in addition, many cases of evolving HLH may not display hemophagocytes on bone marrow examination in the initial stages, and thus, repeat examinations may be required to check for hemophagocytes. Therapy should not be withheld simply for this reason if other criteria laid down for the diagnosis of HLH are met with and clinical condition is fitting with diagnosis of HLH, which generally requires urgent intervention.

Flow chart 53.1 Algorithmic approach to a suspected case of familial hemophagocytic lymphohistiocytosis (HLH)

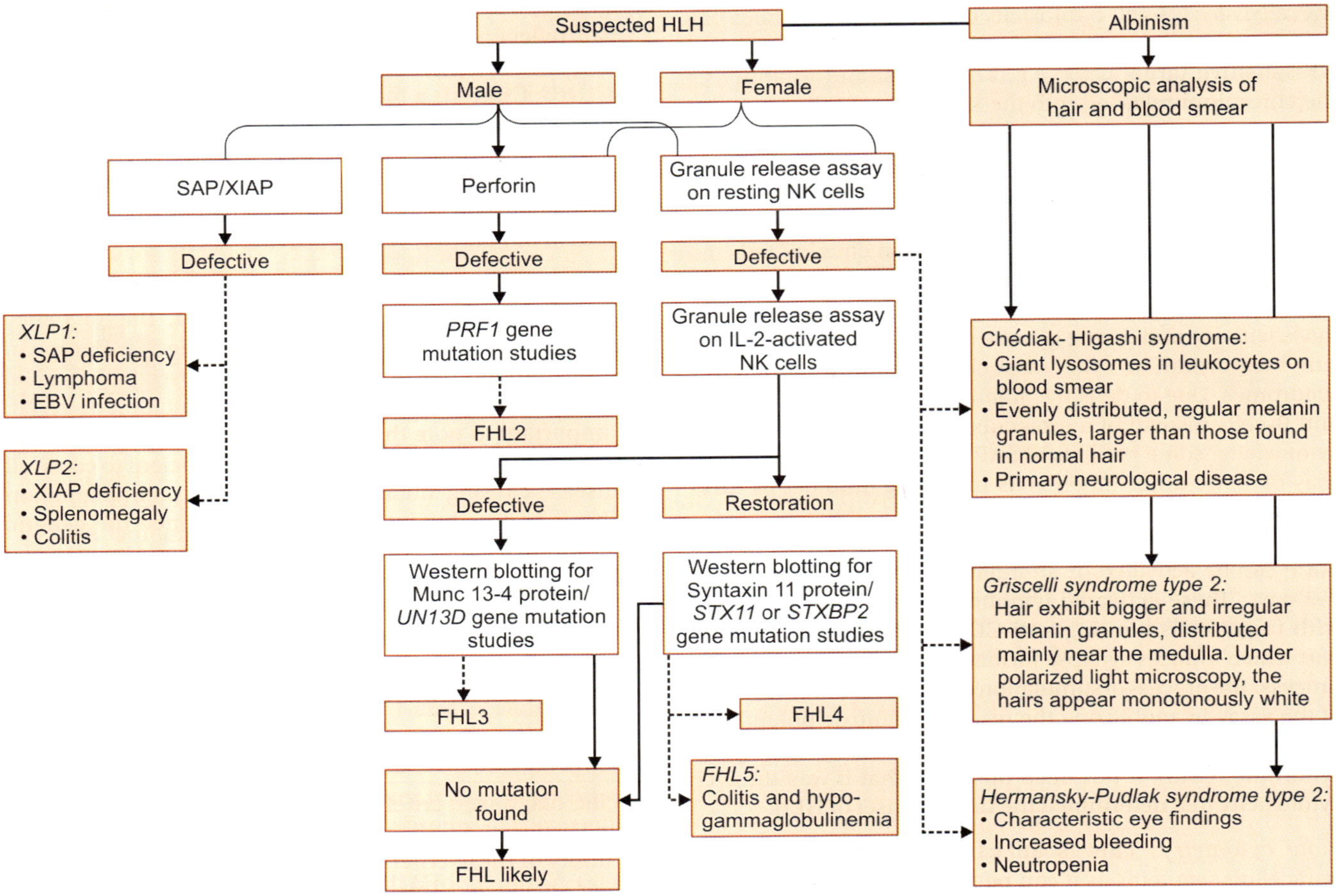

Abbreviations: FHL, familial hemophagocytic lymphohistiocytosis; XLP, X-linked lymphoproliferative; NK cell, natural killer cell; SAP, signaling lymphocyte activating (SLAM) associated protein; XIAP, X-linked inhibitor of apoptosis; HLH, hemophagocytic lymphohistiocytosis; EBV, Epstein-Barr virus

or weeks later. The cytopenias also recover transiently, particularly the thrombocytopenia with nonspecific measures, such as antibiotics and transfusions. In infants, differentials of metabolic disorders because of organomegaly, deranged liver functions and high triglycerides is often considered first. In many cases, presentation with fulminant liver failure with coagulopathy may dominate the presentation thereby delaying the diagnosis of HLH. Isolated CNS HLH can precede systemic manifestations by months and is often treated as chronic encephalitis. Serial studies measuring ferritin, triglycerides, and fibrinogen are many a times required because these may be low to begin with. A high LDH often puts in the doubt of a hemolytic process, but in HLH, the reticulocyte count is often low for the degree of anemia which is compatible with ineffective erythropoiesis. On biopsies, one may not find hemophagocytes. They may only have a megaloblastic picture on the bone marrow. On lymph node biopsy, immature-looking lymphocytes can be seen and be confused with a malignant process, whereas periportal infiltrates in a liver biopsy are interpreted as viral hepatitis. Hematological abnormalities, such as leukemia, myelodysplastic syndromes (MDS), aplastic anemias, and lymphomas may present with features similar to HLH. In addition, certain solid tumors and autoimmune conditions like SLE and systemic-onset juvenile idiopathic arthritis (SoJIA) may be complicated by similar features and the term macrophage activation syndrome (MAS) has been used in such a setting.

Special Considerations in Hemophagocytic Lymphohistiocytosis

Macrophage Activation Syndrome and Hemophagocytic Lymphohistiocytosis[58-62]

Macrophage activation syndrome (MAS) is a major and potentially fatal complication of many autoimmune/autoinflammatory conditions, such as SLE, SoJIA and Kawasaki disease. It can be the first manifestation of the condition and be triggered by infections or represent flares of the underlying condition or with change of medication. Around 10% of patients of SoJIA develop overt MAS, while

Table 53.4 Revised hemophagocytic lymphohistiocytosis (HLH), 2004 diagnostic criteria (Histiocyte society)	
The diagnosis of HLH can be established, if one of either 1or 2 below is fulfilled	
1.	A molecule diagnosis consistent with HLH
2.	Diagnostic criteria for HLH fulfilled (5 of 8 criteria below)
Initial diagnostic criteria	
1.	Fever
2.	Splenomegaly
3.	Cytopenias affecting at least two of the three lineages in the peripheral blood Hemoglobin < 9.0 g% (in neonates <10.0 g%) Platelets <100 × 10^9/L Neutrophils <1.0 × 10^9/L
4.	Hypertriglyceridemia and/or hypofibrinogenemia Fasting triglycerides >/= 3.0 mmol/L (i.e. >265 mg/dL) Fibrinogen ≤ 1.5 mg/dL
5.	Hemophagocytosis in the bone marrow, spleen or lymph nodes; no sign of malignancy
Additional criteria	
6.	Low/absent NK cell activity
7.	Hyperferritinemia; Ferritin >500 µg/L
8.	High soluble IL2R ≥ 2400 U/mL
Additional comments	
1.	If bone marrow aspirate shows no hemophagocytes look for evidence in other organs or perform serial marrow aspirates
2.	Diagnosis would be supported by • Spinal fluid pleocytosis (mononuclear cells) and or elevated spinal fluid protein • Liver biopsy shows findings consistent with chronic persistent hepatitis
3.	Cerebromeningeal symptoms, lymph node enlargement, jaundice, edema, skin rash, transaminitis, hypoproteinemia, hyponatremia, elevated very-low-density lipoprotein (VLDL) and low high-density lipoprotein (HDL)

Table 53.5 Proposed hemophagocytic lymphohistiocytosis (HLH), 2009 diagnostic criteria (Fillipovich et al.)	
1.	Molecular diagnosis of HLH or X-linked lymphoproliferative (XLP)
2.	Or at least 3 of 4 1. Fever 2. Splenomegaly 3. Cytopenias (minimum 2 cell lines decreased) 4. Hepatitis
3.	And at least1 of 4 1. Hemophagocytosis 2. ↑ Ferritin 3. ↑ sIL2Rα (age based) 4. Absent or very decreased NK function
4.	Other results supportive of HLH diagnosis • Hypertriglyceridemia • Hypofibrinogenemia • Hyponatremia

approximately 30% of them have subclinical disease. Mortality in SoJIA with MAS can reach up to 20%. This can be called as a HLH associated with rheumatological diseases and is characterized by features, such as fever, hepatosplenomegaly, lymphadenopathy, altered coagulation profiles and DIC. Since SJIA is likely to be associated with leukocytosis and thrombocytosis, one needs to look for relative cytopenias and trends rather than at absolute values to make an early diagnosis of MAS as frank cytopenia is often the last finding to appear in this setting. Hemophagocytes can often be picked up on microscopic examination of the bone marrow.

The underlying pathophysiology is similar with an exaggerated immune response causing increase T-cell and histiocytes eventually leading to hypercytokinemia. A majority of MAS patients have depressed NK cell functions, depressed perforin expression and elevated levels of sCD163, sIL2Rα and sCD8.

Lately, some parameters have been suggested to distinguish between MAS and HLH as well as MAS and flares of SoJIA. Neutrophils more than 1.8 × 10^9/L, CRP more than 90 mg/L and soluble CD25 less than 7,900 U/mL are indicative of MAS with a high sensitivity and specificity. Besides the above, the dynamics of leukocytes, platelets and fibrinogen help distinctions of MAS from JIA exacerbations.

Although there are no reports associating FHL with SoJIA, polymorphisms and heterozygous mutations in PRF 1 or UNC13D have been identified in a significant number of patients with MAS. Among other findings are polymorphism of TLR9 signaling molecule called interferon regulatory factor 5 (IRF5) which leads to hyperactivation.

Epstein-Barr Virus and Hemophagocytic Lymphohistiocytosis

Epstein-Barr virus is one of the most frequently associated viruses in the infection-associated HLH and can trigger the disease in those with a familial predisposition, particularly in those with XLP syndromes. EBV-associated HLH has been associated with infections not only of the B-cells but also of the NK and T-cells. Serial quantitative PCR of EBV DNA in the NK and T-cells as well as B-cells may help in differentiating progressive HLH with infectious mononucleosis. In cases of HLH, there may be a recurrence of EBV load despite the absence of CD20+ B-cells. Treatment requirements may vary from only steroids to HSCT. It has been found that the use of etoposide significantly improves the outcome in EBV HLH; more so its use becomes inevitable if the HLH is very severe or refractory. Rituximab helps to knock off the EBV infected B-cells and can be put into use in these cases. However, the T and the NK cells still continue to harbor the virus. Alemtuzumab may be administered in such a situation. Cases of aggressive and recurrent HLH after a primary episode of EBV HLH are known to occur.

Neonatal Hemophagocytic Lymphohistiocytosis[63-66]

Hemophagocytic lymphohistiocytosis in neonates needs a special mention because of its overlapping picture with sepsis which can often lead to a misdiagnosis and mismanagement. Also, absence of two cardinal features of HLH, namely fever and splenomegaly, in quite a few cases of neonatal HLH, particularly in the preterms, further delays the diagnosis. HLH presenting in neonatal age can be both familial as well as infection associated. The culprits often implicated in infection-associated HLH include viruses, such as CMV, herpes simplex, rubella, EBV, and adenovirus, as well as bacteria, such as pseudomonas, syphilis and tuberculosis. Features of fetal HLH included hydrops, hepatosplenomegaly, thrombocytopenia and fetal distress; hemophagocytes were found within placental villous capillaries and in many other organs.

A healthy newborn deteriorating in the first few days to months of life with or without fever with thrombocytopenia/pancytopenia with a hepatosplenomegaly or hepatomegaly and deranged liver functions should be thoroughly worked up with bone marrow and other organ biopsies if possible for hemophagocytes, for a trigger (viral and bacterial infections) and tests to confirm or rule out familial nature of the disease. However, in the fetus and neonate LCH, monocytic leukemia, sepsis, and extramedullary hematopoiesis should also be considered in the differential diagnosis of HLH.

A large proportion (around 50%) of neonates present with CNS manifestations ranging from irritability, bulging fontanelle, and neck stiffness to convulsions, cranial nerve palsies, ataxia, hemiplegia/tetraplegia and unconsciousness. So much, so that the neurological features often dominated the clinical presentation and preceded the systemic symptoms; nervous system involvement reflected by an elevated cerebrospinal fluid protein, pleocytosis, and hemophagocytes heralded disease progression.

Treatment includes eliminating the trigger with appropriate antibiotics and antivirals where possible and hitting the HLH activity hard with steroids, cyclosporine and etoposide. This generally helps to tide over the crisis and can keep the disease in check for a period of a year or two. However, those with FHL will eventually require a stem cell transplant (SCT) for survival.

Untreated HLH was found to be universally fatal. Without transplant, the prognosis in cases of FHL is dismal, with average time of death ranging from 1st day to a maximum of 2 years. In cases of infection-associated HLH, the survival with immune-chemotherapy and treatment of the underlying trigger, patients could be sustained for an average of 2.5 months (1 month to 6 months).

TREATMENT OF HEMOPHAGOCYTIC LYMPHOHISTIOCYTOSIS[67-74]

A patient diagnosed with HLH if left untreated has a median survival of only 2 months. As already mentioned, it is a rapidly developing fatal condition with overwhelming multiorgan failure; however, awareness and timely intervention can salvage a large majority of patients.

Principles of Treatment

- To suppress severe inflammation responsible for the clinical syndrome
- To look for the trigger, and if present, give specific therapy directed toward it
- To stop the T-cell reactivation and multiplication
- To consolidate the rescue therapy with a HSCT in cases of familial/persistent/recurred/CNS HLH for permanent cure.

It is important to remember that one need not wait for the molecular diagnosis, confirming the diagnosis of familial HLH because most of the time the patient may not give us the time to confirm, especially given the fact that there are still many lacunae in our knowledge which do not allow us to detect the genetic abnormality of every FHL.

Drugs Used to Suppress the Inflammation

High-dose steroids are used to suppress the inflammation. They act as lymphocytic agents and decrease the cytokine production as well as differentiation of the dendritic cells. Dexamethasone is preferred over prednisolone because of its better CNS penetration. Cyclosporine prevents T-cell activation and acts as IL2 antagonist. Etoposide is a cytostatic drug which not only inhibits the macrophages and the monocytes but also inhibits Epstein–Barr nuclear antigen (EBNA) synthesis in EBV-infected cells.

Hitting the Trigger

Leishmania-associated HLH is probably the only condition where one may get away with treating the leishmaniasis without a primarily HLH-directed therapy with the agents mentioned above. Treatment should be guided only by the severity of the symptoms, although it is essential to take into consideration the contributing factors, and every effort should be made to eliminate or at least control them. For example, antimicrobial therapy for bacterial infections, such as *Staphylococcus*, amphotericin B for *Leishmania* and one may also consider rituximab for EBV elimination and intravenous immunoglobulin (IVIg) for most viral infections.

Hemophagocytic Lymphohistiocytosis (HLH)-94 and HLH-2004 Protocols

Using the backbone of dexamethasone, cyclosporine and etoposide, the Histiocyte Society devised the first protocol to treat HLH in 1994 which led to a reported survival of 55% with a median follow-up of 3 years. It comprised an 8-week induction therapy with dexamethasone and etoposide followed by addition of cyclosporine from 9th week onward in the continuation phase. This was accompanied by a reduction in the dose intensification of the etoposide. This continuation phase was only intended to be a bridge to keep the disease under check while the patient awaits transplantation. It was found that the remission induction rate was 71% with this protocol and that the 5-year post-HSCT survival was 55–56%. To increase the remission rates, an intensification of the initial induction was proposed in the HLH-2004 protocol. This was by adding cyclosporine upfront from the 1st week of induction. Also, addition of intrathecal steroids instead of plain intrathecal methotrexate for patients with CNS involvement further helped dose intensification. Treatment plans for HLH-2004 are shown in **Figures 53.8 and 53.9**.

Induction: As already mentioned, one need not wait for the genetic confirmation of FHL to start treatment. In patients with less severe symptoms, treating with steroids and immunoglobulins may suffice to control the hypercytokinemia and resultant inflammation. However, if there is any hint that the disease is progressing toward a more severe form, switching to the full-blown protocol becomes mandatory and should not be delayed. Etoposide can be life-saving, particularly in EBV-associated FHL, given its property to decrease EBNA production in the EBV-infected cells. Delaying the administration of etoposide has been found to significantly increase the mortality rate. Malignancy- and autoimmune disease-associated HLH are the only two conditions where the induction phase can be modified. For instance, in MAS high-dose steroids form the mainstay of the treatment with cyclosporine being considered in very severe or steroid resistant cases. There are anecdotal reports that immunoglobulin infusions might be useful in MAS but more so in adults.

During the acute phase, patients may require an ICU setting with good supportive care. The standard care consists of a decrescendo course of etoposide, dexamethasone and cyclosporine with or without intrathecal therapy. It is to be highlighted that therapy needs to be initiated even in the face of unresolved infections, cytopenias, and multiorgan dysfunction involving the liver and kidneys. Since etoposide is eliminated by both these routes, required dose adjustments need to be carried out as per the protocol. Isolated hyperbilirubinemia and cytopenia do not warrant etoposide dose reduction. Since we know that the ultimate cure is HSCT, it is important to send HLA typing and start looking for the match while the patient is being pushed into temporary remission. Patients on treatment can follow a highly unpredictable and stormy course and constant monitoring for looking for response or deterioration is essential. In those who respond, improvement in the symptoms and cytopenias is expected in 2–3 weeks. Persistent cytopenias can be attributed to the myelosuppressive effects of etoposide as well as persistence of disease activity. Disappearance of symptoms and bone marrow examination can help distinguish the two. However, it is recommended that one gives at least 3–4 doses of etoposide before interrupting the therapy as hypercytokinemia can

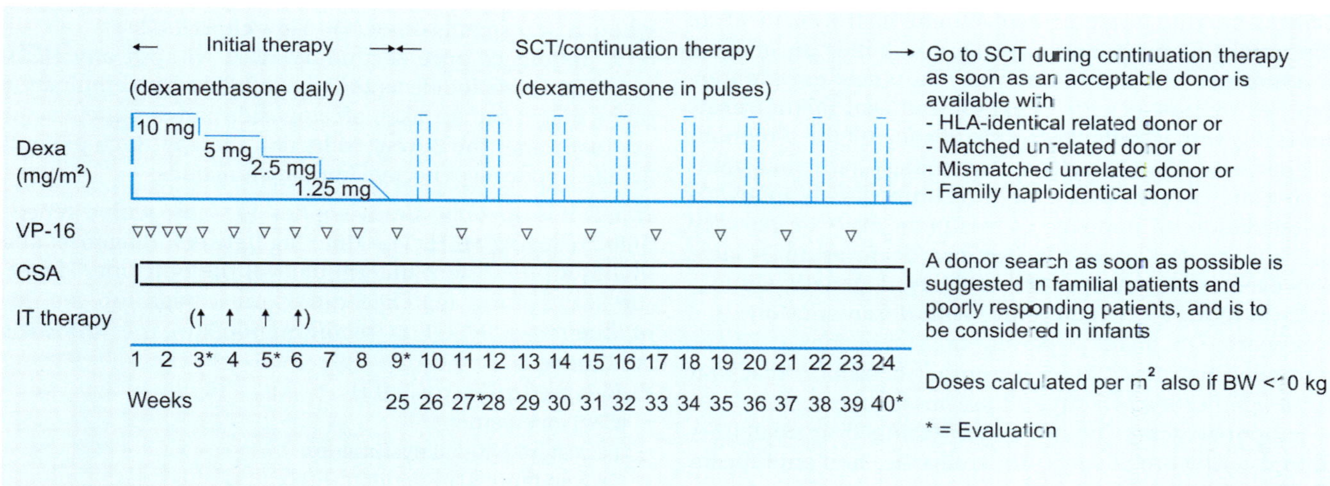

Dexa = Dexamethasone daily with 10 mg/m^2 for 2 weeks, 5 mg/m^2 for 2 weeks, 2.5 mg/m^2 for 2 weeks, 1.25 mg/m^2 for 1 week; and taper then discontinue during 8th week.

Pulses every second week with 10 mg/m^2 for 3 days during the continuation therapy

VP-16 = Etoposide 150 mg/m^2 IV twice weekly for the first two weeks, then weekly during the initial therapy. Every second week during the continuation therapy. Only in certain conditions, such as if ANC < 0.5 × 10^9/L and the bone marrow is hypocellular (which only rarely is the case), can the first two doses be omitted.

CSA = Cyclosporin A aiming at levels around 200 µg/L (monoclonal, trough value). Start with 6 mg/kg daily orally (divide in 2 daily doses), if normal kidney function

IT therapy: ↑ = Methotrexate doses by age: <1 year 6 mg, 1–2 years 8 mg, 2–3 years 10 mg, >3 years 12 mg each dose.

Prednisolone doses by age: <1 year 4 mg, 1–2 years 6 mg, 2–3 years 8 mg, >3 years 10 mg each dose

Maximum four doses are suggested, but start only if progressive neurological symptoms or if an abnormal CSF has not improved

Supporting therapy: Cotrimoxazole, eq 5 mg/kg of trimethoprim, 2–3 times weekly (week 1 and onwards). An oral antimycotic from week 1 to week 9. IvIG (0.5 g/kg IV) q 4 weeks. Gastroprotection suggested week 1–9

Figure 53.8 Treatment protocol overview for hemophagocytic lymphohistiocytosis (HLH), 2004
Abbreviation: SCT, stem cell transplant

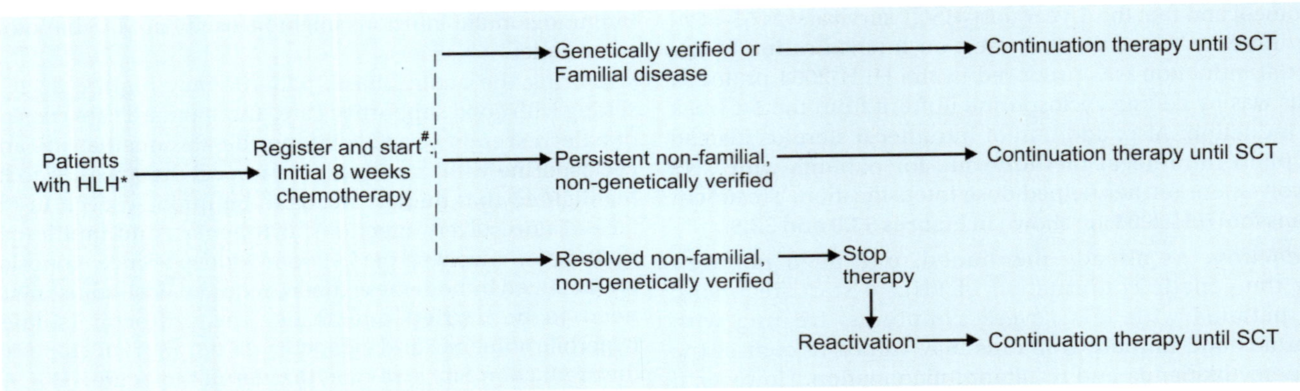

* If there is a treatable infection it should be treated but be aware that this may not be sufficient and the patient may need HLH-treatment in addition. All severe forms should start HLH-treatment. If HLH is persistent or recurring consider that the patient may have an undiagnosed inherited disease. HLH may also develop secondary to a number of other diseases as malignancies, rheumatic diseases and metabolic disorders, requiring a different treatment.

\# Start therapy, if the patient has a genetically verified disease, a familial form of HLH, or if the disease is severe, persistent, or recurrent.

Figure 53.9 Flow chart for children with hemophagocytic lymphohistiocytosis (HLH), 2004
Abbreviation: SCT, stem cell transplant

lead to a hypoplastic marrow as well. Dexamethasone and cyclosporine should, however, be continued.

Central Nervous System Disease

Central nervous system involvement in the form of an abnormal CSF examination or abnormalities on imaging or abnormal CNS symptoms and neurologic examination requires treatment with weekly intrathecal methotrexate preferably with intrathecal hydrocortisone till the symptoms disappear or CSF normalizes. Any change in mental status during the course of treatment or immediately following de-escalation or stoppage of treatment must be pursued and investigated as reactivation can occur as an isolated CNS event. CNS involvement indicates a genetic etiology and will require HSCT for cure. With dexamethasone and cyclosporine on board, hypertension is to be looked for and controlled because PRESS is another condition that may cause significant morbidity to those on treatment.

Supportive care includes monitoring drug toxicities, administering broad-spectrum antibiotics and antifungals, blood product support, prophylactic cotrimoxazole, antivirals and IVIg administration, if indicated.

Cardiac dysfunction resultant to ongoing inflammation or drug toxicities warrants baseline and periodic cardiac evaluation. Kawasaki disease, a vasculitis syndrome that can overlap and be associated with HLH, requires to be kept in mind and appropriate, and timely therapy may prevent permanent damage.

Continuation Therapy

As already mentioned, the continuation therapy acts as a bridge to HSCT. It comprises administration of etoposide once per week alternating with dexamethasone pulse for 3 days in the next week. If the blood pressure and renal functions are stable, cyclosporine should also be continued. HSCT should be planned as soon as possible while the patient is still in remission because of the likelihood of disease reactivation, infection, and etoposide-associated malignancies/MDS if used for a long time. A practical approach to decide when and whom to transplant is shown in **Flow chart 53.2.**

A patient of pure secondary HLH without any HLH-associated genetic defects and who stabilizes after elimination of the trigger can be taken off etoposide and dexamethasone gradually after the 8-week induction therapy. Such patients are likely to recover normal immune functions.

HSCT: It is the only curative option for those with a genetic defect causing HLH. The time lag between diagnosis and SCT is an important determinant of the outcome. Hence, the search for a matched donor must begin on the day of diagnosis. HSCT is recommended in the following conditions:

- Relapsed/refractory HLH
- CNS involvement
- Persistent NK cell dysfunction
- Proven familial or genetic HLH.

While looking for a donor for an affected patient with unknown genetic defect predisposing to FHL, it is to be remembered that there is a possibility that the sibling might be occultly harboring the same defect. Traditionally, myeloablative conditioning (MAC) with cyclophosphamide, busulfan, and etoposide with or without antithymocyte globulin (ATG) has been the standard of care. But high transplant-related mortality (50–65%) was noted in this group, particularly within the first 100 days postinfusion of the stem cells due to fatal inflammatory complications, such as acute respiratory distress syndrome (ARDS), veno-occlusive diseases and multiorgan failure. MAC was poorly tolerated by patients with XIAP. Hence, during the last decade, reduced intensity conditioning (RIC) has been tested

Flow chart 53.2 Treatment strategies of hemophagocytic lymphohistiocytosis (HLH)

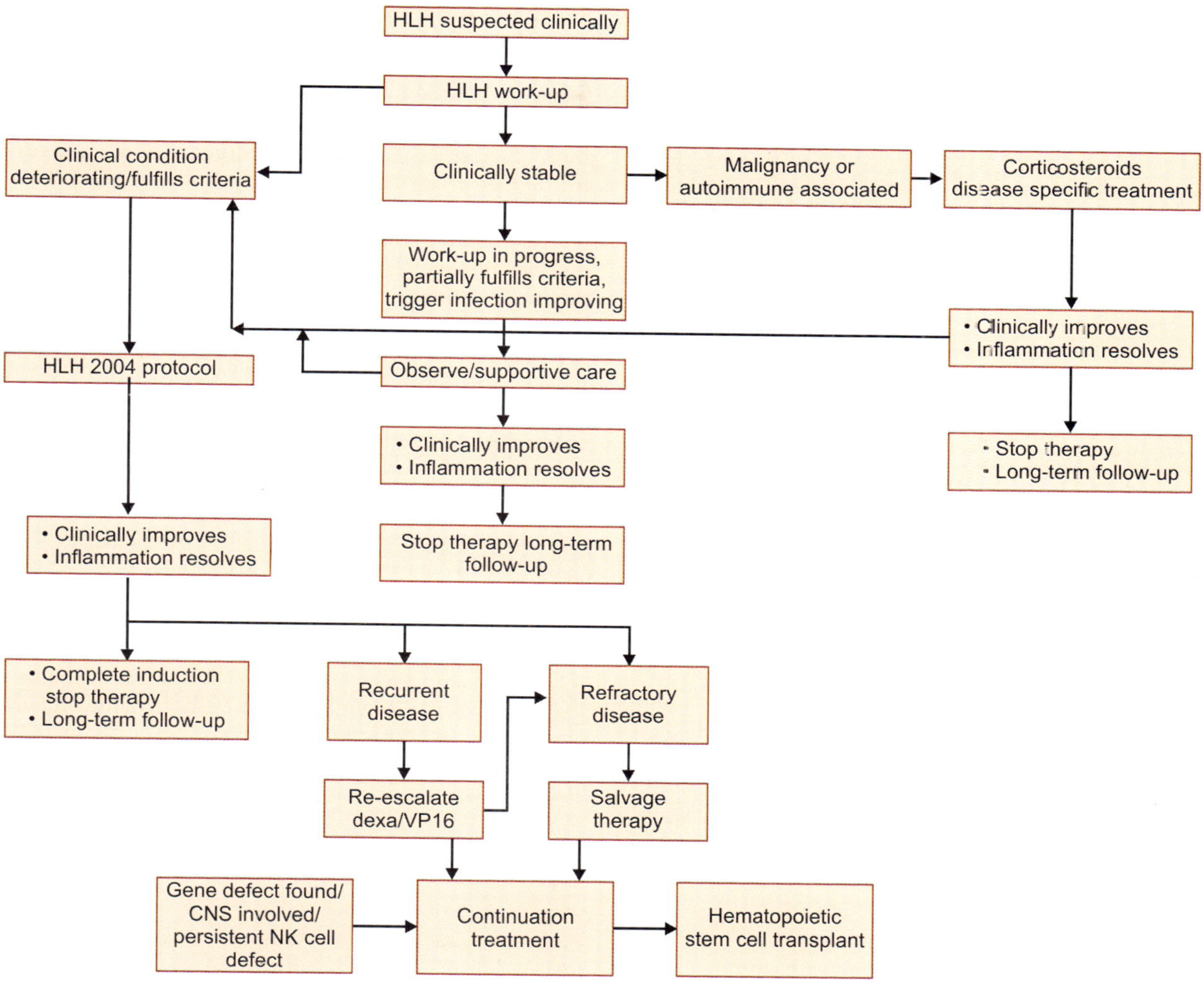

(Adapted from blood journal: review article: how I treat HLH?)

using alemtuzumab, melphalan, and fludarabine. Although a higher incidence of mixed donor chimerism was noted with RIC hematopoietic cell transplantation (HCT), the overall post-transplantation survival was found to be much improved than that following MAC HCT. Marsh et al. reported a 3-year survival of 92% in their RIC cohort as compared to 43% in the MAC cohort. Such and other single institutional reports have gradually led to an increase in the practice of RIC for HCT. Another factor determining the outcome is the disease activity at the time of transplant. In those with active disease at time of transplant, the outcome is only 50%, highlighting the importance of gaining optimum disease control before posting the patient for transplant.

Refractory Disease and Reactivation

If a patient fails to improve by 4th week into the induction of the HLH-2004 protocol, the chance that the patient will benefit from the same combination of drugs is extremely low. Although there is no established salvage therapy for such patients, anecdotal reports have shown some role of alemtuzumab (humanized anti CD 52 antibodies), daclizumab (humanized anti CD25 monoclonal antibody), infliximab, anakinra, vincristine, and fludarabine. ATG has been incorporated in a few trials as a part of salvage therapies and has been reported to give higher complete response rates. However, because of higher relapse rates, the long-term outcome of patients treated on this regimen is not very different.

Reactivation

Once in remission; recurrence of more than three out of eight:

1. Fever
2. Splenomegaly
3. Platelets less than 1 lac
4. Hypertriglyceridemia
5. Hypofibrinogenemia

6. Hemophagocytosis
7. Increased serum ferritin
8. Increase sCD25.

OR

Development of new CNS symptom without other systemic features.

In case of reactivation, it is necessary to re-escalate the doses of steroids and etoposide and restart the induction from week 2 onward. If the symptoms fail to subside, one of the salvage therapies need to be considered. In addition, reactivation becomes a definitive indication to post the patient for HCT.

Follow-up: It is found that most of the patients with primary HLH relapse within the 1st year of stopping treatment. Hence, a blanket advice for all patients off therapy is calling patient for a follow-up examination every month for 1 year and then annual follow-up.

AUTOIMMUNE LYMPHOPROLIFERATIVE SYNDROME

A rare disorder with less than 500 cases described in literature, autoimmune lymphoproliferative syndrome (ALPS) is a difficult diagnosis to make because of the variability of its clinical presentation and overlapping features with many other diseases including lymphomas. Median age at diagnosis is around 2 years, and both sexes are equally affected. A family history may be found, although the manifestations may vary from silent carrier state without any phenotypic disease to mild-to-severe fatal manifestations, all pointing to the role of modifier genes or haploinsufficiency in determining phenotypic expression.

HISTORY

The first glimpses of ALPS in humans were shown by Canale and Smith in 1967 when they described a syndrome with lymphadenopathy, splenomegaly and autoimmune cytopenias in five patients. The identification of what are now called double-negative T-cells by Sneller et al. in 1992 and the lack of cell surface receptor FAS in affected mice models in the same year allowed further insights into this disease. Rieux-Laucat et al. and Fisher et al. were able to establish the mutation in the *FAS* gene were responsible for ALPS in humans as in mice. Over the years, it has been found that other mutations in the genes encoding molecules involved in the apoptotic pathway can also lead to this syndrome.

PATHOPHYSIOLOGY[75-81]

The immune system eliminates autoreactive lymphocytes via central (elimination in the bone marrow and thymus itself) and peripheral (anergy, deletion by apoptosis, suppression by T regulatory cells) tolerance mechanisms to prevent autoimmunity and tissue damage. Apoptosis or programmed cell death, which can occur either by the intrinsic pathway, i.e. through activation of the mitochondrial proteins or extrinsic pathway, i.e. triggered by receptor ligand interactions, plays a key role in the establishing peripheral tolerance. A molecule central to the maintenance of lymphocyte homeostasis is FAS, a membrane-bound member of the TNF family present not only on activated lymphocytes but also on many other cells, such as hepatocytes. Engagement of this receptor by its ligand Fas L leads to conformational changes in its intracellular portion with recruitment of the FADD (FAS associated death domain) to the cytoplasmic tail of FAS which in turn activates the procaspases 8 and 10. Through a series of reactions, this complex eventually leads to cell death as shown in **Figure 53.10**. In ALPS, there is a loss of this peripheral immune tolerance mechanism, and hence, the occurrence of autoimmunity. Also, recent experiments have demonstrated that FAS plays a major role in regulating immune homeostasis during chronic infections rather than controlling acute immune responses in cells.

CLINICAL PRESENTATION[82-88]

Chronic lymphoproliferation in the form of lymphadenopathy (if isolated at least two nodal groups should be involved), splenomegaly, or hepatomegaly in an otherwise healthy child is the most dramatic and common presenting manifestation of this condition. The lymph nodes are often palpable and nontender and often present in the cervical, axillary and inguinal chains, although the involvement of the preauricular, epitrochlear, and submental lymph nodes is also known along with mediastinal and retroperitoneal lymphadenopathy. There can be waxing and waning of the lymph node sizes, so much so that a paradoxical reduction in the lymph node size with intercurrent infections was reported by Canale et al. Over 85% patients may present with mild-to-moderate splenomegaly.

Around 70% of patients suffer autoimmunity of some form with blood cells being one of the most common targets. Cytopenias, which in accordance with the expanding lymphocyte repertoire in children are most severe in early childhood and tend to improve with age although more than often they remain chronic and refractory. Initial presentation may consist of fatigue, pallor and icterus with indirect hyperbilirubinemia (autoimmune hemolytic anemia), spontaneous skin bleeds and mucocutaneous hemorrhages (autoimmune thrombocytopenia) and prolonged fevers and bacterial infections (autoimmune neutropenia).

Other autoimmune manifestations include glomerulonephritis, uveitis, iridocyclitis, autoimmune hepatitis, colitis, mucosal ulcers, arthritis, vasculitis, Guillain-Barré syndrome (GBS), encephalitis, myelitis and autoimmune cerebellar syndromes. Recurrent transient rash can be seen in some cases.

Patients suffering from ALPS are at an increased risk of developing malignancies (around 10–20%), particularly Hodgkin's and non-Hodgkin's lymphoma, although leukemias and solid tumors are also known to occur in these set of patients.

It should be noted that ALPS patients are not likely to present with constitutional symptoms, and their presence

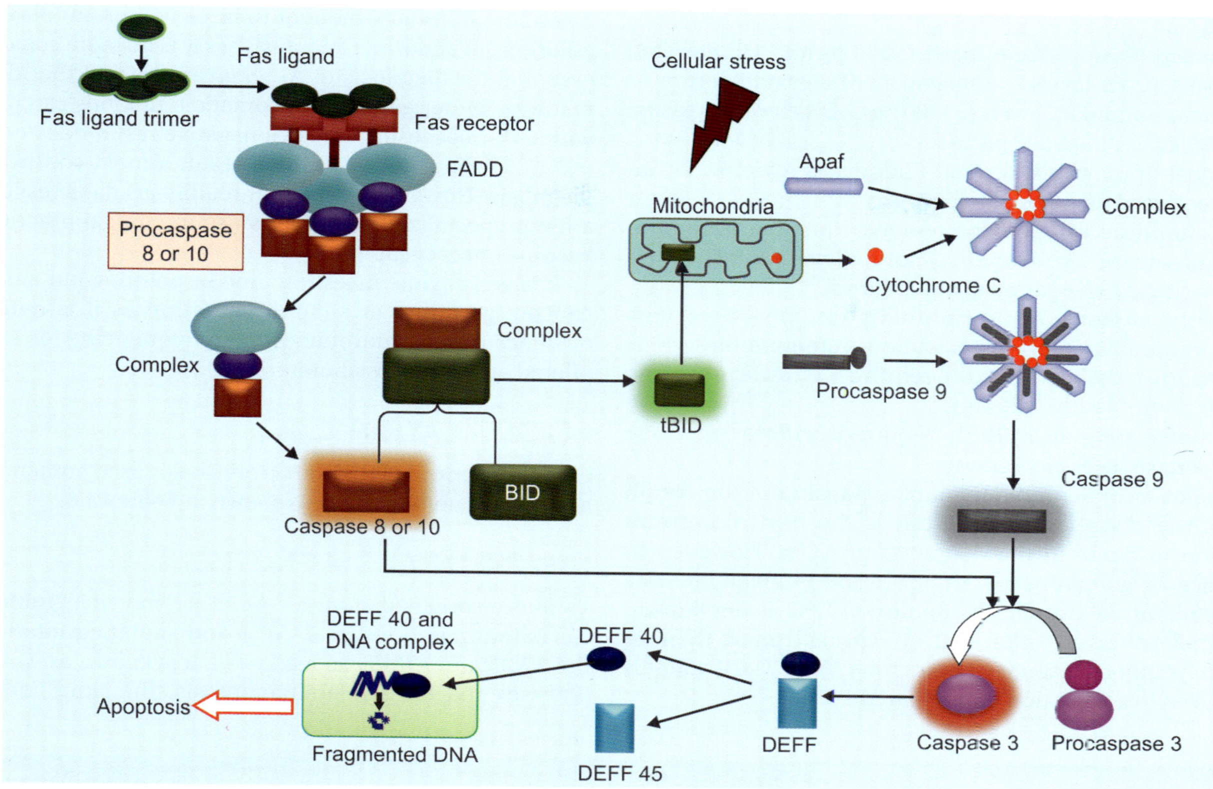

Figure 53.10 Apoptotic pathways

Note: In extrinsic pathway of apoptosis, when Fas is linked to the trimeric Fas ligand, its intracellular death domain transduces signal to cytoplasmic death domain-containing protein FADD (FAS-associated death domain). Caspase protease domain of FADD cleaves the downstream caspases 8 and 10 and triggers the caspase cascade leading to proteolysis, DNA degradation, and ultimately apoptosis. The intrinsic apoptotic pathway is activated by cellular stressors, leading to alterations in mitochondrial membrane permeability and release of apoptosis-inducing substances. Patients with ALPS have defective Fas-mediated apoptosis. Mutations in gene encoding Fas, Fas ligand and caspase 10 are most commonly associated with ALPS.[74]

should prompt one to rule out underlying infections or malignancies.

LABORATORY INVESTIGATIONS[89-93]

Multilineage cytopenias are often the most common laboratory finding. Anemia with a positive Coombs test and also secondary to hypersplenism and iron deficiency is often seen. Unexplained monocytosis and eosinophilia (7%) are also seen. Autoantibodies (92% patients) are more commonly seen than overt disease. Polyclonal hypergammaglobulinemia with positive antinuclear antibody (ANA), anticardiolipin, RA factor as well antiplatelet and antineutrophil antibodies are also seen. Although there is a poor correlation between presence of antibodies and cytopenias, the antibodies so correlate with the presence of lymphadenopathy and the characteristic double negative (DNT) cells ($CD4^-CD8^-$ $TCR\alpha\beta^+$). Lymphocytosis with Th2 cytokine profile, elevated vitamin B_{12}, IL10, IL18 and soluble Fas ligand also help in establishing the diagnosis.

Paracortical expansion of the lymph nodes because of infiltration by the double-negative T-cells along with follicular hyperplasia and polyclonal plasmacytosis can be seen on histopathological review and immunohistochemical examination of lymph node biopsy specimen.

DIAGNOSIS[94]

Revised Diagnostic Criteria for ALPS

Required

- Chronic (>6 months), nonmalignant, noninfectious lymphadenopathy and/or splenomegaly
- Elevated CD3+ TCRab+ $CD4^-CD8^-$ (DNT) cells equal to or greater than 1.5% of total lymphocytes or 2.5% of CD3+ lymphocytes in the setting of normal or elevated lymphocyte counts.

Accessory

Primary

- Defective lymphocyte apoptosis (in two separate assays)
- Somatic or germline pathogenic mutation in FAS, FASLG, or CASP10.

Secondary

- Elevated plasma sFASL levels (>200 pg/mL) OR elevated plasma IL-10 levels (>20 pg/mL) OR elevated serum or plasma vitamin B_{12} levels (>1500 ng/L) OR elevated plasma IL-18 levels above 500 pg/mL
- Typical immunohistological findings as reviewed by an experienced hematopathologist
- Autoimmune cytopenias (hemolytic anemia, thrombocytopenia or neutropenia) and elevated IgG levels (polyclonal hypergammaglobulinemia)
- Family history of a nonmalignant/noninfectious lymphoproliferation with or without autoimmunity
- *Definitive diagnosis:* Both required criteria plus one primary accessory criterion.
- *Probable diagnosis:* Both required criteria plus one secondary accessory criterion.

Besides chronic nonmalignant expansion of the lymph nodes, the presence of DNT cell is the most important criterion to come to the diagnosis of ALPS. However, in presence of lymphopenia, the criterion is invalidated as its impact on the overall distribution of DNT is not known. Nevertheless any elevation of DNT especially more than 3% of total lymphocyte count or more than 5% of T-cell count is rarely seen in a condition other than ALPS.

Although initially thought to be an important diagnostic criterion, an abnormal apoptosis assay is no more considered essential for diagnosis of ALPS given the fact that disease following either germline or somatic mutations can present with a normal result. To say a negative result does not rule out ALPS; however, a positive result almost confirms the diagnosis. However, as it is not readily available except for a few a specialized centers, its use in clinical practice has become impractical.

It is worthwhile investing time in pointing out a disease causing germline or somatic mutation as it is definitive evidence of the syndrome. Genetic sequencing for ALPS is offered only by a few laboratories.

CLASSIFICATION

Classification of ALPS based on previously used nomenclature and revised nomenclature is shown in **Table 53.6**.

DIFFERENTIAL DIAGNOSIS

Various disorders that mimic ALPS are shown in **Table 53.7**. Germline mutations in *CASP 8* and somatic mutations in the *NRAS* and *KRAS* can lead to what is known as ALPS-like illnesses and ALPS-related apoptosis. The latter condition

Table 53.6 Classification of ALPS[74]

Previous nomenclature	*Revised nomenclature*	*Gene*	*Definition*
ALPS Type 0	ALPS-FAS	*FAS*	Patients fulfill ALPS diagnostic criteria and have germline homozygous mutations in FAS
ALPS Type Ia	ALPS-FAS	*FAS*	Patients fulfill ALPS diagnostic criteria and have germline homozygous mutations in FAS
ALPS Type Im	ALPS-sFAS	*FAS*	Patients fulfill ALPS diagnostic criteria and have somatic mutations in FAS
ALPS Type Ib	ALPS-FASLG	*FASLG*	Patients fulfill ALPS diagnostic criteria and have germline mutations in FAS ligand
ALPS Type IIa	ALPS-CASP10	*CASP10*	Patients fulfill ALPS diagnostic criteria and have germline mutations in caspase 10
ALPS Type III	ALPS-U	Unknown	Patients meet ALPS diagnostic criteria; however, genetic defect is undetermined (no FAS, FASL, CASP10 defect)

Abbreviations: ALPS, autoimmune lymphoproliferative syndrome; FASLG, Fas-ligand

Table 53.7 Differential diagnosis of ALPS[74]

Previous nomenclature	*Revised nomenclature*	*Gene*	*Definition*
ALPS Type IIB	CEDS	*CASP8*	Patients present with lymphadenopathy and/or splenomegaly, marginal DNT elevation, recurrent infections, and germline mutations in caspase 8
ALPS Type IV	RALD	*NRAS*	Patients present with autoimmunity, lymphadenopathy and/or splenomegaly, elevated or normal DNTs and somatic mutations in NRAS
		KRAS	Patients present with autoimmunity, lymphadenopathy and/or splenomegaly, normal DNTs and somatic mutations in KRAS
DALD	DALD	Unknwon	Patients present with autoimmunity, lymphadenopathy and/or splenomegaly, normal DNTs and defective *in vitro* FAS-mediated apoptosis
XLP1	XLP1	*SH2D1A*	Patients present with fulminant Epstein-Barr virus infection hypogammaglobulinemia or lymphoma

Abbreviations: CEDS caspase-eight deficiency state; RALD, RAS-associated autoimmune leukoproliferative disease; DALD, Dianzani autoimmune lymphoproliferative disease; XLP1, X-linked lymphoproliferative syndrome; ALPS, autoimmune lymphoproliferative syndrome; DNT, double-negative T-cells has features like lymphadenopathy, splenomegaly and autoimmune phenomena overlapping with ALPS; however, differs in many aspects like absence of paracortical expansion with double negative T-cells, only a slight elevation in peripheral DNTs, affection of the myeloid component leading to monocytosis thereby mimicking JMML. These patients are hence labeled with the diagnosis of RAS-associated leukoproliferative disorders (RALD).

Those with defects in the *CASP 8* have features of lymphadenopathy, autoimmunity and elevated DNTs like ALPS but additionally also have defective NK, B and T-cell activation which in turn results in repeated viral and bacterial infections.

XLP1 or Duncans disease is another close differential presenting with acquired hypogammaglobulinemia and lymphomas following EBV-mediated immune dysregulation.

DALD or Dianzani autoimmune lymphoproliferative disease, which is caused by a yet unknown genetic defect, has all the features of ALPS except increased DNTs.

Castleman disease, Kikuchi-Fujimoto and Rosai Dorfmann disease are a few conditions with benign lymph node enlargements which can have features similar to ALPS but without the characteristic histopathological features.

PRINCIPLES OF TREATMENT[95-112]

Symptomatic management of autoimmune cytopenias and active surveillance for lymphoma are the two main aspects that have to be covered for clinical management of ALPS. A wait and watch policy is now recommended for patients of ALPS especially those having isolated lymphadenopathy without autoimmune manifestations since there is ample evidence available now that most of the manifestations of lymphoproliferation subside with increasing age, nevertheless a significant number of patients need to be treated for the autoimmune phenomena especially the cytopenias with immunosuppressive therapy.

Lymphoproliferation and Splenomegaly

Although massive lymphadenopathy can be socially discerning for the adolescent, it does not warrant any treatment to shrink the size of the lymph node per se. However, it is prudent to monitor the generalized lymph node and spleen sizes longitudinally in order to pick up early malignant transformations, though some amount of waxing and waning of the lymph node sizes over the clinical course of ALPS is expected.

Using clinical examination and measurements as well as CT scans (if required) done twice a year, following grading guidelines with a lymph node matrix covering all groups of nodes (e.g. cervical, axillary, inguinal) are used.

Grade 1	Few shotty lymph nodes
Grade 2	Multiple 1–2 cm nodes
Grade 3	Multiple nodes, few > 2 cm
Grade 4	Extensive visible adenopathy

Similarly, spleen size is documented by measuring its extent below the left costal margin in the midclavicular line. Neither steroids nor any other immunosuppressive therapy shrinks the size of the spleen and lymph nodes. Spleen guards are advisable for active children with huge spleens to prevent the eventuality of trauma and splenic rupture.

Autoimmune cytopenias: IV methyl prednisolone in the dose 10–15 mg/kg/day for 2–4 days followed by oral steroids (1–2 mg/kg) tapered gradually over 8–10 weeks can be used. Alternatively in extremely refractory cases 30 mg/kg of methyl prednisolone has also been tried. It is important to manage the side effects like hypertension, hyperglycemia, osteopenia and immunocompromised status consequent to the prolonged steroid use.

Simultaneous IVIg along with methyl prednisolone may help certain patients with severe autoimmune hemolytic anemia (AIHA) by inhibiting the antibody-mediated red cell destruction and allowing the transfusion of packed red cell in cases of severe anemia causing hypoxia or cardiac failure.

Anti-D use for isolated thrombocytopenia is best avoided because many of these patients are likely to be DCT positive and Anti-D can cause severe hemolysis.

Low-dose granulocyte colony-stimulating factor (GCSF) (1–2 µg/kg) can help in raising the neutrophil count to some extent in autoimmune neutropenias especially during an infective episode.

Rituximab (375 mg/m^2—4 weekly doses) has been tried but is not advisable, the reason being the additional risk of infection that the patient is exposed to as a result of prolonged hypogammaglobulinemia, prolonged neutropenia and no response to pneumococcal polysaccharide vaccine for almost 4 years. The median duration for which the response is sustained is around 21 months.

Mycophenolate mofetil (MMF) at a dose of 600 mg/m^2/dose for two doses per day has been successfully used for the treatment of ALPS-related chronic cytopenias. It is also useful to counter other autoimmune manifestations like uveitis, glomerulonephritis and pulmonary affection. However, it is recommended to use MMF as a steroid sparing agent and not as first line therapy. It is generally started when patients are being treated with corticosteroids for a flare-up of their cytopenia (as reflected by a complete blood count with hemoglobin <8 g%, absolute neutrophil count <500 cells, or platelets <50,000) while they are being slowly tapered off their corticosteroids over 8- to 12-week period. While shifting the patient to MMF, an overlap period of 2 weeks should be kept, which is the time required for the therapeutic levels of MMF to be achieved.

Rapamycin or sirolimus is an mTOR inhibitor which is the only immunosuppressant that helps in bringing down the lymph node enlargements and splenomegaly besides helping with the cytopenias. Again, it should not be used as first line and added only in cases that are refractory to steroids or other steroid sparing agents like MMF. Following a loading dose of 3 mg/m^2 once daily dose of 2.5 mg/m^2 is recommended (up to maximum of 4 mg). A 24-hour trough level of

5–15 ng/mL should be targeted for optimal clinical response and drug levels monitored where facility for the same are available. Since the drug might be needed over a long period of the patients' lifetime, liver and renal toxicities have to be monitored and required dose modifications have to be done. Other side effects include T-cell immunosuppression, hypercholesterolemia and stomatitis.

A few reports have suggested a successful clinical use of other agents, including hydroxychloroquine, cyclosporine, dapsone, azathioprine and 6-mercaptopurine, and they should also be considered as a viable option in some patients with ALPS.

Splenectomy: The new consensus is to keep splenectomy reserved only for those with severe hypersplenism and who fail all the above-mentioned measures to correct the autoimmune cytopenias. Previously, more than 50% of ALPS patients used to undergo splenectomy for their cytopenias but the fatality rate due to sepsis despite proper vaccinations and prophylactic antibiotics was very high, not converting into an survival advantage eventually. If unavoidable the patient should be prevaccinated with both the 13-valent conjugated pneumococcal vaccine and the subsequent 23-valent polysaccharide vaccine. Also, the response of cytopenias is variable and in many patients the cytopenias reappear. Hence, it is best to avoid a splenectomy until it becomes inevitable.

Lymphoma surveillance: Besides cytopenias and infections, what can kill a patient of ALPS is malignant transformation of the nodes especially if they are not picked up early enough and treated accordingly. Clues like fever, night sweats, fatigue, weight loss and loss of appetite should always be enquired, as they may help differential malignant transformation of nodes from ALPS-associated size fluctuations. Fluorodeoxyglucose positron emission tomography (FDG PET) along with CT scan done periodically can and should be used in evaluating and monitoring the lymph nodes besides the clinical grading mentioned previously.

Bone marrow transplant (BMT) can be considered in those with severe refractory disease and in those with homozygous or compound heterozygous mutations. Newer targeted therapies are under investigation and might eliminate the need for BMT eventually.

Genetic counseling: It is likely that a family will have more than one affected member and assessment of relatives of ALPS probands with mutations in genes coding FAS or CASP 10 can identify the member carrying identical heterozygous mutation inherited in an autosomal dominant fashion. However, manifestation depends on the variable penetrance causing gene alteration. Genetic counseling should be an integral part of management of ALPS patients.

ITK DEFICIENCY[113-119]

Epstein-Barr virus is best known to cause infectious mononucleosis in humans. However, in individuals with underlying immune deficiency it can cause severe and fatal immune dysregulation. In the last two decades many PIDs with EBV lymphoproliferation have been discovered (STK4, CD27, MAGT1); ITK i.e. interleukin 2 inducible T-cell kinase deficiency is one such condition. S Ghosh et al. have described eight patients with mutations in the *ITK gene.*

Interleukin-2-inducible T-cell kinase (ITK, also LYK) is one of the five members of the TEC family of kinases which are proteins that function as nonreceptor protein tyrosine kinases in the development and signaling of the lymphoid lineage. Its deficiency can cause a T-cell defect leading to varied manifestations. Once an APC presents the antigen to the T and NK cell, phosphorylation of the ITK takes place which through further downstream pathways eventually causes transcriptional activity for lymphokine production and T-cell proliferation and differentiation. In the absence of this activity, it is difficult to eliminate EBV.

Organomegaly, lymphadenopathy, pancytopenias, opportunistic infections with *Candida* species and *Pneumocystis jirovecii*, pleural and pericardial effusions and autoimmune phenomena can be the presenting symptoms. There is a predisposition to develop EBV-associated malignancies especially Hodgkin's and non-Hodgkin's lymphoma, lymphoproliferative disorders, HLH and other types of monoclonal B-cell expansion and dysgammaglobulinemia. Lymphopenia, progressive hypogammaglobulinemia with progressive loss of CD4+ T-cells form important immunological features. Treatment with rituximab showed some improvement, whole steroids could not be of much help. Chemotherapy and radiotherapy targeted to the malignancy most commonly Hodgkin's lymphoma should be given. Immunoglobulin infusion may be tried to control the viremia. HSCT has been tried in a patient who succumbed following severe graft-versus-host disease (GVHD).

ITCH Deficiency[120-123]

Human ITCH deficiency results in a syndrome characterized by autoimmunity, craniofacial dysmorphisms and altered physical growth. It has been described in an Old Order Amish family in children born out of consanguineous marriage occurring within the family and affecting both sexes, highlighting its autosomal recessive pattern of inheritance.

ITCH attaches ubiquitin to substrate proteins. The primary function of ubiquitin is degradation of target proteins in the proteasome and this process is extremely useful for immune regulation as it affects the antigen processing by the APCs, and by skewing the downstream signaling components toward anergy rather than activation, it helps in the development of immune tolerance. Ubiquitination of the T-cell receptors downregulates its downstream pathways thereby decreasing the IL-2 production and further T-cell proliferation. Dysfunction of the E3 ligase which catalyzes the final step of ubiquitin attachment can hamper this regulation and cause uninhibited T-cell proliferation and activation and loss of self-tolerance resulting in myriad autoimmune phenomena within the body.

Average age of presentation was 4 years. Characteristic clinical features included facial dysmorphisms (frontal bossing, macrocephaly, dolichocephaly, orbital ptosis, small chin, low, posteriorly rotated ears, flat mid face with a prominent occiput), severe failure to thrive, hepatosplenomegaly, global developmental delay with generalized hypotonia, campto- and clinodactyly, a predisposition to recurrent infections and most importantly multisystem autoimmune disease which includes autoimmune hepatitis [antiliver kidney microsomal (LKM) antibodies can be positive, altered AST and Alt, lymphocytic infiltration of the porta hepatis], autoimmune enteropathies leading to malabsorption, autoimmune thyroiditis (often anti-TPO antibodies positive) leading to hypothyroidism and diabetes mellitus type 1. Another fatal affection is due to antibodies against lungs leading to chronic lung disease. No specific abnormalities were found in the complete blood counts.

Unlike in the mice, ITCH is strongly expressed in humans in the gastrointestinal (GI) tract, pancreas, neuronal tissue and lymphoid organs. The associated facial dysmorphism in affected individuals suggests a developmental role for ITCH in nonhematopoietic organs as well.

Treatment consists of immunosuppression with steroids and other steroid sparing agents which include azathioprine, rapamycin and tacrolimus besides supportive care with hormone replacements and diet modifications for malabsorption. Screening for autoimmune phenomenon and instituting early immunosuppressive regimens can halt the damage and salvage the organ function. BMT is being considered as a potential therapy.

APECED[124,125]

Autoimmune **P**oly-**E**ndocrinopathy **C**hronic mucocutaneous candidiasis **E**ctodermal **D**ystrophy or an **A**utoimmune **P**olyendocrinopathy **S**yndrome 1 (APS 1) first detected in 1960s is a autosomally inherited condition with mutation in the *AIRE gene*. Iranian Jews, Finns and Sardinians are the most common populations to be affected by this disease. Despite being a monogenic disease, the clinical heterogeneity of the disease often makes the diagnosis extremely difficult.

The first sign is often chronic *Candida* infections followed by hypoparathyroidism followed by autoimmune Addison's disease. *Candida* infections occur within the first 2 years of life and are found to be associated with oral carcinoma following chronic oral thrush. Autoimmunity to the TH17 regulatory cells leading to defective fungal immunity is thought to be responsible for the chronic candidiasis. Early onset parathyroid affection is the most frequent and often the only endocrine manifestation seen in these patients. No immunological basis for the ectodermal dysplasia affecting skin and nails has been discovered so far. Other autoimmune manifestations are as enlisted in **Table 53.8**.

The diagnosis of APECED is made by the presence of two of the three most common clinical features: chronic mucocutaneous candidiasis (CMC), chronic hypoparathyroidism (CH) and Addison's disease (AD). If a sibling is affected, presence of any one criterion also suffices.

Life expectancy is often determined by the severity of the disease with necrotizing hepatitis, severe malabsorption, tubulointerstitial nephritis and Addisonian crisis due to improper hormone replacement being the most common cause of death.

No disease-specific therapy is available yet and treatment mainly consists of hormone replacement and symptomatic treatment. Immunosuppressive therapy has been tried only in fatal affections like hepatitis and nephritis. Rituximab has been recently tried for pulmonary disease in APECED and has raised some hopes.

IPEX[126-130]

Immunodysregulation, polyendocrinopathy and enteropathy (IPEX) is an X-linked and extremely rare condition resulting from mutations in the *FOXP3* gene and causing aggressive autoimmunity and early death. The most common and striking presenting symptoms are type 1 diabetes mellitus and enteropathy manifesting as secretory diarrhea and hence severe growth retardation. Eczema, Coombs-positive anemia, thrombocytopenia, lymphadenopathy, polyarticular arthritis are less commonly seen symptoms. Severe sepsis occurs frequently and can be the cause of death. Abnormalities of hormones and proteins released in the GI tract, slight increase in the CD4+ cells, increased eosinophils and increased IgE levels are amongst the many abnormalities detected. Treatment mainly consists of immunosuppression with cyclosporine with supportive care; BMT is the only treatment options that is likely to work eventually.

Aicardi-Goutières Syndrome[131-141]

An autosomal recessive condition often seen in children born out of consanguineous marriage Aicardi–Goutières syndrome (AGS); it is an interferonopathy characterized by encephalopathy along with cerebral atrophy, calcifications,

Table 53.8 Components of APECED (**A**utoimmune **P**oly-**E**ndocrinopathy **C**hronic mucocutaneous candidiasis **E**ctodermal **D**ystrophy)[123]

APECED components	*Tissue*
Addison's disease	Adrenals (cortex)
Hypoparathyroidism	Parathyroid glands
Hypothryoidism	Thyroid gland
Type 1 diabetes	Endocrine pancreas
Autoimmune hepatitis	Liver
Vitiligo	Skin
Alopecia	Scalp
Malabsorption	Gastrointestinal tract
Autoimmune gastritis	Stomach
Pernicious anemia	Gastric mucosa, red blood cells

acquired microcephaly and increased CSF lymphocytes and IFN-α. Age at presentation ranges from neonatal period to around 4 months, although rarely the disease might manifest itself for the first time beyond the age of 2 years. Unexplained medium grade fevers accompanied by increased irritability, refusal to feed, disturbed sleep–wake patterns often lead to the erroneous diagnosis of sepsis/meningitis. Microcephaly, neonatal neurological derangement, hepatosplenomegaly (although transitory), anemia and thrombocytopenia often makes TORCH [Toxoplasmosis, Other (syphilis, varicella-zoster, parvovirus B19), Rubella, Cytomegalovirus (CMV) and Herpes] infections a very likely diagnosis. This active phase of disease activity with raised CSF levels of IFNα is followed by a quiescent or stable state. Till date, four disease causing gene mutations have been identified and the syndrome classified accordingly namely *TREX1* on chromosome 3, known as AGS1; *RNaseH2B/FLJ11712* on chromosome 13, known as AGS2; *RNaseH2C/AYP1* on chromosome 11, known as AGS3 and *RNaseH2A* on chromosome 19, known as AGS4. These mutations account for 83% of diagnosed patients. Another, which probably still needs to be looked for, would account for the remaining 17%. A defect in the mechanism of clearance of nucleic acids released from the dead cells results in their accumulation within the cells. These are recognized as foreign proteins probably viral in origin by the innate immunity leading to autoinflammatory response mediated through IFN-α produced by the macrophages.

Below are enumerated criteria for diagnosing AGS:

- Early onset encephalopathy with psychomotor delay, spasticity, extrapyramidal signs and microcephaly, the latter appearing in the course of the 1st year of life
- Calcifications particularly visible at basal ganglia level (putamen, pallidus and thalamus), but also extending to the periventricular white matter.
- Cerebral white matter abnormalities
- Cerebral atrophy
- Exclusion of pre-/perinatal infections, in particular the TORCH complex
- Chronic lymphocytosis (>5 cells/mm^3) on CSF examination, not accompanied by any other sign of an infectious process.
- Raised INF-α in the CSF (>2 IU/mL).
- Elevated neopterins and biopterins in CSF, sometimes associated with decreased folates.
- Important systemic symptoms in the early stages of the disease include irritability, feeding and sleeping difficulties, unexplained fevers and the appearance of chilblain-like skin lesions on the fingers, toes and ears.
- Genetic screening for mutations in the four genes known to cause AGS allows definitive confirmation of the diagnosis in the majority (83%) of cases.

Treatment includes only symptomatic management like control of seizures, physiotherapy. Vasodilators and immunosuppressants do not work effectively for extraneurological symptoms like chilblains. Treatment with folinic acid helps in improving general wellbeing. High-dose corticosteroids have also been tried by some.

CONCLUSION

In the coming years with advances in genetic analysis we look forward into further unravelling the mysteries of the primary immune dysregulation syndromes and finding out the abnormalities at the minutest possible levels. This is likely to help us understand better the pathophysiology and the resulting clinical manifestations. Identification of the possible targets shall allow us to increase the compendium of investigations and therapies that can be used for effective prenatal diagnosis and subsequent prevention as well as early diagnosis and effective treatment for improving the survival and quality of life and even cure these patients.

REFERENCES

1. Al-Herz W, Bousfiha A, Casanova JL, Chatila T, Conley ME, Cunningham-Rundles C, et al. Primary immunodeficiency diseases: an update on the classification from the International Union of Immunological Societies Expert Committee for Primary Immunodeficiency. Front Immunol. 2014;5:162.
2. Aricò M, Janka G, Fischer A, Henter JI, Blanche S, Elinder G, et al. Hemophagocytic lymphohistiocytosis. Report of 122 children from the international registry. FHL study group of the Histiocyte Society. Leukemia. 1996:10(2):197-203.
3. Janka GE, Lehmberg K. Hemophagocytic lymphohistiocytosis: pathogenesis and treatment. Hematology Am Soc Hematol Educ Program. 2013;2013:605-11.
4. Rajagopala S, Dutta U, Chandra KS, Bhatia P, Varma N, Kochhar R. Visceral leishmaniasis associated hemophagocytic lymphohistiocytosis: case report and systematic review. J Infect. 2008;56:381-8.
5. Janka G, Imashuku S, Elinder G, Schneider M, Henter JI. Infection- and malignancy-associated hemophagocytic syndromes. Secondary hemophagocytic lymphohistiocytosis. Hematol Oncol Clin North Am. 1998;12(2):435-44.
6. Risdall RJ, McKenna RW, Nesbit ME, Krivit W, Balfour HH Jr, Simmons RL, et al. Virus-associated hemophagocytic syndrome: a benign histiocytic proliferation distinct from malignant histiocytosis. Cancer. 1979;44:993-1002.
7. Takahashi N, Chubachi A, Miura I, Nakamura S, Miura AB. [Lymphoma-associated hemophagocytic syndrome in Japan]. Rinsho Ketsueki. 1999;40:542-9.
8. Rouphael NG, Talati NJ, Vaughan C, Cunningham K, Moreira R, Gould C. Infections associated with haemophagocytic syndrome. Lancet Infect Dis. 2007;7:814-22.
9. O'Brien MM, Lee-Kim Y, George TI, McClain KL, Twist CJ, Jeng M. Precursor B-cell acute lymphoblastic leukemia presenting with hemophagocytic lymphohistiocytosis. Pediatr Blood Cancer. 2008;50:381-3.
10. Quintanilla-Martinez L, Kumar S, Fend F, Reyes E, Teruya-Feldstein J, Kingma DW, et al. Fulminant EBV(+) T-cell lymphoproliferative disorder following acute/ chronic EBV infection: a distinct clinicopathologic syndrome. Blood. 2000;96:443-51.
11. Janka GE. Familial hemophagocytic lymphohistiocytosis. Eur J Pediatr. 1983;140:221-30.
12. Janka GE. Familial and acquired hemophagocytic lymphohistiocytosis. Eur J Pediatr. 2007;166(2):95-109.
13. Filipovich AH. The expanding spectrum of hemophagocytic lymphohistiocytosis. Curr Opin Allergy Clin Immunol. 2011;11(6):512-6.

14. Kuriyama T, Takenaka K, Kohno K, Yamauchi T, Daitoku S, Yoshimoto G, et al. Engulfment of hematopoietic stem cells caused by down-regulation of CD47 is critical in the pathogenesis of hemophagocytic lymphohistiocytosis. Blood. 2012;120(19):4058-67.
15. Kawaguchi H, Miyashita T, Herbst H, Niedobitek G, Asada M, Tsuchida M, et al. Epstein-Barr virus-infected T lymphocytes in Epstein-Barr virus-associated hemophagocytic syndrome. J Clin Invest. 1993;92(3):1444-50.
16. Beutel K, Gross-Wieltsch U, Wiesel T, Stadt UZ, Janka G, Wagner HJ. Infection of T lymphocytes in Epstein-Barr virus-associated hemophagocytic lymphohistiocytosis in children of non-Asian origin. Pediatr Blood Cancer. 2009;53(2):184-90.
17. Atteritano M, David A, Bagnato G, Beninati C, Frisina A, Iaria C, et al. Haemophagocytic syndrome in rheumatic patients. A systematic review. Eur Rev Med Pharmacol Sci. 2012;16(10):1414-24.
18. Ravelli A, Grom AA, Behrens EM, Cron RQ. Macrophage activation syndrome as part of systemic juvenile idiopathic arthritis: diagnosis, genetics, pathophysiology and treatment. Genes Immun. 2012;13(4):289-98.
19. Karras A. What nephrologists need to know about hemophagocytic syndrome. Nat Rev Nephrol. 2009;5(6):329-36.
20. Gokce M, Unal O, Hismi B, Gumruk F, Coskun T, Balta G, et al. Secondary hemophagocytosis in 3 patients with organic acidemia involving propionate metabolism. Pediatr Hematol Oncol. 2012;29(1):92-8.
21. Duval M, Fenneteau O, Doireau V, Faye A, Emilie D, Yotnda P, et al. Intermittent hemophagocytic lymphohistiocytosis is a regular feature of lysinuric protein intolerance. J Pediatr. 1999;134(2):236-9.
22. Lykens JE, Terrell CE, Zoller EE, Risma K, Jordan MB. Perforin is a critical physiologic regulator of T-cell activation. Blood. 2011;118:618-26.
23. Behrens EM, Canna SW, Slade K, Rao S, Kreiger PA, Paessler M, et al. Repeated TLR9 stimulation results in macrophage activation syndrome-like disease in mice. J Clin Invest. 2011;121:2264-77.
24. Castillo L, Carcillo J. Secondary hemophagocytic lymphohistiocytosis and severe sepsis/systemic inflammatory response syndrome/multiorgan dysfunction syndrome/macrophage activation syndrome share common intermediate phenotypes on spectrum of inflammation. Pediatr Crit Care Med. 2009;10(3):387-92.
25. Henter JI, Elinder G, Soder O, Hansson M, Andersson B, Andersson U. Hypercytokinemia in familial hemophagocytic lymphohistiocytosis. Blood. 1991;78:2918-22.
26. Trizzino A, Zur Stadt U, Ueda I, Risma K, Janka G, Ishii E, et al. Genotype–phenotype study of familial haemophagocytic lymphohistiocytosis due to perforin mutations. J Med Genet. 2008;45:15-21.
27. Stepp SE, Dufourcq-Lagelouse R, Le Deist F, Bhawan S, Certain S, Mathew PA, et al. Perforin gene defects in familial hemophagocytic lymphohistiocytosis. Science. 1999;286:1957-9.
28. Sieni E, Cetica V, Santoro A, Beutel K, Mastrodicasa E, Meeths M, et al. Genotype–phenotype study of familial haemophagocytic lymphohistiocytosis type 3. J Med Genet. 2011;48:343-52.
29. Zhang K, Jordan MB, Marsh RA, Johnson JA, Kissell D, Meller J, et al. Hypomorphic mutations in PRF1, MUNC13-4, and STXBP2 are associated with adult-onset familial HLH. Blood. 2011;118:5794-8.
30. Meeths M, Chiang SC, Wood SM, Entesarian M, Schlums H, Bang B, et al. Familial hemophagocytic lymphohistiocytosis type 3 (FHL3) caused by deep intronic mutation and inversion in UNC13D. Blood. 2011;118(22):5783-93.
31. Dufourcq-Lagelouse R, Jabado N, Le Deist F, Stephan JL, Souillet G, Bruin M, et al. Linkage of familial hemophagocytic lymphohistiocytosis to 10q21-22 and evidence for heterogeneity. Am J Hum Genet. 1999;64:172-9.
32. Feldmann J, Callebaut I, Raposo G, Certain S, Bacq D, Dumont C, et al. Munc13-4 is essential for cytolytic granules fusion and is mutated in a form of familial hemophagocytic lymphohistiocytosis (FHL3). Cell. 2003;115:461-73.
33. Zur Stadt U, Schmidt S, Kasper B, Beutel K, Diler AS, Henter JI, et al. Linkage of familial hemophagocytic lymphohistiocytosis (FHL) type-4 to chromosome 6q24 and identification of mutations in syntaxin 11. Hum Mol Genet. 2005;14:827-34.
34. Zur Stadt U, Rohr J, Seifert W, Koch F, Grieve S, Pagel J, et al. Familial hemophagocytic lymphohistiocytosis type 5 (FHL-5) is caused by mutations in Munc18-2 and impaired binding to syntaxin 11. Am J Hum Genet. 2009;85:482-92.
35. Pagel J, Beutel K, Lehmberg K, Koch F, Maul-Pavicic A, Rohlfs AK, et al. Distinct mutations in STXBP2 are associated with variable clinical presentations in patients with familial hemophagocytic lymphohistiocytosistype 5 (FHL5). Blood. 2012;119:6016-24.
36. Pachlopnik Schmid J, Canioni D, Moshous D, Touzot F, Mahlaoui N, Hauck F, et al. Clinical similarities and differences of patients with X linked lymphoproliferative syndrome type 1 (XLP-1/SAP deficiency) versus type 2 (XLP-2/XIAP deficiency). Blood. 2011;117:1522-9.
37. Nichols KE, Harkin DP, Levitz S, Krainer M, Kolquist KA, Genovese C, et al. Inactivating mutations in an SH2 domain-encoding gene in X-linked lymphoproliferative syndrome. Proc Natl Acad Sci USA. 1998;95:13765-70.
38. Rigaud S, Fondaneche MC, Lambert N, Pasquier B, Mateo V, Soulas P, et al. XIAP deficiency in humans causes an X-linked lymphoproliferative syndrome. Nature. 2006;444:110-4.
39. Berrueco R, Rives S, Camos M, Toll T, Catala A, Estella J. Syndromic albinism and haemophagocytosis. Br J Haematol. 2010;148:815.
40. Stinchcombe J, Bossi G, Griffiths GM. Linking albinism and immunity: the secrets of secretory lysosomes. Science. 2004;305(5680):55-9.
41. de Saint Basile G, Menasche G, Fischer A. Molecular mechanisms of biogenesis and exocytosis of cytotoxic granules. Nat Rev Immunol. 2010;10(8):568-79.
42. Haddad E, Sulis ML, Jabado N, Blanche S, Fischer A, Tardieu M. Frequency and severity of central nervous system lesions in hemophagocytic lymphohistiocytosis. Blood. 1997;89:794-800.
43. Horne A, Trottestam H, Arico M, Egeler RM, Filipovich AH, Gadner H, et al. Frequency and spectrum of central nervous system involvement in 193 children with haemophagocytic lymphohistiocytosis. Br J Haematol. 2008;140:327-35.
44. Ladisch S, Poplack DG, Holiman B, Blaese RM. Immunodeficiency in familial erythrophagocytic lymphohistiocytosis. Lancet. 1978;1:581-3.
45. Zoller EE, Lykens JE, Terrell CE, Aliberti J, Filipovich AH, Henson PM, et al. Hemophagocytosis causes a consumptive anemia of inflammation. J Exp Med. 2011;208:1203-14.
46. Henter JI, Carlson LA, Soder O, Nilsson-Ehle P, Elinder G. Lipoprotein alterations and plasma lipoprotein lipase reduction in familial hemophagocytic lymphohistiocytosis. Acta Paediatr Scand. 1991;80:675-81.
47. Lehmberg K, Ehl S. Diagnostic evaluation of patients with suspected haemophagocytic lymphohistiocytosis. Br J Haematol. 2013;160(3):275-87

by bone marrow transplantation. Bone Marrow Transplant. 1998;22(4):375-80.
113. Ghosh S, Bienemann K, Boztug K, Borkhardt A. Interleukin-2-inducible T-cell kinase (ITK) deficiency—clinical and molecular aspects. J Clin Immunol. 2014;34:892-9.
114. Mansouri D, Mahdaviani SA, Khalilzadeh S, Mohajerani SA, Hasanzad M, Sadr S, et al. IL-2-inducible T-cell kinase deficiency with pulmonary manifestations due to disseminated Epstein-Barr virus infection. Int Arch Allergy Immunol. 2012;158(4):418-22.
115. Stepensky P, Weintraub M, Yanir A, Revel-Vilk S, Krux F, Huck K, et al. IL-2-inducible T-cell kinase deficiency: clinical presentation and therapeutic approach. Haematologica. 2011;96(3):472-6.
116. Serwas NK, Cagdas D, Ban SA, Bienemann K, Salzer E, Tezcan I, et al. Identification of ITK deficiency as a novel genetic cause of idiopathic CD4+ T-cell lymphopenia. Blood. 2014;124(4):655-7.
117. Bienemann K, Iouannidou K, Schoenberg K, Krux F, Reuther S, Feyen O, et al. iNKT cell frequency in peripheral blood of Caucasian children and adolescent: the absolute iNKT cell count is stable from birth to adulthood. Scand J Immunol. 2011;74(4):406-11.
118. Qi Q, Kannan AK, August A. Tec family kinases: Itk signaling and the development of NKTalphabeta and gammadelta T cells. FEBS J. 2011;278(12):1970-9.
119. Chung BK, Tsai K, Allan LL, Zheng DJ, Nie JC, Biggs CM, et al. Innate immune control of EBV-infected B cells by invariant natural killer T cells. Blood. 2013;122(15):2600-8.
120. Lohr NJ, Molleston JP, Strauss KA, Torres-Martinez W, Sherman EA, Squires RH, et al. Human ITCH E3 Ubiquitin Ligase Deficiency Causes Syndromic Multisystem Autoimmune Disease. Am J Hum Genet. 2010;86:447-53.
121. Anandasabapathy N, Ford GS, Bloom D, Holness C, Paragas V, Seroogy C, et al. GRAIL: An E3 ubiquitin ligase that inhibits cytokine gene transcription is expressed in anergic CD4þ T cells. Immunity. 2003;18:535-47.
122. Mueller DL. E3 Ubiquitin ligases as T cell anergy factors. Nat Immunol. 2004;5:883-90.
123. Safford M1, Collins S, Lutz MA, Allen A, Huang CT, Kowalski J, et al. Egr-2 and Egr-3 are negative regulators of T cell activation. Nat Immunol. 2005;6:472-80.
124. Peterson P, Pitkänen J, Sillanpää N, Krohn K. Autoimmune polyendocrinopathy candidiasis ectodermal dystrophy (APECED):a model disease to study molecular aspects of endocrine autoimmunity. Clin Exp Immunol. 2004;135:348-57.
125. Capalbo D, Martino LD, Giardino G, Mase RD, Donato ID, Parenti G. Autoimmune polyendocrinopathy candidiasis ectodermal dystrophy: Insights into genotype-phenotype correlation. Int J Endocrinol. 2012;2012:353250.
126. Myers AK, Perroni L, Costigan C, Reardon W. Clinical and molecular findings in IPEX syndrome. Arch Dis Child. 2006;91:63-4.
127. Wildin RS, Smyk-Pearson S, Filipovich AH. Clinical and molecular features of the immunodysregulation, polyendocrinopathy, enteropathy, X linked (IPEX) syndrome. J Med Genet. 2002;39:537-45.
128. Eisenbarth GS, Gottlieb PA. Autoimmune polyendocrine syndromes. N Engl J Med. 2004;350:2068-77.
129. Wildin RS, Ramsdell F, Peake J, Faravelli F, Casanova JL, Buist N, et al. X-linked neonatal diabetes mellitus, enteropathy and endocrinopathy syndrome of the mouse scurfy. Nature Genet. 2001;27:18-20.
130. Bennett CL, Christie J, Ramsdell F, Brunkow ME, Ferguson PJ, Whitesell L, et al. The immune dysregulation, polyendocrinopathy, enteropathy, x-linked syndrome (IPEX) is caused by mutations of FOXP3. Nat Genet. 2001;27:20-1.
131. Chatila TA, Blaeser F, Ho N, Lederman HM, Voulgaropoulos C, Helms C, et al. JM2, encoding a fork head-related protein is mutated in X-linked autoimmunity-allergic dysregulation (sic) syndrome. J Clin Invest. 2000;106:R75-81.
132. Orcesi S, Piana RL, Fazzi E. Aicardi–Goutières syndrome. IAGSA (International Aicardi-Goutières Syndrome Association), Department of Child Neurology and Psychiatry, IRCCS 'C. Mondino Institute of Neurology' Foundation, Pavia, Italy. Br Med Bull. 2009;89(1):1-6.
133. Aicardi J, Goutieres F. A progressive familial encephalopathy with calcifications of the basal ganglia and chronic cerebrospinal fluid lymphocytosis. Ann Neurol. 1984;15:49-54.
134. Lebon P, Badoual J, Ponsot G, Goutières F, Hémeury-Cukier F, Aicardi J, et al. Intrathecal synthesis of interferon-alpha in infants with progressive familial encephalopathy. J Neurol Sci. 1988;84:201-8.
135. Bönnemann CG1, Meinecke P. Encephalopathy of infancy with intracerebral calcification and chronic spinal fluid lymphocytosis—another case of the Aicardi–Goutieres syndrome. Neuropediatrics. 1992;23:157-61.
136. Goutieres F, Aicardi J, Barth PG, Lebon P. Aicardi–Goutieres syndrome: an update and results of interferon-alpha studies. Ann Neurol. 1998;44:900-7.
137. Aicardi J. Aicardi–Goutie`res syndrome: special type early-onset encephalopathy. Eur J Paediatr Neurol. 2002;6(Suppl A):A1-7.
138. Lanzi G, Fazzi E, D'Arrigo S. Aicardi–Goutières syndrome: a description of 21 new cases and a comparison with the literature. Eur J Paediatr Neurol. 2002;6 (Suppl A):A9-22.
139. Rice G, Patrick T, Parmar R, Taylor CF, Aeby A, Aicardi J, et al. Clinical and molecular phenotype of Aicardia-Goutières syndrome. Am J Hum Genet. 2007;81:713-25.
140. Goutières F. Aicardi–Goutières syndrome. Brain Dev. 2005;27:201-6.
141. Crow YJ, Livingston JH. Aicardi–Goutières syndrome: an important Mendelian mimic of congenital infection. Dev Med Child Neurol. 2008;50(6):410-6.

CHAPTER 54

Complement Disorders

Ankur Jindal, Surjit Singh

INTRODUCTION

Complement system constitutes a major component of the innate immunity and, as the name suggests, it helps both innate and adaptive immune systems to fight against various pathogens.

Complements were first identified in the year 1890 when Jules Bordet found that for bacteriolysis two different substances were required—the heat stable-specific antibodies and a second heat-labile component responsible for lytic activity. Paul Ehrlich carried out similar work independently and coined the term complement.

Complement system works via interaction among a complex group of more than 30 glycoproteins. Most of these proteins are synthesized in the liver, although blood monocytes, tissue macrophages, fibroblasts and epithelial cells of gastrointestinal tract and genitourinary tract also contribute to some extent. Complement components constitute around 15% of total globulin fraction of plasma. A simplified nomenclature of complements is given in **Table 54.1**.

Various components of the complement system are given in **Flow chart 54.1**.

Complement pathway can be activated by any of the following three pathways as given in **Figure 54.1**.

Classical pathway is activated when C1q component binds to Fc portion of antibody (which is attached to antigen).

Alternative pathway is having continuous turnover in body at a low level (due to labile thioester bond in C3). Antibody is not required for activation of alternative pathway.

Lectin pathway resembles classical pathway in its activation except that the lectins are there in place of antibodies.

All three pathways lead to the formation of the membrane attack complex (MAC), which by disturbing the cell membrane integrity leads to lysis of the microbe. All three pathways result in release of anaphylatoxins (C3a, C4a and C5a) which help in inflammation.

Complement system plays many useful roles in the body which include destruction of microbes, clearance of apoptotic cells and cellular debris, promotion of inflammation, tissue regeneration and clearance of immune complexes from many tissues.

Table 54.1 Terminology of complement system

Components	*Designation and nomenclature*
Classical pathway and membrane attack complex	Capital letter C combined with a number, e.g. C1–C9. Numbers are in order of reactivity except that C4 is activated before C2 and C3 in the classical and lectin pathways.
Alternative pathway	Factors such as factor B and factor D.
Liberated fragments after proteolytic activation	Smaller fragment with "a" (such as C3a or Ba), larger fragment with a "b" as in C3b or Bb.
Receptors and regulators	By their function (e.g. immune adherence receptor, C1 esterase inhibitor), order of discovery [e.g. complement receptor type 1 (CR1)], or ligands to which they bind (e.g. C3b/C4b receptor).
Membrane receptors and regulators (present on hematopoietic cells)	"Cluster of differentiation" (CD) (e.g. the designation of CR1 as CD35)

Disorders of complement system will produce two major problems in the body. One, related to impaired defense against infections, which will make the individual more prone for recurrent infections and secondly, the impairment of clearance of immune complexes leads to various autoimmune manifestations.

Complement system is regulated by a set of proteins which prevents its overactivation and minimizes collateral damage to normal healthy tissue. These regulatory proteins may be membrane bound [e.g. decay accelerating factor (DAF), CR1 (CD35) etc.] or they may be free in the circulation (e.g. C1 esterase inhibitor, factor H, factor I). Deficiency of individual regulatory proteins is associated with a particular clinical syndrome.

Flow chart 54.1 Various components of complement system

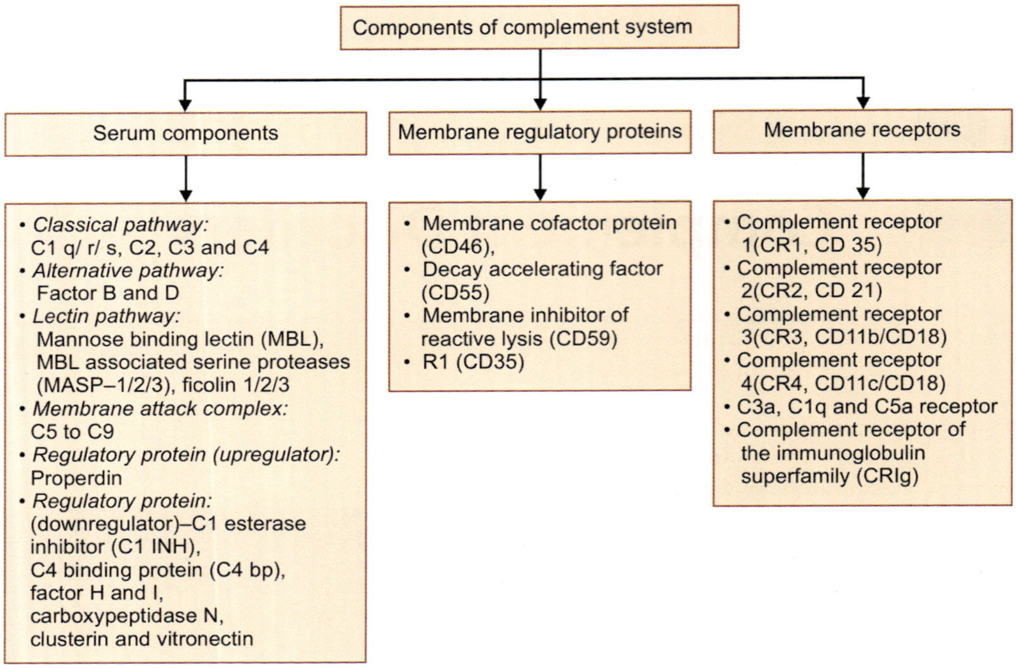

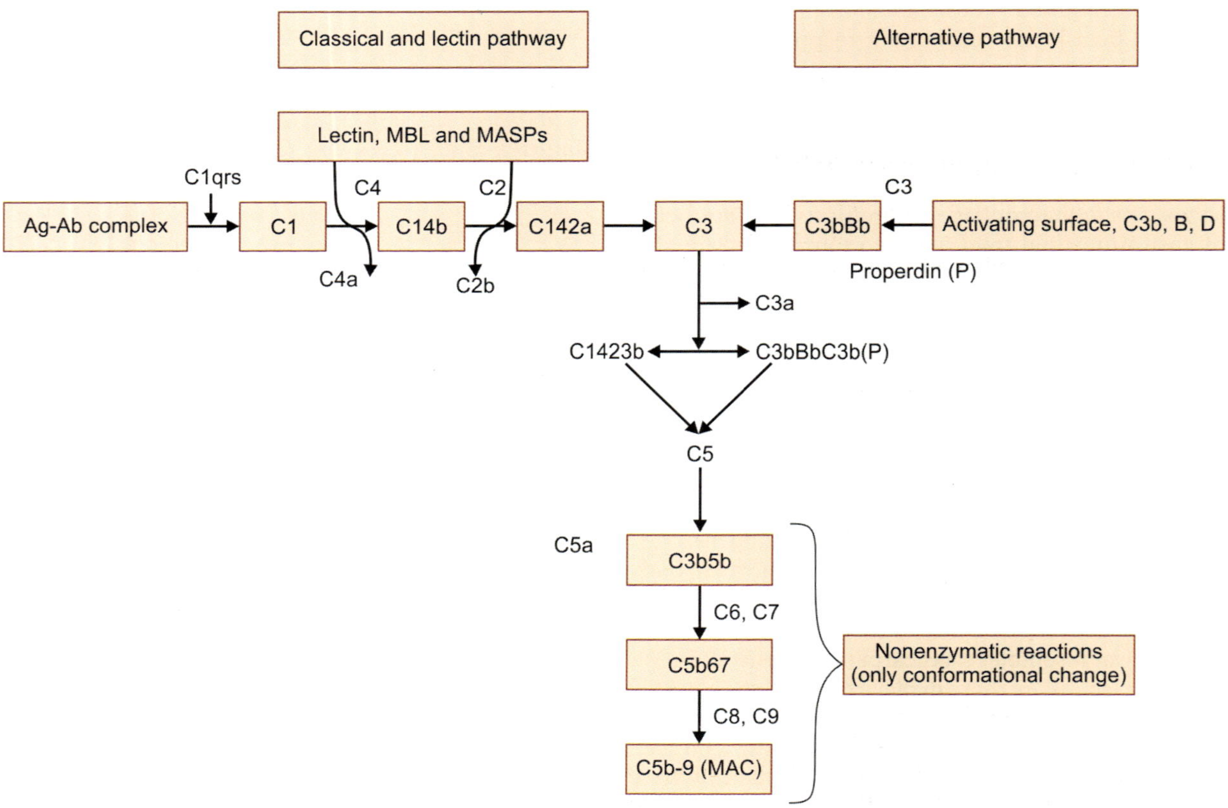

Figure 54. 1 Pathways of complement activation

Abbreviations: MAC, membrane attack complex; MBL, mannose binding lectin; MASP, MBL associate serine proteases

EPIDEMIOLOGY

Primary immune deficiency resulting from disorders of the complement system is not very common. The report of Latin American Group for Primary Immunodeficiency Diseases (LAGID) found complement deficiency in 2.8% of all patients with diagnosed primary immunodeficiency. Amongst complement deficiencies, C1 esterase inhibitor deficiency was the most common identified disorder.[1] Nationwide survey of primary immunodeficiency disorders in Japan found the complement deficiency in 3% of all patients with diagnosed primary immunodeficiency.[2] Prevalence data of complement deficiency disorders are available from several other populations. These show prevalence rates varying between 0.4% (Turkey) and 6% (Brazil) of all cases of primary immunodeficiency.[3-5]

In a survey of primary immunodeficiency disorders (PIDs) in India (2007–2010), in which two centers (Mumbai and Chandigarh) were identified to look for immunodeficiency profile. Complement deficiencies were found in 3.2% of all cases of PIDs (all had C1 esterase inhibitor deficiency) from Chandigarh and none from Mumbai.[6] In another survey of PIDs from India, complement deficiency was not found in any of the 27 children with PID.[7] This probably highlights lack of awareness and availability of investigations for complement deficiency disorders in our country.

ETIOLOGY AND PATHOGENESIS

Causes of complement deficiency can be hereditary or acquired, with acquired causes being more common.

Acquired Causes of Complement Deficiency

They may result from either increased consumption by immune complexes or because of reduced hepatic synthesis or because of loss of complement components in the urine. The increased consumption by immune complexes is more common than reduced synthesis and urinary losses.

Systemic lupus erythematosus (SLE) is characterized by activation of complement system and immune complexes formation. Usual pattern is the activation of classical pathway by activating C142 and hence deposition of C3 in various tissues, but alternate pathway activation also occurs. Microorganisms along with their byproducts also lead to immune complex formation by fixation of C1 and classical pathway activation. This can also be seen in conditions like bacterial endocarditis, infected ventriculoperitoneal shunts, dengue fever, acute viral hepatitis B, malaria, infectious mononucleosis and lepromatous leprosy. Nephritis or arthritis may develop due to immune complexes deposition and complement pathway activation in these conditions.

Some forms of glomerulonephritis, some of the vasculitic disorders and partial lipodystrophy are primarily associated with the activation of alternative pathway of complement activation.

Some degree of C1q deficiency develops in patients with severe combined immunodeficiency (SCID) and hypogammaglobulinemia, probably due to low immunoglobulin G (IgG) (IgG normally binds to C1q reversibly and prevents its breakdown).

C3 nephritic factor (NeF, an IgG antibody) stabilizes the C3 cleaving enzyme (C3bBb) of the alternative pathway and leads to its overactivation and decreased level of C3. This may be responsible for glomerulonephritis and if levels of C3 fall below 10%, it may predispose to recurrent pyogenic infections. IgG NeF may also lead to overactivation of classical pathway by inhibiting the breakdown of C42, the C3 convertase. This may be responsible for disorders like postinfectious glomerulonephritis and SLE.

In some patients with sickle cell disease, there can be defect in the alternative pathway of complement system. The deoxygenation of red blood cells (RBCs) leads to increased exposure of phospholipids on their membrane and hence activation of complement pathway. Thus, the components of alternative pathway are reduced. This activation is more during the painful crisis phase.

Factor B and D may be reduced in patients with nephrotic syndrome because of increased loss.

Patients with cirrhosis of liver, hepatic failure or malnutrition may have significantly depressed levels and activity of complement components.

Mild-to-moderate deficiency of complements is common in neonatal period and more so in premature neonates. The opsonization and chemotactic activity may be significantly depressed.

Hereditary Causes of Complement Deficiency

Majority have autosomal recessive mode of inheritance (needs two abnormal alleles to produce complete deficiency and most symptomatic patients have complete deficiency) except properdin deficiency which has X-linked recessive inheritance, C1 esterase inhibitor deficiency has autosomal mode of inheritance and factor I and mannose-binding lectin deficiency is transmitted as autosomal codominant trait.[8]

As a general rule, deficiency of early components of the complement system is associated with autoimmune manifestations predominantly SLE while deficiency of the late components of complement system is associated with predisposition to infections especially recurrent meningococcal infections. But, this is not always true in the sense that deficiency of early complement components like C1q or C4b deficiency may sometimes be associated with severe infections and the late complement components deficiency like C5, C6, C7, or C8 deficiency may have SLE-like presentation.

The pathogenesis of autoimmunity in early complement deficiency can be explained by two mechanisms. First, the early components of complement system (C1q, C3) help in clearance of necrotic and apoptotic cells, which may act as source of autoantigens. Second, C3 deposits on immune complexes and facilitates their removal from the circulation by binding to complement receptor 1 (CR1) on RBCs and transport to the spleen and liver. In absence of C3, these complexes will remain in the circulation for longer time and will cause autoimmunity.

Hereditary Deficiency of Regulatory Components

Factors H and I are important regulatory proteins of complement pathway and their deficiency leads to continuous activation of alternative pathway due to the prolonged persistence of C3 convertase in the circulation. This predisposes individuals to recurrent infections and some forms of glomerulonephritis and atypical hemolytic uremic syndrome (HUS). Properdin has role in stabilizing C3 convertase of alternative pathway and its deficiency predisposes to meningococcal infection. Properdin has role in clearing early necrotic and apoptotic cells from tissues and hence also prevents autoimmune diseases. [9]

C1 esterase inhibitor (C1 INH) controls the complement system by suppressing C1rs and MASP-2 and also inhibits the components of the fibrinolytic, clotting, and kinin pathways (factor XII, activated factor XI, plasma thromboplastin antecedent, and kallikrein). It acts as a "suicide inhibitor" in this process. C1 INH deficiency (hereditary angioedema) leads to over activity of C1 and kallikrein which leads to breakdown of C4 and C2 and also releases bradykinin. Bradykinin is the main molecule responsible for producing localized, nonpitting edema by inducing leakage of postcapillary venules. Hereditary angioedema has autosomal mode of inheritance but some cases may develop secondary to autoantibody to C1 INH or may be associated with B-cell cancer.

Absence of expression of decay accelerating factor (DAF) and CD59 (membrane inhibitor of reactive lysis) on RBCs membrane leads to paroxysmal nocturnal hemoglobinuria (PNH). DAF is a membrane-complement control protein which prevents formation of C3 cleaving enzyme (C3Bb) and CD59 prevents full development of MAC. These molecules are anchored to the RBC surface via glycosylphosphatidylinositol (GPI) molecule. In PNH, a somatic mutation in *PIG-A* gene on the X chromosome prevents the normal synthesis of this molecule.

Clinical Manifestations of Complement Deficiency

As the complement system forms an important component of innate immunity so one of the main manifestations of complement deficiency is predisposition to recurrent and severe infections, sometimes with unusual organisms also. Patients with complement deficiency are also more prone for autoimmune diseases such as SLE, due to the mechanisms explained above. Other clinical manifestations include recurrent urticaria, angioedema, glomerulonephritis, atypical forms of HUS and paroxysmal nocturnal hemoglobinuria.

Association of complement deficiency with autoimmune diseases is best exemplified by SLE. Deficiency of various complement components is associated with SLE and SLE-like diseases. Deficiency of C1q and C1r/C1s is associated with a very high risk (more than 90%) followed by a slightly lower risk with C4 deficiency and much lower risk with C2 deficiency (10–20%).[10]

Systemic lupus erythematosus is common among families with hereditary complement deficiency but familial SLE patients do not have more prevalent complement deficiency. Complete complement deficiency is rare among families with two or more SLE patients, but is concentrated among families with onset of SLE prior to age of 18 years.[11]

Specific Complement Deficiency and Associated Clinical Manifestations

C1q Deficiency

C1q molecule is responsible for initiating the classical pathway and hence its deficiency predisposes the individual for increased susceptibility to infections with encapsulated organisms.

C1q deficiency is among the most common complement deficiency associated with SLE, with equal male and female prevalence. Antinuclear antibody (ANA) is positive in 75% patients but anti-dsDNA is usually negative. Discoid rash and oral ulcers occur significantly more frequent in C1q deficiency-associated SLE/SLE-like disease than in sporadic SLE, whereas arthritis and anti-dsDNA occur less frequently **(Figs 54.2 and 54.3)**. Renal and neurological manifestations usually occur at a similar frequency to the sporadic cases of SLE.[12]

C1q-deficient lupus should be suspected when there is onset at very early age (in infancy or very young childhood); there are predominant cutaneous manifestations and frequent infections.

In our experience of lupus due to C1q deficiency, all children (n = 3) had disease onset below 3 years of age with predominant cutaneous manifestations, ANA was positive with speckled pattern (on indirect immunofluorescence) with consistently negative anti-dsDNA, normal C3 and C4 even during disease activity. We suspected C1q deficiency based on these features and two of these three children were found to have mutation in C1qA gene.

C1r/C1s Deficiency

Similar to C1q deficiency patients with C1r/C1s deficiency have susceptibility to infections with encapsulated organisms and systemic lupus. C1r/s deficiency is less common than C1q deficiency, otherwise the clinical and laboratory profile is almost similar.

C2 Deficiency

This is the most common homozygous complement deficiency with a prevalence of 1:10,000 to 1:20,000 individuals.[13]

C2-deficient patients are more prone for development of SLE, membranoproliferative glomerulonephritis (MPGN), Henoch-Schönlein purpura (HSP) and dermatomyositis. Risk of SLE in C2 deficiency is much less as compared to C1 and

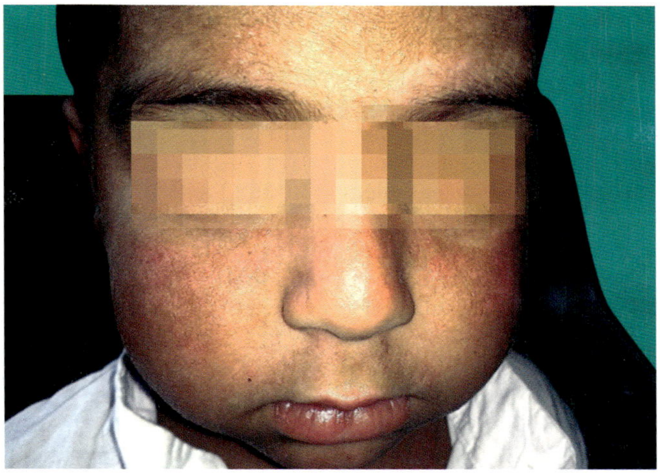

Figure 54.2 Erythematous rash involving cheeks and bridge of nose with mild scarring in a 3-year-old boy, case of C1q deficient systemic lupus erythematosus (SLE)
Note: Sparing of nasolabial folds and extension onto forehead

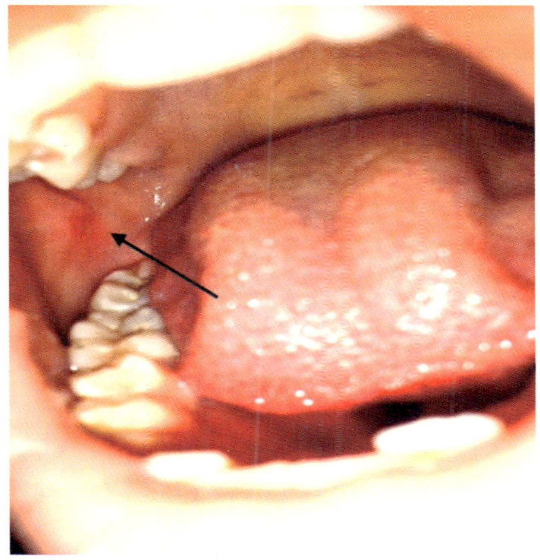

Figure 54.3 Oral ulcer involving the buccal mucosa (opposite the upper molar tooth) in a 3-year-old boy, case of C1q deficient systemic lupus erythematosus (SLE)

C4 deficiency and rare in C3 deficiency, thus maintaining the hierarchy of the classical pathway of complement system.[14] There is a female predominance; ANA and anti-dsDNA are not elevated in many patients. They have high prevalence of anti-Sjögren's-syndrome-related antigen A (SSA) antibodies and also anticardiolipin antibodies without antiphospholipid syndrome.[15]

Homozygous C2-deficient individuals are also more susceptible to infection with encapsulated organisms (because of impaired opsonization).[16]

C3 Deficiency

Its deficiency is extremely rare and predisposes to recurrent bacterial infections of the respiratory tract. *H. influenzae, N. meningitidis, Enterobacter aerogenes* and *Escherichia coli* are the common organisms. SLE-like disease is rare. MPGN and mesangiocapillary glomerulonephritis may develop in ¼th of patients.[17]

C4 Deficiency

C4 is the most polymorphic complement protein (components of C4, C4A and C4B are encoded by separate genes located in the MHC class III region). Complete C4 deficiency or low C4A gene copy numbers predispose to SLE.[18] C4 deficiency particularly C4B deficiency also predisposes to increased risk of recurrent infections by encapsulated bacteria like *N. meningitidis, H. influenzae* and *S. pneumoniae.*[19]

Terminal Component (C5-C9) Deficiencies

Inherited deficiency of each of these terminal complements has been described. C9 deficiency is relatively common in Japanese population; rest complement deficiencies are very rare. Patients are predisposed to have recurrent meningococcal infections with uncommon serotypes of *Neisseria meningitidis* such as Y and W135. For unclear reasons, these infections are less severe and usually not lethal. One postulated mechanism for lesser severity of infections in this deficiency is that lack of MAC formation will prevent bacterial lysis and hence lesser release of lipopolysaccharide and hence mild inflammation.[20] Various autoimmune disorders have been reported with terminal complement deficiency like SLE, MPGN, scleroderma and rheumatoid arthritis but there is no definite association.[14]

Factor B Deficiency

Very few case reports of factor B deficiency associated with meningococcal infection are available. Gain of function mutation may lead to atypical HUS.[21]

Factor D Deficiency

Opsonizing activity is impaired in its absence. Deficiency is rare with only few case reports. Neisseria infections predominate, but *Streptococcus pneumoniae* infections have also been reported.[22] There is no known autoimmunity associated with factor D deficiency.

Properdin Deficiency

Properdin stabilizes the complex of C3b with Bb (C3bBb). There is impaired function of alternative pathway in its absence. More than 100 cases reports of properdin deficiency are available. Three types have been recognized: Type 1 is most common and has total absence of properdin; type 2 has 1–10% of normal properdin and type 3 has normal levels but dysfunctional properdin. Patients are prone for *Neisseria meningitidis*[23] and there is no known autoimmunity. Recently properdin deficiency in combination with factor H mutation has been shown to produce severe C3 glomerulopathy.[24]

Lectin-binding Pathway Deficiency

Mannose-binding lectin (MBL) deficiency is fairly common, seen in around 10–15% of Caucasians population and is associated with recurrent infections in children and adults. C2 and properdin-deficient patients are more prone for infections if they have coexisting MBL deficiency.[25] Similarly presence of MBL deficiency in cystic fibrosis, CVID patients[26] and in stem cell transplant patients[27], makes them more susceptible to infections and decreases their overall survival. There is susceptibility to encapsulated organisms in MBL-deficient patients in form of meningococcal meningitis or community-acquired pneumonia. There is greater prevalence of autoimmune manifestations predominantly SLE and increased risk of cardiovascular complications.

Mannose-binding lectin associated serine protease-2 (MASP-2) cleaves C4 and C2 to form C4B2a, which subsequently cleaves C3. Patients with MASP-2 deficiency present with recurrent respiratory infection and autoimmunity. Course of the disease is more severe as compared to MBL deficiency.

Ficolin-3 deficiency also predisposes to recurrent respiratory tract infections and cerebral abscess formation.[28]

Factor H Deficiency

Factor H regulates alternate pathway by degrading and inhibiting the synthesis of C3Bb (C3 convertase of alternative pathway). In factor H deficiency, there is uncontrolled activity of C3Bb and hence depletion of C3. This predisposes to recurrent pyogenic infections with *Streptococcus pneumoniae* and *Haemophilus influenzae*. Factor H deficiency is the most common genetic cause of atypical aHUS.[29] Other disease associations include dense deposit disease, C3 glomerulopathy and age-related macular degeneration (ARMD).

Factor I Deficiency

It controls the alternative pathway by inhibiting C3b and its deficiency leads to uncontrolled conversion and depletion of C3. Patients are prone for recurrent pyogenic infections (mainly involving the respiratory tract) with *S. pneumoniae, H. influenzae, N. meningitidis* and *S. pyogenes*. Immune-complex-related diseases [glomerulonephritis (GN), vasculitis, arthralgia and SLE] may also develop.[30]

C1 Esterase Inhibitor (C1INH) Deficiency

Its deficiency is responsible for hereditary angioedema which is characterized by recurrent episodes of acute localized increase in vascular permeability in skin or mucous membrane leading to edema at these sites. Common mucosal sites involved are oropharynx and gastrointestinal tract. Involvement of laryngeal mucosa is most troublesome and may lead to death. Typically, the edema is nonpruritic and nonpitting and there is no urticaria. Sudden appearance of nonpitting edema not associated with itching is virtually pathognomonic for hereditary angioedema (HAE). Various clinical manifestations seen in HAE includes extremity edema (in 87–100%), abdominal symptom in form of colicky pain, nausea, vomiting and diarrhea (in 74–93%), facial edema (in 65–85%), laryngeal edema (50–55%) and oropharyngeal edema (in 30–64%).[31-33] Erythema marginatum is a common presentation in pediatric patients. Trigger can be variable from a traumatic or emotional event to sometimes spontaneously. Edema of bowel wall may produce pain abdomen with guarding and may have associated vomiting and loose stools.[34] The severity of this disease decreases after the age of 20 years and this disease may remain undiagnosed for years together. We have seen cases where following the diagnosis of HAE in a child and on probing the history, many of the parents had history of similar complaints. On further evaluation of parents, they were diagnosed as HAE.

Complement Receptor (CR3/CR4) Deficiency

Both CR3 (CD11b/ CD18) and CR4 (D11c/CD18) help in opsonization and enhance the binding of monocytes and neutrophils at endothelial surface at site of inflammation. Inherited deficiency leads to leukocyte adhesion deficiency (LAD) type 1. Patients usually present soon after birth with recurrent infections typically involving skin, lung and bowel. They may have history of delayed fall of umbilical cord and omphalitis. Characteristic feature is absence of neutrophils at site of infection and hence absence of pus formation but there is striking neutrophilia in peripheral blood.[35]

CD59/CD55 Deficiency

Deficiency of these membrane-bound complement regulators leads to paroxysmal nocturnal hemoglobinuria. The RBCs and leukocytes lacking these molecules on their surface are prone for complement-mediated lysis. PNH is characterized by intravascular hemolysis, increased risk of venous thrombosis and bone marrow failure.[36] Acute exacerbations of hemolysis usually occur on background low levels of hemolysis. Acute hemolysis leads to hemoglobinuria and may also produce dysphagia, abdominal pain and severe lethargy. Venous thrombosis occurs in about 50% of patients with hemolytic disease with predilection for involvement of intra-abdominal and cerebral veins. A proportion of patients may develop progressive pancytopenia.

The clinical manifestations of common complement disorders are summarized in **Table 54.2**.

INVESTIGATIONS

Indications of Screening

A high index of suspicion for screening for complement deficiencies should be kept in mind whenever a patient presents with above-mentioned clinical signs, symptoms and characteristic laboratory findings such as presence of ANA in a young child with autoimmune manifestations and absent

Table 54.2 Salient features of common complement factor deficiencies

Deficient complement components	*Clinical correlate*
C1q, r, s	Meningitis, pneumonia and sepsis with *S. pneumoniae* and *N. meningitidis*. Lupus is very common
C2	Sepsis, pneumonia, meningitis and osteitis with *S. pneumoniae*, *S. aureus* and *N. meningitidis*. Lupus may develop
C3	Respiratory tract infections, meningitis with *N. meningitidis, S. pneumoniae, H. influenzae, S. pyogenes, S. aureus, Enterobacter aerogenes* and *E. coli*. Lupus/immune complex-mediated diseases like glomerulonephritis may develop
C4	Sepsis, meningitis and pneumonia caused by *S. pneumoniae* and *N. meningitidis* and *H. influenzae*. Lupus and glomerulonephritis are common associates
C5, C6, C7, C8, C9	Meningitis, sepsis due to *Neisseria* (*N. meningitidis* Y and W135 serotypes)
Factor B	Meningococcal infection, gain of function mutation may lead to aHUS
Factor D	Meningitis, sepsis due to *Neisseria*
Properdin	Meningitis, sepsis due to *Neisseria*, C3 glomerulopathy may develop in association with factor H mutation
MBL (common, present in 10–15% population)	Meningococcal meningitis or community acquired pneumonia (increases the severity of other coexisting diseases such as CVID, cystic fibrosis, etc.). Lupus may develop
Factor H	Recurrent pyogenic infections with *N. meningitidis* and *H. influenzae*. MPGN and aHUS may develop
Factor I	Recurrent pyogenic infections of respiratory tract with *N. meningitidis, H. influenzae, S. pneumoniae, S. pyogenes*. Lupus and other immune complex mediated diseases like glomerulonephritis and vasculitis may develop.
C1INH	Hereditary angioedema
CR3/CR 4	Leukocyte adhesion defect type1, infections with *S. aureus* and gram-negative bacteria
CD 59/55	PNH. Infections mostly develop in setting of cytopenias.

Abbreviations: aHUS, atypical hemolytic uremic syndrome; C1 INH, C1 esterase inhibitor; CR, complement receptor; CVID, common variable immunodeficiency; MBL, mannose binding lectin; PNH, paroxysmal nocturnal hemoglobinuria

dsDNA has very high chances of having deficiency of early components of complement pathway. Certain warning signs, which warrant investigations for underlying complement deficiency, are summarized as:

- Meningococcal meningitis especially with serotypes Y and W135
- Recurrent infections with other encapsulated organisms
- Angioedema without urticaria
- Lupus in infancy or early childhood
- Inflammatory disorders of kidney and eye.

Laboratory evaluation of complement system begins with some screening tests for functional evaluation of each pathway followed by more specialized laboratory tests with characterization of the defect at individual molecular level and further genetic testing.

Before we begin the discussions of various laboratory investigations, it is essential to know that the sample has to be processed immediately or if not performed immediately, it must be frozen or transported on dry ice. Repeated freezing and thawing must be avoided because there is a risk of in vitro activation. For quantification of activation products of complement, EDTA sample is required while for most of the analysis, a serum sample is more suitable; and serum sample is mandatory for analysis of C3 nephritic factor.

CH50

The total hemolytic component (THC) or CH50 assesses the ability of serum to lyse sheep RBCs optimally sensitized with rabbit IgM antibody. To produce a normal result in this assay, all nine components of classical pathway (C1-C9) are required, so this is a useful screening test for function of classical pathway. This assay is not useful for assessment of complete alternative pathway because many of the complements like properdin, factor B and D are not necessary for classical pathway. Low CH50 value will result from either a genetic defect with total absence of one or more complement components or it may result from acquired deficiency of complement components in certain autoimmune diseases with immune complex formation. CH50 value will be zero or markedly reduced in one or more of the genetic defect in complement components, while in acquired deficiency there will be a relatively lesser degree reduction.

There are chances of laboratory error, most common being improper handling of sample which may result in low CH50 value and hence a low value should always be rechecked. Another cause for false positive result could be the presence of mixed cryoglobulins or cold reacting complexes that do not precipitate in cold.

AH50

AH50 is analyzed by lysis of unsensitized rabbit RBCs under conditions that allow only alternative pathway to activate. It measures total functional activity of the alternative pathway. It is not widely available and useful for evaluation of conditions like thrombotic microangiopathy.

Measurement of Specific Components

Antigenic levels of C3 and C4 are easily available and very useful tests for many of the disorders **(Table 54.3)**. They are usually measured by nephelometric immunoassay.

Measurement of C3 and C4 levels are very useful in diagnosis and follow-up of many diseases. SLE is the prototypic disease for the assessing the usefulness of measurement of these complement levels. In SLE, C3 or C4 level is usually decreased and they usually normalize with effective therapy. They are also useful for predicting disease relapse, much before the clinical relapse occur.

Table 54.3 Interpretation of C3 and C4 values

Complement level	*Interpretation*
↓ C3, ↓ C4	Activation of classical pathway
↓ C3, normal C4	Activation of alternative pathway Seen in nephritis secondary to nephritic factor (NeF) (Difference from immune complex nephritis) Also in deficiency of factor I or H (due to consumption of factor B)
↓ C4, normal C3	Hereditary and acquired angioedema (deficiency of C1INH). C4 is low even during asymptomatic periods

Other disease where measurement of complement level is useful includes differentiation of immune complex-mediated disorders in a child presenting with acute nephritis like presentation. Level of C3 will be low in postinfectious glomerulonephritis, MPGN, cryoglobulinemic nephritis, shunt nephritis and subacute bacterial endocarditis while a normal level suggests pauci-immune GN, HSP nephritis, IgA nephropathy and Goodpasture syndrome.

Individual components of complement pathway (C1-C9, factor B, D, MBL, etc.), their activation products (C1q, C3a, c4a, etc.) and regulator proteins (factor H, factor I, properdin, etc.) can be measured by immunochemical method. ELISA has been devised for rapid identification of individual components of complement pathway.[37]

Antifactor H antibody measurement is very useful test for diagnosis and deciding management of patients with atypical HUS. Antifactor H antibody positive HUS is now a well-defined entity with different management protocol and prognosis as compared to HUS secondary to hereditary deficiency of one of the complement components.

For diagnosis of angioedema (both hereditary and acquired), C4 level should be measured first **(Flow chart 54.2)**.[38-40]

Flow cytometry analysis of GPI anchored proteins (GPI-AP) on RBCs membrane is the most sensitive and informative

Flow chart 54.2 Suggested algorithm for laboratory diagnosis of angioedema

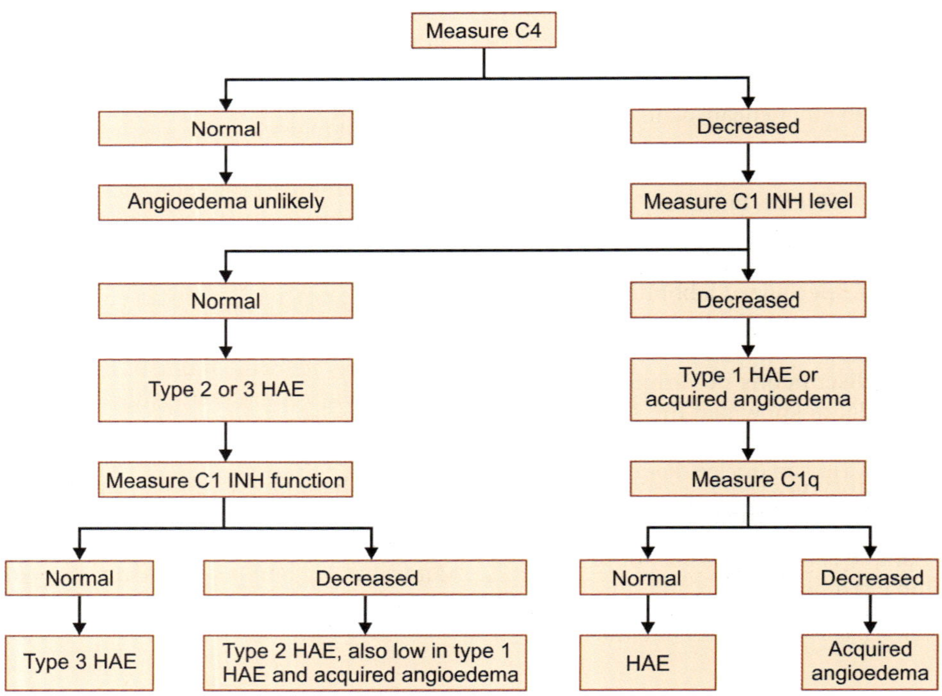

Abbreviations: C1 INH, C1 esterase inhibitor; HAE, hereditary angioedema

assay for the diagnosis of PNH. The flow cytometry not only determines the percentage of abnormal cells, it also provides information about degree of deficiency. PNH III has complete deficiency of GPI-APs on RBCs, PNH II has subtotal deficiency, PNH I is those with normal expression. This differentiation is useful in guiding the management. Flow cytometry should be performed before transfusion or at least a month after the transfusion.

Following a screening test and more definitive specific component estimation, a genetic analysis should be done if available.

DIFFERENTIAL DIAGNOSES

Patients presenting with recurrent infections need to be differentiated from other immunodeficiency diseases, e.g. T cells, B cells and phagocytic defects. These immunodeficiency disorders are more common than complement deficiency. Complete blood counts may provide useful information. Absolute lymphocyte count, if normal, rules out most of the T-cell defect; absolute neutrophil count, if in normal range, rules out congenital or acquired neutropenia and leukocyte adhesion deficiency (has very high total leukocyte with neutrophilic predominance, even between infections), normal platelet count excludes Wiskott-Aldrich syndrome and absence of Howell-Jolly bodies in peripheral smear rules out asplenia. Simple screening tests for B-cell defects should be done by measuring IgA, IgG and IgM.

A diagnostic evaluation for complement deficiency can be considered upfront if there is history of recurrent meningococcal meningitis especially with uncommon serotypes of *N. meningitidis*; disseminated meningococcal and gonococcal infections; when there is a family history of a complement disorder and during evaluation of immunodeficiency, no other specific defect could be identified.

In patients presenting with autoimmune manifestations, there can be certain clues which will lead us to think about an underlying complement deficiency, as discussed in clinical presentation, e.g. autoimmunity at a very early age, suggestive family history and certain laboratory features like in a young child with lupus like presentation, if ANA is positive with negative dsDNA, one may think of C1q deficiency.

In patients presenting with acute GN-like presentation, initial evaluation with C3 and C4, will differentiate complement mediate from noncomplement-mediated GN in almost all cases.

In HUS-like presentation, if there is young age at presentation, family history of similar cases in the past, no forthcoming history of diarrhea, and other causes like cobalamin pathway defect (pancytopenia is usually present and by measuring homocysteine and methionine in blood and methylmalonic acid in urine) and *Streptococcus pneumoniae* infection has been ruled out, one must think of complement-mediated HUS.

Hereditary angioedema needs to be differentiated from idiopathic angioedema and hypocomplementemic urticarial vasculitis. In HAE, symptoms begin at very early age as compared to other two conditions, family history is present in 70–80% patients, there is no urticaria, gastrointestinal mucosal involvement can occur, C4 is typically low with normal CH50 and there is no response to steroids and antihistamines. In idiopathic angioedema, C4 and CH50 both are normal, while in hypocomplementemic urticarial vasculitis, CH50 is low with normal. Both these diseases are associated with urticaria and do respond to steroids and antihistamines.

MANAGEMENT

There is no definitive management available for most of the disorders of complement deficiency. Three disorders of complement system in which a specific treatment is available include:

- Hereditary angioedema (C1 esterase inhibitor deficiency)
- Paroxysmal nocturnal hemoglobinuria
- Atypical HUS

The infections in patients with complement deficiency should be aggressively managed. Fever or any other signs of infection should be taken seriously and must be evaluated extensively to find out the focus. Appropriate antibiotic coverage should be given to cover common infecting organisms. Knowledge about previous culture and sensitivity report is helpful in deciding the choice of antibiotics.[41]

Drug prophylaxis and vaccination is described with prevention strategy.

Management of Hereditary Angioedema

Management of hereditary angioedema is divided in two parts—one, management of acute attack and second, a long-term therapy to prevent the attacks. Acute attack can be aborted by plasma-derived C1 esterase inhibitor, inhibition of kallikrein and antagonist of bradykinin receptor while for both long-term and short-term prophylaxis attenuated androgens and plasma-derived C1 esterase inhibitor therapy is useful. Short-term prophylaxis means that treatment is given to prevent attack during some stress or procedure, while long-term prophylaxis is intended to reduce the life-time burden of disease.

Four drugs have been approved by the Food and Drug Administration (FDA) for management of acute attacks of C1 INH deficiency which includes one human plasma-derived C1-INH therapy (Berinert), a recombinant human C1-INH product (rhC1-INH, Ruconest), a plasma kallikrein inhibitor (Ecallantide) and a bradykinin B2 receptor antagonist (Icatibant). These agents are approved for adolescents and adults. FDA has also approved two agents for prophylaxis for this disease which includes one human C1 INH (Cinryze) and one attenuated androgen, danazol.[40]

Use of these therapies in pediatric population is still controversial with country-specific recommendations.

Among the attenuated androgens, stanozolol is the recommended drug in pediatric age group in USA. Tranexamic acid (antifibrinolytic) is recommended for children in certain countries (at 30–50 mg/kg/day in 2–3 divided doses) and one human C1 INH (Berinert, 20 U/kg, for acute attack in children) is approved in USA and Europe.[42] Berinert is also useful in providing short-term prophylaxis in pediatric age group and has been found to be safe.[43] Though other drugs in C1INH group is not recommended for pediatric age group but there are encouraging results of its use in pediatric age group also. A recent consensus group has given its recommendations for the management of HAE in pediatric population.[42,44] For acute attack, Berinert (at dose of 20 U/kg) is recommended therapy and for long-term prophylaxis, Cinryze (at dose of 1000 U twice weekly) is recommended, there is no weight-based dosing for Cinryze. The group recommends no other therapy for management of either an acute attack or for prophylaxis in pediatric age group. When C1-INH therapy is not available for long-term prophylaxis, antifibrinolytics (20–40 mg/kg) are preferred over androgens because of their better safety profile.[44]

Though androgens are not recommended therapy for long-term use in children, but they are being used, sometime has shown more benefits than risk. The dose of danazol equivalent is 2.5 mg/kg/day (initial maximum dose of 50 mg/day). Dosage interval should be reduced to every other day or every third day (maximum single dose is 200 mg for >10 years age).

Fresh frozen plasma contains C1INH and can be used for both acute management and for prophylaxis before any procedure but because of presence of high-molecular-weight kininogen (HMWK), there can be worsening after administration, which is a limiting factor for its use.

Management of Paroxysmal Nocturnal Hemoglobinuria

Supportive management in form of transfusions, folic acid supplementation and management of thrombosis should be given to all patients. Iron therapy should be given if required.

Allogeneic stem cell transplant is the only curative treatment but in view of 15% chance of spontaneous remission and with the availability of complement directed therapy, the use of transplant should be individualized. Following a thromboembolic event, indefinite anticoagulation is recommended and for acute hepatic vein thrombosis (Budd-Chiari syndrome), thrombolysis should be considered.

Role of steroids and androgens in PNH is controversial.

Eculizumab is a humanized monoclonal antibody which blocks complement activation at C5 level and hence blocks the synthesis of MAC. Various trials on the use of eculizumab in PNH have found that this treatment significantly reduces the frequency of hemolytic episodes, transfusion requirement, and episodes of thrombosis and improves the overall quality of life.[45] The dose is 600 mg weekly for 4 weeks (induction) followed by 900 mg twice weekly as maintenance.

In resource-limited settings, a combination of danazol and cyclosporine has been found useful.[46] There is concern for increase in risk of thrombosis with the use of danazol. Danazol is useful for features of bone marrow failure but not useful for hemolytic manifestations.[47]

Management of Complement-mediated Hemolytic Uremic Syndrome

Management options include plasma exchange/plasmapheresis, plasma infusions, immunosuppressive therapy, eculizumab (monoclonal humanized anti-C5 antibody) and supportive treatment (dialysis, transfusions, management of complications).

Plasmapheresis is a useful therapy for both acquired (antifactor H antibody-mediated) and hereditary causes (factor deficiency). It should ideally be started within first 24–48 hours. Plasmapheresis should be done daily for at least first 5 days and further therapy to be decided depending on the response.

Immunosuppression is useful if antifactor H antibody is positive. Prednisolone (1–2 mg/kg/day) should be added if there is poor response to plasmapheresis. Methylprednisolone pulses (30 mg/kg/dose) may be given during the induction phase of the treatment depending on the clinical condition. In more severe and unresponsive cases, cyclophosphamide (500 mg/m^2 per dose) should be used during the induction phase. After achieving remission, these patients require prolonged maintenance dose of immunosuppressant to prevent the relapse. Mycophenolate mofetil (MMF, 25–30 mg/kg/day) with or without low-dose steroids is useful for maintenance therapy. Other immunosuppressive drugs which are found to be useful are rituximab, azathioprine and IVIg.[48]

Since the introduction of eculizumab, this treatment has become the standard of treatment in resource-rich nations. For best results, therapy should be started within first 24–48 hours and prolonged maintenance needs to be given for nearly 2 years. This therapy has been found to be very useful for induction of remission and for maintenance of remission. The limitation is its cost and availability.[49]

In resource limited settings like in India, the treatment of choice will remain plasmapheresis in all cases and immunosuppression if antibody is present along with other supportive treatments. A proposed protocol for management of aHUS is given in **Flow chart 54.3**.

Prevention Strategy[41]

Patient should be vaccinated against encapsulated organisms including pneumococcus, *H. influenzae* and meningococcal vaccine.

- The tetravalent meningococcal conjugate vaccine (A, C, W135, Y) should be given to children more than 1 year old. Conjugate C vaccine can be given in less than 1 year of age.
- Annual influenza vaccination is also recommended.
- There is no contraindication for live vaccines in patients with complement deficiency.

Flow chart 54.3 Suggested management protocol for atypical hemolytic uremic syndrome (aHUS) in resource limited settings

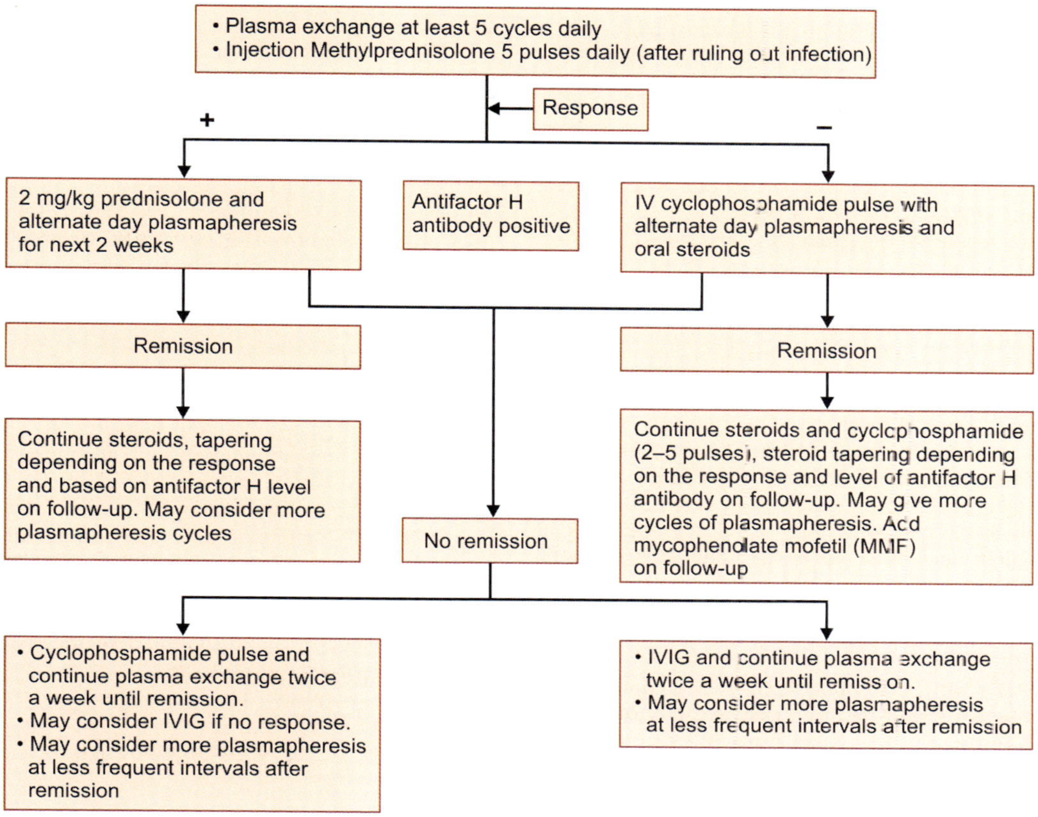

Note: Immunosuppression in antifactor H antibody positive patients, repeated plasma therapy in suspected factor deficiency

- All other vaccine should be given as per the national immunization schedule.

Antibiotic prophylaxis should be given to all patients except those with terminal complement deficiency because infections are of moderate severity in terminal complement deficiency. The recommended regimen is oral penicillin (at 50,000 IU/kg/day in two divided doses, adult dose of 1 million units twice daily). Injectable penicillin (1.2–2.4 million units every 3–4 weeks) is an alternative.

CONCLUSION

- Complement system is a major part of innate immune system.
- Complement deficiency disorders are not as common as other primary immunodeficiency diseases but with increasing awareness, these disorders are being diagnosed more frequently.
- They may have varied presentation from recurrent infections (especially with encapsulated organisms) to various autoimmune manifestations (predominantly early onset SLE)
- A high index of suspicion, especially among pediatricians, is must for the identification of these disorders
- Screening tests for complement deficiency disorders are easily available these days.

REFERENCES

1. Leiva LE, Zelazco M, Oleastro M, Carneiro-Sampaio M, Condino-Neto A, Costa-Carvalho BT, et al. Primary immunodeficiency diseases in Latin America: the second report of the LAGID registry. J Clin Immunol. 2007;27(1):101-8.
2. Ishimura M, Takada H, Doi T, Imai K, Sasahara Y, Kanegane H, et al. Nationwide survey of patients with primary immunodeficiency diseases in Japan. J Clin Immunol. 2011;31(6):968-76.
3. Rezaei N, Mohammadinejad P, Aghamohammadi A. The demographics of primary immunodeficiency diseases across the unique ethnic groups in Iran, and approaches to diagnosis and treatment: PIDs in Iran. Ann N Y Acad Sci. 2011;1238(1):24-32.
4. Kilic SS, Ozel M, Hafizoglu D, Karaca NE, Aksu G, Kutukculer N. The prevalences [correction] and patient characteristics of primary immunodeficiency diseases in Turkey--two centers study. J Clin Immunol. 2013;33(1):74-83.

5. Grumach AS, Duarte AJ, Bellinati-Pires R, Pastorino AC, Jacob CM, Diogo CL, et al. Brazilian report on primary immunodeficiencies in children: 166 cases studied over a follow-up time of 15 years. J Clin Immunol. 1997;17(4):340-5.
6. Gupta S, Madkaikar M, Singh S, Sehgal S. Primary immunodeficiencies in India: a perspective. Ann N Y Acad Sci. 2012;1250:73-9.
7. Verma S, Sharma PK, Sivanandan S, Rana N, Saini S, Lodha R, et al. Spectrum of primary immune deficiency at a tertiary care hospital. Indian J Pediatr. 2008;75(2):143-8.
8. Pettigrew HD, Teuber SS, Gershwin ME. Clinical significance of complement deficiencies. Ann N Y Acad Sci. 2009;1173:108-23.
9. Kemper C, Hourcade DE. Properdin: New roles in pattern recognition and target clearance. Mol Immunol. 2008;45(16):4048-56.
10. Giles BM, Boackle SA. Linking complement and anti-dsDNA antibodies in the pathogenesis of systemic lupus erythematosus. Immunol Res. 2013;55(0):10-21.
11. Aggarwal R, Sestak AL, D'Sousa A, Dillon SP, Namjou B, Scofield RH. Complete complement deficiency in a large cohort of familial systemic lupus erythematosus. Lupus. 2010;19(1):52-7.
12. Stegert M, Bock M, Trendelenburg M. Clinical presentation of human C1q deficiency: How much of a lupus? Mol Immunol. 2015;67(1):3-11.
13. Lewis MJ, Botto M. Complement deficiencies in humans and animals: links to autoimmunity. Autoimmunity. 2006;39(5):367-78.
14. Chen M, Daha MR, Kallenberg CGM. The complement system in systemic autoimmune disease. J Autoimmun. 2010;34(3):J276-86.
15. Jönsson G, Sjöholm AG, Truedsson L, Bengtsson AA, Braconier JH, Sturfelt G. Rheumatological manifestations, organ damage and autoimmunity in hereditary C2 deficiency. Rheumatol Oxf Engl. 2007;46(7):1133-9.
16. Jönsson G, Truedsson L, Sturfelt G, Oxelius V-A, Braconier JH, Sjöholm AG. Hereditary C2 deficiency in Sweden: frequent occurrence of invasive infection, atherosclerosis, and rheumatic disease. Medicine (Baltimore). 2005;84(1):23-34.
17. S Reis E, Falcão DA, Isaac L. Clinical aspects and molecular basis of primary deficiencies of complement component C3 and its regulatory proteins factor I and factor H. Scand J Immunol. 2006;63(3):155-68.
18. Yang Y, Chung EK, Wu YL, Savelli SL, Nagaraja HN, Zhou B, et al. Gene copy-number variation and associated polymorphisms of complement component C4 in human systemic lupus erythematosus (SLE): low copy number is a risk factor for and high copy number is a protective factor against SLE susceptibility in European Americans. Am J Hum Genet. 2007;80(6):1037-54.
19. Jaatinen T, Lahti M, Ruuskanen O, Kinos R, Truedsson L, Lahesmaa R, et al. Total C4B deficiency due to gene deletion and gene conversion in a patient with severe infections. Clin Diagn Lab Immunol. 2003;10(2):195-201.
20. Tedesco F. Inherited complement deficiencies and bacterial infections. Vaccine. 200830;26 Suppl 8:I3-8.
21. Loirat C, Frémeaux-Bacchi V. Atypical hemolytic uremic syndrome. Orphanet J Rare Dis. 2011;6:60.
22. Ram S, Lewis LA, Rice PA. Infections of people with complement deficiencies and patients who have undergone splenectomy. Clin Microbiol Rev. 2010;23(4):740-80.
23. Fijen CA, van den Bogaard R, Schipper M, Mannens M, Schlesinger M, Nordin FG, et al. Properdin deficiency: molecular basis and disease association. Mol Immunol. 1999;36(13-14):863-7.
24. Lesher AM, Zhou L, Kimura Y, Sato S, Gullipalli D, Herbert AP, et al. Combination of factor H mutation and properdin deficiency causes severe C3 glomerulonephritis. J Am Soc Nephrol JASN. 2013;24(1):53-65.
25. Bathum L, Hansen H, Teisner B, Koch C, Garred P, Rasmussen K, et al. Association between combined properdin and mannose-binding lectin deficiency and infection with *Neisseria meningitidis*. Mol Immunol. 2006;43(5):473-9.
26. Fevang B, Mollnes TE, Holm AM, Ueland T, Heggelund L, Damås JK, et al. Common variable immunodeficiency and the complement system; low mannose-binding lectin levels are associated with bronchiectasis. Clin Exp Immunol. 2005;142(3):576-84.
27. Mullighan CG, Heatley SL, Danner S, Dean MM, Doherty K, Hahn U, et al. Mannose-binding lectin status is associated with risk of major infection following myeloablative sibling allogeneic hematopoietic stem cell transplantation. Blood. 2008;112(5):2120-8.
28. Munthe-Fog L, Hummelshøj T, Honoré C, Madsen HO, Permin H, Garred P. Immunodeficiency associated with FCN3 mutation and ficolin-3 deficiency. N Engl J Med. 2009;360(25):2637-44.
29. Vernon KA, Ruseva MM, Cook HT, Botto M, Malik TH, Pickering MC. Partial complement factor H deficiency associates with C3 glomerulopathy and thrombotic microangiopathy. J Am Soc Nephrol. 2016;27(5):1334-42.
30. Alba-Domínguez M, López-Lera A, Garrido S, Nozal P, González-Granado I, Melero J, et al. Complement factor I deficiency: a not so rare immune defect: characterization of new mutations and the first large gene deletion. Orphanet J Rare Dis. 2012;7:42.
31. Kemp JG, Craig TJ. Variability of prodromal signs and symptoms associated with hereditary angioedema attacks: a literature review. Allergy Asthma Proc. 2009;30(5):493-9.
32. Kesim B, Uyguner ZO, Gelincik A, Mete Gökmen N, Sin AZ, Karakaya G, et al. The Turkish Hereditary Angioedema Pilot Study (TURHAPS): the first Turkish series of hereditary angioedema. Int Arch Allergy Immunol. 2011;156(4):443-50.
33. Nanda MK, Elenburg S, Bernstein JA, Assa'ad AH. Clinical features of pediatric hereditary angioedema. J Allergy Clin Immunol Pract. 2015;3(3):392-5.
34. Davis AE, Lu F, Mejia P. C1 inhibitor, a multi-functional serine protease inhibitor. Thromb Haemost. 2010;104(5):886-93.
35. van de Vijver E, Maddalena A, Sanal Ö, Holland SM, Uzel G, Madkaikar M, et al. Hematologically important mutations: Leukocyte Adhesion Deficiency (first update). Blood Cells Mol Dis. 2012;48(1):53-61.
36. Mastellos DC, Ricklin D, Yancopoulou D, Risitano A, Lambris JD. Complement in paroxysmal nocturnal hemoglobinuria: exploiting our current knowledge to improve the treatment landscape. Expert Rev Hematol. 2014;7(5):583-98.
37. Seelen MA, Roos A, Wieslander J, Mollnes TE, Sjöholm AG, Wurzner R, et al. Functional analysis of the classical, alternative, and MBL pathways of the complement system: standardization and validation of a simple ELISA. J Immunol Methods. 2005;296(1-2):187-98.
38. Gompels MM, Lock RJ, Morgan JE, Osborne J, Brown A, Virgo PF. A multicentre evaluation of the diagnostic efficiency of serological investigations for C1 inhibitor deficiency. J Clin Pathol. 2002;55(2):145-7.

39. Hemperly S, Agarwal N, Xu Y-Y, Zhi Y-X, Craig T. Recent advances in the management of hereditary angioedema. J Am Osteopath Assoc. 2013;113(7):546-55.
40. Riedl MA. Hereditary angioedema with normal C1-INH (HAE type III). J Allergy Clin Immunol Pract. 2013;1(5):427-32.
41. Aguilar C, Malphettes M, Donadieu J, Chandesris O, Coignard-Biehler H, Catherinot E, et al. Prevention of infections during primary immunodeficiency. Clin Infect Dis. 2014;59(10):1462-70.
42. Wahn V, Aberer W, Eberl W, Faßhauer M, Kühne T, Kurnik K, et al. Hereditary angioedema (HAE) in children and adolescents: a consensus on therapeutic strategies. Eur J Pediatr. 2012;171(9): 1339-48.
43. Bork K, Hardt J, Staubach-Renz P, Witzke G. Risk of laryngeal edema and facial swellings after tooth extraction in patients with hereditary angioedema with and without prophylaxis with C1 inhibitor concentrate: a retrospective study. Oral Surg Oral Med Oral Pathol Oral Radiol Endod. 2011;112(1):58-64.
44. Craig T, Pürsün EA, Bork K, Bowen T, Boysen H, Farkas H, et al. WAO guideline for the management of hereditary angioedema. World Allergy Organ J. 2012;5(12):182-99.
45. Sahin F, Ozkan MC, Mete NG, Yilmaz M, Oruc N, Gurgun A, et al. Multidisciplinary clinical management of paroxysmal nocturnal hemoglobinuria. Am J Blood Res. 201515;5(1):1-9.
46. Ghosh K, Madkaikar M, Gupta M, Jijina F. Evaluation of danazol, cyclosporine, and prednisolone as single agent or in combination for paroxysmal nocturnal hemoglobinuria. Turk J Haematol. 2013;30(4):366-70.
47. Risitano AM, Rotoli B. Paroxysmal nocturnal hemoglobinuria: pathophysiology, natural history and treatment options in the era of biological agents. Biologics. 2008;2(2):205-22.
48. Sinha A, Gulati A, Saini S, Blanc C, Gupta A, Gurjar BS, et al. Prompt plasma exchanges and immunosuppressive treatment improves the outcomes of anti-factor H autoantibody-associated hemolytic uremic syndrome in children. Kidney Int. 2014;85(5):1151-60.
49. Loirat C, Fakhouri F, Ariceta G, Besbas N, Bitzan M, Bjerre A, et al. An international consensus approach to the management of atypical hemolytic uremic syndrome in children. Pediatr Nephrol. 2016;31(1):15-39.

CHAPTER

55

Autoinflammatory Syndromes

Latika Gupta, Amita Aggarwal

INTRODUCTION

Autoinflammatory syndromes or periodic fever syndromes are a group of disorders characterized by recurrent systemic and organ-specific inflammation. Most of these occur in childhood while a few can present later in life. The patients present with repeated bouts of fever associated with rash, arthritis or other symptoms for which no infectious or malignant cause can be found. The pathogenesis of these disorders was initially thought to be akin to the autoimmune diseases found in adults like lupus and rheumatoid arthritis. However, in 1999 Kastner et al. proposed that inflammatory pathways distinct from those in autoimmune diseases are operative in these syndromes.[1] It was later established that the innate rather than adaptive immune system mediates aberrant immune stimulation in these diseases. Single gene defects have been identified in most of them. Also unlike the other autoimmune diseases, they do not have female predisposition nor are they associated with certain HLA alleles.

EPIDEMIOLOGY

As these are rare disorders, their prevalence and incidence are not known. Case reports and case series have been published from most parts of the world. Euro Fever Project survey which involved all centers linked to the Paediatric Rheumatology International Trial Organisation (PRINTO), a nonprofit organization devoted to collaborative studies on pediatric rheumatic disease has been a major effort in collating data from different countries. By July 2011, 1,880 patients from 67 centers in 31 countries had been entered in the registry. Of these, 1,049 patients had a diagnosis of a monogenic autoinflammatory disease; and the gene defect had been identified in 703.

Among the monogenic periodic fever syndromes, familial Mediterranean fever (FMF) has been reported most often; more so in the Middle East.[2]

PATHOGENESIS

Role of Innate Immune System

The generation of immune response in humans involves innate and adaptive immune system. The innate system, consisting of neutrophils, macrophages, mast cells and natural killer cells, is the first line of defense. It recognizes conserved molecular patterns on pathogens and results in release of proinflammatory cytokines. In addition, macrophages process the antigens of the invading agents and present them to T cells for activation of the adaptive immune response. The adaptive response is mediated by T and B cells. Immune activation abates as the microbial agent gets cleared from the body. The autoinflammatory syndromes occur when inappropriate activation of the innate immune machinery occurs in the absence of an inciting agent or there is lack of regulation of the immune response.

What is the Inflammasome?

Inflammasomes are multimolecular complexes that oligomerize to form a scaffold that activates caspase 1. This in-turn converts precursor proinflammatory cytokines like proIL1-beta and proIL-18 to their active forms **(Fig. 55.1)**. These then serve to eliminate the foreign agent from the host. Another mechanism of causing inflammation via inflammasome is through pyroptosis. This is induction of death in macrophages which serve as hosts for invading pathogens.

How is the Inflammasome Activated?

When the host is attacked by an infections agent pathogen associated molecular patterns (PAMPs) present on their cell surface or secreted by them are identified by receptors present on cells of the innate immune system called the pattern recognition receptors (PRRs). Various families of

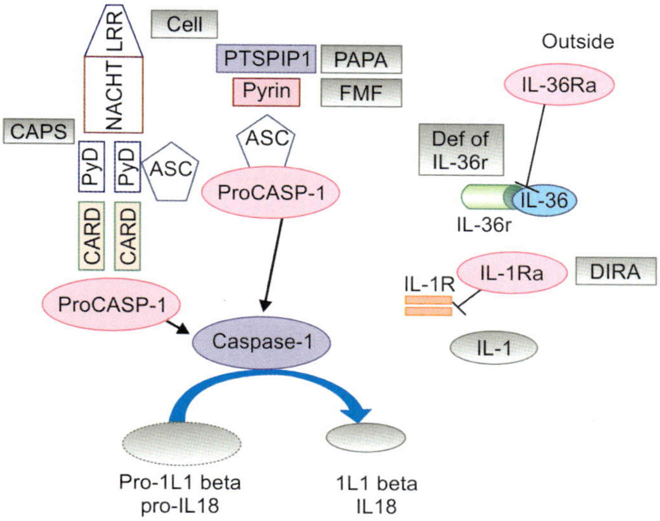

Figure 55.1 The inflammasome pathway and the autoinflammatory diseases associated with it

Abbreviations: ProCASP-1, procaspase 1; PyD, pyrin domain; NACHT domain, domain present in NAIP, CIITA, HET-E (plant het product involved in vegetative incompatibility) and TP-1 (telomerase-associated protein 1); LRR, leucine rich repeat; ASC, apoptosis-associated speck-like protein containing CARD; PTSPIP1, proline-serine-threonine phosphatase interacting protein 1; IL1Ra, interleukin 1 receptor antagonist; PAPA, pyogenic arthritis, pyoderma gangrenosum and acne; FMF, familial Mediterranean fever; CAPS, cryopyrin-associated periodic syndromes; IBD, inflammatory bowel disease; DIRA, deficiency of the interleukin-1 receptor antagonist

PRRs proteins have been described, one of which is the nucleotide oligomerization domain (NOD)-like receptors (NLR) which form part of the inflammasome complex. This inflammation ceases once infectious source is eliminated. However at times, gain of function mutations in the genes encoding inflammasome components can lead to constitutive activation or episodic over activity in the absence of triggers. This manifests as autoinflammatory syndrome. Research in the field of innate immunity and disorders related to it is ongoing and new mutations are still being described.[3]

Other Mechanisms of Autoinflammatory Syndromes

Apart from inflammasome activation, defects in the downstream signaling pathways can lead to similar manifestations. A host of *Cytokinopathies* is being described, including defects in IL1 receptor antagonist, IL-10 and IL-36 **(Fig. 55.1 and Table 55.1)**.

A separate group of clinical syndromes called *Interferonopathies* has been described recently. These have upregulation of transcripts induced by interferon 1 (IFN1) signaling.

Some disorders have defects of nuclear factor-kappa beta (NF-κβ)/Rel the final common pathway for execution of multiple cytokine functioning. These have come to be known as the *Relopathies*.[4]

Table 55.1 Classification of autoinflammatory syndromes

Inflammasomopathies Familial Mediterranean fever Cryopyrinopathies Pyogenic arthritis, pyoderma gangrenosum, and acne	*Interferonopathies* STING-associated vasculopathy with onset in infancy Chronic atypical neutrophilic dermatosis with lipodystrophy and elevated temperature Aicardi-Goutières disease
Relopathies Blau syndrome Hyperimmunoglobulin D syndrome	*Cytokinopathies* Deficiency of IL-1 receptor antagonist Deficiency of interleukin 36–receptor antagonist Majeed syndrome

CLASSIC AUTOINFLAMMATORY SYNDROMES[1,5]

Familial Mediterranean Fever

Familial Mediterranean fever is most often seen in the Middle East in Sephardic Jews, Armenians, Turks, and, to a lesser extent, Ashkenazi Jews, Greeks, and Italians. Children present with episodic attacks of fever lasting 1–3 days. Most patients also experience serositis and arthritis. They may have an erysipeloid eruption which usually begins on the lower limbs near the ankle. Persistent inflammation leads to amyloidosis in a significant majority of cases; though the incidence has fallen after colchicine was introduced for treatment of this disease.

TNF Receptor-1 Associated Periodic Syndrome

Tumor necrosis factor (TNF) receptor-1 associated periodic syndrome (TRAPS) was earlier known as the familial Hibernian fever. In most patients, the disease starts in the first decade of life though cases have been reported at all ages due to autosomal dominant nature with incomplete penetrance. It was first reported in the Irish population.

Attacks commonly last for 5 days to 2 weeks. The child often has conjunctivitis and periorbital edema with typical focal migratory myalgia with overlying erythema. They may have arthritis and abdominal pain also. The rash is migratory and characteristic with single or multiple erythematous patches that spread distally down an extremity.

Hyperimmunoglobulin D Syndrome

Hyperimmunoglobulin D syndrome (HIDS) or mevalonate kinase deficiency (MKD) often manifests in infancy with episodic fever lasting 3–7 days, accompanied, in most cases, by chills, cervical lymphadenopathy, abdominal pain and vomiting or diarrhea. Arthritis, pleomorphic rash and

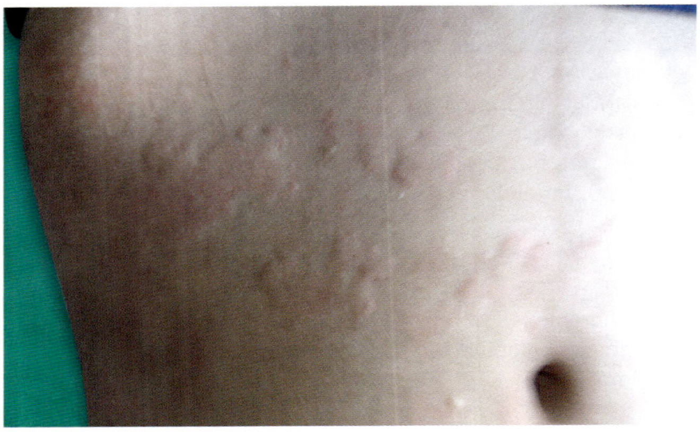

Figure 55.2 Urticarial rash in a child with Muckle-Wells syndrome

splenomegaly may be seen. Attacks may be precipitated by vaccination, viral infection, trauma or stress. Amyloidosis is rare in HIDS and the attacks may reduce with age.

Cryopyrin-associated Periodic Syndromes

Cryopyrin-associated periodic syndromes (CAPS) represent a family of syndromes associated with mutations in cryopyrin, a protein in the inflammasome assembly. All of these manifest with urticarial rash and fever.

Patients with CAPS typically fall into one of three clinical syndromes depending on the severity and age of manifestation:

1. The mildest, familial cold autoinflammatory syndrome (FCAS) has short episodes of fever lasting less than a day and urticarial rashes triggered by exposure to cold.
2. Muckle-Wells syndrome (MWS) presents with fevers and urticarial rashes that are not typically associated with cold exposure **(Fig. 55.2)**. Over time, some patients develop sensorineural hearing loss, and if not treated adequately systemic amyloidosis may develop.
3. The most severe of these is neonatal-onset multisystem inflammatory disorder (NOMID), also called chronic infantile neurologic cutaneous and articular syndrome (CINCA). It manifests at birth with fever, urticarial rashes and chronic meningitis. They may have cartilage or bony deformities as well especially large patellae.

Periodic Fevers with Aphthous Stomatitis, Pharyngitis and Adenitis

Periodic fevers with aphthous stomatitis, pharyngitis, and adenitis (PFAPA) is the most common of all autoinflammatory syndromes though the underlying gene defect has not been identified. Children often present with fever lasting 3–6 days every 3–4 weeks. The periodicity is classical and the next attack can often be predicted. They have pharyngitis with aphthous ulcerations and cervical lymphadenopathy. The throat swabs do not isolate any organism and the child's febrile spells can be terminated by a single dose of oral corticosteroid. The response is so dramatic that it is often considered diagnostic. Most patients with PFAPA outgrow the febrile episodes with time, and no long-term consequences have been identified.

Other Autoinflammatory Syndromes Deficiency of the Interleukin-1 Receptor Antagonist

Deficiency of the interleukin-1 receptor antagonist (DIRA) presents in early infancy with a diffuse pustular skin rash simulating psoriasis, sterile osteomyelitis and periostitis with articular pain in the absence of fever. It is a rare syndrome with very few cases described worldwide.[6]

Pyogenic Arthritis, Pyoderma Gangrenosum and Acne

Pyogenic arthritis, pyoderma gangrenosum and acne (PAPA) syndrome is a rare, autosomal dominant condition that presents in the first decade of life with oligoarticular, destructive arthritis, typically involving the elbow, knee, and/or ankle. Severe cystic acne is absent at the onset and manifests only when the child grows to adolescent age. Disfiguring pyoderma gangrenosum and pathergy-like abscesses can occur at injection sites in a subset of patients. Pus from all sites is sterile on multiple occasions. Some patients have a tendency to sulfonamide-induced bone marrow suppression.[7]

Blau Syndrome

Blau syndrome is the childhood counterpart of adult sarcoid; albeit with slight differences in clinical presentation. It is a monogenic syndrome with autosomal dominant inheritance; so most patients have strong family history. The classic presentation includes skin rash, uveitis and oligoarthritis with boggy joints. These features occur due to granulomatous inflammation of the skin, eye and joints. Lung involvement is rare. Atypical manifestations include fever, cranial neuropathies, arteritis and granulomatous involvement of visceral organs.[8]

NEWER SYNDROMES

Chronic Atypical Neutrophilic Dermatosis with Lipodystrophy and Elevated Temperature

Chronic atypical neutrophilic dermatosis with lipodystrophy and elevated temperature (CANDLE) syndrome is also called as the Nakajo-Nishimura disease. It results from defects in the proteasome complex. The patients present with fever, panniculitis and eyelid swelling. They often have basal ganglia calcification and hepatomegaly and may have myositis and arthritis. The defect in proteasome results in defective disposal of protein leading to protein overload which triggers unfolded protein response in the cells. This leads to upregulation of the IFN gene signature. The disease course is progressive and mortality is high.[9]

STING-associated Vasculopathy with Onset in Infancy

STING-associated vasculopathy with onset in infancy (SAVI) syndrome manifests with vasculopathy, vasculitis and interstitial lung disease (ILD), usually in infancy. Vascular manifestations include small dermal vasculitis and microvascular thrombosis. The affected children have telangiectasia, purpura or ulcerations of the fingertips, ear lobes and the tip of the nose. Digital ischemia can sometimes be severe and surgical amputation may be needed. Most patients later develop fatal progressive ILD. A study to block IFN-alpha pathway by Janus kinase (JAK) inhibitor (downstream signaling molecule), baricitinib is ongoing as these patients have evidence of increased IFN-alpha signature.[10]

Deficiency of Adenosine Deaminase 2

Deficiency of adenosine deaminase 2 (ADA2) presents with heritable polyarteritis nodosa like disease. The children have fever, livedoid or urticarial rash and small vessel vasculitis. The vasculitis may present with stroke or involvement of the kidney or bowel.[11,12]

Phospholipase C Gamma 2 Associated Antibody Deficiency and Immune Dysregulation

Phospholipase C gamma 2 associated antibody deficiency and immune dysregulation (PLAID) is also called FCAS3 presents with urticaria and sometimes angioedema induced by evaporative cooling (exposure to the air or wind) rather than touching cold objects. Neonates present with ulcers on the ear lobes and tip of the nose or fingers. Granulomatous lesions of the skin occur classically sparing the warmer flexural areas and skin folds. They may have arthralgia, bowel and lung infections as part of partial immunodeficiency.[11]

When to Suspect Autoinflammatory Syndromes[13]

Clinicians often suspect autoinflammatory syndromes when a child has recurrent fever or rash in which infection has been ruled out or seems unlikely. The episode of fever often abates on their own only to reappear at a later time; or persists despite antibiotics. The attacks are characterized by marked inflammation and the child is completely fine in between attacks. A careful evaluation often reveals other salient markers which may help classify the disease into the various syndromes. They have multisystem involvement and the duration of attacks is usually shorter than that due to infections.

Periodic fever syndromes manifest as recurrent bouts of fever which contrary to their name, do not manifest with periodicity. Episodes may be interspersed with normal periods of growth lasting months to years. The only exception is PFAPA syndrome which occurs at intervals of 3–4 weeks; with fever lasting 3 days to a weeks' time.

Often fever is accompanied by a host of other manifestations including rash, serositis, arthritis, meningitis or uveitis. The child may have hepatosplenomegaly and lymphadenopathy and acute phase reactants are often raised. All manifestations normalize in between attacks and child gains height and weight appropriately.

Since these disorders are rare, the most important task is to rule out infection and malignant process. Autoimmune connective tissue diseases can also present in a similar fashion rarely. It is prudent to confirm the diagnosis before embarking on treatment as immunosuppressant medicines often mask the underlying disease.

Most of these manifest in the first decade of life. Severe cold-associated periodic syndromes (CAPS) manifest in infancy, while TRAPS and FMF can sometimes appear in the second decade or later. Subtle family history of attenuated manifestations of a similar disease can often be elicited. Sometimes complications from underlying disease, like renal failure from inflammation-induced amyloidosis may be present in the family. TRAPS is an autosomal dominant disease, while most of the others are recessive in inheritance.

Ethnicity may offer a clue to FMF, as it is common in the Mediterranean and the Middle East region.

Differentiation Based on Age at Presentation

Chronic infantile neurologic cutaneous and articular syndrome and DIRA present at birth, though at times may appear up to 4 weeks of life. HIDS starts in infancy though may present late due to mild features. FCAS also occurs in the 1st year of life. Blau syndrome presents in the age of 1–4 years in most patients. In PFAPA syndrome the attacks start in the first decade of life; the attacks tend to attenuate with age and the child grows into a healthy adult without any deficit.

When the disease is first suspected in an adult, FMF is the most likely diagnosis, though TRAPS also has been diagnosed as late as the age of 54 years.

Differentiation Based on Ethnicity

Most cases in the Eurofever Registry belong to Western Europe as data collection from those centers has been most robust. FMF is most common in the Mediterranean region, while PFAPA cases have been reported in good proportions from all areas.

Differentiation Based on Fever (Table 55.2)

Fever spells lasting 1–2 days with arthritis serositis and erysipeloid eruption on the legs is seen in FMF. Fever spells of 4–7 days with hepatosplenomegaly and lymphadenopathy along with gastrointestinal manifestations (vomiting, diarrhea and abdominal pain) are seen in HIDS or mevalonate kinase deficiency. It is a partial deficiency, complete absence of enzyme associates with mevalonate aciduria. These patients have a rash which also involves the palms and soles.

Tumor necrosis factor (TNF) receptor-1 associated periodic syndrome has fever spells lasting much longer; from 1–3 weeks. They have painful erythema with underlying fasciitis or focal myositis and periorbital edema. On the other

Table 55.2 Diagnostic chart for a child with recurrent fever

Duration of fever attack (days)	
< 2	Familial Mediterranean fever Familial cold autoinflammatory syndrome Muckle–Wells syndrome
4–6	Hyperimmunoglobulin D syndrome
>14	TNF receptor associated periodic syndrome
Continuous	Chronic infantile neurological cutaneous and articular syndrome Deficiency of the interleukin-1 receptor antagonist

Table 55.3 Approach based on rash

Type of rash	*Disease*
Urticarial rash	Cryopyrinopathies
Morbilliform rash	Hyperimmunoglobulin D syndrome
Migratory erythema	TNF receptor-1 associated periodic syndrome
Erysipeloid eruption	Familial Mediterranean fever
Lipodystrophy	Chronic atypical neutrophilic dermatosis with lipodystrophy and elevated temperature
Sterile pustulosis Acne Pyoderma gangrenosum	Pyogenic arthritis, pyoderma gangrenosum, and acne
Generalized pustulosis	Deficiency of IL-1 receptor antagonist
Maculopapular to ichthyosiform	Blau syndrome

hand, PFAPA manifests at intervals of 3–4 weeks, such that the parents can almost predict when it is going to come again. The child has tonsillitis with aphthous ulcers and painful cervical lymphadenopathy with sterile cultures on multiple occasions. Around 90% respond dramatically to a single dose of oral corticosteroid such that it is almost considered diagnostic.

Differentiation Based on Rash (Table 55.3 and Fig. 55.2)

Cryopyrin-associated periodic syndromes are associated with rash that is critical to their diagnosis. Most of these have urticarial rashes. These urticarial lesions are nonpruritic and respond poorly to antihistaminics. However, they fade in a few hours like classic urticaria. They differ from vasculitic urticarial as they do not leave postinflammatory hyperpigmentation. In FCAS, the rash appears on cold exposure with fever and arthralgia. It differs from contact cold urticaria; the ice cube test is negative. These patients do not have angioedema.

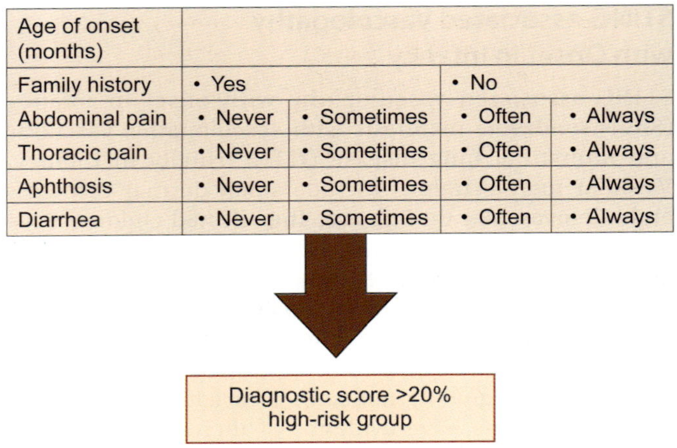

Figure 55.3 Gaslini diagnostic score for determination of risk for carrying gene mutations

MWS has a more chronic course with persistent urticaria unrelated to cold exposure and prominent arthritis. Neonatal onset multisystem inflammatory disease or chronic infantile neurological, cutaneous and articular syndrome (NOMID or CINCA) is the most severe with onset at birth and has an urticarial rash.

Familial Mediterranean fever has erysipeloid eruption which dominates on the lower limbs while TRAPS has fasciitis with overlying erythema that is often migratory. Rash in MKD involves the palms and soles. Patients suspected to have FMF clinically can be subjected to Gaslini risk scoring for presence of genetic mutations. Testing may be justified when a high-risk score is obtained **(Fig. 55.3)**.

Differentiation Based on Arthritis

Pyogenic arthritis, pyoderma gangrenosum and acne syndrome has recurrent destructive oligoarthritis of the knees, ankles or elbows. Pus aspirate from the joint is sterile on multiple occasions. In the second decade, the children often develop disfiguring pyoderma gangrenosum, sometimes at the aspiration site with acne and pustulosis. They may have suppurative hidradenitis as well. Autosomal dominant pattern of inheritance supports a positive family history in most cases.

Blau syndrome is the childhood counterpart of sarcoidosis; though lung involvement is rare. The involved children often are under 4 years old with involvement of one parent with granulomatous affection of the eyes, skin and arthritis. The arthritis is polyarticular and resistant to treatment. Tenosynovitis of the hands characteristically leads to painless swelling of the digits which leads to contractures and has come to be known as camptodactyly.

Deficiency of the IL1 Receptor antagonist or DIRA leads to multifocal sterile pustulosis with osteolytic lesions and overlying periostitis. Often infection is first suspected in a neonate with such symptoms, but cultures are sterile and then the diagnosis is thought of.

Pustular psoriasis without bone lesions occurs in two related syndromes; deficiency of IL 36 receptor antagonist (DITRA) and CARD 14-mediated pustular psoriasis (CAMPS).

Differentiation Based on Multifocal Osteolytic Lesions

The most common autoinflammatory condition affecting the bones in older children and adults is complex regional multifocal osteomyelitis (CRMO). No genetic mutation has been identified so far. It usually occurs after the age of 8 years with pain in various bones and sterile osteolytic lesions. Malignancy needs to be excluded. Often they have family history of psoriasis or Crohn's disease which also are disorders of defective innate immunity.

Older young males often present with acne and pustular lesions on the trunk along with axial or peripheral oligoarthritis. Often the sternoclavicular joint may be affected. They have hyperostosis as well, and this constellation of manifestations is called as the synovitis, acne, pustulosis, hyperostosis and osteitis (SAPHO) syndrome.

Confirmation of the Diagnosis

Most of these disorders are monogenic in inheritance and the gene defects have been found. However, newer mutations and their associated syndromes continue to be described.

The most common of all autoinflammatory syndromes are the *PFAPA* and *FMF*. No gene has been found for PFAPA yet and FMF most commonly affects *FMF* gene (MEFV).[12] It encodes a protein called pyrin which regulates IL-1 β production via the inflammasome **(Fig. 55.1 and Table 55.4)**.

A few cases with onset in adulthood have mutations in *TNFSF1A* gene instead, and testing for these is recommended to confirm the diagnosis. Since genetic analysis for these is available at specialized laboratories only, a prediction score has been devised by Gaslini et al. **(Fig. 55.3)**. It consists of five variables scores from which are summated to give a percentage risk of having a positive test. A risk more than 20% justifies testing.[14,15]

Patients with TRAPS often have a defect in the *TNFR1* gene which encodes the 55 kDa subunit of TNF receptor. HIDS results from mutation in *MVK* gene encoding mevalonate

Table 55.4 Gene defects in autoinflammatory syndromes

Syndrome	*Gene*	*Protein*	*Mode of inheritance*
FMF	*MEFV*	Pyrin	AR
MKD/ HIDS	*MVK*	Mevalonate kinase	AR
TRAPS	*TNFR1*	55 kDa subunit of TNF receptor	AD
CAPS FCAS1 FACS2 FACS2 MWS NOMID/CINCA	 *NLRP3* *NLRP12* *PLCG2* *NLRP3* *NLRP3*		AD
CANDLE	*PSMB8*	Proteasome	AR
SAVI	*TMEM173*	STING	
DIRA	*IL-1RN*	IL1 receptor antagonist	AR
DITRA	*IL36RN*	IL36 receptor antagonist	
CAMPS	*CARD14*		
Blau syndrome	*NOD2/CARD15*		AD
PAPA	*PSTPIP1*	Proline serine threonine phosphatase interacting protein 1	AD
PFAPA	Not identified	Nucleotide-binding oligomerization domain protein 2	
NLRC4 MAS	*NLRC4*		
LUBAC deficiency	*IRP2*	Heme oxidized iron responsive element binding protein 2	
SPENCDI	*ACP5*	TRAP	
Majeed syndrome (subtype of CRMO)	*LIP2*	Lipin2	AR

Abbreviations: FMF, familial Mediterarrean fever; MKD/HIDS, mevalonate kinase deficiency/hyperimmunoglobulin D syndrome; TRAPS, TNF receptor-associated periodic syndrome; CAPS, cryopyrin-associated periodic syndromes; FCAS, familial cold autoinflammatory syndrome; MWS, Muckle-Wells syndrome; NOMID/CINCA, neonatal-onset multisystem inflammatory disorder/chronic infantile neurologic cutaneous and articular syndrome; CANDLE, chronic atypical neutrophilic dermatosis with lipodystrophy and elevated temperature; SAVI, STING-associated vasculopathy with onset in infancy; DIRA, Deficiency of the interleukin-1 receptor antagonist; DITRA, deficiency of IL36 receptor antagonist; CAMPS, CARD 14 mediated pustular psoriasis; PAPA, pyogenic arthritis, pyoderma gangrenosum and acne; PFAPA, periodic fevers with aphthous stomatitis, pharyngitis, and adenitis; MAS, macrophage activation syndrome; LUBAC, linear ubiquitin chain assembly complex; SPENCDI, spondyloenchondrodysplasia with immune dysregulation ; CRMO, complex regional multifocal osteomyelitis kinase. They also have high IgD levels (>100 IU/mL) and 80% have elevated IgA also.

Cryopyrin-associated periodic syndromes comprises of three different syndromes; all involve different mutations of the same gene *NLRP3* which encodes a protein called cryopyrin. Hence, they are also called as the cryopyrinopathies. NLRP3 is a PRR for DAMPs and PAMPs. Gain of function mutations lead to constitutive IL1-β production.

Familial cold autoinflammatory syndrome has been now proposed to consist of three types, type 1 being the first described variety with defect in *NLRP3*, while *FCAS2* and 3 have defects in *NRRP12* and *PLCG2*.

Around 40% of the patient are negative for NLRP3 mutation analysis and may have somatic mosaicisms, testing for which is available at a few centers only. Blau syndrome often has a defect in *NOD2/CARD15* gene. This gene is also implicated in Crohn's disease, though a different part of it is mutated.

Assessment of Disease Activity

The autoinflammatory diseases activity index (AIDAI) **(Table 55.5)** is a validated tool to assess disease activity in FMF, TRAPS, CAPS and MKD. It has 12 items, each of which is scored from 0–1. A score of 9 or more identifies patients in whom the disease is active. It has a sensitivity and specificity of 89% and 92%, respectively. It is a simple questionnaire-based tool which can be used by the patients to self-report disease activity and record it for future visits. The use of AIDAI can standardize assessment of disease activity and facilitate comparison in trials.[15]

The symptoms need to be answered as yes (1) or no (0) for each day of the month. Symptoms due to cause other than autoinflammatory disease are not reported.

Table 55.5 Autoinflammatory disease activity index

Features	*1 (Yes)/0 (No)*
Fever > 38°C or 100.4°F	
Overall symptoms	
Abdominal pain	
Nausea/vomiting	
Diarrhea	
Headache	
Chest pain	
Painful nodes	
Arthralgia/myalgia	
Swelling of joints	
Eye manifestations	
Skin rash	
Pain relief medicines taken	Entered but not scored

TREATMENT

The rarity of these disorders makes it difficult to develop treatment recommendations. Most of the evidence is based on case series and personal experiences. Very few randomized control trials are available. Most of the common clinical practice experience has been published as a large cohort registered under the Eurofever Registry.

For the treatment of FMF, colchicine is the drug of choice. Ample evidence suggests that complete remission can be induced in two-thirds and partial in one-third. Around 5–10% fail on it or develop adverse events. They do well with on-demand corticosteroids. Anakinra has been tried in a few patients successfully.

Cryopyrin-associated periodic syndromes responds well with canakinumab and rilonacept. Anakinra is the second line drug now. For TRAPS, nonsteroidal anti-inflammatory drugs (NSAIDs) and corticosteroids are the first line of management. Surprisingly, the disease responds better with anti-IL1 therapy than with anti-TNF therapy. MKD responds poorly to most therapies, corticosteroids are used in most patients. Anti-IL1 and anti-TNF therapy is reserved for nonresponders.

In PFAPA syndrome, the response to a single dose of oral steroid is almost universal (90%) and dramatic. But, in some steroids may lead to more frequent attacks. Tonsillectomy has been proposed to be therapeutic in a good number of patients.

Pyogenic arthritis, pyoderma gangrenosum and acne syndrome leads to disfiguring skin lesions and destructive arthritis which responds poorly to NSAIDs and partially to steroids. Good results have been documented with anakinra in small series. DIRA responds to anakinra. *NLRP12* associated FCAS responds to steroids. The drugs used are summarized in **Table 55.6**.[16]

CONCLUSION

Autoinflammatory syndrome are rare monogenic disorders that present with multisystem involvement and fever usually in young age. Early recognition can prevent organ damage by use of specific drugs like colchicine in FMF. These syndromes have also helped us improve our understanding of innate immune system.

KEY POINTS

- Autoinflammatory syndromes are a family of disorders with aberrant activation of the innate immune system
- Most of these are monogenic defects in the inflammasome pathway though defects in alternative pathways of inflammation have been described recently
- The classification now includes interferonopathies, cytokinopathies and relopathies
- They are suspected when recurrent episodes of fever with inflammation occur in the absence of infection or malignancy
- Prediction scores delineate the cases where gene mutation testing is advisable

Table 55.6 Recommended treatment of different autoinflammatory syndrome

Disease	*Drug*
FMF	Colchicine
Colchicine resistant	Corticosteroids Interferon-α Anakinra, anti-TNF
CAPS	Canakinumab, rilonacept Anakinra
TRAPS	Corticosteroids Anakinra, etanercept
MKD	NSAIDs, corticosteroids Anakinra Etanercept
PAPA	Corticosteroids, anakinra, anti-TNF
DIRA	Anakinra
NLRP12	NSAIDs, corticosteroids
PFAPA	(Adeno)tonsillectomy
	Corticosteroids

Abbreviations: FMF, familial Mediterarrean fever; MKD, mevalonate kinase deficiency/hyperimmunoglobulin D syndrome; TRAPS, TNF receptor-associated periodic syndrome; CAPS, cryopyrin-associated periodic syndromes; DIRA, Deficiency of the interleukin-1 receptor antagonist; PAPA, pyogenic arthritis, pyoderma gangrenosum and acne; PFAPA, periodic fevers with aphthous stomatitis, pharyngitis, and adenitis; NSAIDs, nonsteroidal anti-inflammatory drugs

- *PFAPA* and *FMF* are the most common autoinflammatory syndrome
- Some present with predominant skin rash or osteolytic bone lesions
- Newer mutations and their syndromes continue to be described in literature.

REFERENCES

1. Stojanov S, Kastner DL. Familial autoinflammatory diseases: genetics, pathogenesis and treatment. Curr Opin Rheumatol. 2005;17:586-99.
2. Toplak N, Frenkel J, Ozen S, Lachmann HJ, Woo P, Koné-Paut I, et al. An international registry on autoinflammatory diseases: the Eurofever experience. Ann Rheum Dis. 2012;71:1177-82.
3. Ozkurede VU, Franchi L. Immunology in clinic review series; focus on autoinflammatory diseases: role of inflammasomes in autoinflammatory syndromes. Clin Exp Immunol. 2012;167:382-90.
4. Moghaddas F, Masters SL. Monogenic autoinflammatory diseases: Cytokinopathies. Cytokine. 2015;74:237-46.
5. Federici S, Sormani MP, Ozen S, Lachmann HJ, Amaryan G. Woo P, et al. Evidence-based provisional clinical classification criteria for autoinflammatory periodic fevers. Ann Rheum Dis. 2015;74:799-805.
6. Minkis K, Aksentijevich I, Goldbach-Mansky R, Magro C, Scott R, Davis JG, et al. Interleukin 1 receptor antagonist deficiency presenting as infantile pustulosis mimicking infantile pustular psoriasis. Arch Dermatol. 2012;148:747-52.
7. Lindor NM, Arsenault TM, Solomon H, Seidman CE, McEvoy MT. A new autosomal dominant disorder of pyogenic sterile arthritis, pyoderma gangrenosum, and acne: PAPA syndrome. Mayo Clin Proc. 1997;72:611-5.
8. Manouvrier-Hanu S, Puech B Piette F, Boute-Benejean O, Desbonnet A, Duquesnoy B, et al. Blau syndrome of granulomatous arthritis, iritis, and skin rash: a new family and review of the literature. Am J Med Genet. 1998;76:217-21.
9. Tüfekçi Ö, Bengoa Ş, Karapinar TH, Ataseven EB, İrken G, Ören H. CANDLE syndrome: A recently described autoinflammatory syndrome. J Pediatr Hematol Oncol. 2015;37:296-9.
10. Liu Y, Jesus AA, Marrero B, Yang D, Ramsey SE, Montealegre Sanchez GA, et al. Activated STING in a vascular and pulmonary syndrome. N Engl J Med. 2014;371:507-18.
11. Canna SW, Goldbach-Mansky R. New monogenic autoinflammatory diseases a clinical overview. Semin Immunopathol. 2015;37:387-94.
12. Rigante D, Vitale A, Lucherini OM, Cantarini L. The hereditary autoinflammatory disorders uncovered. Autoimmun Rev. 2014;13:892-900.
13. Federici S, Gattorno M. A practical approach to the diagnosis of autoinflammatory diseases in childhood. Best Pract Res Clin Rheumatol. 2014;28:263-76.
14. Gattorno M, Sormani MP, D'Osualdo A, Pelagatti MA, Caroli F, Federici S, et al. A diagnostic score for molecular analysis of hereditary autoinflammatory syndromes with periodic fever in children. Arthritis Rheum. 2008;58:1823-32.
15. Piram M, Frenkel J, Gattorno M, Ozen S, Lachmann HJ, Goldbach-Mansky R, et al. A preliminary score for the assessment of disease activity in hereditary recurrent fevers: results from the AIDAI (autoinflammatory diseases activity index) consensus conference. Ann Rheum Dis. 2011;70:309-14.
16. Ter Haar N, Lachmann H, Özen S, Woo P, Uziel Y, Modesto C, et al. Treatment of autoinflammatory diseases: results from the Eurofever Registry and a literature review. Ann Rheum Dis. 2013;72:678-85.

CHAPTER

56

Management of Specific Immunodeficiencies

Vinod Gunasekaran, Nita Radhakrishnan, Anupam Sachdeva

INTRODUCTION

Primary immunodeficiencies (PIDs) are a broad group of disorders encompassing more than 230 various diseases.[1] These are conditions where one or more of the components of immune system are defective leading to predisposition to certain infections such as viruses, bacteria, fungi and protozoa. Due to poorly regulated immune system, these children are also prone to develop autoimmunity and malignancies. In the absence of definitive treatment and proper supportive care to these children, infections, autoimmunity and malignancies affect the quality of life and may be fatal in children with PIDs.[1]

IMMUNE SYSTEM OF HUMAN BODY

Immunity may be nonspecific or specific to infectious agents. Nonspecific immunity may be cellular [natural killer (NK) cells, macrophages and neutrophils take part in innate immunity] or soluble proteins (complement system). Specific immunity may be humoral (antibodies produced by plasma cells) or cellular (T lymphocyte-mediated).

CLASSIFICATION OF PRIMARY IMMUNODEFICIENCY[2,3]

- Combined T-cell and B-cell immunodeficiencies (Severe combined immunodeficiency, Omenn syndrome)
- Predominantly antibody deficiencies (Agammaglobulinemia, hyper IgM syndrome, selective IgA deficiency, common variable immunodeficiency, IgG2 subclass deficiency)
- Other well-defined immunodeficiency syndromes (Wiskott-Aldrich syndrome, ataxia telangiectasia, DiGeorge anomaly, hyper-IgE syndrome, chronic mucocutaneous candidiasis)
- Diseases of immune dysregulation (Familial hemophagocytic lymphohistiocytosis, autoimmune lymphoproliferative syndrome, Chediak-Higashi syndrome, Griscelli syndrome II)
- Congenital defects of phagocyte number and function (Chronic granulomatous disease, leukocyte adhesion deficiency I, severe congenital neutropenia, cyclic neutropenia)
- Autoinflammatory disorders (TRAPS: TNFR-associated periodic fever syndrome)
- Complement deficiencies (C1 esterase inhibitor deficiency).

IMPORTANCE OF EARLY DIAGNOSIS

Primary immunodeficiencies are rare and chronic disorders, which are increasingly diagnosed, in recent years during to increased awareness regarding the genetic predisposition to certain infections. Still, it is frequently diagnosed at a stage when an irreversible damage (like bronchiectasis, malabsorption, etc.) has occurred.[1] Early diagnosis and quick referral to specialized centers help to provide the best outcome in PID. It decreases the complications and morbidity to a great extent. It also plays significant role in prevention by appropriate genetic counseling and antenatal diagnosis. Despite all, lack of infrastructure and financial aids hinder in improving the outcome in developing countries.

Warning Signs

Ten warning signs have been suggested which are suspicious of underlying primary immunodeficiency.[2] They are as follows:

1. More than or equal to 4 ear infections in a year.
2. More than or equal to 2 serious sinus infections in a year.
3. More than or equal to 2 months on antibiotics with little effect.
4. More than or equal to 2 pneumonia in a year.
5. Failure to thrive.
6. Recurrent deep skin or organ abscesses.

7. Persistent oral or cutaneous fungal infection.
8. Requiring intravenous antibiotics for clearing infections
9. More than or equal to two deep-seated infections (including septicemia)
10. Family history of PID.

MANAGEMENT OF SPECIFIC PRIMARY IMMUNODEFICIENCIES

The management of common PIDs encountered in practice is discussed briefly as:

Severe Combined Immunodeficiency

Severe combined immunodeficiency (SCID) is rare but fatal disorder if untreated. It is characterized by inadequate T-lymphocyte production with a varying combination of defects in B and NK cell production. Presence of lymphopenia, decreased immunoglobulin levels and flow cytometry for lymphocyte subsets showing decrease in T-cells with or without decrease in B and NK cells help in reaching the diagnosis. A diagnosis of SCID is incompatible with life beyond 1 year of life, unless treated by hematopoietic stem cell transplantation (HSCT) to reconstitute the immune system. Various screening methods have been tried to diagnose these children before they clinically manifest. Detection of T-cell receptor excision circles (TRECs) on the neonatal blood spot (Guthrie card) is the commonly used one. X-linked inheritance with mutations in *IL2RG* gene (T-B+NK-) constitutes around 69% of the cases. The underlying genetic defects identified so far include the following:

- Cytokine signaling defects—γc, JAK3, IL-7Ra defects
- T-cell receptor (TCR) defects—CD3, ZAP-70, lck, Orai1 defects
- VDJ recombination defects—RAG1/2, artemis, DNA ligase IV, Cernunnos-XLF, DNA PKcs defects
- *Defects of metabolism*: Adenosine deaminase deficiency, AK2 (reticular dysgenesis)
- Other—CD45, coronin 1A, RMRP defects.

Treatment

Infants with combined T-cell and B-cell immunodeficiencies should receive only irradiated cytomegalovirus (CMV) negative blood products. Except for those patients with SCID due to deficiency of adenosine deaminase (ADA), for which a replacement enzyme exists, the only curative therapy for SCID is allogeneic HSCT. The overall survival at 5 years in a 10-year retrospective study of 240 SCID transplants was found to be 74%. Most deaths were in the first year of transplantation, mostly due to infections and pulmonary complications. Presence of active infection at transplantation and age more than 3.5 months are found to be associated with a lower survival rate. Around 94% of children with age less than 3.5 months at presentation survived at 5 years after transplant, whereas only 50% of children with age more than 3.5 months along with active infection at transplantation survived. Survival rate among recipients of matched sibling donors was found to be 97%. Survival rate among cord-blood recipients was found to be 58%. B+ SCID was found to have better immune reconstitution, whereas NK+ SCID had poorer immune recovery. These data clearly indicate that early diagnosis and performing a HSCT before catching an infection and having a matched sibling donor are the key predictors of having a successful transplant.

Agammaglobulinemia

Due to abnormalities is B-cell development, these children have absent or decreased B-cells and consequently, immunoglobulin levels are decreased or absent. Disease is characterized by recurrent bacterial infections starting beyond 4–6 months of age and predisposition to enteroviral infections. X-linked mutation in *BTK* gene (encoding Bruton's tyrosine kinase) is the most common defect (85%) leading to X-linked agammaglobulinemia (XLA).[4] Autosomal recessive patterns are also seen and are more severe.

Treatment

Management mainly depends on replacement of intravenous immunoglobulins (IVIG) on frequent intervals. IVIG is manufactured from tens of thousands of plasma of screened healthy donors. The vast majority of immunologists prescribe IVIG at 400 mg/kg every 4 weeks. Infusions are given every 3 to 4 weeks at an initial dose of 400–600 mg/kg titrating the dose and interval to achieve IgG trough level greater than 500 mg/dL. However, the target should be prevention of infections rather than maintaining a trough IgG level. The threshold level differs in different patients. A higher trough level is maintained in patients with preexisting permanent damage like bronchiectasis, chronic gut diseases, etc. A recent meta-analysis has found a 27% decrease in the incidence of pneumonia for every 100 mg/kg/28 days increase in IVIG administration. Some centers use antibiotic prophylaxis in addition to IVIG therapy. Gene therapy for *BTK* gene mutation is under research.

Intravenous Immunoglobulins

The WHO has established the following production criteria for IVIG (1982):[5]

- Each lot should be derived from plasma pooled from at least 1,000 donors.
- It should contain at least 90% intact IgG with the subclasses present in ratios similar to normal pooled plasma.
- IgG molecules should maintain biological activity such as complement fixation.
- It should be free from contaminants of prekallikrein activator kinins, plasma proteases and preservatives.
- It should be free from infectious agents.

Adverse Reactions

Headache is the most common adverse event. Other mild reactions include back or abdominal pain, nausea, rhinitis, wheezing, chills, low-grade fever, myalgia and transient self-limiting neutropenia. Serious reactions include aseptic meningitis, meningism, exacerbation of chronic renal failure, painful erythema at the infusion, anaphylaxis, Stevens-Johnson syndrome, hypotension, myocardial infarction, thrombosis, cytopenia, hemolysis, stroke, seizure, loss of consciousness, acute respiratory distress syndrome, pulmonary edema, acute bronchospasm, and transfusion-associated lung injury.

Hyperimmunoglobulin M Syndrome

The defect is in the class-switch recombination (via CD40 and CD40 ligand in B and T-cells) during immunoglobulin synthesis, thereby leading to normal or increased IgM levels along with decrease in other Ig levels (G and A). Studying the expression of CD40 and CD40 L (CD154) clinches the diagnosis. It manifests with recurrent bacterial infections (respiratory and intestinal) and predisposition to CMV, *Pneumocystis carinii*, giardiasis and Cryptosporidium infections.

Treatment

The treatment remains lifelong IVIG replacement. Children with severe neutropenia may require G-CSF. Boiling of drinking water should be emphasized to prevent Cryptosporidium infections. HSCT is curative. An overall survival rate of 68–71% was reported, which is slightly better than the survival rate of nontransplanted patients at the age of 20 years. Early age at transplant and absence of organ damage are predictors of good outcome.

Common Variable Immunodeficiency

Common variable immunodeficiency (CVID) is a heterogeneous group of disorder diagnosed by exclusion.[4] The age of first manifestation ranges from late childhood to adulthood. A family history of recurrent infections or autoimmunity may be present (10–20%). Characteristic features include recurrent infections, decreased IgG and other immunoglobulins and absence of specific antibody response to vaccines and infections.[4] Secondary causes like protein losing conditions must be excluded. Infectious spectrum usually includes bacterial sinopulmonary infections and giardiasis. In children, transient hypogammaglobulinemia and hypomorphic SCID may mimic CVID. In adults, lymphoid malignancies should be excluded.

Treatment

Management includes IVIG replacement, antibiotic prophylaxis and management of complications. Infectious complications include chronic suppurative otitis media, bronchiectasis and malabsorption. Noninfectious complications include autoimmunity and malignancies (especially lymphoid). HSCT may be necessitated in difficult cases.

Management of Bronchiectasis

Permanent complications like bronchiectasis are best prevented (though not completely) by early diagnosis of B-cell defects (especially XLA and CVID) and prompt initiation of IVIG replacement therapy. In established cases, the requirement of IVIG is nearly doubled and a higher trough IgG levels (600 to >1000 mg/dL) are targeted. The other standard measures for management of bronchiectasis including antibiotics for prophylaxis (fluoroquinolones) and exacerbations (as indicated) and chest physiotherapy should be instituted.

Wiskott-Aldrich Syndrome

It is a X-linked disorder characterized by thrombocytopenia (with small-sized platelets) leading to bleeding manifestations, recurrent infections and eczema. Other features include raised IgA and IgE levels with variable IgM and IgG levels. Wiskott-Aldrich syndrome (WASP) protein codes for a cytoskeletal protein in hematopoietic cells, which helps in their maturation, activation and transportation.[6] The clinical spectrum of mutation in this gene varies from isolated thrombocytopenia (termed X-linked thrombocytopenia) to a complete spectrum of WAS. Diagnosis is confirmed by mutation analysis.

Treatment

The only curative treatment is hematopoietic stem cell transplantation. As soon as a diagnosis of WAS is made, a search for human leukocyte antigen (HLA)-matched donor must be initiated. HLA-matched sibling transplantation carries a success rate of 80–90%. Matched unrelated HSCT have also been performed with high success rate (especially in <5 years of age).[7] Early diagnosis helps in early initiation of supportive care including antibiotic prophylaxis, IVIG therapy (for children with low IgG or recurrent infections), managing eczema and platelet transfusions as required. Iron supplementation is required due to chronic blood loss. Infections must be treated with effective antimicrobials. Eczema/dry skin can be managed with bath oils, moisturizing creams and judicious use of steroids. Specific allergens if identified need to be avoided. Splenectomy has been found to improve platelet counts in more than 90% cases, however, it should be reserved for refractory cases considering the risk of infections. Autoimmunity is managed with steroids and IVIG.

Hyperimmunoglobulin E Syndrome (HIES or Job's Syndrome or Buckley Disease)

Eosinophilia, elevated IgE levels, eczema and recurrent infections are hallmarks of Hyper-IgE syndrome (HIES). Recurrent cold abscesses caused by *Staphylococcus aureus* are a typical finding. Other infections include recurrent sinopulmonary infections (pneumococcus, *H. influenza* and *Pneumocystis jirovecii*) and chronic mucocutaneous candidiasis. Mutation in *STAT3* gene is causative in autosomal dominant HIES and is associated with other nonimmunological features like craniosynostosis, high-arched palate, vascular anomalies and risk for malignancies.[8] DOCK8 mutation leads to HIES with associated typical features including specific allergies and predisposition to viral infections.[8] Tyk2 mutation is associated with mycobacterial infections.

Treatment

Management includes antibacterial (especially against *Staphylococcus*) and antifungal (against *Candida* and *Aspergillus*) prophylaxis to prevent infections. Other supportive measures include oral hygiene (antiseptic mouthwash) and skin hygiene, treatment of active infections and IVIG replacement (only in cases with hypogammaglobulinemia). Management of bronchiectasis may be required as indicated. Role of HSCT is controversial in HIES.

Familial Hemophagocytic Lymphohistiocytosis

It is characterized by fever, organomegaly, cytopenias, hyperferritinemia, hypertriglyceridemia, hypofibrinogenemia and evidence of hemophagocytosis in the bone marrow. An autosomal recessive defect in genes encoding perforin or Munc13, causes reduced NK and T-cell cytotoxicity, resulting in widespread accumulation of lymphocytes and mature macrophages with hypercytokinemia.

Treatment

Allogeneic HSCT is the only curative approach in familial hemophagocytic lymphohistiocytosis (HLH). A report from a multicenter prospective trial, HLH-94 demonstrated 62% 3-year event-free survival (EFS) in 65 children undergoing allogeneic HSCT with a variety of stem cell sources.[9]

Chronic Granulomatous Disease

It is a heterogeneous disease occurring due to defect in one of the subunits of NADPH oxidase enzyme complex in phagocytic cells.[10] Such defects lead to impaired production of super oxides and reactive oxygen intermediates thereby leading to impaired killing of intracellular microbes. Common infections include Aspergillus, *Staphyloccocus aureus*, *Burkholderia cepacia*, *Serratia marcescens* and *Nocardia*.[10] Both X-linked and autosomal recessive inheritance are noted. Nitroblue tetrazolium dye test and dihydrorhodamine test are used in diagnosis.

Treatment

Use of life-long antibiotic (co-trimoxazole) and antifungal (itraconazole/voriconazole) prophylaxis have significantly improved the short-term survival rate of these patients. Colitis and other inflammatory complications are managed medically with steroids and aminosalicylates. However, the underlying genetic defect is not corrected by these measures and the quality of life is significantly impaired. The survival rate at 30 years is around 50% even with the best supportive care. HSCT is curative in chronic granulomatous disease (CGD). A European study of 23 CGD transplants reported a survival rate of more than 80%, with deaths confined to high-risk children with active fungal infection.[11] Recent studies report a better outcome using a matched donor and performing HSCT at an earlier age, before developing serious infections.

Leukocyte Adhesion Deficiency I

It is characterized by delayed separation of umbilical cord, omphalitis, leukocytosis and recurrent mucocutaneous infections since infancy with no pus formation. It occurs due to mutation in gene coding CD18 (β2 integrin) leading to defective adhesion of leucocytes to endothelium. Absence of CD18 expression in leukocytes by flow cytometry is diagnostic.

Treatment

It includes management of infections, antibiotic prophylaxis and HSCT in severe cases.

VACCINATION IN PATIENTS WITH PRIMARY IMMUNODEFICIENCIES

The routine immunization program in children suspected of PID needs a careful attention as some of the routine vaccines are contraindicated in PID patients. However, in certain PIDs these vaccines can be safely given. A decision regarding which vaccine should be avoided and which can be administered depends on the category of PID. For example, infants with SCID are at a great risk of problems with live vaccines and they have to be strictly avoided, whereas patients with complement deficiencies can safely receive all the routine vaccines.

A guidance on which vaccines should be avoided and recommended in patients with PID is given in the following table **(Table 56.1)**.

CONCLUSION

Primary immunodeficiencies are often fatal as they are detected late before specific therapy can be instituted. Early diagnosis and quick referral to specialized centres help to provide the best outcome in PID. It decreases the complications and morbidity to a great extent. It also plays significant role in prevention by appropriate genetic counselling and antenatal diagnosis.

KEY POINTS

- Early detection of primary immunodeficiencies is vital in providing a cure to the illness. Most patients are unfortunately diagnosed very late in the course of illness.

Table 56.1 Vaccination in patients with primary immunodeficiencies (PID)

Category of PID	*Specific immunodeficiency*	*Contraindicated vaccines*	*Recommendations*
Combined T-cell and B-cell immunodeficiencies • T-lymphocytes	SCID, complete DiGeorge syndrome, Wiskott-Aldrich syndrome, ataxia telangiectasia	All live vaccines BCG OPV Contraindication for rotavirus vaccine associated with severe combined immunodeficiency	IPV instead of OPV should be given
Predominantly antibody deficiencies • B lymphocytes	X-linked agammaglobulinemia CVID Selective IgA deficiency IgG subclass deficiency	OPV Live influenza (inhaled) BCG Ty21a (live oral typhoid) Yellow fever	IPV instead of OPV should be given All other live vaccines safe. Annual inactivated influenza vaccine is essential, as IVIG may not protect against rapidly changing virus strains[4] Pneumococcal vaccines are also important[12]
Complement deficiencies	C2, C3, C4, C8, C9 deficiencies properdin, or factor B deficiency	None	All routine vaccines can be given
Phagocytic function	CGD LAD	BCG Live *Salmonella typhi* vaccine	All other live vaccines can be given

Abbreviations: SCID, severe combined immunodeficiency; BCG, bacillus Calmette-Guérin; OPV, oral polio vaccine; IPV, inactivated polio; CGD, chronic granulomatous disease; LAD, leukocyte adhesion deficiency

- Severe combined immunodeficiencies can be definitively cured by gene therapy as well as hematopoietic stem cell transplantation.
- Shared care from pediatricians is vital in long-term management of these patients.

REFERENCES

1. Chapel H, Prevot J, Gaspar HB, Español T, Bonilla FA, Solis L, et al. Primary immune deficiencies–principles of care. Front Immunol. 2014;5:627.
2. Madkaikar M, Mishra A, Ghosh K. Diagnostic approach to primary immunodeficiency disorders. Indian Pediatr. 2013;50:579-86.
3. Gupta S, Madkaikar M, Singh S, Sehgal S. Primary immunodeficiencies in India: a perspective. Ann NY Acad Sci. 2012;1250;73-9.
4. Hoernes M, Seger R, Reichenbach J. Modern management of primary B-cell immunodeficiencies. Pediatr Allergy Immunology. 2011;22:758-69.
5. World Health Organization. Appropriate uses of human immunoglobulin in clinical practice: Memorandum from an IUIS/WHO meeting. Bull World Health Organ. 1982;60(1):43-7.
6. Suri D, Singh S, Rawat A, Gupta A, Kamae C, Honma K, et al. Clinical profile and genetic basis of Wiskott-Aldrich syndrome at Chandigarh, North India. Asian Pac J Allergy Immunol. 2012;30:1-8.
7. Filipovich AH, Stone JV, Tomany SC, Ireland M, Kollman C, Pelz CJ, et al. Impact of donor type on outcome of bone marrow transplantation for Wiskott-Aldrich syndrome: collaborative study of the International Bone Marrow Transplant Registry and the National Marrow Donor Program. Blood. 2001;97(6):1598-603.
8. Mogensen TH. STAT3 and the hyper-IgE syndrome: Clinical presentation, genetic origin, pathogenesis, novel findings and remaining uncertainties. JAKSTAT. 2013;2(2):e23435.
9. Henter J, Samuelsson-Horne A, Aricò M, Egeler R, Elinder G, Filipovich A, et al. Treatment of hemophagocytic lymphohistiocytosis with HLH-94 immunochemotherapy and bone marrow transplantation. Blood. 2002;100:2367-73.
10. Rawat A, Singh S, Suri D, Gupta A, Saikia B, Minz RW, et al. Chronic granulomatous disease: two decades of experience from a tertiary care centre in North-West India. J Clin Immunol. 2014;34(1):58-67.
11. Seger RA, Gungor T, Belohradsky BH, Blanche S, Bordigoni P, Di Bartolomeo P, et al. Treatment of chronic granulomatous disease with myeloablative conditioning and an unmodified hemopoietic allograft: a survey of the European experience, 1985-2000. Blood. 2002;100(13):4344-50.
12. Principi N, Esposito S. Vaccine use in primary immunodeficiency disorders. Vaccine. 2014;32:3725-31.

CHAPTER

57

Neonatal Screening and Prenatal Diagnosis of Primary Immunodeficiency Disorders

Manisha Madkaikar, Jahnavi Aluri, Maya Gupta

INTRODUCTION

The newborn screening (NBS) program is aimed at identifying treatable inherited diseases which are life-threatening or affect long-term health, before they become symptomatic. Initiation of early treatment in these disorders significantly reduces the mortality and morbidity in the affected patients. Primary immunodeficiency disorders (PIDs) are heterogeneous group of inborn errors of immune system. All the severe forms of PID meet the criteria for inclusion in NBS. However, currently only severe combined immunodeficiencies (SCID) and X-linked agammaglobulinemia (XLA) are included in NBS.

WHY SHOULD WE INCLUDE PRIMARY IMMUNODEFICIENCY DISORDERS IN NBS?

Till date more than 200 distinct PID have been described.[1] Majority of these are single gene defects. The estimated combined incidence of these disorders is as high as 1 in 1,200.[2] The common manifestations of PID include recurrent, life-threatening infections and/or susceptibility to autoimmunity, inflammation and malignancy.[3] Clinical severity varies from mild to life-threatening disease depending on the underlying immune defect. PIDs are classified according to underlying immune defect into nine major categories which include—combined immunodeficiencies (due to impairment in both T and B-cell function), combined immunodeficiencies with associated syndromic features (varying degree of T and B-cell defects with syndromic features), predominantly antibody deficiencies (to impaired production of antibody by B-cells), diseases of immune dysregulation, congenital defects of phagocyte number, function, or both, defects in innate immunity, autoinflammatory disorders, complement deficiencies and phenocopies of PID (inherited immuno-deficiencies arising from acquired mechanisms).

Early diagnosis of PID is important to prevent the significant morbidity and mortality associated with these diseases. Treatment consists of antimicrobial therapy to treat and prevent the infections, immunoglobulin supplements for antibody deficiencies and hematopoietic stem cells transplantation (HSCT) for severe forms of PID.

The first group of PID which was included under NBS was SCID. Other severe forms of PID also have been suggested as screening candidates for NBS are familial hemophagocytic lymphohistiocytosis (FHL), severe antibody deficiencies (XLA or other agammaglobulinemia), etc.

NEED FOR NEWBORN SCREENING FOR SCID AND OTHER T-CELL IMMUNODEFICIENCIES

The term “SCID” encompasses a genetically heterogeneous group of inherited disorders characterized resulting from defects in T-cell development and/or function. There are more than 18 distinct genetic defects leading to SCID.[4] It represents the most severe form of PID and is a life-threatening pediatric emergency. However, the affected infants are generally healthy at birth as they are partially protected by the transplacentally acquired maternal immunoglobulin G (IgG) antibodies in the first few months of life. As this protection wanes, these infants develop severe and recurrent infections especially opportunistic infections, chronic diarrhea, and poor weight gain leading to significant morbidity and mortality. Unless treated early for reconstitution of a functioning immune system, these infants die of severe infection by 1 year of age. Hematopoietic cell transplantation (HCT) has been shown to be an effective treatment for SCID, particularly if performed early in infancy, before the development of recurrent and increasingly severe infections. Only about 20% of infants with SCID have a family history that prompts early testing.[5] Early data from pilot screening programs in the USA suggest that one in 30,000–50,000 infants may be born with SCID, whereas data from Turkey, Saudi Arabia and Kuwait indicate higher rates.[6] Thus, SCID being a clinically severe disease, diagnosis being not apparent at birth, availability of definitive therapy and significant improvement of quality life with early intervention makes it an ideal candidate for NBS program.

TREC ASSAY AND ITS UTILITY AS A SCREENING TEST FOR SCID

Severe combined immunodeficiency is molecularly heterogeneous condition with a variety of genetic defects leading to the same clinical phenotype. However, majority of these defects are associated with an abnormality of T-cell development in the thymus.[4] All the T-cells after generation in the bone marrow undergo a process of receptor gene splicing and rearrangement in the thymus. During this process of recombination the T-cell antigen receptor (TCR) genes; which are composed of large numbers of alternate segments, called variable (V), diversity (D) and joining (J) regions that lie upstream of constant regions, are randomly cut and rejoined to generate a unique rearrangement in each cell. The excised DNA fragments that are not incorporated into the mature TCR locus are joined at their ends to form a great variety of circular DNA byproducts, called T-cell receptor excision circles (TRECs) **(Fig. 57.1)**. These DNA circles are stable but do not replicate during cell division. They get diluted with T-cell division. Since TRECs are found only in naïve T-cells that have recently left thymus, it provides a surrogate marker for the T-cell development in the thymus and is useful as a screening test for SCID. TREC copy number in the peripheral blood varies significantly depending on the age of the individual. Normal newborns have about 1 TREC per 10 T-cells, reflecting high numbers of naïve T-cells that have not yet proliferated extensively; whereas older children and adults have about 1 per 100 and 1 per 1,000 T-cells, respectively, reflecting peripheral expansion.[7] Infants with SCID have very low or undetectable TRECs.[8] Even maternal T-cells present in an infant with SCID do not falsely raise the TREC count, because maternal cells have few TRECs.

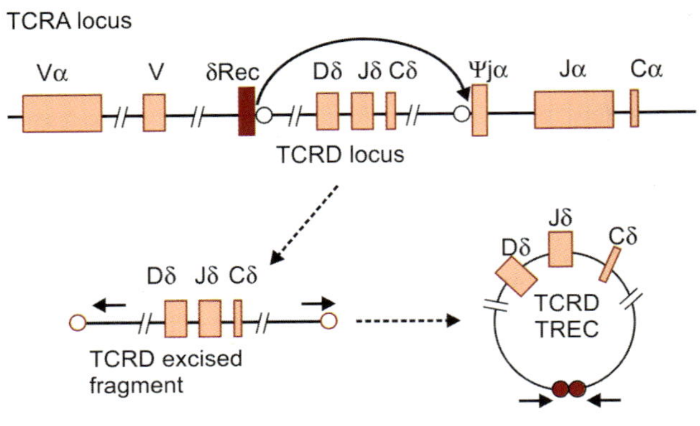

Figure 57.1 Generation of T-cell receptor excision circles (TRECs). The germline configuration of the TCRA locus, with TCRD embedded, is shown embedded at the top of the figure, which also shows the points (gray dots) at which the DNA is cut to excise the TCRD locus in T lymphocyte progenitors destined to express the α and β T-cell antigen receptors (TCRs). After excision, lower left, and ligation, lower right, of the δRec-ψJα fragment to form a TREC. Polymerase chain reaction (PCR) primers can amplify a DNA junction fragment containing the joint (from Puck JM, 2012)

In the year 2005, dried blood samples (DBS) screening method for SCID using TRECs as the biomarker for native T-cells was published by Chan and Puck. This method relies on quantitative real-time polymerase chain reaction (qPCR) on the genomic DNA extracted from DBS for measuring the delta-Rec and psi-Joining segment-alpha signal joint. As TRECs are stable in dried blood collected on filters, the TREC copy number reflects the number of recently formed T-cells in the peripheral blood.[8]

International Status

In 2008, Wisconsin became the first state to implement mandatory NBS for T-cell deficiency[9] followed by Massachusetts in February 2009[10,11] and later by New York, the Navajo Nation, California, Puerto Rico and Louisiana. All these states employ an in-house modification of the TREC assay and have established a TREC cutoff value to efficiently pick up true positive cases. Now many other states are conducting TREC screening for SCID, and still more are in the planning stages of offering this testing. These programs have successfully identified SCID and related conditions, allowing infants to receive prompt treatment without the burden of devastating infections. The incidence of SCID previously estimated at 1 in 100,000 births is now 1 in 58,000 infants, as reported from the NBS for SCID in 11 programs in the United States from January 2008–2013.[12]

Conditions that are picked up TREC screening assay

- *Typical SCID:* This form of SCID is characterized by less than 300 autologous T-cells/μL of blood and less than 10% of normal proliferation to mitogens [e.g. phytohemagglutinin (PHA)].[13]
- *Leaky SCID or Omenn syndrome,* due to mutations in typical SCID genes that do not completely affect the gene function. These forms of SCID are characterized by 300–1,500 autologous T-cells/μL. Patients with Omenn syndrome may have normal or elevated CD3 T-cell counts, but they have restricted TCR diversity (oligoclonality) of T-cell.[13]
- Variant SCID, with persistently low T-cells but no defect in a known SCID gene.[13]
- Conditions with primary T-cell lymphopenia (CD3 T-cells ≤1,500 cells/μL):
  - Complete DiGeorge syndrome or partial DiGeorge syndrome with low T-cells
  - CHARGE syndrome
  - Jacobsen syndrome
  - Trisomy 21
  - RAC2 dominant interfering mutation
  - DOCK8 deficient hyper-IgE syndrome
  - Cartilage hair hypoplasia.
- *Secondary T-cell lymphopenia:* This is diagnosed in a subset of infants with recognized congenital conditions, such as intestinal lymphangiectasia, hydrops, gastroschisis, a congenital heart defect, chylothorax, or neonatal leukemia. It can also occur due to prenatal administration of glucocorticoids or inflammatory conditions (e.g. sepsis).

- Premature infants presenting with T-cell lymphopenia, T-cells less than or equal to 1,500 cells/μL. However, this may resolve with age.[13]

T-cell defects that cannot be picked up by the TREC screening assay: Diseases in which T-cells develop in the thymus to the point of production of the TRECs but have impaired functions cannot be picked up by the TREC assay. This includes newborns with Zap70 deficiency,[14] major histocompatibility complex (MHC) class II deficiency,[15] CD40 ligand deficiency, NF-kappa-b essential modulator (NEMO) deficiency and patients with a late-onset of adenosine deaminase (ADA) deficiency.

Interpreting TREC Results

Low or undetectable TREC levels indicate T-cell lymphopenia condition. However, as this assay is a PCR based technique, low number may also arise due to artifacts such as inadequate sample, poor elution of DNA from the DBS or due to presence of PCR inhibitors such heparin. In order to avoid false positive results, amplification of a conserved gene sequence from a reference gene is carried out. The general strategies employed are:

- *Singleplex TREC assay:* This involves parallel amplification of a reference gene and TRECs in samples where the initial TREC qPCR reaction gives result below the predetermined TREC cutoff. If the reference gene is not detected, the test is termed inconclusive. If detected, the replicate TREC values are used as the final TREC values.
- *Multiplex Real-time qPCR:* This involves the simultaneous amplification of TREC and reference gene. Samples with the abnormal multiplex result are retested using the same multiplex assay. If the reference gene is not detected, the test is termed inconclusive. If detected, the replicate TREC values are used as the final TREC values.

Unless the infant begins to show any signs of PID, no further testing is recommended if the SCID NBS is normal.

RECENT ADVANCEMENT

Implementing NBS protocols for combined quantification of TRECs and kappa-deleting recombination excision circles (KRECs), a biomarker of mature B-cells, hold a great promise of identification of SCID and agammaglobulinemia at birth.

Triplex Real-time PCR Protocol

Similar to quantification of TRECs, quantification of KRECs provides early assessment of B-cell development in primary B-cell immunodeficiencies. KRECs are formed during the process of Vk-Jk rearrangement in the bone marrow. A single uniform qPCR strategy can be applied to determine the presence and number of copies of TRECs and KRECs in DBS together with a control gene, the TCRA constant gene (TCRAC) **(Flow chart 57.1)**.[11]

Flow chart 57.1 Generalized procedure for T-cell receptor excision circles (TREC)/kappa-deleting recombination excision circle (KREC) assay

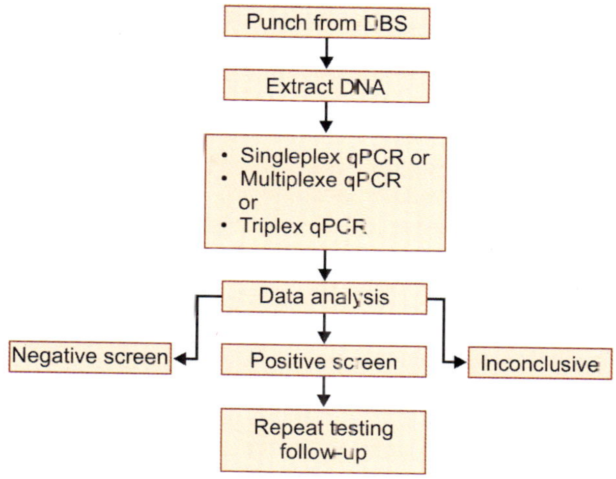

Abbreviations: qPCR, quantitative real-time polymerase chain reaction; DBS, dried blood samples; DNA, deoxyribonucleic acid

Management of Patients Detected with TRECs/KRECs Lower than the Normal Cut-off

Diagnosis of SCID is incomplete with just an abnormal qPCR screen. Follow-up testing involves:

- Flow cytometry using antibodies to CD3, CD4, CD8, CD19 and CD16/56 to determine whether the infant has normal percentages of T-cells and subsets, B-cells and NK cells.
- Additional markers may include CD45RO/RA for memory and naïve T-cells respectively; CD62L (L-selectin); CD27 and CCR7 for characterization of naïve T-cells.
- Assessment of the proliferative response of T-cells *in vitro* to mitogens to determine the T-cell function.

Abnormal flow cytometry results that confirm a T-cell and/or B-cell lymphopenia necessitate immediate measures to be put in place for all patients. These include immunoglobulin replacement therapy and prophylactic antibiotics, avoidance of live vaccines, protection from exposure to infections. Optimal transplant protocols for very young infants with SCID remain controversial, but with newborn screening these protocols can be established by multicenter studies.[13]

NATIONAL STATUS

The awareness of PID in India which was lacking few years back has gradually started increasing, with many centers initiating the basic immunophenotypic assays for diagnosis of PID. However, NBS programs for early diagnosis of SCID is yet to be initiated in India. Once the NBS is implemented, the true incidence and proportions of each type of SCID can be determined in India. It will help significantly in improving the mortality and morbidity seen with PIDs in India. However in order to achieve this, clinicians have to play an active role in promoting NBS for PID and other T- and B-lymphocyte abnormalities and work closely with laboratories that are developing the new techniques. The NBS-positive results should be followed up by appropriate diagnosis for confirmation and best possible and most appropriate treatment for the affected children.

Also, with the advent of modern molecular technologies, newborn screening for other severe immune system defects such as leukocyte adhesion deficiency, chronic granulomatous disease (CGD) should be available soon.

PRENATAL DIAGNOSIS

Prenatal diagnosis enables early diagnosis of congenital anomalies and genetic disorders in the unborn fetus.[16] The pediatrician who diagnoses a child with a genetic defect or a birth defect also has a responsibility of counseling the family about the possibility of recurrence of the same or similar problem in future offspring. A number of techniques are used for providing prenatal diagnosis (PND). Knowledge about the mode of inheritance of the disease, availability of the knowledge of the genetic defect underlying the disease and accuracy, reliability and safety of the various procedures is essential before counseling the family members.

Primary immunodeficiency disorders are a group of single gene disorders of immune system resulting from defects in different components of immune system. More than 200 distinct PID have been described till date. Despite rapid progress in the understanding of the underlying molecular basis of PID, its optimum management still remains a challenge. Patients affected with severe form of PID are highly susceptible to severe and recurrent infections and do not survive unless treated with immune reconstituting therapies like HSCT or gene therapy.[17,18] HSCT from a HLA matched sibling is an option only available to less than 20% of cases. Other form of supportive therapy like regular intravenous Ig transfusions and prophylactic antibiotics especially for patients with XLA and CGDs may result in long-term survival but is still associated with morbidity, poor quality of life and prohibitively high expenses of therapy.[19] Therefore, in families having a severely affected child, genetic counseling and PND is an important part of management.

Modes of Inheritance of Primary Immunodeficiency Disorders

Different modes of inheritance are seen in patients with PID depending on the gene affected and the type of mutation and the residual activity of the mutant protein. In PID, patients with same clinical phenotype like CGDs have different modes of inheritance depending on the underlying genetic defect like X-linked CGD resulting from defect in the *CYBB* gene encoding the enzymatic center of the NADPH oxidase gp91phox whereas defect in the *CYBA, NCF1, NCF2* and *NCF4* gene encoding $p22^{phox}$, $p47^{phox}$, $p67^{phox}$ and $p40^{phox}$ respectively result in autosomal recessive form of CGD.[20] The common modes of inheritance seen in PID are:[21]

X-linked inheritance: This is the most common inheritance pattern of PID. The responsible genes for these disorders are located on the X chromosome that predominantly affects males. Some example of this inheritance pattern are agammaglobulinemia (XLA), Wiskott-Aldrich syndrome, SCID, caused by mutations in the common gamma chain, hyper-IgM syndrome, due to mutations in CD40 ligand, X-linked lymphoproliferative disease and CGD.

Autosomal recessive inheritance: In this pattern of inheritance both male and female are affected equally. Few examples are SCID due to adenosine deaminase deficiency (ADA-SCID), RAG1/RAG2 deficiency SCID, CGD $p47^{phox}$, and Ataxia-telangiectasia. Some autosomal recessive disorders are complicated by the involvement of several different genes with similar clinical manifestation. In such cases, immunophenotypic characterization is the only robust way to provide a clue towards the underlying genetic defect.

Autosomal dominant inheritance: Some PID follows autosomal dominant inheritance affecting both males and females. These mutations can be presented as de novo and have complicated phenotypic expression due to the variable degree of penetrance. Examples of autosomal dominant PID are hyper-IgE syndrome, due to mutations in STAT3 (Jobs syndrome), hypogammaglobulinemia, DiGeorge syndrome and some rare forms of inborn errors of IL12-23/IFNγ loop defects. Over the last few years, the clinical phenotype and molecular basis of the various immunological defects has been characterized. The patient's clinical and immunological characteristics guide selection of the candidate gene to be screened. However, diagnosis of PID remains complicated due to the complexity of the diseases and requirement of an array of specialized tests like flow cytometry, cytotoxicity assays, lymphocyte proliferation assays, complement assays followed by DNA sequencing of a candidate gene. Moreover, the centers providing the diagnosis are very few which often delay the detection of underlying molecular defect. However, every attempt should be made to reach to a molecular diagnosis as it is extremely important for providing the PND.

Prenatal Diagnosis Techniques

A number of invasive and noninvasive techniques are used for PND for the chromosomal, genetic and structural abnormalities in the fetus. This chapter will focus on the PND techniques that are most commonly used for PID which are essentially single gene disorders. If the genetic defect is known in the index case then molecular genetic diagnostic tools are used to detect the same mutation in the fetal sample obtained either by chorionic villous sampling (CVS) or amniocentesis. However, sometimes though a phenotypic diagnosis in the index case is clear [like abnormal nitroblue tetrazolium (NBT) test or dihydrorhodamine (DHR) in case of CGD] but underlying genetic defect has not been identified phenotypic diagnosis using flow cytometry can be performed on fetal blood sample obtained by cordocentesis. The advantages of each technique and the risks involved are discussed here.

Chorionic villus sampling: It is performed at 10–12 weeks of gestation. A sample of fetal chorionic tissue is removed by aspiration by either transabdominal or transcervical route. After aspiration fetal villi are dissected from the decidual tissue and then genetic testing is performed on the DNA extracted from the same. The main advantage of this procedure is the earlier diagnosis which allows sufficient time for counseling, decision making and safe termination of pregnancy. Though in some studies CVS is associated with a higher miscarriage rate than amniocentesis (0.5–1%), other studies have shown comparable results between CVS and second trimester amniocentesis.[22] The procedure should be avoided before the 10 weeks of gestation as it is shown to be associated with higher risk of limb reduction defects.[23] The chances of maternal contamination with this procedure are 10 times higher than amniocentesis.[23]

Amniocentesis: In amniocentesis exfoliated fetal cells in amniotic fluid are studied for molecular analysis. This can be performed at 13–15 weeks gestation, however, the preferred timing is 16–17 weeks of gestation. Amniocentesis is associated with very low rate of complications and provides adequate sample for analysis in more than 99% of the cases.[22] The risk of miscarriage with amniocentesis procedure is about 0.25–0.50%. If performed at earlier gestation period, it is associated with a high rate of amniotic fluid leakage, higher risk of fetal loss and talipes. The presence of maternal cell contamination with this procedure is only 0.1–0.2.[24]

Sampling of fetal blood or cordocentesis: This is also called as percutaneous umbilical cord blood sampling (PUBS), or umbilical vein sampling. It is a diagnostic test performed in the second trimester to check for phenotypic and genotypic defects in the developing baby. Compared to other diagnostic tests, it has slightly high risk of miscarriage of 2%.[25] The major complications for cordocentesis are associated with amniocentesis, fetal bradycardia, umbilical cord laceration and thrombosis. Cordocentesis is usually performed only when CVS, amniocentesis fail to provide the definite diagnosis. The maternal contamination in fetal blood is ruled out by many approaches. The fetal blood shows a high mean corpuscular volume (MCV) value (>110fL) with narrow, single red cell distribution curve hence, a simple and rapid way is to observe MCV of fetal blood. The other confirmatory methods are the Kleihauer-Betke test, flow cytometry, and/or by variable number tandem repeat (VNTR). A VNTR is a location in a gene where a short nucleotide sequence is organized as a tandem repeat that often show variations in length between individuals. Each variant acts as an inherited allele, allowing them to be used for personal or parental identification. To rule out the maternal contamination parental allele with different sizes are considered as an informative short tandem repeat (STR) marker.

Once a specimen is collected, a variety of laboratory techniques may be used for diagnosis. This includes molecular analysis and phenotypic analysis.[26,27]

Molecular analysis: PND by molecular study involves two approaches—direct or indirect method. The direct analysis is typically performed if the gene mutation has been characterized in the family, whereas indirect analysis by linkage studies is done in cases where disease gene is unknown. The direct method is rapid and provides 100% accuracy, however, the accuracy of indirect mutation analysis depends on the distance of the DNA marker to the disease locus and is time consuming.

Phenotypic analysis: Diagnosis of PID is sometimes complicated due to molecular heterogeneity and overlapping clinical manifestation. Molecular diagnostic facilities for each of these diseases are not available and possible in all cases. In such cases, PND by phenotypic analysis of the fetal white blood cells can be offered for families with index case having immunophenotypically well characterized PID. Phenotypic evaluation of PIDs provides an important clue for diagnosis of these disorders.

Flow cytometry is a rapid and simple technique but there are some technical limitations of flow cytometry that need to be taken into consideration before using it for PND.

- Before offering this facility, it is essential to establish the normal ranges for lymphocyte subsets, expression of CD18 and CD11 on leukocytes,[28] NBT test and DHR activity and HLA-DR on fetal sample as it differs from the normal ranges in peripheral blood. For example, normal expression of DHR ranges in from 70% to 95% in fetal blood whereas it is 95–100% in peripheral blood.
- Significant phenotypic variations are observed in certain categories of PID. For example, leaky SCID or Omenn syndrome may have normal or even increased T-cells at birth or shortly thereafter due to oligoclonal expansion.[29] Similarly in some forms of XLA, expression of B-cells and immunoglobulin production is associated with an age-related loss.[30] In such cases, relying only on T and B-cell numbers for PND is not advisable as in such patients the status of T, B counts is unclear at 18 weeks of gestation.
- For the ease of PND by flow cytometry, it is recommended that the diagnostic marker should be expressed on a relatively large cellular subset at the appropriate gestational age.
- Marker showing low expression in normal fetal cells in comparison to adult cells owing to the immaturity of the immune cells cannot be used as a marker for PND.
- In some cases of missense mutation, normal protein expression does not rule out an underlying molecular defect in the respective gene as these mutations may result in expression of a defective protein. Hence, it is recommended that the PND by flow cytometry should be offered only in cases where index case shows absent protein expression.[31]
- It has been observed that neutrophils count in the fetal blood is often less than the full term cord blood and adult peripheral blood. Scoring enough neutrophils for NBT and LAD-I test is challenging in fetal blood sample at

18 weeks. Hence, it is advisable that phenotypic PND of CGD should not be based on only NBT test. The diagnosis has to be confirmed by DHR assay which is more sensitive, specific and quantitative. Alternatively, one can look for other available cell population of WBC which are present in higher number with a high expression of diagnostic marker. For example, in PND of LAD-I the lymphocyte represents a better cell population for analysis as both the diagnosis markers (CD18 and CD11a) are highly expressed on lymphocytes.[31]

- RBC lysis for leukocyte enrichment in assay can be difficult due to high fetal hemoglobin content. Also, high number of nucleated RBCs present in fetal blood can complicate the analysis. Thus, for accurate analysis, live gating of leukocytes using CD45 becomes essential.[28,31] For neutrophil gating, addition of CD15 to the panel provides a better separation of neutrophils compared to CD45 gating alone.

ADVANCES IN PRENATAL DIAGNOSIS TECHNIQUES

Two recent advancements in noninvasive technique for PND are isolation of fetal cells [nucleated red blood cells (NRBC)] circulating in the blood between 11 weeks and 15 weeks of gestation based[32] and use of cell free fetal DNA (cff) circulating in the maternal blood from 7th week of gestation. These are extensively investigated for single gene mutations, fetal chromosomal abnormalities and even entire fetal genome. However, these techniques have some limitation in discriminating the amplified fetal DNA from maternal DNA, hence currently it is applied for diagnosis of fetal sex (for X-linked diseases), detection of fetal chromosomal aneuploidy and Rhesus (Rh) antigen status.[33] Apart from testing known single gene mutations, technological advances will soon make noninvasive prenatal assessment of the entire genome a reality. In addition to information about chromosomal abnormality or single gene mutations, these methods also reveal other gene mutation with polymorphisms. Under these circumstances, data interpretation and genetic counseling will be a major challenge. With the advancement of *Next Gen sequencing techniques*, it would be possible to screen the entire fetal genome cost effectively in coming years.

CONCLUSION

Management of severe PID is still far from satisfactory and results in significant financial and emotional burden on the family and the society. Hence, once a patient is diagnosed with PID it is extremely important to provide genetic counseling to the family members. Knowledge of pattern of inheritance of the particular PID and the underlying genetic defect as well as different PND procedures available and their limitations is important for guiding the families. Molecular diagnosis is on sample obtained from CVS or amniocentesis is preferred in families with a known genetic defect. However, phenotypic analysis of fetal blood sample can be considered in cases where molecular diagnostic facilities are not available.

KEY MESSAGE

Implementation of newborn screening program for PIDs like SCID would help in improving the mortality and morbidity associated with these disorders. This can be achieved only by a close association of pediatricians and laboratories to set up techniques for early diagnosis and facilities for providing prompt treatment to the affected children.

REFERENCES

1. Ochs HD, Hagin D. Primary immunodeficiency disorders: general classification, new molecular insights, and practical approach to diagnosis and treatment. Ann Allergy Asthma Immunol. 2014;112(6):489-95.
2. Boyle JM, Buckley RH. Population prevalence of diagnosed primary immunodeficiency diseases in the United States. J Clin Immunol. 2007;27:497.
3. Al-Herz W, Bousfiha A, Casanova JL, Chatila T, Conley ME, Cunningham-Rundles C, et al. Primary immunodeficiency diseases: an update on the classification from the international union of immunological societies expert committee for primary immunodeficiency. Front Immunol. 2014;5:162.
4. Borte S, von Döbeln U, Hammarström L. Guidelines for newborn screening of primary immunodeficiency diseases. Curr Opin Hematol. 2013;20(1):48-54.
5. Brown L, Xu-Bayford J, Allwood Z, Slatter M, Cant A, Davies EG, et al. Neonatal diagnosis of severe combined immunodeficiency leads to significantly improved survival outcome: the case for newborn screening. Blood. 2011;117:3243-6.
6. Verbsky J, Thakar M, Routes J. The Wisconson approach to newborn screening for severe combined immunodeficiency. J Alergy Clin Imunol. 2012;129:622-7.
7. Douek DC, McFarland RD, Keiser PH, Gage EA, Massey JM, Haynes BF, et al. Changes in thymic function with age and during the treatment of HIV infection. Nature. 1998;396:690.
8. Chan K, Puck JM. Development of population-based newborn screening for severe combined immunodeficiency. J Allergy Clin Immunol. 2005;115:391.
9. Routes JM, Grossman WJ, Verbsky J. Statewide newborn screening for severe T-cell lymphopenia. JAMA. 2009;302: 2465-70.
10. Comeau AM, Hale JE, Pai SY, Bonilla FA, Notarangelo LD, Pasternack MS, et al. Guidelines for implementation of population-based newborn screening for severe combined immunodeficiency. J Inherit Metab Dis. 2010;33(Suppl 2):S273-81.
11. Gerstel-Thompson JL, Wilkey JF, Baptiste JC. High-throughput multiplexed T-cell-receptor excision circle quantitative PCR assay with internal controls for detection of severe combined immunodeficiency in population-based newborn screening. Clin Chem. 2010;56:1466-74.
12. Kwan A, Abraham RS, Currier R, Brower A, Andruszewski K, Abbott JK, et al. Newborn Screening for Severe Combined Immunodeficiency in 11 Screening Programs in the United States. JAMA. 2014;312(7):729-38.
13. Puck JM. Laboratory technology for population-based screening for severe combined immunodeficiency in neonates:

the winner is T-cell receptor excision circles. J Allergy Clin Immunol. 2012; 129:607

14. Grazioli S, Bennett M, Hildebrand KJ, Vallance H, Turvey SE, Junker AK. Limitation of TREC-based newborn screening for ZAP70 Severe Combined Immunodeficiency. Clin Immunol. 2014;153:209-10.
15. Kuo CY, Chase J, Garcia Lloret M, Stiehm ER, Moore T, Aguilera MJ, et al. Newborn screening for severe combined immunodeficiency does not identify bare lymphocyte syndrome. J Allergy Clin Immunol. 2013;131:1693.
16. Hulten A, Dhanjal S, Pertl B. Rapid and simple prenatal diagnosis of common chromosome disorders: advantages and disadvantages of the molecular methods FISH and QF-PCR. Reproduction. 2003;126:279-97.
17. Sponzilli I, Notarangelo D. Severe combined immunodeficiency (SCID): from molecular basis to clinical management. Acta Biomed. 2011;82:5-13.
18. Sokolic R, Kesserwan C, Candotti F. Recent advances in gene therapy for severe congenital immunodeficiency diseases. Curr Opin Hematol. 2008;15:375-80.
19. Wood P, Stanworth S, Burton J, Jones A, Peckham DG, Green T, et al. UK Primary Immunodeficiency Network. Recognition, clinical diagnosis and management of patients with primary antibody deficiencies: a systematic review. Clin Exp Immunol. 2007;149:410-23.
20. Matute D, Arias A, Wright A, Wrobel I, Waterhouse C, Li J, et al. A new genetic subgroup of chronic granulomatous disease with autosomal recessive mutations in p40 phox and selective defects in neutrophil NADPH oxidase activity. Blood. 2009;114:3309-15.
21. Lim MS, Elenitoba-Johnson KS. The molecular pathology of primary immunodeficiencies. J Mol Diagn. 2004;6(2):59-83.
22. Tabor A, Alfirevic Z. Update on procedure-related risks for prenatal diagnosis techniques. Fetal Diagn Ther. 2010;27(1):1-7.
23. Lippman A, Tomkins J, Shime J, Hamerton L. Canadian multicentre randomized clinical trial of chorion villus sampling and amniocentesis. Final report. Prenat Diagn. 1992;12: 385-408.
24. Gosden C, Tabor A, Leck I, Grant A, Alfirevic Z, Wald N. Amniocentesis and chorionic villus sampling. In: Wald N, Leck I (Eds). Antenatal and Neonatal Screening. London: Oxford University Press; 2000. pp. 470-517.
25. Durandy A, Oury C, Griscelli C, Dumez Y, Oury JF, Henrion R. Prenatal testing for inherited immune deficiencies by fetal blood sampling. Prenat Diagn. 1982;2:109-13.
26. Linch DC, Beverley PC, Levinsky RJ, Rodeck CH. Phenotypic analysis of fetal blood leucocytes: potential for prenatal diagnosis of immunodeficiency disorders. Prenat Diagn. 1982;2:211-8.
27. Weening S, Bredius G, Wolf H, van der Schoot CE. Prenatal diagnostic procedure for leukocyte adhesion deficiency. Prenat Diagn. 1991;11:193-7.
28. Madkaikar R, Gupta M, Rao M, Ghosh K. Prenatal diagnosis of LAD-I on cord blood by flow cytometry. Indian J Pediatr. 2012;79(12):1605-9.
29. Avila M, Uzel G, Hsu A, Milner D, Turner L, Pittaluga S, et al. Highly variable clinical phenotypes of hypomorphic RAG1 mutations. Pediatrics. 2010;126(5):e1248-52.
30. Sigmon JR, Kasasbeh E, Krishnaswamy G. X-linked agammaglobulinemia diagnosed late in life: case report and review of the literature. Clin Mol Allergy. 2008;6:5.
31. Mishra A, Gupta M, Dalvi A, Ghosh K, Madkaikar M. Rapid flow cytometric prenatal diagnosis of primary immunodeficiency (PID) disorders. J Clin Immunol. 2014;34(3):316-22.
32. D'Souza E, Sawant PM, Nadkarni AH, Gorakshakar A, Mohanty D, Ghosh K, et al. Evaluation of the use of monoclonal antibodies and nested PCR for noninvasive prenatal diagnosis of hemoglobinopathies in India. Am J Clin Pathol. 2008; 130(2):202-9.
33. Chiu RW, Lo YM. Clinical applications of maternal plasma fetal DNA analysis: translating the fruits of 15 years of research. Clin Chem Lab Med. 2013;51(1):197-204.